Manual of Pediatric Therapeutics

Manual of Pediatric Therapeutics

Third Edition

Department of Medicine
The Children's Hospital, Boston

Edited by John W. Graef, M.D.,
and Thomas E. Cone, Jr., M.D.

Editorial Board:
Alex F. Flores, M.D.
Margaret Hostetter, M.D.
Jeffrey M. Lipton, M.D., Ph.D.
Janice Lowe, M.D.
William I. Murphy, M.D., Ph.D.

Foreword by
Mary Ellen Avery, M.D.
Thomas Morgan Rotch Professor of Pediatrics,
Harvard Medical School; Physician-in-Chief,
The Children's Hospital, Boston

Little, Brown and Company
Boston/Toronto

Dedicated to our children: Alison, Andrea, Barbara, Barbara, Benjamin, Bryan, David, Elizabeth, Emily, Jack, Joshua, Katherine, Kathryn, Margaret, Mayme, Sarah, and William

Contents

Foreword

House staff have a way of knowing what information is useful and jotting it down in the fewest possible words. The previous editions of the *Manual of Pediatric Therapeutics* have been written primarily by house officers and fellows in training at The Children's Hospital, Boston, with advice from practicing pediatricians and a few members of the senior staff. This is indeed a house staff manual aimed at providing the specific and useful information that is required in the day-to-day management of children.

The editors of this new edition have recruited some of the current group of young staff members to update previous chapters and to add three new ones—on well child care, behavioral disorders, and metabolic diseases. A chapter on acute care management includes some of the information contained in the previous edition's chapter on emergencies, child abuse, and sudden infant death syndrome.

Drs. Graef and Cone continue their leadership in editing the many contributions from their colleagues to produce a well-organized and indexed presentation of an enormous amount of information.

The editors and contributors have kept the focus on therapy, as the title indicates. This manual thus supplements other available handbooks and textbooks. It is the kind of book that every pediatrician will want to have within easy reach when confronted with the need to make a therapeutic decision.

Mary Ellen Avery

Preface

The third edition of the *Manual of Pediatric Therapeutics* has been almost 3 years in production. In a departure from the plan of previous editions, we have been fortunate in securing the assistance of five gifted young pediatricians to form an editorial board in addition to our overall supervision of the material. This has provided additional perspective, fresh insight, and, most importantly, up-to-date editorial judgment since all of our editorial board members are recent graduates of The Children's Hospital training programs.

As with the second edition, this third edition is really a new book. A number of chapters have been discarded, and the material from those chapters deemed necessary has been incorporated into existing chapters. Three new chapters have been added: Well Child Care, Behavior, and Metabolic Diseases. The chapter on emergencies has been broadened to include the discipline of intensive care and renamed Acute Care.

The book's organization remains basically the same, that is, from general principles to specific therapeutic recommendations. Thus, the first portion of the book can be used to apply broadly to general pediatric practice, and the second portion is organized by traditional (and not so traditional) subspecialties.

Chapter 1 contains two new essays on principles of therapeutics and on the pediatric consultation. Chapter 2, our new and badly needed section on well child care, was contributed to by three practicing pediatricians from a busy group practice in Boston. They are truly pediatricians' pediatricians in that they provide care for several of the editors' children. Chapter 3, Acute Care, was written by the staff of both our emergency services and multidisciplinary intensive care unit. Thus, it is almost a "submanual" on acute care.

So, too, are Chapters 5 and 6 on their subject—the care of well and sick newborns. Once again, Dr. John Cloherty has contributed his expertise along with Dr. William Murphy from the Joint Program in Neonatology, Harvard Medical School. They have provided us with a précis of the popular *Manual of Neonatal Care* by Dr. Cloherty and Dr. Ann Stark (Little, Brown, 1980).

The remaining chapters are grouped roughly by topic. Thus, Chapter 7, Fluid and Electrolytes, is followed by Renal Disorders, Cardiac Disorders, and Gastroenterology; Disorders of the Endocrine System, Prepubertal and Adolescent Gynecology, and Diabetes Mellitus are next to each other, followed by our new chapter, Metabolic Diseases.

The next section of the book focuses on problems of inflammation in the chapters titled Antibiotics and Infectious Diseases, Parasitic Infections, Blood Disorders, Inflammatory and Immunodeficiency Disorders, and Allergic Disorders. Chapter 20, Neurology, has been completely rewritten and adjoins our new chapter on behavioral disorders. The text concludes with two important subspecialties of pediatrics, Skin Disorders and Eye Disorders.

The *Manual* is extensively cross-referenced to either the specific page number or to the outline section if the material is in close proximity. A large and detailed index provides further access to specific entries. Finally, the front and back covers contain a quick and handy reference for dosages needed in emergency situations.

As always, production of such a text requires the assistance of many people. Our grateful thanks must go to Annette Cardillo Luongo, Florence Stikeleather, and

Lisa Kenn for assistance in manuscript preparation. Our thanks, too, to Dr. Jose L. Suescun for his critical review of the text and helpful comments, and especially to Carol Snarey of Little, Brown, who continued a long tradition of listening patiently to the editors' excuses for delays in delivering finished manuscripts while we fussed over details.

To our astonishment, the demand for this book has been so great that it has been translated into seven languages, and we receive comments from readers from such diverse countries as Iran and Peru. We have generally aimed the book for use by those who have an interest in pediatrics and access to texts that can clarify diagnostic questions. A particularly useful companion is Dr. Kenneth Roberts' *Manual of Clinical Problems in Pediatrics* (Little, Brown, 1979).

As before, our therapeutic recommendations reflect practice here at Children's Hospital. Other centers may have different and equally valid and undoubtedly sometimes better approaches. That is the nature of medicine; science gives us only a structure within which to practice our art. We hope you will find this text helpful.

J. W. G.
T. E. C., Jr.

Manual of Pediatric Therapeutics

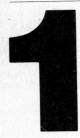

General Care of the Patient

I. **Caring for children.** Illness can be a frightening and unpleasant experience, particularly for children. Children can feel and react even at times when they might appear uninterested or are absorbed by fear about their illness and the attendant hospital procedures. For this reason, care must be taken to respect the modesty, integrity, and privacy of each child. And because children are likely to be afraid of situations they do not understand, they need to be told about their illness and its treatment in terms they can comprehend. Insincerity is a quality children quickly recognize, and deceiving a child is an abuse of trust that only serves ultimately to alienate him or her.

It should not be surprising if a child reacts angrily to painful procedures or is frustrated at his or her own lack of progress. An understanding physician views this anger as a normal reaction and should not feel threatened by it. It is the quiet and passive infant or child who may be a cause for concern. Older children, particularly, understand pain and even death and can be made unnecessarily anxious by bedside staff conversations that may be misinterpreted or misunderstood.

Both parents, but particularly the mother, are seen by the child uniquely, especially when the child is sick. Parents, in turn, know their children far better than those trying to help care for them. Listening to parents, carefully noting their observations, putting them at ease, and hearing out their worries even if they appear unrelated can help to provide them with the emotional resources needed to help their child. Impatience with or misunderstanding parents can impede their inclusion in the therapeutic process, particularly because parents will continue to care for the child after the illness—a point easily overlooked during the time of acute intervention.

To make their meaningful participation easier, parents need objective advice from the physician. While they should not be asked to make medical judgments, they have a legal and ethical right to be informed of the benefits and risks of therapy and to be included in the decision-making process.

Finally, a pediatrician's responsibility to a child does not end when the child has been cured of a physical illness. It is the unique role of those who care for children to help them fulfill their potential and take their rightful place as responsible adults. This may require the pediatrician to go far beyond traditional medical intervention into the area of schools, environment, and economic circumstances in the effort to assist the child.

II. **Principles of therapeutics.** Because of the considerable recuperative capacities of infants, children, and adolescents, it has been observed by experienced pediatric clinicians that, in the large majority of patients, therapeutic intervention is either irrelevant or worse. The remaining patients can be divided into those for whom an intervention would be helpful if only more were known about the disease and those for whom an appropriate intervention can, in fact, affect the outcome beneficially. Thus, the appropriate therapeutic choice for the pediatrician is most often reassurance. The most difficult decision is not which therapy, but whether to intervene at all.

In considering possible intervention, the clinician must assess the following, in order of importance: accuracy of diagnosis; relative effectiveness of possible therapies; risks to the patient of toxic effects; discomfort to the patient; and costs. These factors must be balanced against the risks and benefits of not intervening. Finally, follow-up and long-term observation should be provided.

A. Accuracy of diagnosis

1. After initial assessment is completed, a **working diagnosis** is established. As new information becomes available, the working diagnosis should be constantly reassessed.
2. No therapy should be completed simply because it has been started. It is better to recognize an error in diagnosis than to continue a therapeutic regimen based on flawed data or conclusions.
3. The most common error in diagnosis is attributing pathogenicity to an associated, but not causative, finding.
4. When a diagnosis depends on a laboratory test, the clinician should be aware of the relative accuracy of **that** test in **that** laboratory.
5. It is prudent to obtain the results of diagnostic tests at first hand.

B. Effectiveness of therapies

1. Few therapeutic regimens are **completely** effective in **all** cases.
2. Data on effectiveness are usually comparative. The clinician should assess the relevance of available studies to the case at hand.
3. "Cures" are usually a combination of therapy and the patient's own defenses. Thus, the underlying condition of the patient may be the most important single variable in effectiveness.
4. Even an effective therapy such as hemodialysis may not be more effective than the patient's own physiology (e.g., renal clearance of a particular substance). Thus, the general application of an effective technique is not necessarily appropriate in all cases.

C. Risks to the patient are sometimes overlooked. This is particularly true when multiple pharmacologic agents are used.

1. Drug interactions should be known and anticipated.
2. Any worsening of the patient's condition should prompt a reevaluation of the therapy.
3. Do not **assume** that the patient has received the dose or the drug prescribed. Compliance studies indicate that patients may not participate as fully as expected in prescribed therapy. For hospitalized patients, daily routine should include careful checking of nurses' notes and medication orders.
4. The appearance, taste, and odor of a medication may have a profound effect on compliance. The clinician should be familiar with the available preparations, flavors, and unpleasant characteristics of particular medications.
5. Therapeutic advice should be realistic. If a particular therapy is necessary despite adverse side effects, patients may need reinforcement and support to comply.
6. Potential side effects should be discussed fully with parents and, if appropriate, patients. **Avoid medical jargon.** Simple listing of effects is not sufficient. Be sure they are **understood.**

D. Discomfort for the patient is difficult to assess, but should be considered.

1. Physicians who have been patients testify to the discomfort of procedures considered routine. These include nasogastric suction, some intravenous medications, and gastrointestinal discomfort associated with some drugs.
2. Given the choice of two therapies, relative discomfort should be weighed in the choice.
3. Discomfort is not, per se, a contraindication to a particular regimen.
4. When an uncomfortable regimen is chosen, parents and patients should be informed of the discomfort in optimistic terms. Reassurance regarding the duration of discomfort and steps to minimize it are helpful.

E. Costs must be considered.

1. A hospital or local pharmacist can usually provide costs of a pharmaceutical regimen.
2. Generic drugs are cheaper than trade preparations, particularly if the pharmacist has permission to interchange.
3. Prescribe enough medication to avoid repeated trips to the pharmacy but not so much as to be wasteful.
4. There may be hidden costs to a particular regimen. These include monitoring

laboratory tests (e.g., serum levels), instability in storage and thus waste of a prescribed drug, or use of preparations that provide less drug per unit cost.

5. Clinical decisions by physicians can add enormously to health care costs. Thus, a system that keeps the physician informed of these costs should be encouraged.

F. Follow-up and long-term care. After a therapeutic regimen has been completed, whether in or out of the hospital, a follow-up visit should be scheduled to begin the process of continuing observation. Physicians should be alert to recurrent symptoms as well as possible sequelae. Frequently, therapeutic regimens may produce their own sequelae, such as an alteration in renal and/or hepatic function, that could pose problems for care. Most important, if acute care has been provided by a person or persons other than the patient's primary provider, an orderly return of responsibility to the primary provider should occur with the full knowledge of the patient and parents. Periodic follow-up by acute care providers is appropriate and is enhanced by communication between the acute care and primary care providers.

III. The hospitalized patient

A. Medical orders. Written medical orders are the physician's instructions to the nursing staff concerning the care and treatment of the patient. They should be written clearly and accurately, with special consideration to dosage calculation and decimal points. Orders are the **legal responsibility** of the physician; each entry as well as each page (if there is more than one) should be correctly labeled with the time and date and properly signed. An incorrect entry should be canceled by drawing a single line through it, and *error* should be written nearby, so that there will be no confusion at a later time. Unusual orders should be discussed with the nurse at the time they are written and individualized for each patient. Properly written orders should cover diagnosis and treatment and provide for the patient's comfort and dignity. The following schemes may be utilized:

1. **Diagnosis.** List the diagnostic findings in order of significance. Indicate the condition of the patient, whether critical, fair, or satisfactory. When a patient's condition is listed as critical, the family should be informed **by the physician** to avoid misunderstanding.

2. **Disposition.** This includes the frequency of monitoring vital signs and weighing the patient, permitted activities, special observations, isolation procedures, and environmental conditions.
   a. Unnecessarily frequent determination of vital signs overburdens the nursing staff and may unnecessarily discomfit the patient.
   b. Bed rest for an ill child is often more constraining than limited activity, and the social environment will also affect the degree of activity. Hospitalized children, particularly those in isolation, should not be denied social interaction.

3. **Diet.** Choose the diet with these considerations in mind: age, caloric needs, ability to chew, and special requirements necessitated by problems of absorption, intestinal irritation, residue, and transit time (see Chap. 10).

4. **Diagnostic tests.** Group in logical sequence (e.g., blood, radiographic). List all tests and the dates they are to be done. Diagnostic tests should be ordered after careful consideration of the costs, risks, and potential benefits, particularly regarding therapeutic implications.

5. **Drugs.** Include generic name, dose, route, frequency, and length of time to be administered. Review orders for narcotics *daily*. In general, separate drugs for specific therapy from drugs for symptomatic relief. Orders for respiratory or physical therapy must also be explicit as to duration, frequency, type, anatomic site of administration, and associated medication. Oxygen and aerosols require specific orders as well.

B. Analgesia and sedation (see also Chap. 3)
1. **Analgesia**
   a. **General principles.** The following guidelines may be helpful:
      (1) If pain is present in multiple sites, only the *single* most severe source will be recognized by the patient.

Table 1-1. Narcotic and nonnarcotic analgesics and dosages for pediatric use

Name	Dose
Nonnarcotic Acetylsalicylic acid (aspirin)	65–100 mg/kg/24 hr in 4–6 doses
Acetaminophen	Under 1 year 60 mg 1–3 years 60–120 mg 3–6 years 120 mg Over 6 years 240 mg
Pentazocine	30 mg q3–4h prn in adults. Not for children under 12
Narcotic Codeine phosphate	3 mg/kg/24 hr in 6–8 divided doses. Antitussive: 1 mg/kg/24 hr
Meperidine	6 mg/kg/24 hr
Methadone	0.7 mg/kg/24 hr
Morphine sulfate	0.1–0.2 mg/kg/dose
Camphorated opium tincture (Paregoric)	0.25–0.5 ml/kg/dose

(2) Although it is sometimes assumed that pain is not felt in children, particularly in small infants, or is easily forgotten, local anesthesia should be provided for diagnostic procedures whenever feasible.

(3) True analgesics such as morphine may mask pain, while sedatives such as phenobarbital will not. For this reason, sedatives may be helpful in elucidating pain and tenderness, particularly in the acutely disturbed abdomen.

(4) Postoperative pain, although generally of shorter duration in children than in adults, may still be severe enough to require medication for several days.

(5) Neonates also feel pain, but are less able to express it. Do not forget to order analgesia for neonates when pain is expected to be present. When not otherwise contraindicated, pain relief can be achieved with smaller amounts of narcotics when combined with a sedative ("lytic cocktail," sec. **2.b.(3)**).

  b. Specific therapeutics
  (1) Nonnarcotic analgesics. See Table 1-1.
    (a) Acetylsalicylic acid (aspirin) is the most frequently used analgesic and has antipyretic properties as well (see Chap. 2, p. 26) for the dose and route of administration).
      (i) Its analgesic properties are most suitable for the pain of headache, arthralgia, dysmenorrhea, or muscular ache. Doses in patients with acute rheumatic fever and juvenile rheumatoid arthritis are considerably higher (see Chap. 18, pp. 464ff.) than for simpler analgesia.
      (ii) Enteric-coated preparations are available to reduce gastric irritation, but absorption of these preparations is variable.
      (iii) Toxic effects include salicylism (see Chap. 4, p. 105), GI bleeding, iron deficiency anemia, abnormal clotting, altered thyroid function, decreased fasting blood sugar in diabetes, and increased cardiac load, which can aggravate incipient congestive heart failure and hemolysis in patients with glucose 6-phosphate dehydrogenase (G-6-PD) deficiency.
    (b) Acetaminophen. Although this drug is more valuable for antipyresis than for analgesia, its advantage is its availability in liquid

form. It is also more expensive. Peak blood levels are achieved in 2 hr (see Chap. 2, p. 26). **Toxic effects** include methemoglobinemia, anemia, and liver damage, but it does not cause hemolysis in G-6-PD deficiency. Overdose can produce fulminant liver failure (see Chap. 6, p. 106). **Phenacetin,** a sister drug, has similar properties, although it is probably more toxic. It is often used with aspirin and caffeine (Empirin Compound), but there is no evidence that this combination is more effective than aspirin alone.

(c) **Pentazocine,** a morphine-related drug, produces weak morphine antagonism and morphinelike subjective effects. **It is not approved for use in children under 12,** and because of its adverse effects on the CNS, **its use should be reserved for hospitalized patients.** For an extensive discussion of this preparation, see *Med. Lett. Drugs Ther.* 18:45, 1976.

(2) **Narcotic analgesics.** See Table 1-1.

(a) **Codeine,** a morphine derivative, is more effective than aspirin but less so than morphine itself. It is also less addictive than morphine and causes less disturbance of GI function, although seizures have been reported with its use. Its antitussive properties are well known, and it is frequently used for this purpose; however, there is risk of its abuse for this indication. Prolonged use of any narcotic is constipating. This may be especially significant postoperatively.

(b) **Meperidine (Demerol)** is probably a more effective analgesic than codeine, partly because higher doses are tolerated. It is highly addictive but less constipating and less depressing to the respiratory center than is morphine. It is widely used as an obstetric analgesic. *Because it does not constrict smooth muscle,* meperidine can be used in the presence of asthma, although sedation in any case of respiratory distress is extremely dangerous. In combination with promethazine (Phenergan) and chlorpromazine (Thorazine), it can be used as a "lytic cocktail" to produce rapid sedation with analgesia for painful diagnostic procedures (see Table 1-1 and sec. **2.b.(3)**).

(c) **Methadone** is included because of its widespread use in antiaddiction programs and in cancer patients with ongoing severe pain. Its analgesic potency is roughly equivalent to that of morphine, and it is effective PO. Its respiratory depressant effect is considerable, but it causes less GI disturbance than does morphine. When an addict can substitute it for morphine or heroin, withdrawal may ultimately be eased, if more prolonged. Nevertheless, **methadone is addictive.** It merely produces less euphoria than morphine or heroin; thus, the psychological component of addiction is undermined by its use.

(d) **Morphine** is perhaps the most important and widely used narcotic analgesic and is effective in any age group. It has little sedative effect and produces concomitant euphoria, with the risk of addiction.

(i) Because PO and PR preparations, although effective, are somewhat unreliable in absorption and metabolism, parenteral use is generally advised, either SQ (20 min), IM (20 min), or IV (immediate but dangerous). Analgesia usually lasts 3–4 hr.

(ii) Morphine is excreted via the liver and **should be administered with caution to a newborn or a patient with liver disease.**

(iii) **Paregoric** or **camphorated opium tincture** makes use of the constipating properties of morphine to aid in relieving symptoms of diarrhea with spasm of the colon. **Camphorated**

opium tincture should never be confused with tincture of opium, which is 25 times more powerful.

(iv) Because morphine is so addictive, its administration in the pediatric age group should be limited to patients with pulmonary stenosis and infundibular spasm, congestive heart failure, severe visceral pain of known origin, intractable pain, severe postoperative pain, and the pain of terminal disease. Although up to 14 days of administration is usually required to produce addiction, some adolescents may become addicted on only 1 or 2 doses.

(v) Tolerance to morphine includes tolerance to its CNS depressive properties, so that increasing the dose does not increase the likelihood of respiratory toxicity. The physician should remember that when a patient's dose is missed, an amount smaller than normal may suffice at the next dose. Death frequently occurs in addicts who administer *their usual high dose* after a few days off the drug, when tolerance is less.

(vi) Toxic effects include respiratory depression, increased intracranial pressure, arterial hypotension, nausea and vomiting, hyperglycemia, antidiuresis, urinary retention, addiction, and constipation.

2. Sedation

a. General principles. Among the most important characteristics of childhood are curiosity and the drive to explore and learn. Sedation can interfere with the child's capacity to interact with and learn from the environment. It narrows the child's experience, which, like childbirth for the mother, may be painful, but with help and support, can also be rich and memorable.

(1) Indications for sedation in children are few. They include preanesthesia (Table 1-2); painful diagnostic procedures such as bone marrow aspiration; agitation that contributes to morbidity, as in respiratory diseases such as asthma or croup (in which sedation should be used only with **extreme caution**); intubation or tracheostomy for respiratory assistance; intractable pain; and occasionally in the evaluation of severe visceral pain (e.g., acute appendicitis). In this last case, sedation short of general anesthesia does not mask pain but permits its elucidation by reducing surrounding anxiety and factitious tenderness.

Any child who is paralyzed, either iatrogenically or by disease, may still be aware of his or her surroundings with all of the fear and pain as well as the loss of control entailed. Sedation in such a case is an important part of acute care.

In children, sedation is *not* the treatment of choice in insomnia or hyperactivity and is used only as a last resort.

(2) The reaction of children to sedatives, particularly barbiturates, is unpredictable. At the toddler stage, sedatives may cause agitation. In addition, children have a higher incidence of idiosyncratic reactions to sedatives than do adults. For most purposes, the *weakest* effective sedative, such as hydroxyzine, is safe and least liable to cause unwanted side effects.

b. Specific therapeutics. See Table 1-3.

(1) Alcohol is an old-fashioned sedative, especially useful in infants; 10 ml brandy in 30 ml water PO or by gavage is usually effective.

(2) Chloral hydrate is probably the safest sedative and is inexpensive. It has a wide margin of safety, with the acceptable dose from 20–40 mg/kg/24 hr. Although the aftertaste is bitter, it seems to be well tolerated by children, particularly if offered in a small glass of juice; it is also available in PR form. Peak activity usually occurs within 30–60

Table 1-2. Preoperative medication for infants and children[a]

Age	Average weight (kg)	Pentobarbital[b] (Nembutal) (mg)	Morphine[c] (mg)	Atropine (mg)
Newborn	3.3			0.15
6 months	8.1	30 PR		0.2
1 year	10.6	45 PR	1.0	0.2
2 years	14.0	60 PR	1.5	0.3
3 years	15.0	60 PR	2.0	0.3
4 years	17.1	90 PR	3.0	0.3
5 years	19.4	90 PR	3.0	0.3
6 years	22.0	90 PR	4.0	0.4
7 years	24.7	90 PR	5.0	0.4
8 years	27.9	100 PO	6.0	0.4
9 years	31.4	100 PO	6.0	0.4
10 years	35.2	100 PO	7.0	0.4
11 years	39.6	100 PO	7.0	0.4
12 years	44.4	100 PO	7.0	0.4
13 years	49.1	100 PO	8.0	0.4
14 years	54.4	100 PO	8.0	0.4
15 years	58.8	100 PO	8.0	0.4
16 years	61.9	100 PO	8.0	0.4

[a]This guide is for average, well-developed patients. Increases or reductions in medication must be made for patients who do not fall into the guidelines, that is, hyperactive, obese, or poor-risk patients.
[b]The suggested guide for pentobarbital when followed by morphine is 4.0 mg/kg for rectal use (maximum, 120 mg) and 3.0 mg/kg for oral use (maximum, 100 mg). Pentobarbital should be given at least 90 min before surgery.
[c]The suggested guide for morphine is 0.75 mg/year of age. Morphine should be given 35–45 min (IM or SQ) before surgery.

Table 1-3. Sedatives and dosages for pediatric use

Drug	Dose
Alcohol	10 ml brandy in 30 ml/H_2O in infants
Chloral hydrate	15–40 mg/kg/24 hr in 2–3 divided doses
Paraldehyde	0.15 ml/kg/dose
Antihistamine	Diphenhydramine 5 mg/kg/24 hr Promethazine 0.5 mg/kg/dose Hydroxyzine 2 mg/kg/24 hr
Chlorpromazine	2 mg/kg/24 hr
Barbiturates	
Amobarbital (Amytal)	6 mg/kg/24 hr in 3 divided doses
Secobarbital (Seconal)	6 mg/kg/24 hr in 3 divided doses
Pentobarbital (Nembutal)	6 mg/kg/24 hr in 3 divided doses
Phenobarbital	6 mg/kg/24 hr in 3 divided doses
Demerol compound	
25 mg meperidine	1 ml/15 kg IM, not to exceed 2 ml
6.25 mg chlorpromazine	per dose
6.25 mg promethazine in 1 ml	

min of administration. **Caution should be used in patients with live disease. Aspiration can produce fatal laryngospasm.**

(3) Paraldehyde (see also Chap. 3, pp. 59ff) has the advantage of rapic action and is relatively safe. Used primarily for alcohol withdrawal ir adults, it is particularly valuable in the management of seizures ir children. **Caution should be exercised in patients with liver dis ease,** but it can be used in those with renal insufficiency. It is ad ministered in corn oil PR; **IV administration has been associatec with polyethylene emboli from dissolved tubing.**

(4) Antihistamines have a variety of clinical uses that have varying degrees of success. (For a more complete discussion of these agents see *Med. Lett. Drugs Ther.* 19:1, 1977.)

(a) Antihistamines with the most effective sedative properties in clude promethazine (Phenergan), diphenhydramine (Benadryl) and hydroxyzine (Atarax). Cyclizine, meclizine, and pro methazine are also clinically useful as antiemetics. Trimeprazine and diphenhydramine may reduce pruritus, possibly due to their sedative properties. Promethazine, chlorpromazine, and meperi dine form a sedative compound (see **3**), which produces rapid analgesia with sedation and is particularly useful for painful diagnostic procedures.

(b) Serious side effects are few, and the drugs are well tolerated PO.

(c) Because of the occasional stimulating effect of barbiturates in children under 2, antihistamines may be used to achieve a seda tive effect, but in many children no effect at all is seen.

(5) Tranquilizers. With the exception of the phenothiazines, these drugs have little use in pediatrics (see *Can. Anaesth. Soc. J.* 5:177, 1958). Chlorpromazine is the most widely used phenothiazine and is the third component of the lytic cocktail. It has a relatively wide margin of safety and can be used effectively in agitated adolescents. It is one of the effective agents in the management of the infant of the heroin addicted mother.

(6) Barbiturates are true hypnotic agents.

(a) Phenobarbital is used most widely in the control of seizure disor ders and to antagonize stimulants such as caffeine or amphetamines (see Chap. 3, p. 60; Chap. 20, pp. 504, 508).

(b) Secobarbital and pentobarbital are probably more useful sedative hypnotics because of their rapid action and are widely used as preoperative medication. They are not analgesics, so that pen tobarbital in particular can be helpful in evaluating abdominal pain in the anxious small child.

(c) All three agents are available for use PO, PR, or parenterally.

(d) For PR administration of barbiturates a suppository should be used; even then, effective absorption is variable. IM or IV injec tion is more reliable, but the individual reactions to a given dose preclude prediction of its effect.

(e) Because of respiratory depression, extreme caution should be used in administering barbiturates IV, although pentobarbital produces relatively little respiratory depression for the hypnotic dose used.

3. Combined analgesia and sedation (lytic cocktail, Demerol compound). To supply rapid analgesia and sedation, a compound preparation of meperidine, chlorpromazine, and promethazine has found wide acceptance at our institu tion. Ampules of 10 ml are made up in the proportions listed in Table 1-3.

IV. The pediatric consultation. Pediatricians may be asked to consult with colleagues from other medical specialties (e.g., surgery, internal medicine), other pediatric pro viders (e.g., family practitioners, child psychologists), or other pediatricians. The guidelines in **A–G** may be helpful.

A. Respond as soon as possible. A colleague seeking consultation is usually in need of prompt assistance unless otherwise specified. If necessary, a suitable substitute should be offered. Do not provide a substitute without the knowledge of the requesting colleague, since this may create confusion.

B. Determine what questions require your assistance and respond specifically to them.

C. Your colleague has asked for assistance, not replacement. Explain the limits of your role to patients and parents at the onset and maintain those limits, particularly if the consultation requires follow-up.

D. Successful consultation is best accomplished by meticulous attention to detail. Do not assume you have more knowledge than a requesting colleague. You may, however, have more time. Frequently, the answer to a clinical dilemma lies in elucidating the temporal relationships of illness events or in finding an overlooked detail on physical examination.

E. Do not comment on a colleague's management in the presence of the patient or parents. Such comments are frequently misunderstood, blown out of proportion, or both.

F. The best consultation provides the requesting colleague with information on which to base clinical decisions. Inform—do not attempt to dictate patient care.

G. Discuss your findings with the requesting colleague **before** discussing them with patient and family.

Medical practice is, at best, inexact. Part of good medical judgment is knowing when to ask for help. Consultation provided in a prompt and helpful manner assures a patient of an extra measure of knowledge and concern, with the added benefit of enhancing the knowledge of all participants.

V. Death of a child (see also *Pediatrics* 62:96, 1978). In the first week of life, more deaths occur than in any subsequent period of childhood. Between the first week of life and 1 year of age, the sudden infant death syndrome is the most common cause of death. (For a complete discussion of this syndrome see Chap. 3, p. 69). After 1 year of age, accidents exceed all other acquired causes.

The strongest of all grief reactions occurs when parents have lost a child. Much of parental grief is based on the concept of parent-infant bonding. The reciprocal interaction between a parent and a young infant results in early involvement and mutual investment of growing intensity. The death of a child brings a sudden and drastic end to that relationship. Parents react to the death of their child in a manner that reflects their family life, emotional structure, individual attachment, and the degree of specific circumstances associated with the loss. What health professionals do during this period is usually based on their own feelings as well as on assumptions that arise from customs, traditions, state and hospital health rules, and even research interests. Thoughtful and caring medical personnel can share and help to lighten the family's burden.

When a child has a fatal disease, the parents and immediate family face the loss of all their expectations for the child and an extended period of sadness. After learning of the diagnosis, parents usually cannot absorb the detailed information they are given about the disease and its clinical course. They require sufficient time and privacy to formulate their questions, and they need guidance to establish realistic expectations, especially if referral to a large medical center is to be made. Often, their questions are repetitious; sometimes they completely avoid certain topics. Fathers may sometimes have less insight into the mechanisms of child rearing and child health risks than do mothers, and they may be less prepared to accept the fragility of life and the constraints on their own control over their children's environment or destiny. Fathers seem to limit their requests for help, or, even more often, such requests after the loss of their child are not recognized by health professionals. Given a chance to express their feelings, fathers can utilize support constructively. If possible, the same physician should talk with both parents together and/or separately about the child's progress and remain aware of their individual needs.

Following a child's death the physician's first responsibility is to inform the parents in a direct, sensitive manner; warmth and understanding provide a closeness with the family. Unless there are exceptional circumstances, a parent should *never* be informed of a child's death by telephone.

An important prerequisite in talking to parents about their child's death is knowledge of the circumstances in which it occurred. Not being given this information may serve to reinforce parents' doubts and guilts.

It may be helpful to provide sedation or a quiet place for the parents, who may prefer to be alone. The hospital staff can also help with funeral arrangements, inform other family members, or arrange transportation.

Similarly, viewing and touching the body may be important, to help the parents grasp the actuality of their child's death. They may need time alone to hold and talk to the deceased child as their last gestures of caring. In the case of a newborn, seeing the body is especially important to the parents. Though these parents have had little physical contact with their child, they have experienced pregnancy and have formulated plans and expectations that are suddenly ended. During the pregnancy they may also have had the normal fears about deformed infants, and mothers may often recall incidents during pregnancy that they feel could have influenced the eventual outcome. To quiet those fears, they may need to see that their baby was not grossly abnormal.

Not only the parents but surviving children may need help with their grief. Children under the age of 5 years view the death as a temporary and reversible situation. Children between 5 and 10 years of age may look at death in terms of responsibility—something or someone was responsible. By the time children are about 10 years old, they are able to understand that death is inevitable and irreversible. Surviving older children appear to be able to resolve the problem of loss, and do substantially better when they are included in the grief process. For this reason parents can be advised to be as open as possible with their explanations and their own reactions. Clinicians may need to clarify that a sibling died of a special illness or one that affects only infants and not older children or parents. Children may also need to be reassured that their health is good and that the same event will not happen to them.

In the course of normal sibling rivalry, children might wish an infant brother or sister to die. Small children indulge in magical thinking; they believe they can cause events to occur by wishing them. In this way they may implicate themselves and need assurance that they did nothing to cause the death.

Some children mourn losses for a long time. Their grief may be exhibited in school difficulties or sleep problems or special fears. These should be addressed individually, with the knowledge that sibling loss almost certainly plays a significant role in these behavior changes.

Follow-up visits with parents are important. If an autopsy has been performed, a visit to discuss the findings should follow its completion. Irrespective of an autopsy, visits should be made at 6 weeks and 6 months to gauge the progress of grieving, anticipate unusual problems in adjusting to the child's death, and answer the many questions about the circumstances of the death and how to help siblings adjust to their feelings. Friends and relatives usually tire of discussing the death long before parents have worked through their own feelings.

When parents have lost a child, the decision to have another is complex. If they are able to complete the grief process, the psychological environment for the subsequent newborn will be healthier. Parents are too often advised to have a "replacement" child quickly. There is no replacement for a lost child, and it may be better advice to parents to allow more time following a loss before a subsequent pregnancy. The physician who was so intimately involved can not only be open to such discussions but also can help to correct the inevitable distortions of events caused by grief.

Finally, physicians must be aware of and deal with their own feelings about the death of a patient. A feeling of failure is often present, particularly when complicated management did not suffice. There may be a desire to "make it up" to the family because of possible uncertainty surrounding the physician's participation. There is nothing wrong with feeling a sense of loss at the death of a patient or with the need to grieve, but it is the physician's hard task to put his or her own grief aside until the needs of the parents and family have been met.

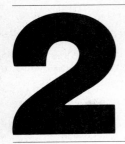

Well Child Care

I. **General principles.** The term *well child care* describes an ongoing relationship with a provider of pediatric care intended to assure good health by providing **early intervention, preventive care, and follow-up.** Repeated visits to the office by the child and his or her parent permit mutual trust and respect to be established and routine screening tests (Table 2-1) to be carried out.

II. **Specific considerations**

  A. **Growth and development**

    1. **Height and weight charts.** Several types of height and weight charts that provide a graphic record of physical growth are available, the most recent having been compiled by the National Center for Health Statistics, U.S. Public Health Service. These charts cover the ages from birth to 36 months and from 2–18 years. **Sequential measurements** are much more useful than single determinations of height and weight in giving an overall picture of the child's growth pattern (Figs. 2-1, 2-2, 2-3, and 2-4). When weight or height appears to deviate from the norm, incremental growth curves can be helpful in differentiating pathologic from nonpathologic patterns (see Figs. 2-5 and 2-6).

    2. **Developmental milestones.** There are several printed graphs, such as the Denver Developmental Screening Test, which can be used to plot development in gross motor, fine motor, language, and social capacities over a period of time.

  B. **Feeding**

    1. **General principles**

      a. A **flexible approach** should be used to allow parents and their infants and children choices in both feeding patterns and content of diet.

      b. **Breast milk** is the preferred source of nutrition for either low-birth-weight or full-term infants and can be continued through 18–24 months of age. Failure, when it occurs, is most commonly due to maternal anxiety about the quantity of intake, an unsatisfied infant, fears of cosmetic effects, cultural pressures, and lack of adequate instructions.

      c. Concerns likely to arise in the first few weeks are best discussed at a prenatal visit or at hospital visits after the child's birth. The early discussion of variability in feeding patterns, both in quantity and in quality, helps to allay future concerns and anxieties. These discussions include demand versus scheduled feedings, how and when to supplement, fussiness as a sign of hunger, "sleeping through" feedings, introduction of solids, patterns of bowel movements, vitamin and fluoride supplements, the role of the father in feedings, and medical assessment of adequacy of intake.

      d. Parents are encouraged to call during the first few weeks after birth with questions pertaining to feeding.

      e. Parents of infants with **family histories of allergy** should be aware of the more troublesome foods in the first year of life (orange juice, nuts, fish, strawberries, chocolate, and egg whites). Delaying exposure to these foods has been shown to result in fewer sensitivity reactions.

      f. **Protein requirements** are proportionately higher during childhood because of rapid growth rates. If protein sources are largely vegetable, foods

Table 2-1. Routine screening in well child care[a]

Test	Frequency
Hemoglobin and hematocrit	Once between 9–12 months Once between 4–5 years Once between 12–14 years

Sickle cell	For all at-risk patients (e.g., blacks, Hispanics)
	    Infants: Either mother or father to be screened for hemoglobin SS or hemoglobin SS trait
	    All children ages 9 months–6 years, at time of first well child checkup
	    All children who present with anemia who have no documented screen

Tuberculin	Once between 9–12 months Once between 4–5 years Once between 12–14 years
Urinalysis and urine culture	Once in both sexes when a clean spontaneously voided sample can be obtained, then only if genitourinary symptoms are present. Present medical evidence suggests the need for reevaluation of the frequency and timing of additional routine urinalysis and culture.
EP (lead and iron deficiency)	**High risk:** Once between 9–12 months; then every 6 months to age 3 years; then yearly to age 6 years **Low risk:** Once between 9–12 months and again at 2 years
Cholesterol	Only if positive family history of hypercholesterolemia or premature cardiovascular disease
Hearing	Every 3 years from age 3 years
Vision	Yearly from 3–5 years[b]; then every 2 years
Dental	Every checkup; first referral age 2½–3 years
Hypertension	Every checkup from age 3 years

[a]It is at the discretion of the provider, if warranted, to do more frequent testing.
[b]May modify according to accuracy, detail, and frequency of school screening program.

    must be more varied to ensure an adequate intake of amino acids and vitamins (for recommended daily dietary allowances, see Table 2-2).

    g. A child's food intake is seldom constant and varies daily in quantity and quality. In general, parents can be reassured that a child will take in enough to grow. A special period of apparent, decreased intake seems to occur at 7–9 months, along with the desire of babies to feed themselves; at 2–3 years, along with the further need for independence; and at 5–6 years. Since these behaviors are normal developmental processes, it is important for pediatricians to ally themselves with the parents in staying calm about these periods despite the pressure from concerned relatives.

    h. New foods may be refused initially because of their unfamiliarity.

    i. Forced feedings are never useful at any age.

  2. Breast-feedings. See also Chap. 5, pp. 123ff.

    a. Breast milk alone is adequate as the sole source of nutrition for the first 6–9 months of life, assuming a supply adequate to meet caloric and volume needs.

    b. Demand feeding is strongly encouraged. It is important to discuss the normal changing requirements for calories and fluid as babies grow, as this is reflected in increased milk production and a subsequent decrease in the frequency of nursings.

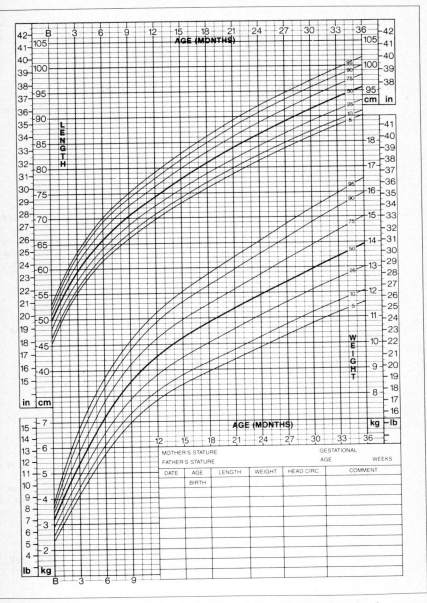

Fig. 2-1. Physical growth of girls from birth to 36 months of age. NCHS percentiles. (Adapted from P.V.V. Hamill et al., Physical growth: National Center for Health Statistics percentiles. *Am. J. Clin. Nutr.* 32:607, 1979. Data from the Fels Research Institute, Wright State University School of Medicine, Yellow Springs, Ohio. © 1982 by Ross Laboratories, Columbus, Ohio.)

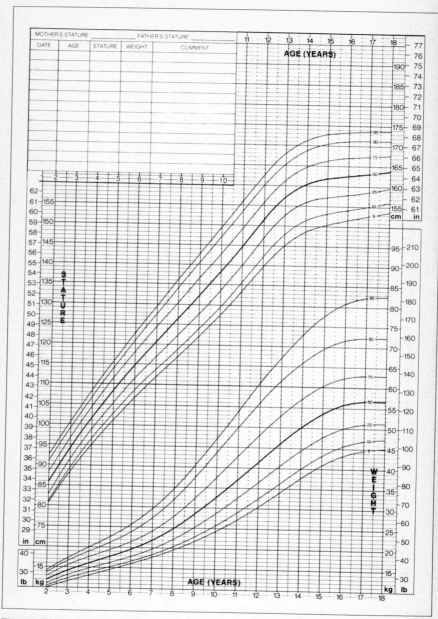

Fig. 2-2. Physical growth of girls from 2 to 18 years of age. NCHS percentiles. (Adapted from P.V.V. Hamill et al., Physical growth: National Center for Health Statistics percentiles. *Am. J. Clin. Nutr.* 32:607, 1979. Data from the National Center for Health Statistics, Hyattsville, Maryland. © 1982 by Ross Laboratories, Columbus, Ohio.)

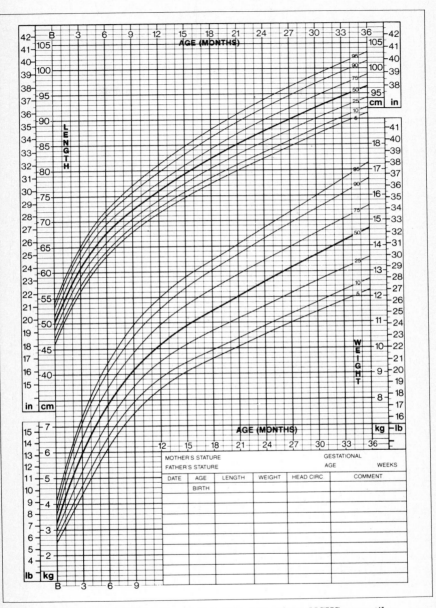

Fig. 2-3. Physical growth of boys from birth to 36 months of age. NCHS percentiles. (Adapted from P.V.V. Hamill et al., Physical growth: National Center for Health Statistics percentiles. *Am. J. Clin. Nutr.* 32:607, 1979. Data from the Fels Research Institute, Wright State University School of Medicine, Yellow Springs, Ohio. © 1982 by Ross Laboratories, Columbus, Ohio.)

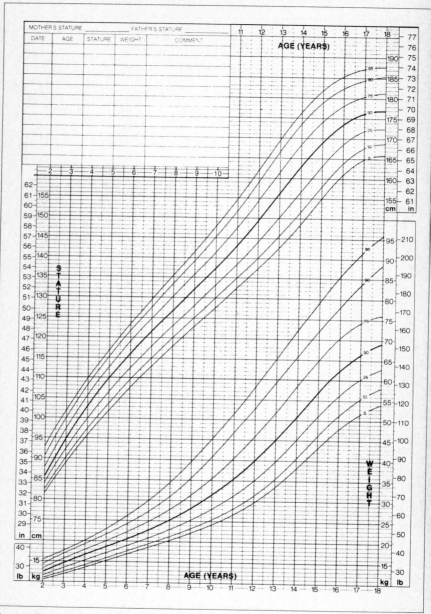

Fig. 2-4. Physical growth of boys from 2 to 18 years of age. NCHS percentiles. (Adapted from P.V.V. Hamill et al., Physical growth: National Center for Health Statistics percentiles. *Am. J. Clin. Nutr.* 32:607, 1979. Data from the National Center for Health Statistics, Hyattsville, Maryland. © 1982 by Ross Laboratories, Columbus, Ohio.)

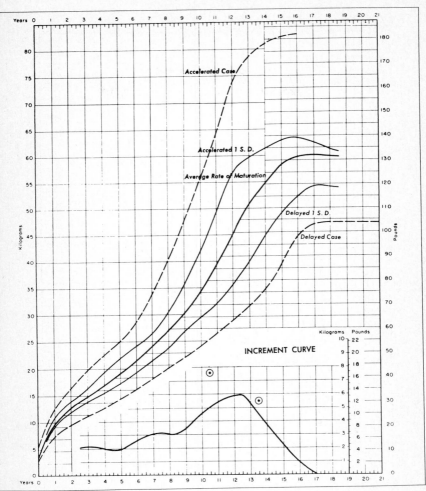

Fig. 2-5. Growth curves of weight by age for girls. (Reproduced with permission from L. Bayer and N. Bayley, *Growth Diagnosis*. Chicago: University of Chicago Press, 1959. Courtesy of Ross Laboratories.)

c. Mothers who are planning to nurse should take steps to prepare their breasts and particularly their nipples. Prenatal exposure to air, manipulation, and application of emollients such as lanolin may help to "toughen" the nipples and prevent cracking.

d. To assess the adequacy of breast-feeding, an initial visit is scheduled at 2 weeks of age for first-time mothers and their babies. A weight gain of half an ounce per day or more is indicative of a successful beginning. Subsequent visits may be scheduled as needed depending upon the amount of support required.

e. Supplementation with formula may be used after nursing is established on either a sporadic or a regular basis to meet the needs of both mother and baby. Many new mothers have the misconception that one must either breast-feed completely or not breast-feed at all.

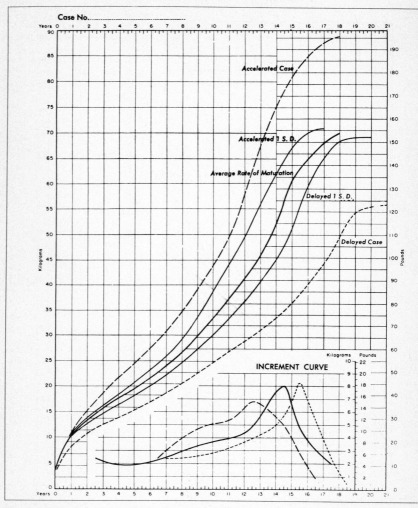

Fig. 2-6. Growth curves of weight by age for boys. (Reproduced with permission from L. Bayer and N. Bayley, *Growth Diagnosis*. Chicago: University of Chicago Press, 1959. Courtesy of Ross Laboratories.)

  f. Breast-feeding is encouraged for as long as mother and infant find it mutually satisfying.
3. Formula feeding. See also Chap. 5.
  a. Choice of cow's milk–based formula (Similac, Enfamil, or SMA) is usually determined by current nursery use or by prior experience. Soy-based products may be used initially for babies with strong family histories of true milk allergy.
  b. Iron-containing formula is recommended for preterm babies or those with anticipated iron needs (e.g., perinatal blood loss, twin pregnancy, maternal anemia). Powdered or concentrated formula mixed with water is recommended for babies in communities with fluoridated water.

4. Introduction of solids

    a. A flexible approach to the introduction of solid foods is helpful. A 2- to 4-day period should separate the introduction of each new food to mark the occurrence of specific food intolerance or allergy.

    b. Increasingly, babies are being fed blended or strained table foods or soft finger foods rather than commercially available strained or junior foods.

    c. Rarely does the introduction of solid foods prior to 3–4 months significantly alter the feeding and sleeping patterns of babies.

    d. Some babies who resume night feedings after having given them up will again sleep through the night with the judicious use of an evening solid feeding.

    e. A source of iron should be added at 4 months of age, with the introduction of iron-containing formula, cereals or other iron-containing solids, or an iron supplement. Further solids may then be introduced.

    f. Formula or breast milk should be continued through the first year of life.

    g. Although specific food intolerance or allergy is unusual during the first year of life, one may want to avoid "allergenic" foods, such as whole eggs and citrus fruits, until the second year.

5. Vitamin and fluoride supplements. See also Chap. 5.

    a. Breast-fed infants are given 400 IU/day of vitamin D. This requirement can be met with vitamin D alone or with a commercially available preparation that contains 1500 IU of vitamin A and 50 mg of vitamin C as well.

    b. The fluoride dosage schedule (Table 2-3) follows the recommendations of the American Academy of Pediatrics Committee on Nutrition and is adapted from guidelines proposed by the American Dental Association Council on Dental Therapeutics. In communities with fluoridated water, a fluoride supplement is given to breast-fed babies until they begin to drink water.

C. Immunizations. The American Academy of Pediatrics and the Public Health Service Advisory Committee on Immunization Practices have recommended a schedule for routine, active immunization of normal infants and children (see Table 2-4), to begin at age 2 months. This schedule is appropriate for premature and low-birth-weight infants and for breast-fed and bottle-fed infants. Table 2-5 includes a schedule for primary immunization of children not immunized in infancy. In children more than 6 years of age, adult-type diphtheria-tetanus toxoid (DT) is preferred over diphtheria-pertussis-tetanus (DPT) except in unusual circumstances.

1. General contraindications to immunization

    a. Acute febrile illness. Minor infection without fever is **not** a contraindication.

    b. Immunodeficiency disorders

    c. Leukemia, lymphoma, or generalized malignancy

    d. Immunosuppressive therapy, including radiation therapy, corticosteroids, or antimetabolites. Children receiving alternate-day corticosteroids for suppression of respiratory inflammation are not at risk during immunization.

    e. Pregnancy. Live virus preparations—measles, mumps, rubella, oral poliomyelitis, and yellow fever vaccines—are contraindicated.

    f. Gamma globulin, plasma, or blood transfusion within the preceding 8 weeks

    g. Prior allergic reaction to the same or related vaccine

        (1) Children who are allergic to eggs should not receive vaccines grown on chick or duck embryos (e.g., influenza, yellow fever, and duck embryo rabies vaccines). These children can safely receive vaccines grown on chick or duck fibroblasts (e.g., measles, rubella, and mumps).

        (2) Some vaccines—e.g., rubella—are available from several cell systems, among them duck, human, and rabbit cells. An appropriate, nonallergenic choice may be made from among these preparations.

Table 2-2. Recommended daily dietary allowances, revised 1980

Group	Age (years)	Weight (kg)	Energy (kcal)	Protein (gm)	Vitamin A† (RE)	Fat-soluble vitamins Vitamin A activity (IU)	Vitamin D (IU)	Vitamin E activity (IU)
Infants	0.0–0.5	6	kg × 117	kg × 2.2	420	1400	400	4
	0.5–1.0	9	kg × 108	kg × 2.0	400	2000	400	5
Children	1–3	13	1300	23	400	2000	400	7
	4–6	20	1800	30	500	2500	400	9
	7–10	28	2400	34	700	3300	400	10
Males	11–14	45	2800	45	1000	5000	400	12
	15–18	66	3000	56	1000	5000	400	15
	19–22	70	3000	56	1000	5000	400	15
Females	11–14	46	2400	46	800	4000	400	10
	15–18	55	2100	46	800	4000	400	11
	19–22	55	2100	44	800	4000	400	12
Pregnant			+300	+30	+200	5000	400	15
Lactating			+500	+20	+400	6000	400	15

Group	Age (years)	Weight (kg)	Ascorbic acid (mg)	Folic acid (µg)	Water-soluble vitamins Niacin (mg)	Riboflavin (mg)	Thiamine (mg)	Vitamin B$_6$ (mg)	Vitamin B$_{12}$ (µg)
Infants	0.0–0.5	6	35	30	6	0.4	0.3	0.3	0.5*
	0.5–1.0	9	35	45	8	0.6	0.5	0.6	1.5
Children	1–3	13	40	100	9	0.8	0.7	0.9	2.0
	4–6	20	40	200	11	1.0	0.9	1.3	2.5
	7–10	28	40	300	16	1.4	1.2	1.6	3.0

Males	11–14	45	45	400	18	1.6	1.4	1.8	3.0
	15–18	66	45	400	18	1.7	1.4	2.0	3.0
	19–22	70	45	400	19	1.7	1.5	2.2	3.0
Females	11–14	46	45	400	15	1.3	1.1	1.8	3.0
	15–18	55	45	400	14	1.3	1.1	2.0	3.0
	19–22	55	45	400	14	1.3	1.1	2.0	3.0
Pregnant			60	+400	+2	+0.3	+0.4	+0.6	+1.0
Lactating			60	+100	+5	+0.5	+0.5	+0.5	+1.0

			Minerals					
	Age (years)	Weight (kg)	Calcium (mg)	Phosphorus (mg)	Iodine (μg)	Iron (mg)	Magnesium (mg)	Zinc (mg)
Infants	0.0–0.5	6	360	240	40	10	50	3
	0.5–1.0	9	540	360	50	15	70	5
Children	1–3	13	800	800	70	15	150	10
	4–6	20	800	800	90	10	200	10
	7–10	28	800	800	120	10	250	10
Males	11–14	45	1200	1200	150	18	350	15
	15–18	66	1200	1200	150	18	400	15
	19–22	70	800	800	150	10	350	15
Females	11–14	46	1200	1200	150	18	300	15
	15–18	55	1200	1200	150	18	300	15
	19–22	55	800	800	150	18	300	15
Pregnant			+400	+400	+25	†	+150	+ 5
Lactating			+400	+400	+50	†	+150	+10

*The allowances are intended to provide for individual variations among most persons as they live in the United States under usual environmental stresses. Diets should be based on a variety of common foods in order to provide other nutrients for which human requirements have been less well defined.

†Retinol equivalents: 1 retinol equivalent = 1 μg retinol or 6 μg β-carotene.

Source: Modified from Committee on Dietary Allowances and Committee on Interpretation of the Recommended Dietary Allowances. Food and Nutrition Board, National Research Council, 9th rev. ed. Washington, D.C.: National Academy of Sciences, 1980.

Table 2-3. Supplemental fluoride dosage schedule (mg/day*)

Age	Concentration of fluoride in drinking water (ppm)		
	<0.3	0.3–0.7	>0.7
2 weeks–2 years	0.25	0	0
2–3 years	0.50	0.25	0
3–16 years	1.00	0.50	0

*Fluoride content of 2.2 mg of sodium fluoride is 1 mg fluoride.
Source: Adapted from *Pediatric Nutrition Handbook*. Evanston, Ill.: American Academy of Pediatrics 1979.

Table 2-4. Recommended schedule for active immunization of normal infants and children

Recommended age	Vaccine(s)	Comments
2 months	DTP, OPV	Can be initiated earlier in areas of high endemicity
4 months	DTP, OPV	2-month interval desired for OPV to avoid interference
6 months	DTP (OPV)	OPV optional for areas where polio might be imported
15 months	Measles, mumps, rubella (MMR)	MMR preferred
18 months	DTP, OPV	DTP essential
4–6 years*	DTP, OPV	
14–16 years	Td	Repeat every 10 years for lifetime

DTP = diphtheria and tetanus toxoids with pertussis vaccine; OPV = oral, attenuated poliovirus vaccine which contains poliovirus types 1, 2, and 3; MMR = live measles, mumps, and rubella viruses in a combined vaccine; Td = adult tetanus toxoid (full dose) and diphtheria toxoid (reduced dose) in combination.
*Up to the seventh birthday.
Note: For all products used, consult manufacturer's brochure for instructions for storage, handling, and administration.
Source: Adapted with permission from the Report of the Committee on Infectious Diseases, American Academy of Pediatrics, 1982.

2. **Contraindications to live virus vaccines** (poliomyelitis, measles, mumps, and rubella)
   a. In general, live virus vaccines are contraindicated in patients who are pregnant, immunosuppressed, or immunodeficient. Other considerations include the following:
      (1) A diagnosis of immunodeficiency in a child should prompt a screening of the immunocompetency of all siblings before any immunizations are given. Normal siblings of immunosuppressed or immunodeficient patients should receive **killed** poliomyelitis vaccine (IPV).
      (2) It is permissible to give rubella vaccine to the child of a pregnant woman.
      (3) When a primary series of oral poliomyelitis vaccine (OPV) is completed at or beyond the fourth birthday, a booster dose is not required. Children who have received primary immunization with IPV should receive a booster dose of IPV every 5 years until the age of 18 years unless a primary series of OPV is completed. Routine primary

Table 2-5. Recommended immunization schedules for infants and children not initially immunized at usual recommended times in early infancy

Timing	Preferred schedule	Recommended schedules — Alternatives #1	#2	#3	Comments
First visit	DTP #1, OPV #1	MMR	DTP #1, OPV #1	DTP #1, OPV #1, MMR	MMR should be given no younger than 15 months old
1 month after first visit	MMR	DTP #1, OPV #1	MMR, DTP #2	DTP #2	
2 months after first visit	DTP #2, OPV #2		DTP #3, OPV #2	DTP #3, OPV #2	
3 months after first visit	(DTP #3)	DTP #2, OPV #2			In preferred schedule, DTP #3 can be given if OPV #3 is not to be given until 10–16 months
4 months after first visit	DTP #3 (OPV #3)		(OPV #3)	(OPV #3)	OPV #3 optional for areas for likely importation of polio (e.g., some southwestern states)
5 months after first visit		DTP #3 (OPV #3)			
10–16 months after last dose	DTP #4, OPV #3 or OPV #4	DTP #4, OPV #3 or OPV #4	DTP #4, OPV #3 or OPV #4	DTP #4, OPV #3 or OPV #4	
Preschool	DTP #5, OPV #4 or OPV #5	DTP #5, OPV #4 or OPV #5	DTP #5, OPV #4 or OPV #5	DTP #5, OPV #4 or OPV #5	Preschool dose not necessary if DTP #4 or #5 given after fourth birthday
14–16 years old	Td	Td	Td	Td	Repeat every 10 years

Alternative #1 can be used in those more than 15 months old if measles is occurring in the community.
Alternative #2 allows for more rapid DTP immunization.
Alternative #3 should be reserved for those whose access to medical care is compromised by poor compliance.
Source: Adapted with permission from the Report of the Committee on Infectious Diseases, American Academy of Pediatrics, 1982.

poliomyelitis virus vaccination of adults (18 years and older) residing in the United States is not necessary (see *M.W.R.* 31:22–33, 1982).

(4) Children with static, unchanging neurologic disorders may be immunized against pertussis, measles, mumps, and rubella. These vaccines afford protection against even more damaging neurologic sequelae.

3. **Side effects.** The side effects of immunizations may be local or systemic but are usually mild and self-limited. Fever and/or minor erythema or swelling in the extremity used for the injection are the most common. Parents should be advised that such reactions may occur, but that the incidence and severity of these reactions are far exceeded by the risks and dangers of the diseases against which they afford protection.

4. **Recommendations for specific nonroutine immunizations**
   a. **Smallpox.** In the United States, routine vaccination of children or adults, including health workers, has been discontinued.
   b. **Influenza.** Vaccination with **killed** virus vaccine is recommended for those at high risk of severe influenzal illness because of underlying cardiac, renal, or pulmonary disease, diabetes, sickle cell anemia, or malignancy. Allergy to previous influenza vaccinations or hypersensitivity to eggs or egg products is a contraindication to immunization. At present, the subvirion (split virus) preparation is recommended for persons less than 12 years old.
   c. **Meningococcal polysaccharide vaccines.** Three meningococcal polysaccharide vaccines (monovalent A, monovalent C, and bivalent AC) are currently licensed in the United States for the following indications:
      (1) Travel to countries having epidemic meningococcal disease
      (2) As an adjunct to antibiotic prophylaxis (see Table 15-9) for household contacts of a person with meningococcal disease caused by serogroup A or C
      (3) Control of epidemic meningococcal disease caused by serogroup A or C
   d. **Pneumococcal vaccine.** A vaccine containing polysaccharide antigens from the pneumococcal serotypes most prominent in human disease (American types 1–4, 6, 8, 9, 12, 14, 19, 23, 51, and 56) has been licensed in the United States. Infants and toddlers may have a poor or unpredictable antibody response; hence, the vaccine is not recommended for children under age 2 years. Patients with splenic dysfunction (e.g., sickle hemoglobinopathies or splenectomy patients) and those whose chronic diseases have an increased susceptibility to pneumococcal infection (e.g., patients with diabetes, hepatic disease, cardiopulmonary disease, and chronic renal failure and hemodialysis patients) should receive the accepted single-dose injection of pneumococcal vaccine and should in addition be maintained on daily antibiotic prophylaxis with penicillin, ampicillin, or erythromycin.

D. **Screening.** See Table 2-1 for frequency of screening visits. See also Chaps. 5 and 14.

E. **Accident prevention.** See Table 2-6 for guidance in accident prevention by age group.

III. Common management problems
A. **Organic problems in the infant or young child**
   1. **Fever**
      a. **General considerations**
         (1) Fever should be considered a sign of infection in most children. Fever, unless exceptionally high—over 41.1°C (106°F)—does no specific harm to the patient. Indeed, in some cases the presence of fever may be of biologic value.
         (2) Factors that should arouse the physician's concern are fevers that fail to respond to specific antipyretic measures or patients who fail to act and look better when less febrile.

Table 2-6. Accident prevention in childhood

Age and cause of morbidity	Prevention
0–6 Months	
Auto accidents	Use authorized car seat until child is 3 years old, then use seat belts
Crib injuries	Be sure that crib meets consumer protection specifications; refrain from using pillow in crib
6–12 Months	
Falls	Use child-proof barriers for stairs and doors; have screens and locks on windows
Foreign body ingestions	Check toys for small removable parts and discard; keep floors clear of coins, buttons, nails, tacks, etc.
Shocks	Insert plastic covers into electric outlets
Pica	Remember that paint on walls and ceilings—and yard dirt—may contain lead
Crib injuries (from falling)	Ascertain that height from the mattress to the top of the crib rail is 21 inches or more
12–24 Months	
Burns	Keep hot beverages away from table edge; use rear burners of stove whenever possible; keep matches out of reach
Ingestions	Keep all medicines, cleaners, and chemicals out of reach in a locked cabinet; have Ipecac on hand at home
Car accidents (as pedestrian)	Buy suitable toys—two-wheelers, skateboards, roller skates, and even some tricycles cannot be controlled by the typical toddler; supervise play near streets, or have the child play in a fenced-in area
24–48 Months	
Same as for 12–24 months	
School age	
Sports injuries	Maintain adult supervision in contact sports; buy appropriate protective equipment for contact sports

      (3) The presence of fever in an infant under 3 months of age should prompt the physician to see that child without delay.

      (4) In the neonatal period a temperature below normal is probably of as much concern as an elevated temperature.

      (5) The height of the fever does not necessarily correlate directly with the severity of its cause.

      (6) Attempts to reduce a fever should **never** interfere with efforts to ascertain its cause.

   b. Management

      (1) The treatment of the temperature elevation should be aimed at making the patient comfortable. **The mere presence of fever does not always mandate treatment.**

      (2) Adequate hydration of the patient with oral fluids and increased ambient fluid content of the air help prevent dehydration.

      (3) Exposure of the skin to the air by removal of the clothing and sponging the body with tepid water promote heat loss. Alcohol or ice water should not be used for this purpose, since they cause a rapid lowering of the skin temperature with resulting vasoconstriction and prevention of heat loss.

      (4) Antipyretics. See Table 2-7.

Table 2-7. Some antipyretics useful in pediatrics

Drug	Analgesic	Antiinflammatory*	Suggested antipyretic oral dose (mg/kg q4h)
Aspirin and other salicylates	+	+	10–12
Acetaminophen	+	–	10–12

*Specifically, antirheumatic.
Source: Modified from A. K. Done and D. D. Done, *Pediatr. Clin. North Am.* 19:171, 1972.

(a) **Acetylsalicylic acid (aspirin).** The most widely used medication available, aspirin still has side effects and toxicity that necessitate caution in its use. Cumulative levels occur, and the half-life of the drug is long. Because of insolubility it is available only as a tablet or suppository. Children's preparations are flavored tablets of 75 mg each and are now limited by law to bottles of 36 tablets. The ordinary dosage for fever in children is 60 mg/year of age q4h. **Side effects and toxic reactions** include GI upset, GI bleeding, interference with platelet activity, and prolongation of prothrombin time. The rectal preparation can irritate the mucosa, and a toxic reaction is known to occur from this route due to variable absorption. For **management of overdose**, see Chap. 4, p. 105. For discussion of aspirin and Reye syndrome, see *Pediatrics* 69:810, 1982.

(b) **Acetaminophen,** a widely used liquid alternative to aspirin, has the advantage of somewhat greater accuracy of dosage and less gastric irritation. It lacks antirheumatic properties, but is equal to aspirin in effectiveness as an antipyretic. The dose is 10–12 mg/kg q4h. For management of overdose, see Chap. 4, p. 106.

(c) **Chlorpromazine** in small doses (0.1 mg/kg/24 hr) helps reduce fever by surface vasodilation and inhibition of shivering (thermogenesis). Its use in this manner is generally reserved for hospitalized patients with core temperatures > 40°C (104°F). It should not be used routinely.

(d) **Salicylamide** is unrelated to aspirin, does not have antirheumatic properties and is not as effective an antipyretic as aspirin or acetaminophen. Because it is a liquid it is still often used in infants, but is rarely useful and has little to recommend it.

2. **Colic and crying.** Although *colic* refers to paroxysmal abdominal pain of intestinal origin, the symptom in infancy is used loosely and includes moderate-to-severe and otherwise unexplained bouts of crying. Infants in the first 3–4 months of life appear to be most susceptible. Once begun, the persistence of the intense, inconsolable crying can be distressing to parents.

a. **Etiology.** There is no single cause, but persistent crying should stimulate efforts for an explanation. Hunger is one of the most frequent causes of crying and must be differentiated from other possible causes such as failure to eructate swallowed air, otitis media, corneal abrasions, and milk intolerance. The condition is less frequent in breast-fed babies. However, specific foods ingested by a mother who is breast-feeding can produce intestinal distress in the infant.

b. The **typical pattern** is that of a usually calm and placid baby either gradually or suddenly appearing in apparent pain with screaming, flexed lower extremities, often with a distended and tense abdomen. Exhaustion usually terminates the episode. Sometimes there is some relief with the passage of flatus or feces.

c. Management. If a specific cause of colic is present, preventive measures should be directed at that cause.

(1) Underfeeding and overfeeding can be properly relieved. Air swallowing, which may be responsible in part for discomfort, may be aided by altering feeding and burping techniques. Lengthening feeding times and either thickening feedings or changing supplies may help.

(2) Listening and lending support is the cornerstone of management. The baby that is often fussy and crying provokes tremendous anxiety and tension, and the parents need an outlet for their own concern and feelings, often of inadequate parenting.

(3) Parents need reassurance that many babies whose basic needs have been met simply have a need to "let off steam" and cry and that this crying will not harm them physically or psychologically. This simple giving of permission to parents to let their baby cry may lessen parental anxiety and family tensions and may eventually result in a quieter, calmer baby.

(4) The use of sedative and anticholinergic agents has not been effective, and the hazards of overdosage and toxicity are such that use of these drugs is not recommended in small infants.

3. Constipation

a. Diagnosis

(1) Constipation may be diagnosed by history with the findings of fecal contents on abdominal or rectal examination. Abdominal pain may suggest it.

(2) Although constipation may accompany many syndromes (see Chap. 21, pp. 519ff), it more often represents too little free water in the diet, inadequate intake of high-residue food, disruption of the child's daily habits, or a painful anal fissure that causes withholding of the stool.

(3) Passing a daily stool does not exclude constipation as a problem. Large, hard, or painful stools, sometimes large enough to clog the toilet, are significant signs even if they occur daily by history. Similarly, infrequent stools, even once every 1–7 days, can be normal in breast-fed infants.

b. Treatment. A stepwise approach follows.

(1) To assist the child to pass a hard stool:

(a) Glycerine or bisacodyl (Dulcolax) suppository (one only)

(b) *Pediatric* Fleet's enema (may be repeated once)

(c) Mineral oil, 15 ml PO. Magnesium sulfate or sodium sulfate may help in passing a hard stool and softening a forming stool.

(d) Manual disimpaction, which is unpleasant for both child and physician, may be necessary. There is no known simple or pleasant way to perform this time-honored physician's chore.

(e) Soapsuds or milk and molasses slurry enemas are helpful in resistant cases. Gastrografin or Mucomyst enemas can be useful in the impaction of cystic fibrosis, but have serious potential side effects, including electrolyte disturbances, intravascular depletion, and toxic absorption, and are expensive.

(2) To increase bulk and soften the stool:

(a) An increase in intake of free water.

(b) Natural dietary lubricants (e.g., prune juice, olive oil, tomatoes, and tomato juice).

(c) High-residue foods (e.g., green vegetables and fruits). The addition of bran and whole grain products is optimal for lifelong dietary changes.

(d) Pharmacologic stool softeners such as dioctyl sodium sulfosuccinate (Colace), 5 mg/kg/24 hr, malt soup extract (Maltsupex), or senna concentrate (Senokot). The dosage of stool softeners is as follows: age 1 month–1 year, ½ tsp bid; 1–5 years, 1 tsp bid; 5–15 years, 2 tsp bid. Large initial doses are essential; when the stools become soft, the dosage can be reduced. Regular daily dosage is continued for about 2–3 months and slowly reduced as bowel tone and regular bowel habits are reacquired. Relapses are common and prolonged follow-up is advisable. Initially, Senokot, in particular, may produce cramping.

(e) To assist the child with anal fissures:
- **(i)** A glycerine or bisacodyl suppository may be necessary (one only).
- **(ii)** Soften the stool as described.
- **(iii)** Sitz baths tid for small children.

(f) If anatomic lesions have been ruled out:
- **(i)** Establish a pattern of bowel movement after meals (gastrocolic reflex) or at other times—but at the same time each day—by sitting the child on the toilet whether or not a bowel movement results.
- **(ii)** Be sure that emotional stress and anxiety have been carefully excluded as causes.

(g) If constipation persists and encopresis occurs, a psychiatric evaluation is indicated, and long-term management by the pediatrician is required (see Chap. 10, pp. 519ff).

4. Cough
a. General considerations
- **(1)** A cough is a reflex directed at clearing the upper and lower airway of irritating secretions or foreign material. Many parents have the misconception that cough itself is harmful and **must** be treated. An explanation can be offered of the usefulness and protective benefits of coughing in lieu of a prescription.
- **(2)** Only in a few specific conditions (croup, perhaps foreign bodies, pertussis) do the characteristics of the cough itself help to make the diagnosis.

b. Management
- **(1)** Treatment should be directed at the underlying cause, e.g., infection, allergy, foreign body, irritants such as cigarette smoke.
- **(2)** Humidification of an otherwise dry environment may be beneficial.
- **(3)** One may consider use of a codeine-containing (or dextromethorphan) cough suppressant for the irritative cough that interferes with sleep.
- **(4)** See Table 2-8 for symptomatic medications.

5. Teething
a. General considerations
- **(1)** *Teething* is defined as the natural eruption of teeth. The symptoms that accompany the process begin from the first to the fifteenth month and may continue off and on into the third year of life.
- **(2)** Teething is rarely, if ever, directly responsible for **significant** fever, rhinorrhea, rashes, or diarrhea.
- **(3)** The normal appearance at age 4 months of oral exploration and consequent salivation and drooling is frequently attributed to, but rarely due to, teething. The gingival inflammation that occurs with the actual eruption of a tooth may produce an increase in this activity, as well as periods of irritability.
- **(4)** The lower central incisors are generally the first teeth to erupt and usually do so at 5–7 months of age. For an approximate chronology of deciduous tooth eruption, see Table 2-9.

b. Management
- **(1)** Rubbing swollen gums or giving the infant a cold, hard object to bite may provide relief of discomfort.
- **(2)** Application of commercially available topical analgesics at best provides limited and very transient relief.
- **(3)** When discomfort and irritability are clearly related to teething, aspirin or acetaminophen may be useful.

Table 2-8. Symptomatic medications

Antitussives	
Dextromethorphan hydrobromide, N.F.	
Available as: syrup (15 mg/ml)	1 mg/kg/24 hr
	30 mg/M^2/24 hr
	Divide into 3–4 doses
Codeine phosphate, U.S.P.	
Available as: syrup (10 mg/5 ml); tablets (15 and 30 mg)	0.3 mg/kg/dose
	Repeated every 4–6 hr
Expectorant	
Guaifenesin, glyceryl guaiacolate, N.F. (Robitussin)	
Available as: syrup (100 mg/5 ml)	12 mg/kg/24 hr
	350 mg/M^2/24 hr
	Divide into 6 doses
Decongestant	
Pseudoephedrine hydrochloride, N.F. (Sudafed)	
Available as: syrup (30 mg/5 ml); tablets (30 and 60 mg)	4 mg/kg/24 hr
	125 mg/M^2/24 hr
	Divide into 4 doses
Antihistamines	
Brompheniramine maleate, N.F. (Dimetane)	
Available as: tablets (4 mg); tablets, prolonged action, (8 and 12 mg); elixir (2 mg/5 ml)	0.5 mg/kg/24 hr
	15 mg/M^2/24 hr
	Divide into 3–4 doses
Chlorpheniramine maleate, U.S.P. (Chlor-Trimeton, Teldrin)	
Available as: tablets (4 mg); capsules, prolonged action, (8 and 12 mg); syrup (2 mg/5 ml)	0.35 mg/kg/24 hr
	10 mg/M^2/24 hr
	Divide into 4 doses
	0.2 mg/kg
	6 mg/M^2
	As single dose (prolonged action)

Source: H. C. Shirkey (ed), *Pediatric Therapy*, St. Louis: Mosby, 1975.

Table 2-9. Chronology of eruption of deciduous teeth

Deciduous tooth	Eruption (mean age in months ± SD)
Maxillary	
Central incisor	10 (8–12)
Lateral incisor	11 (9–13)
Canine	19 (16–22)
First molar	16 (13–19, boys; 14–18, girls)
Second molar	29 (25–33)
Mandibular	
Central incisor	8 (6–10)
Lateral incisor	13 (10–16)
Canine	20 (17–23)
First molar	16 (14–18)
Second molar	27 (23–31, boys; 24–30, girls)

Source: Adapted from John M. Davis et al., *An Atlas of Pedodontics* (2nd ed.). Philadelphia: Saunders, 1979.

Table 2-10. Common causes of vomiting in infancy, childhood, and adolescence

Infants	Children	Adolescents
Formula intolerance	Food poisoning	Food poisoning
Overfeeding	Drug ingestion	Drug ingestion
Infection (bacterial or viral)	Infection (bacterial or viral)	Infection (bacterial or viral)
Neuromuscular incoordination	Cyclic vomiting	Pregnancy
Esophageal dysfunction	Esophageal dysfunction	Esophageal dysfunction
Intestinal obstruction	Intestinal obstruction	Intestinal obstruction
Increased intracranial pressure	Increased intracranial pressure	Increased intracranial pressure
Peptic ulcer disease	Peptic ulcer disease	Peptic ulcer disease
Reye syndrome	Reye syndrome	Reye syndrome
Inborn error of metabolism	Heavy-metal poisoning	Neurosis (i.e., self-induced)
Uremia		Inflammatory bowel disease
Rumination		

Source: Developed by Jeffrey Hyams, M.D., Department of Pediatrics, Hartford General Hospital, Hartford, Conn.

6. Coryza (upper respiratory infection)
   a. General considerations
      (1) The symptom of persistent mucous drainage from the nose is most often called a "cold" and is by far the most frequent illness encountered in pediatric practice.
      (2) The illness is most often caused by a virus, produces a clear nasal discharge, and, when uncomplicated, lasts 3–5 days and disappears.
      (3) Such viral infections may lower local resistance in the nose and throat, which may in turn lead to secondary bacterial invasion.
      (4) Coryza can be due to excessively dry air or irritants such as allergens.
   b. Management in the infant
      (1) Remove mucus with a suction bulb. A 3-oz bulb is most efficient.
      (2) Increase the humidity in the environment by using a cold mist humidifier or by placing a pan of water on the radiator.
      (3) Thin nasal mucus with a few drops of saline solution made by dissolving ¼ tsp of salt in a cup of water.
      (4) If the discharge becomes purulent and is associated with fever, consider secondary bacterial infection.
      (5) Decongestants contain cardiotonic agents and should not be used in infants under 6 months of age. In any case their value remains unproven.
   c. Management in the older child
      (1) Treat as for the infant, except that gentle nose blowing can also be used.
      (2) A vasoconstricting nosedrop may be prescribed, but should not be used chronically.
      (3) Oral decongestants or antihistamines have not been established as effective drugs; however, in some children they may relieve profuse coryza. The benefits must be weighed against the possible side effects of irritability and drowsiness. Occasionally, paradoxical hyperactivity may occur.
      (4) See Table 2-8 for symptomatic medications.

7. **Vomiting.** See also Chap. 10.
   a. **General considerations**
      (1) Vomiting is a common symptom. Table 2-10 includes the differential diagnosis for the causes of vomiting in infants, older children, and adolescents.
      (2) Common causes of vomiting are viral gastroenteritis, formula intolerance, and improper feeding technique. Hence, an adequate **history** is important.
      (3) In monitoring the adequacy of hydration, the physician should question the parents as to the frequency of urination, degree of the moistness of the mucous membranes, and the presence or absence of tears with crying. The parental perception of how sick the child is between episodes of vomiting will help in determining how soon the child needs to be seen.
      (4) Always be alert for intestinal obstruction, either partial or complete, or for increased intracranial pressure as causes of vomiting.
   b. **Management of nonobstructive vomiting**
      (1) Initiate frequent (every 30–60 min) small (1–2 oz) amounts of easily digested clear fluids. The volume may be increased as the symptom decreases.
      (2) Formula intolerance may be due to the sugar or to the protein in the formula. A change to a soy product that does not contain lactose or to a casein-based formula may be helpful.
      (3) The assessment of improper feeding technique requires first-hand observation in the office and continuing follow-up by telephone.
      (4) If vomiting is due to simple gastroenteritis, a **single** dose of an antiemetic such as prochlorperazine IM or PR may provide relief.

8. **Diarrhea.** See also Chap. 10, pp. 268ff.
   a. **General considerations**
      (1) Causes include local intestinal factors; viral, bacterial, and parasitic infections; antibiotics; inflammatory bowel disease; or extraintestinal infections such as otitis media and pneumonia.
      (2) Important facts in the history include the general condition of the patient; presence of fever; number, consistency, and size of the stools; presence or absence of blood in the stool; and diarrhea in family members. When seeing a child with gastroenteritis, always **record a weight,** noting the clothing worn.
      (3) Evaluate the state of hydration (skin turgor, mucous membranes, fullness of the fontanelles, presence of tears), activity level of the child, and the presence or absence of infection other than in the GI tract.
   b. **Treatment**
      (1) Since most cases of gastroenteritis are self-limiting viral infections, an initial period of dietary treatment is helpful, with daily telephone contact to follow the patient's progress. Initially (for the first 12–24 hr), clear liquids, such as oral electrolyte solutions and flat Coca-Cola or ginger ale, are given—in small amounts if the child is vomiting.
      (2) After 12–24 hours, when the vomiting has stopped and diarrhea alone is present, early refeeding with breast milk, a gradually strengthened soy-based formula, or lactase-treated cow's milk, in addition to the oral electrolyte solution, will prevent starvation, stooling, and a deficit of protein and calories and will stimulate repair of intestinal mucosa.
      (3) After 24–48 hr, a bland diet (banana, rice cereal, applesauce, and toast) may be introduced.
      (4) **Kaopectate and antispasmodics should not be used.** Such medications make many parents lose sight of the importance of a restrictive, clear-fluid diet. Even with a decrease in the number of stools, continual fluid loss into the gut may persist.

9. Thrush

a. General considerations

(1) Thrush is an infection of the mouth caused by *Candida albicans*. It commonly occurs in infants who have been intimately exposed to the fungus during passage through the birth canal. It may often be associated with a diaper rash caused by the same organism and in such cases may well imply stool colonization with the fungus. A nursing mother may have concomitant surface infection of the nipples and areolae.

(2) Persistence of extensive oral candidiasis after the age of 3–4 months is distinctly unusual and should prompt an evaluation of cell-mediated immunity.

b. Management

(1) Thrush is most easily treated with nystatin (Mycostatin) solution (100,000 units/ml), given as 1 ml in each cheek qid after meals. Treatment is continued for 10–14 days.

(2) Nystatin ointment (occlusive) or cream (nonocclusive) can be used on the diaper rash. In many cases it may take several weeks to eradicate this condition.

B. Functional problems

1. Sleeping habits

a. General considerations. After the first few months of life, sleeping patterns are, in large part, learned responses. By 3–4 months of age, most babies have learned to sleep in an apparently uninterrupted stretch of 6–8 hr, generally at night if their feeding, bathing, and play time are scheduled in the daytime. By 7–12 months, babies should be accustomed to taking their long sleep period at the family's convenience, namely, at night.

b. Management

(1) It is best to remove the baby's crib from the parents' room at 4–6 months or even earlier, so that the periodic awakening of most young infants at night does not escalate into a prolonged wakeful time.

(2) After 6–9 months of age, the baby's waking at night, despite having been fed, tucked in, and diapered, needs to be handled with a resolute firmness and consistency, so that by experience the baby learns that there is a quiet time for **all** members of the family.

(3) Letting the child cry for some period of time after a bedtime has been established will usually result in the child's falling into a new pattern of sleep.

(4) Nightmares and night terrors (3–4 years of age) are common and need to be handled with reassurance and gentle comforting in the dimly lit bedroom. Frequent episodes should be investigated with regard to possible daytime environmental factors that might be precipitating these frightening nighttime dreams.

(5) The young child should grow up with the firm conviction that he or she is to stay in his or her bed until morning. This is a safe habit and also allows the parents the privacy and comfort of their own bed and bedroom. Be firm about **not** allowing the child to come into the parents' bed. If the child must be comforted for a special reason, it should be done in his or her own room and bed.

(6) Many children are able to give up their crib by 2 years of age, and some even by 18 months. Do not advise parents to make the change too early, because they might be losing a "safe place" for the child at night.

2. Eating habits or "the picky eater"

a. General considerations. Concerns about feeding, especially pertaining to the amount and variety of food, commonly arise during the second year. Children are now feeding themselves, have become discriminating, and are beginning to respond to behavioral feedback from parents who feel they should exercise control over the amount and type of food eaten. In general, children eat only when they are hungry. The child who refuses to eat a given meal will not become ill or hypoglycemic or be undernourished by the next meal—merely hungry. Therefore, the child need not be permitted to manipulate and thus dictate his or her diet.

b. **Management**

(1) To ensure that a child is likely to try more than one food at a meal, offer reasonable (usually small) portions of a variety of foods, including milk. The latter is often offered in quantity sufficient to meet total caloric needs.

(2) Milk is not essential beyond 1 year of age, provided protein, calcium, and vitamin D are available from other sources. Fortunately, the same is true of vegetables in a diet containing fruit, grains, and meats. Vitamin supplements are generally not necessary in children who are growing well except in instances of the most restrictive diets.

(3) The caloric gains achieved do not usually justify the playing of games with foods: for example, "If you don't eat your peas, there will be no dessert." Such bargaining merely provides the child with more opportunity to manipulate and gain attention. The throwing of food should consistently result in the end of that meal for the child.

(4) Growth charts may be useful in reassuring the parents that the child who "doesn't eat enough to keep a bird alive" actually eats enough to keep a child alive, permitting normal growth and development at the same time.

(5) The use of between-meal snacks may help to allay parental anxiety, but will most likely result in a "snacker" who continues to eat poorly at mealtime.

(6) Anticipating and discussing normal eating patterns prior to the development of parental anxiety and mealtime tension is time well spent.

3. **Toilet training**

a. **General considerations.** All normal children will toilet train themselves. Most parents, however, have difficulty in waiting for this to happen. The parents can **help** the child achieve this goal and should think of it in this manner, not that they are actually training the child. Remind parents that there is no earthly way for them to keep their child from becoming toilet trained, but unfortunately they can do all sorts of things to delay the process.

b. **Management**

(1) The best time to start is between **2 and 3 years** of age, which is the time when many children begin to train themselves. Before this age, they have to learn by association, coincidence, luck, and fleet parental feet.

(2) **Bowel control** is much simpler for a child to master than control of urination because the former involves much less complicated muscle coordination and occurs far fewer times during the day. It might help to put the child on the potty or toilet just after a meal when the gastrocolic reflex occurs.

(3) **Urine training** should begin when the frequency of urination decreases and the child begins to awaken dry after a nap, usually around 2.5–3 years of age.

4. **Fears**

a. **General considerations.** Expression of fear, either in action or in words, is part of normal development. Fears become abnormal only when they interfere with or severely inhibit the child's day-to-day functioning.

b. **Management**

(1) Fear of **strangers** may appear at age 5 to 8 months. Gently remind strangers to keep at a distance until the child becomes used to their presence.

(2) Fear of the **bathtub** or of bathing may arise between 1 and 2 years of age and may occasionally derive from a negative experience, e.g., soap in the eyes or slipping in the water. Advise parents not to insist on a bathtub bath, but to try an alternative—a dishpan bath or sponge bath.

(3) Fear of **separation** is one of the most common and—for parents—most distressing developmental reactions of childhood. It appears around 2 years of age when a sensitive, dependent child is suddenly separated from his or her major caretaker. The manifestations usually worsen at bedtime. Encourage the parents to allow the child to develop independence, in carefully controlled circumstances, at an early age. Accustom the child to a baby-sitter gradually; a half-hour "warm-up period" before the parents leave may be helpful. Above all, when it is time to leave, parents should act with confidence.

(4) Imaginary worries arise at 3–5 years of age. Dogs, the dark, fires, and death all figure prominently. Such patterns may be seen in children who are tense from battles over toilet training or feeding, but need not be ascribed to these causes. Frightening stories, warnings, or television shows may also stimulate these fears. Management involves parental reassurance and an understanding acceptance of the child's aversions. Above all, never force the child to face fears abruptly. Instead, encourage him or her to play games about the fears.

(5) The fear of **injury** occurs at or beyond 3 years of age and is often triggered by seeing crippled or deformed people. The child is quick to perceive that something is wrong and quickly puts himself or herself in the injured person's place. A child may interpret the physical differences between the sexes as an injury. The best treatment is simply to offer an explanation appropriate to the child's age and comprehension.

5. Thumb and finger sucking
a. General considerations
(1) Sucking is an instinctual behavioral pattern. Most young infants suck on their fingers for varying periods of time. This behavior should be considered normal.

(2) Thumb sucking is strongly related to the emotional satisfaction of the infant or young child. Finger sucking will not have any detrimental effect on the position of the permanent teeth, as long as the habit is discontinued **before** the second teeth have erupted.

b. Management.
The majority of children give up the habit of finger sucking, except in moments of severe stress, by the time they reach school age. In most cases, thumb sucking represents a **greater problem to the parents than to the child.** The history usually reveals that the child does not do an unusual amount of thumb sucking; it is the parent who is made anxious by the behavior. Ordinarily, information, reassurance, and support will relieve the parents and thus prevent secondary emotional problems in the child.

6. Self-stimulation
a. General considerations.
What parents report as "self-stimulation" usually consists of the normal self-soothing habits of children that arise in early infancy. Such behaviors appear in two forms:

(1) Rhythmic habits, including rocking, head rolling, and head banging. Appearing in the second half of the first year, these behaviors usually occur at times of fatigue, sleepiness, or frustration and serve to comfort the child.

(2) Genital exploration or manipulation. The extent of this behavior is directly correlated with age. In an infant or young child, genital manipulation is a manifestation of wholesome curiosity, while in the 3- to 6-year old, it is an expression of a normal interest in sex. At this stage, genital stimulation should arouse no concern if the child is outgoing and sociable and not preoccupied with the activity. A common cause of excessive stimulation is a fear of something happening to the genitals. In the latent stage, from 6 years to puberty, such behavior is generally naturally suppressed.

b. Management

   (1) Management of concerns regarding rhythmic behavior is directed toward averting injury and reducing noise. No attempt should be made to discipline or restrain the young child.

   (2) In the management of masturbatory behavior the physician must consider the parents' religious and moral feelings. Parents should be advised that gentle inhibition of the activity or distracting the child is far more appropriate than calling attention to the activity. Attempts to suppress the behavior actively, especially if punitive, may produce potentially damaging psychological sequelae.

C. Common complaints in the older child

1. Headache. See also Chap. 20, pp. 508ff.

a. General considerations. Headache is a common complaint of children, and repeated evaluations may be needed. Associated symptoms and signs that mandate evaluation are vomiting, nocturnal awakening, school absence, abnormal neurologic findings, hypertension, or any motor or visual abnormality.

   (1) Depending on the location and pattern of symptoms, occult sinusitis should be ruled out.

   (2) Poor vision is a rare cause of headache.

   (3) The majority of headaches described by children are accompanied by absolutely no other symptoms or signs, as reported by the patient or parent.

   (4) The most common headache not associated with acute infection, trauma, systemic illness, or a space-occupying lesion is migraine.

b. Management

   (1) A thorough neurologic examination, blood pressure check, and funduscopic examination are essential for the evaluation of headache.

   (2) If associated symptoms are lacking, and if significant abnormalities are not present on physical examination, the headache may be treated with the judicious use of aspirin or acetaminophen. Stronger analgesics or caffeine or ergotamine preparations are not warranted as the initial treatment of uncomplicated headache.

   (3) If a history of school absence is elicited, the possibility of school avoidance should be considered.

2. Abdominal pain

a. General considerations. Abdominal pain is most frequent in the school-age child. In no more than 5% of cases of recurrent abdominal pain is an organic cause identified; the diagnosis is usually suggested by the clinical presentation, and appropriate investigation and treatment are indicated when the cause is organic (see Chap. 10).

b. Management

   (1) The diagnosis of pain of emotional origin should be supported by evidence of emotional disturbance, not merely by lack of an organic cause. In this respect the history tends to be more revealing than the physical examination or laboratory tests.

   (2) Commonly, evidence of other emotional disturbances such as school or sleep problems or difficulties with family or peers is found. Frequently, the family history will reveal other members with emotional or psychosomatic problems, often taking similar form.

   (3) Laboratory investigations should be kept at a minimum and should be reasonable (e.g., urine and stool examinations), so as not to create further anxiety. A CBC may be warranted to allay the fears of the child or parent who suspects malignancy.

    (4) For the child or adolescent with pain of short duration, the reassurance afforded by normal findings may be curative.

    (5) In cases of more severe, chronic, and incapacitating pain, management should be directed at the underlying emotional disturbance.

D. Common complaints of parents of older children and adolescents

  1. Television

    a. General considerations

      (1) The physician should include questions about the television habits of his or her patients and their families in the general checkup.

      (2) There is some evidence that watching violent scenes produces aggressive behavior in young people.

      (3) Television advertisements encourage conflict and confrontation between parent and child.

    b. Management

      (1) Parents should be encouraged to set limits on television viewing by their children and should monitor their own viewing habits.

      (2) Excessive television viewing is potentially a mental and physical health hazard and can significantly compromise the child's functioning in school and in the social sphere. As for any health hazard, the key is prevention.

      (3) Guidelines for television viewing can be obtained from the San Francisco Committee on Children's Television, Inc., or Action for Children's Television, Newton, Mass.

  2. Cigarettes

    a. General considerations

      (1) The pediatrician can influence behavior patterns and growth through repeated encounters with the child, and early and repeated discussions of drug issues, including cigarette smoking, may influence future usage patterns.

      (2) Areas to be emphasized are the effects of prenatal usage on the unborn baby, including low birth weight for gestational age and its concomitant problems; the effects on the incidence and severity of respiratory infection and pulmonary function in children exposed to smoking parents; and the known increase in cigarette usage among the children of smoking parents.

    b. Management

      (1) Physicians and nurses can obviously act as examples by not smoking and by not permitting smoking in their offices.

      (2) The key is **prevention.**

  3. Alcohol and drugs. See also Chap. 4.

    a. General considerations

      (1) Attitudes toward alcohol and drugs are learned first at home. Children later apply these attitudes in peer groups.

      (2) When parents are in agreement, they constitute a powerful and important factor affecting the child's point of view.

      (3) Adolescents consider the use of alcohol and drugs as the mark of an adult. Thus, getting deliberately intoxicated for the first time is seen as an act of autonomy and independence.

      (4) Factors in the history that are indicators of alcoholism and/or drug abuse include:

        (a) Drunkenness at an early age; drinking to become drunk

        (b) Truancy, school expulsion, dropping out of school, job problems

        (c) An alcoholic parent

        (d) Automobile accidents or arrests

    b. Management

      (1) The subject should always be approached as an issue of health, not of morals. A nonthreatening discussion of chemical use and abuse should begin at least by age 12.

    (2) As the patient grows older, any problems with alcohol or drugs should be discussed openly and directly as the pediatrician becomes aware of high intake or frequent use.

    (3) Discussion should include the effects of alcohol and drugs on others' lives and how drug or alcohol abuse affects one's ability to relate to family and friends.

    (4) Make appropriate referrals for drug counseling when necessary.

    (5) Confidentiality is important. If the patient's parents are to be involved, the patient should be so informed.

    (6) The patient's needs are the physician's first consideration. However, a distinction should be made between caring for a "user" and a "dealer." Dealing in drugs is a federal offense carrying severe penalties; the use of drugs, antisocial though it may be, can be managed as an illness. The pediatrician should be informed of legal constraints in his or her locality.

4. Sex education and activity
a. General considerations

    (1) The parents are the natural people to educate their child about sex, but many are reluctant or unable to do so. Under these circumstances the roles of the pediatrician and school become important.

    (2) Sex education should begin when first questions arise, usually at age 3–4 years. The child should be thoroughly educated before puberty in the anatomic and physiologic functions of the sexes.

    (3) While understanding the goals of parents to maintain family morals and social standards, the physician should help parents realize that the main tasks of adolescence are separation from the family and adjustment to sexuality.

    (4) Adolescent behavior is influenced by peers and in many ways reflects prevalent subcultural values and practice. Every adolescent must come to terms with the pressure of sexuality; his or her response may range from attempts at total suppression to indiscriminate promiscuity.

    (5) The importance of sexuality can be either underestimated or highly exaggerated by the adolescent, the parent, or the physician.

b. Management
(1) Helping to relieve sources of anxiety
(a) Early adolescence

    (i) Somatic changes. Breast development, nocturnal emission, erections

    (ii) Anticipatory concerns about sexual intercourse and contraception

    (iii) Masturbation and its consequences

    (iv) Homosexuality and its manifestations

(b) In later adolescence

    (i) Contraception

    (ii) Venereal disease

    (iii) Sexual preference

    (2) Many concerns can be discussed as an accepted part of a routine physical examination.

    (3) When the physician is faced with the dilemma of dispensing contraceptives without parental knowledge, this situation is best handled by working within the value constraints of the family. However, the physician has the responsibility to challenge the attitudes and values of either or both parties when the welfare of the patient is at stake.

    (4) Fear or suspicion of homosexuality must be differentiated from its actual presence. When homosexual commitment is absent, the patient can be reassured. In the presence of homosexual commitment, referral for psychological counseling for the adolescent **and** for the parents

Table 2-11. Indicators of significant language delays*

Age (months)	Indicators
12	Limited babbling; quiet child
18	Does not understand specific words, his name, or names of common objects; cannot follow simple commands such as "Come here," "Sit down"
24	Uses few single words; is not imitating words
30	Does not know names of common objects or simple body parts; cannot point on command to familiar objects or get an object on request not directly in visual field; no true two word combinations such as "No cookie," "More milk"; child is often misunderstood
36	No simple sentences (subject, verb, object); does not seem to understand simple explanations or discussions of events in past or future

*Children with these findings would be significantly behind normal developmental expectations.

may be warranted, particularly when parental and social disapproval creates a fundamental conflict for the adolescent within the family.

IV. Speech and language delay

A. The **etiology** includes hearing deficit, overall development delay, oral motor planning problems (dyspraxia), autism, environmental deprivation, and primary language disorder.

B. Diagnosis and evaluation. See Table 2-11.

 1. All children with language delay should have their hearing formally evaluated. This can be done at any age in specialized facilities.
 2. Developmental evaluation should be done using age-appropriate tools (i.e., Denver Developmental Tests, Bayley Scales of Infant Development). Language delay must be regarded as a part of overall development delay.
 3. History and observations should include the child's means of communicating his or her needs without language. Those with a hearing deficit, oral motor planning problems, and primary language disorders may act out their needs, whereas children with developmental delay and autism will not.
 4. Feeding problems and inability to imitate tongue movements should be examined in evaluating for oral motor planning problems.
 5. Comparison between levels of receptive and expressive language may be helpful.
 6. The history should involve a description of the home environment and child's interactional style (to look for environments with low levels of language stimulation).
 7. **Caution**—many children will not show their best language skills with strangers. Diagnosis often must be suggested by the history.

C. Treatment

 1. Referral to a speech pathologist for isolated language delay or to an audiologist for hearing problems is often appropriate after the initial workup.
 2. Mild delays can be treated in many cases by educating and encouraging parents to use language more pervasively in a play context, with frequent modeling of words.
 3. Early intervention (under 3 years old) or language-centered classrooms in public schools (over 3 years) may be helpful for these children.

Acute Care

I. Cardiopulmonary resuscitation (CPR)

A. The **diagnosis** of cardiorespiratory arrest must be rapid (absent pulse and respirations, cyanosis). Prompt and orderly resuscitative efforts are vital, and assignment of responsibilities is mandatory.

    1. The **first person** at a cardiorespiratory arrest must establish the diagnosis. If the patient is unresponsive, the airway is cleared; four **crescendo** breaths are given, and then the carotid-axillary-apical pulse is palpated. If the patient remains unresponsive, help is called and the "ABCs" of resuscitation are started.

    2. **The resuscitation team** includes the following:

        a. The **leader** (the most experienced person) is in charge, makes **all** therapeutic decisions, assigns others their roles, and continually reassesses the quality of the resuscitation. The leader should immediately appoint persons for **airway management** and **cardiac compression.**

        b. **Vascular access** should be accomplished by the next available person.

        c. **Medications** and **recording.** Appropriate doses of medications are prepared. The dosages and times of giving medications, as well as any procedures or diagnostic tests, are documented.

        d. The **help-all/circulator** obtains and monitors the blood pressure, adequacy of cardiac compressions, and chest movement during ventilation and assists wherever help is needed.

        e. **Historian.** One person must obtain a history from the parents or caretakers and keep them informed of events.

        f. The **ECG** should be monitored. Persons responsible for CPR must know how to change ECG recorder paper.

B. The following equipment *must* be available:

    1. **Airway.** Oxygen, suction and suction catheters, adult and pediatric-size masks, endotracheal tubes, laryngoscopes with pediatric and adult blades, oral airways, self-inflating and anesthesia bags, McGill forceps, and tape

    2. **Drugs.** See Table 3-1.

    3. **Vascular access.** Syringes, catheters, cutdown tray, tourniquet, and tape

    4. **Other.** Blood pressure cuff, thermometer, ECG machine and leads, defibrillator, chest tubes and Pleurivacs, Foley catheter, nasogastric tubes, and cardiac pacemaker

C. **The ABCs of resuscitation** (adapted from the American Heart Association recommendations)

    1. **Airway (A)**

        a. Clear with a suction catheter, bulb, or finger sweep.

        b. The jaw thrust maneuver removes obstruction caused by the tongue and soft tissues of the neck.

        c. The head must be in the midline. Because the larynx in a child is more anterior and superior than in an adult, the child should be put in the "sniffing" position by placing a small pillow under the occiput; extreme hyperextension of the neck can obstruct the airway.

    2. **Breathing (B).** Begin mouth-to-mouth or bag-to-mouth ventilation at the rate of 20/min with the highest available oxygen concentration. **Watch the motion of the chest wall with each breath to assess the adequacy of**

Table 3-1. Drugs used in a resuscitation*

Drug	Dose (adult dose)	Preparation	Route	Indication
Atropine	0.03 mg/kg (0.4 mg)	0.4 mg/ml	IV, IC, IM, ETT	To treat bradycardia and to block vagally mediated bradycardia
Bicarbonate	1–2 mEq/kg every 10 min (same)	1 mEq/ml	IV, IC	Metabolic acidosis
Elemental calcium	10 mg/kg (300 mg)	CaCl = 27 mg/ml; calcium gluconate = 9 mg/ml	IV, IC	Electromechanical dissociation: for positive inotropy and to increase vasomotor tone
Dextrose	0.5 gm/kg (same)	25% D/W and 50% D/W	IV, IC	Presumed hypoglycemia
Epinephrine	0.1 ml/kg (10 ml)	Epinephrine 1 : 10,000 (10 ml = 1 mg)	IV, IC, ETT	Asystole, bradycardia, hypotension, to coarsen ventricular fibrillation before countershock
Lidocaine	1 mg/kg (50–100 mg)	100 mg/10 ml	IV, IC, ETT	Ventricular ectopy
Naloxone hydrochloride (Narcan)	0.01 mg/kg (0.4 mg)	0.4 mg/ml	IV, IC	Opiate intoxication

IC = intracardiac; ETT = via endotracheal tube.
*See sec. **II** for a discussion of cardiotonic infusions.

the ventilation. **The chest wall must move!** If the chest does not move, assess the patency of the airway (sec. **III.A**, p. 43). An endotracheal tube is occasionally required to maintain the airway (e.g., in epiglottitis). Rarely, an emergency tracheostomy is indicated.

3. **Circulation (C)**
    a. The patient is placed on a hard, solid surface, and external cardiac compression is started.
    b. The respiratory and cardiac resuscitation efforts must be synchronized: one breath to five compressions. Counting should be done aloud by the person doing the compressions. Each breath is given on the upstroke of the fifth cardiac compression. The rate of cardiac compressions for adults is 60/min, whereas 100 compressions/min is appropriate for infants.
    c. If the patient is more than 4 years of age, the "adult-style," two-handed chest massage can be used. In **infants** there are two correct hand placements: (1) both thumbs are placed over the sternum while the fingers are curved around the back over the spine or (2) one hand can be placed behind the back for support while sternal compressions are done with two fingers of the other hand. This second procedure can also be used for **toddlers.** Pressure should always be completely released between forceful compressions to allow filling of the heart chambers.
    d. Palpate the femoral pulse to assess the adequacy of cardiac compressions.
    e. An ECG monitor can be attached when help arrives.

4. **Drugs**
    a. Vascular access should be accomplished when help arrives. A central line is preferable, but a peripheral line is acceptable. If no line is available, *atropine, epinephrine,* and *lidocaine* can be given via the endotracheal tube. **The intracardiac route is dangerous and should be used only when no other route is available.** See Table 3-1 for drug doses and indications.
    b. If there is asystole, the usual order of medication is bicarbonate, epinephrine, calcium, and glucose. Atropine is given if there is a bradyarrhythmia.

5. **Countershock therapy (cardioversion) for ventricular fibrillation or ventricular tachycardia**
    a. In ventricular tachycardia, use the synchronized mode; in ventricular fibrillation, use defibrillation, or nonsynchronized mode.
    b. The **dose** is 2–3 watt-sec/kg, or 10–15 watt-sec/year of life.
    c. **Paddle placement**
        (1) **Anterior-posterior placement** is preferable. Gel is applied to the paddles, the posterior paddle is placed behind the heart, and the anterior paddle is placed over the precordium.
        (2) **Anterior chest wall.** One paddle is placed over the apex and the other over the sternal notch at the base of the heart.
    d. Be certain that "**all hands are off the bed and off the patient**" prior to discharge.
    e. Cardiopulmonary resuscitation is immediately reestablished until effective cardiac output is achieved.
    f. If ventricular tachycardia or ventricular fibrillation continues, repeat countershock at a higher voltage; increase the voltage by 50% or by 50 watt-sec. Lidocaine, 1 mg/kg, should be given as an IV bolus before the cardioversion.

D. If the resuscitation does not establish cardiac output, the cause of the "arrest" should be evaluated for correctable mechanical and/or metabolic insults such as the following:
    1. **Hypothermia.** The patient may appear dead and/or unresponsive to pharmacologic management if the temperature is less than 30°C. Rewarming must accompany meticulous CPR (see sec. **VII.G.**).
    2. **Tension pneumothorax or hemothorax**
    3. **Cardiac tamponade**

4. Profound **hypovolemia** (see Chap. 7)
5. Profound **metabolic imbalance** (see Chap. 11)
6. **Toxin ingestion** (see Chap. 4)

E. **Common iatrogenic complications** include:
   1. **Trauma** from closed chest massage: rib fracture causing pneumothorax or hemothorax; splenic and hepatic rupture
   2. **Pneumothorax** from subclavian and internal jugular cannulation or from positive pressure ventilation
   3. **Bleeding** and **pericardial tamponade** from intracardiac injections

F. After successful resuscitation the patient must be **closely monitored.** The following should be constantly assessed:
   1. **Cardiovascular system**
      a. Central venous pressure (CVP) catheter to assess the intravascular volume status
      b. Continuous ECG monitoring and a 12-lead ECG
      c. Swan-Ganz catheter to measure cardiac output
   2. **Pulmonary system**
      a. Arterial blood gases (ABGs) to document the adequacy of ventilation and oxygenation
      b. Chest x-ray for evidence of aspiration, pneumothorax, and rib fracture
   3. **Central nervous system.** Observe for seizures and signs of increased intracranial pressure.
   4. **Renal system.** The renal lesion most commonly seen is acute tubular necrosis (see Chap. 8, pp. 209ff).
   5. **Miscellaneous injuries**
      a. **Hypoxic injuries to the GI tract.** Monitor stool guaiac and liver function tests.
      b. Disseminated intravascular coagulation (see Chap. 17, pp. 209ff)
      c. If trauma is suspected, evaluate with appropriate radiographs and serial hematocrits.
      d. Sepsis or serious local infection may be a precipitating cause of the original arrest and can be anticipated from emergency "dirty" procedures.

II. Shock

A. **Definition.** Failure of cardiac output to meet the metabolic demands of the body
B. **Etiology.** See Table 3-2.
   1. **Hypovolemic** shock due to
      a. Loss of volume (blood, plasma, free water) *or*
      b. Loss of vascular resistance (sepsis, anaphylaxis, drug)
   2. The terms **hypervolemic shock** and **normovolemic shock** describe **cardiogenic shock** resulting from pump failure, arrhythmias, outflow obstructions, and hypermetabolic states.
C. **Evaluation**
   1. The **history** includes:
      a. The presence of underlying disease
      b. The duration of the illness
      c. Temperature
      d. Medications past and present
      e. Recent oral intake
      f. Output (vomiting, stool, urine)
      g. Level of activity
   2. **Physical examination** includes particular attention to the cardiovascular system. An **accurate** weight and temperature should be obtained.
   3. **Laboratory studies** include:
      a. ABGs
      b. CBC
      c. Electrolytes, blood sugar, calcium, BUN, creatinine, cardiac enzymes, liver function tests, toxic screen, prothrombin time, partial thromboplastin time, and fibrin split products
      d. A chest x-ray to evaluate cardiac size and pulmonary vasculature

D. Monitoring
1. **Vital signs.** The following must be continuously monitored and recorded on flow sheets:
    a. Temperature
    b. Respiratory rate
    c. Continuous ECG
    d. **Blood pressure.** In infants and children, arterial cannulation is the best way to monitor blood pressure continually. If this method is not possible, blood pressure can be obtained with a blood pressure cuff; often, a Doppler is required for auscultation.
    e. **Intake and output records.** Measurement of hourly urine output, as well as nasogastric losses, and iatrogenic blood losses
2. Swan-Ganz catheterization and CVP measurement may be required (see sec. **VIII.C** and **D.**).

E. Treatment of shock
1. **Oxygen** should be administered to every patient in shock. Intubation and ventilatory support may be necessary. ABGs should be obtained.
2. **Volume resuscitation.** In shock without congestive heart failure, rehydrate with a total of 20 ml/kg volume replacement in two separate aliquots of 10 ml/kg. (Table 3-3 lists available volume expanders.)
    a. If this volume replacement produces no clinical improvement, a CVP catheter is placed before further therapy is begun.
        (1) For a CVP less than 5 mm Hg, further volume resuscitation is continued until the CVP is greater than 5 mm Hg.
        (2) For a CVP greater than 5 mm Hg with no clinical improvement, the following procedures should be considered:
            (a) ABGs to assess the adequacy of ventilation and oxygenation and degree of metabolic acidosis
            (b) An ECG to evaluate the possibilities of myocarditis, pericardial tamponade, metabolic imbalance, or arrhythmias
            (c) An echocardiogram to evaluate ventricular function
            (d) A Swan-Ganz catheter (see sec. **VIII.D.**)
    b. **General rules for volume resuscitation**
        (1) If possible, warm the blood or infusate to prevent a decrease in the patient's temperature.
        (2) Infusions of 10 ml/kg can be given as an IV push over 5–10 min in emergency situations, but 15- to 30-min infusion is preferable.
3. **Drugs.** See Table 3-4
4. Evaluate and treat the precipitating event.

III. Respiratory emergencies
A. **Upper airway obstruction** may be caused by infectious processes (epiglottitis, croup, abscess, and diphtheria) that cause swelling of intrinsic tissues or by extrinsic objects.
1. **Evaluation**
    a. **History**
        (1) **Onset.** Acute or gradual
        (2) The nature and course of symptoms, including fever, dyspnea, stridor, wheezing, dysphagia, dysphonia or aphonia, and cough
        (3) Precipitating event or condition, including choking on a foreign body, trauma to the upper airway, and an acquired or congenital abnormality of the airway
        (4) Current medications
        (5) Allergies
    b. The **physical examination** is aimed at quickly assessing the adequacy of ventilation and oxygenation and identifying the cause and site of airway obstruction.
        (1) **General appearance,** including alertness, distress, anxiety. Restlessness, altered mental status, pallor, or cyanosis suggests hypoxia.
        (2) Vital signs

Table 3-2. Causes of shock in infants and children

Type of shock	Newborn	Older child
Hypovolemic		
Loss of intravascular volume		
Blood	Intracerebral hemorrhage, placental hemorrhage, twin-twin, fetal-maternal transfusion	Trauma: Hemophilia, splenic-hepatic rupture, pelvic or long bone fracture Epistaxis, ectopic pregnancy, GI hemorrhage, sickle cell sequestration crisis
Fluid	Gastroenteritis, gastroschisis, omphalocele, meningonyelocele	Gastroenteritis, severe burn, diabetes mellitus and insipidus, cystic fibrosis with profound sweat loss, nephrotic syndrome
Loss of vascular resistance	Sepsis, adrenengenital syndrome, CNS injury	Sepsis, anaphylaxis, adrenal crisis, CNS injury, drug ingestion
Hypervolemic, normovolemic		
Myocardial failure	Endocardial fibroelastosis, viral infections, congenital heart disease, sepsis, hypoglycemia	Viral infections, cardiotropic drugs, coronary insufficiency, sepsis, hypoglycemia, hypocalcemia
Outflow obstructive lesions	Coarctation, critical aortic stenosis, malignant hypertension	Coarctation, aortic stenosis or idiopathic hypertrophic subaortic stenosis, pulmonary embolism, cor pulmonale as seen with asthma, cystic fibrosis, malignant hypertension
Arrhythmias	Paroxysmal atrial tachycardia and other arrhythmias, drug intoxication, sepsis	Paroxysmal atrial tachycardia and other arrhythmias, drug intoxication
Increased metabolic demands	Severe anemia, hyperthyroidism	Severe anemia, hyperthyroidism

Table 3-3. Fluids for volume resuscitation

Fluids	Type	Advantages	Disadvantages
Normal saline	Crystalloid	Safe, available, effective	
Lactated Ringer's	Crystalloid	Safe, available, effective	Contains potassium
Albumisol[b] (5% albumin)	Colloid	Effective, does not require cross-match, no risk of hepatitis	Expensive
Fresh frozen plasma	Colloid	Effective, replaces trace elements and clotting factors	Hepatitis risk, expensive
Blood	Colloid	Effective, increases oxygen-carrying capacity	Hepatitis risk, expensive

[a]The available fluids are summarized in this table. There are many discussions and disagreements regarding the use of colloid versus crystalloid. Although the main argument is that colloids stay in the intravascular compartment longer than do crystalloids, in the acute situation any of these volume expanders is adequate and effective.

[b]Salt-poor albumin (25%) is not an appropriate rapid-volume expander and should not be used in acute shock.

Table 3-4. Drugs used in the treatment of shock

Drug	Dose	Maximum adult dose	Mechanisms of action	Indications	Limitations
Epinephrine	0.01–0.5 µg/kg/min	1–4 µg/min	α- and β-adrenergic: increases heart rate, increases systemic vasc. resistance, positive inotropy	Anaphylaxis, hypotension, diminished cardiac contractility, bradycardia	Ventricular arrythmias, decreases coronary blood flow, decreases renal blood flow
Norepinephrine	0.01–0.5 µg/kg/min	1–4 µg/min	α- adrenergic, increases heart rate, increases systemic vascular resistance	Hypotension without preexisting vasoconstriction	Ventricular arrhythmias, decreases coronary blood flow, decreases renal blood flow
Isoproterenol	0.01–0.5 µg/kg/min	1–4 µg/min	β-adrenergic, increases heart rate, positive inotropy, decreases vasomotor tone	Bradycardia, diminished cardiac contractility	Ventricular arrhythmias, hypotension if the patient was hypovolemic
Dopamine	1–5 µg/kg/min	Same	Dopaminergic; increases renal, coronary, and splanchnic flow	Poor tissue perfusion, to attempt to increase renal perfusion	
	5–15 µg/kg/min	Same	β-adrenergic, increases heart rate, positive inotropy	Bradycardia, decreased myocardial contractility	Ventricular arrhythmias
	15–30 µg/kg/min	Same	α- and β-adrenergic, increases heart rate, increases systemic vascular resistance, positive inotropy	Hypotension, bradycardia, decreased myocardial contractility	Ventricular arrhythmias, decreases coronary blood flow, decreases renal blood flow

(3) Cardiorespiratory findings. The nature and adequacy of air movement and adventitious sounds, including stridor, dysphonia, and wheezing. Tachycardia is often present in the child with a compromised airway. Hypotension and bradycardia occur in association with severe impairment of air movement.

2. Specific conditions
a. Epiglottitis is a rapidly progressive bacterial cellutitis of the supraglottic tissues that causes a narrowing of the airway inlet, with the impending risk of total obstruction. **It is a true medical emergency.**
   (1) Etiology. *Haemophilus influenzae* type B is the cause in 95% of cases. Rarely, group A streptococci, pneumococci, diphtheria, or tuberculosis has been incriminated as the causal agent.
   (2) Evaluation and diagnosis. To prevent death the diagnosis must be made and definitive airway maintenance established quickly. The onset of respiratory difficulty is usually acute, with rapid progression over several hours, most often in children 3–6 years old. Drooling dysphagia, fever, toxicity, inspiratory stridor, protruding jaw, and extended neck are seen. However, if the airway is substantially compromised, definitive airway placement should preclude all diagnostic studies.
      (a) No attempt should be made to visualize the epiglottis or to carry out any other procedure until nasotracheal intubation or tracheotomy is accomplished. Any manipulation, including aggressive physical examination or venipuncture, may precipitate complete obstruction.
      (b) The presumptive diagnosis can be made on clinical grounds alone. If the child is in little distress, lateral neck x-rays may assist in the definitive diagnosis. These should be done under controlled conditions, with the required staff and equipment for immediate intubation or tracheostomy in attendance.
   (3) Therapy
      (a) The definitive treatment is the placement of a secure artificial airway. Under controlled conditions and in skilled hands, nasotracheal intubation is effective and safe. Intubation may be required from 1–4 days. When intubation cannot be carried out, tracheostomy is indicated. Visualization of the epiglottis should occur once the airway has been secured.
      (b) After intubation the epiglottis can be examined and swabs for culture can be taken. Once the artificial airway has been secured, blood cultures can be drawn and IV fluids begun.
      (c) Antibiotic therapy. See Chap. 15, p. 389.
      (d) Other foci of infection should be ruled out. Meningitis, pneumonia, pericarditis, and septic arthritis have all been reported in association with epiglottitis.
b. Croup, or viral laryngotracheobronchitis, is characterized by subglottic edema that can cause abnormal vocalization and airway compromise.
   (1) Etiology. Parainfluenza, respiratory syncytial virus, adenovirus, and measles virus are the most common causes. Bacterial infection has been increasingly recognized but remains unusual.
   (2) Evaluation and diagnosis
      (a) History. A coryzal prodrome is common, with increasing barking cough and hoarseness. Often, it is worse at night and usually occurs in children under 3 years of age.
      (b) Physical examination is directed at assessing the extent of airway narrowing. Inspiratory stridor, tachypnea, retractions, and diminished breath sounds indicate critical narrowing. Restlessness, tachycardia, altered mental status, or cyanosis suggests hypoxia.
      (c) Laboratory data. A lateral neck x-ray will rule out epiglottitis.

An anteroposterior neck film will show subglottal narrowing (the classic steeple sign). ABGs will help assess the adequacy of ventilation and oxygenation.

(3) Therapy

(a) Home care. Most cases of croup are mild and can be managed at home. Therapeutic measures include a cool mist vaporizer, increased fluids, and careful observation. Parents should be instructed to call their usual health care provider if the child's respiratory distress worsens.

(b) Humidified oxygen should be administered if hypoxia is suspected.

(c) A quiet room where parent may stay with the child and elimination of all but the most necessary procedures will help reduce the child's anxiety and increased respiratory work.

(d) Aerosolized racemic epinephrine is usually effective; 0.25–0.5 ml of racemic epinephrine can be diluted with 2 ml of normal saline (NS) and administered by standard passive aerosal equipment. However, rebound worsening often occurs approximately 30–60 min after use. Therefore, its use **requires** hospitalization.

(e) The use of steroids remains somewhat controversial. However, in many centers, their use in moderate to severe cases is advocated. Dexamethasone, 1 mg/kg q6h IV for 3 doses, or a single bolus of 2 mg/kg IV, are suggested regimens.

(f) When respiratory compromise is severe and respiratory failure is present or imminent, intubation under controlled conditions is indicated.

c. Foreign body aspiration is the leading cause of injury-related death in toddlers. The sequelae of aspiration depend on the relative compromise of air movement.

(1) The etiology is usually related to the tendency for young children to place small objects in the mouth. Poorly designed or age-inappropriate toys or food products, including peanuts, hard candy, and gum, are usually involved. Obstruction of the upper airway from foreign bodies usually occurs at the laryngeal level.

(2) Evaluation and diagnosis are directed at assessing the adequacy of air movement and locating the site of obstruction.

(a) The **history** should identify the acuteness of onset and the circumstances surrounding aspiration. Choking, gagging, high-pitched wheezing, dysphonia, or aphonia may be noted. A history of fever and the clinical course will help differentiate aspiration from an infectious obstructive process (epiglottitis, croup).

(b) The **physical examination** should first establish the adequacy of the airway.

(c) Laboratory data. ABGs should be measured if respiratory distress is present. Anteroposterior and lateral neck and chest roentgenograms will reveal radiopaque foreign bodies and occasionally provide information as to the location of radiolucent objects. Inspiratory and expiratory films and fluoroscopy are very useful in patients with negative radiographic findings.

(3) Therapy should be responsive to the acuteness and severity of the obstruction.

(a) If the child is in stable condition—pink, coughing, and vocalizing well—attempts to remove the foreign body (laryngoscopy or bronchoscopy) should await controlled conditions.

(b) A conscious, actively choking, aphonic child with minimal air movement requires immediate noninvasive procedures.

(i) Deliver four back blows between the scapulae while supporting the infant face down on the rescuer's forearm, or across the rescuer's thighs.

(ii) If back blows are not successful, four chest thrusts (as in standard CPR) are administered.

(iii) Abdominal thrusts (Heimlich maneuver) are not generally recommended in children less than 8 years of age because of the potential injury to abdominal organs. Blind finger sweeps are usually contraindicated since they often advance a foreign body further down the airway. Instead, if back blows and chest thrusts prove unsuccessful, the jaw should be lifted and the mouth opened, first to visualize, and then to remove, the object.

(iv) An unconscious child with inadequate respirations should receive 100% O_2 by face mask. When staff members experienced in laryngoscopy are present, immediate direct laryngoscopy may allow visualization and removal of the foreign body. When this is not possible, or if laryngoscopy is difficult or prolonged, then emergency cricothyrotomy with a large-bore (e.g., 4-gauge) catheter, or tracheostomy, is indicated. If neither laryngoscopy, cricothyrotomy, nor tracheostomy is available, then mouth-to-mouth or bag-and-mask ventilation should be instituted immediately until an artificial airway has been placed.

d. Peritonsillar abscess

(1) Etiology. Gram-positive bacteria, especially streptococci

(2) Evaluation and diagnosis

(a) Usually occurs in children over age 8. If spontaneous rupture occurs, aspiration pneumonia or death may follow.

(b) A soft-palate bulge is usually seen, with deviation of the uvula to the opposite side.

(c) The tonsil is inflamed and pushed medially.

(d) There is marked trismus with drooling because of the obstructive enlargement of the tonsils.

(e) A "hot-potato" voice is characteristic.

(f) There are signs and symptoms of infection.

(3) Therapy

(a) Hospitalization is required in children and most adolescents.

(b) Incision and drainage or large-bore needle aspiration. Incision and drainage through the soft palate above the tonsil (not lateral to the tonsil, since the internal carotid artery may be punctured) is preferable to aspiration. Obtain bacterial cultures at this time.

(c) IV antibiotics. Give penicillin G, 100,000 units/kg/day in 4 divided doses. When cultures are available, select an appropriate antibiotic on the basis of culture results (see Table 15-2).

(d) Give nothing by mouth.

(e) Give IV fluids.

(f) Administer a cool mist via face mask or croup tent.

(g) Elevate the head of the bed 30 degrees.

(h) Because of the frequency of recurrence, tonsillectomy is indicated after the acute episode.

e. Diphtheria pharyngitis

(1) Etiology. *Corynebacterium diphtheriae*

(2) Evaluation and diagnosis

(a) Intense inflammation of the tonsils and pharynx is seen. The structures may be covered by a thick, dirty-gray pseudomembrane that is densely and tenaciously adherent to underlying structures. Its removal yields brisk bleeding.

(b) The membrane can occlude the airway.

(c) Involvement of the larynx must be ruled out.

(d) Microscopic examination of smears and cultures is necessary for diagnosis.

(3) Treatment
  (a) Assure an **airway.** If the larynx is involved, tracheotomy is necessary to minimize laryngeal stenosis.
  (b) IV antibiotics. Give penicillin G (see Table 15-2).
  (c) Antitoxin must be given early to prevent tissue fixation by the toxin (see Table 15-8).
  f. Retropharyngeal abscess is suppurative adenitis of the nodes of Henle in the buccopharyngeal and prevertebral fascia. Since these nodes atrophy after the age of 5, the abscesses occur prior to this age.
  (1) Etiology. Gram-positive cocci and anaerobes are the causative organisms. Retropharyngeal abscess often follows otitis media.
  (2) Evaluation and diagnosis
  (a) The abscess is almost always unilateral and does not spread across the midline.
  (b) A bulge of the posterior lateral pharyngeal wall may be seen.
  (c) The head and neck may be extended or the neck flexed with prevertebral muscle spasm; the head is extended for a better airway.
  (d) Drooling and swallowing difficulties are present.
  (e) The retropharynx should not be palpated because of the risk of rupture, aspiration, and death.
  (f) Anteroposterior and lateral soft tissue neck x-rays will support the diagnosis, especially if gas is seen in the retropharyngeal area. Fluoroscopy may be helpful.
  (3) Therapy
  (a) Surgical drainage under general anesthesia
  (i) The anesthesiologist must be careful not to rupture the abscess during intubation.
  (ii) The neck is hyperextended, and the neck and head are held below the level of the chest to prevent drainage of pus into the larynx and the trachea. Bacterial cultures are obtained at this time.
  (b) IV antibiotics. See Table 15-2.
B. Lower airway disease includes impaired gas exchange in the lung, or a portion of the lung, caused by viral and bacterial infections, foreign bodies, or intrinsic bronchospastic disease.
  1. Evaluation
  a. History. Review the nature and course of the onset. A history of choking or gagging may raise a suspicion of foreign body aspiration. Fever, the nature and frequency of coughing, tachypnea, and pain, or a past medical history of asthma, recurrent infection, neurologic abnormalities, or other chronic disease may also guide therapy.
  b. Physical examination. The adequacy of air exchange should be determined and the location and nature of any abnormality identified. Irritability, anxiety, or altered mental status may signify hypoxia or hypercapnia. Vital sign measurements, particularly temperature, respiratory rate, and pulses paradoxicus, should be obtained. Finding altered breath sounds, wheezing, rales, retractions, and abnormal diaphragmatic excursions provides useful diagnostic information.
  c. Laboratory data. ABGs, CBC, chest x-ray, and other selected radiographic studies may be helpful.
  2. Specific conditions
  a. Asthma is a condition in which bronchospasm, mucosal edema, and mucous secretion and plugging contribute to significant narrowing of the airways and subsequent impaired gas exchange.
  (1) Evaluation and diagnosis
  (a) The **history** includes age, duration, and course of the present attack, the course and severity of previous attacks, and a list of all medications (with doses) previously administered. A history con-

sistent with foreign body aspiration and anaphylaxis should be ruled out.

(b) The **physical examination** should assess the adequacy of air exchange.

(i) Altered mental status is a sign of marked impairment of gas exchange.

(ii) Vital signs should be measured often. Tachypnea and tachycardia are common. An abrupt decline in respiratory rate may indicate impending respiratory failure.

(iii) Measure and follow pulsus paradoxicus.

(iv) **Ventilatory status.** Assess the quality of breath sounds, degree of dyspnea, and retractions. Pallor and cyanosis may be observed in severe cases.

(v) Assess the severity of dehydration.

(vi) Palpate for the presence of subcutaneous emphysema in the neck and upper chest.

(c) Laboratory tests and ancillary studies

(i) Measurement of ABGs is critical in assessing the adequacy of gas exchange in a severe attack, both on presentation and in response to therapy.

(ii) When fever or other signs of infection are present, a CBC may prove helpful. To avoid an artificially elevated WBC, blood should be drawn before epinephrine therapy is given.

(iii) Spirometry, particularly peak expiratory flow rate and 1-sec forced expiratory volume (FEV_1), may provide a good indication of impairment of respiratory function.

(iv) Chest roentgenograms are useful only when the cause is in question (e.g., foreign body aspiration), when an associated pneumonia is considered likely, or when complications such as pneumothorax or pneumomediastinum are suspected.

(v) Serum theophylline levels in children taking theophylline should be followed.

(2) Therapy

(a) Oxygen. Give humidified O_2 by nasal canula or face mask to deliver a 30–40% concentration in inspired air. Patients with an acute asthma attack will uniformly present with some degree of hypoxemia secondary to perfusion of nonventilated, atelectatic segments of the lung and maldistribution of gas within the lung (ventilation/perfusion abnormalities).

(b) Hydration. The acutely ill asthmatic child will have increased fluid requirements.

(i) Oral fluids are usually adequate in mild attacks.

(ii) In severe attacks, oral fluid may precipitate vomiting, and a stable IV line should be placed. Generally, infusion of 5% D/W in 1/4 NS with 20–40 mEq/L of KCl at 1.5 times maintenance for the first 12 hr is used with adjustments that depend on clinical status.

(c) General supportive care. An asthmatic attack is a frightening experience for both child and parents. Fatigue, pain, hypoxemia, and medication may contribute to an agitated state. Effort should be made to comfort and reassure the child and the parents.

(d) Subcutaneous medication

(i) **Epinephrine.** Give 0.01 mg/kg (1:1000 dilution) SQ, with a maximum of 0.4 mg/dose. If a beneficial effect is obtained, the injection can be repeated twice at 20-min intervals. When complete clearing of the attack is achieved, give 0.005 mg/kg of Sus-Phrine (epinephrine in 1:200 thioglycolate suspension) 20 min after the last dose for action of longer duration. If the patient is still suffering from significant bronchospasm

after 3 doses of epinephrine or deteriorates after its adminis
tration, **do not give further doses. Excessive or inappro
priate use of epinephrine can induce serious cardia
arrhythmias and cause increased restlessness and anx
iety.**

(ii) **Terbutaline.** When adverse effects of epinephrine are pro
hibitive for further use in older children, terbutaline, 0.0
mg/kg SQ, with a maximum dose of 0.30 mg, can be used.

(e) **Aerosols**

(i) **Isoetharine (Bronkosol),** 0.25–0.5 ml diluted in 2 ml of N
should be delivered by an O_2-driven nebulizer. Treatment
may be repeated in the same manner as SQ epinephrine.

(ii) **Isoproterenol,** 0.25–0.5 ml of a 1:200 preparation with 2 m
of NS via O_2-driven nebulizer.

(iii) Metaproterenol, salbutamol, terbutaline, and other mor
selective beta-2–specific agents may play a role in the man
agement of severe attacks. However, at present, they are no
considered first-line drugs in *severe, acute* asthma. **Note: In
termittent positive pressure breathing administration o
aerosal medication has not been found to be more effec
tive than passive systems and is more likely to caus
paradoxical bronchospasm and pneumothorax.**

(f) **Intravenous infusions** are indicated when SQ or aerosol trea
ment has failed, when the initial presentation is one of sever
distress, or when oral medications are not tolerated (e.g., vomit
ing).

(i) **Aminophylline** is the mainstay of IV therapy for sever
asthmatic attacks. Before administration, previous doses
theophylline preparations should be ascertained, with a care
ful estimate of their effect on serum levels. A serum leve
determination prior to therapy may also give some indicatio
of past compliance with oral therapy. In **bolus therapy,** 5–
mg/kg in 30–50 ml of fluid is infused over 20 min. This ca
be repeated q4–6h. Serum levels should be followed and dos
age adjusted thereafter. Postinfusion peak levels should b
determined approximately 30–60 min after infusion ha
ended. A **constant infusion,** after a loading dose of 5–8 m
kg in 30–50 ml of IV fluid, is run in over 20 min. A constar
infusion requires starting with 1.1 mg/kg/hr and increasin
to 1.7. Serum levels can be measured any time during th
constant infusion. **Note: When aminophylline is adminis
tered in combination with beta agonists, constant cardia
monitoring and vital sign measurement are essentia
Rapid IV infusion of aminophylline can lead to cardia
arrhythmias, hypotension, and death.** The dosage of th
infusion should be adjusted according to last oral dose give
aiming for a therapeutic range of between 10–20 µg/L.
Signs of theophylline toxicity include severe headache
tachycardia, tremors, gastritis with frequent vomiting, an
seizures. For management see Chap. 4, p. 108.

(ii) **Isoproterenol** infusion should be reserved for cases of im
pending respiratory failure. A constant infusion of 0.15–0.
mcg/kg/min will usually provide a therapeutic response. I
**infusion of isoproterenol has been associated with m
ocardial ischemia, arhythmias, and death.** Careful vita
sign and cardiac monitoring are essential. The rate of infu
sion should be titrated with the degree of resultant tachyca
dia. Heart rates over 150–200/min generally require a redu
tion in infusion rate.

      (iii) The role of corticosteroids in the management of acute severe attacks is controversial. However, a short, high-dose course of tapered corticosteroids may be attempted in any child with a severe attack or in those who have responded well to such a regimen in the past. **Methylprednisolone** (Solu-Medrol), 0.25–0.5 mg/kg IV, or **hydrocortisone,** 5–10 mg/kg IV q6h may be used. Serious toxicity is minimized by the use of a short-term regimen.

b. Bronchiolitis is a syndrome of acute, small airway obstruction in young infants, with the risk of respiratory failure.

    (1) Etiology. It is usually viral in origin (most commonly, respiratory syncytial virus).

    (2) Evaluation should include assessments of hydration and respiratory exchange.

    (3) The **diagnosis** is suggested by the onset in an infant of coryza, cough, and dyspnea and by prominent wheezing, hyperinflation of the lungs, and retractions. Fever may not be present.

    (4) Therapy

        (a) Humidified O_2 (40% or more). In severe cases, ABGs should be monitored.

        (b) Adequate hydration is important. Whether fluids are administered PO or IV depends on the severity of the respiratory distress. **In severe respiratory distress, administration of oral fluids may induce vomiting and aspiration pneumonia and is contraindicated.**

        (c) In severe cases, assisted ventilation may be required.

        (d) Antibiotics are not routinely given, but are indicated if associated otitis media or pneumonia is present.

        (e) Glucocorticoids have not been shown to be beneficial.

        (f) Bronchodilators given parenterally or by inhalation may be worth trying, but are not reliably effective (see pp. 482ff).

c. Foreign body aspiration must always be considered in children presenting with an initial episode of wheezing or recurrent or unresponsive pneumonia.

    (1) Evaluation. Roentgenographic studies will identify radiopaque foreign bodies.

        (a) Tracheal foreign bodies that are not radiopaque can still often be seen from anteroposterior chest films, since they may be outlined by lucency of the air in the tracheal lumen.

        (b) Bronchial foreign bodies are suggested by paradoxical movement of the diaphragms or ipsilateral obstructive emphysema with a mediastinal shift to the contralateral side. Inspiratory and expiratory anteroposterior chest films or fluoroscopy will reveal this picture. Lateral decubitis radiographs may be helpful in documenting unilateral air trapping.

        (c) A foreign body caught in the esophagus can cause significant respiratory symptoms.

    (2) Therapy. Aspirated foreign bodies should be regarded as true emergencies **only** when air exchange is significantly compromised or when the foreign body may imminently migrate into a more dangerous position. Emergent mechanical efforts to dislodge a foreign body should be attempted only when air exchange is inadequate to sustain life. In all other cases, no attempt to mobilize the foreign body should be made until bronchoscopy can be performed.

        (a) Bronchoscopy is the definitive therapy. It should be done under optimal conditions in the operating room by skilled personnel.

        (b) Chest percussion, postural drainage, or bronchodilators are not recommended, since the foreign body may be dislodged and become positioned in the trachea, causing complete obstruction.

(c) Antibiotics are useful when infection complicates foreign body aspiration (see Chap. 15).

(d) After successful removal of a foreign body by bronchoscopy, inflammatory changes may produce fibriotic changes, which in turn may cause impaired airflow. However, persistent atelectasis, pneumonitis, pneumonia, or emphysema should raise the question of a remaining fragment or second foreign body.

d. Pneumonia may present with significant respiratory distress secondary to impaired gas exchange.

(1) General supportive measures include 30–40% O_2 by face mask, and intubation if respirations are inadequate.

(2) For specific information regarding etiology, evaluation, and therapy, see Chap. 15.

e. Pneumothorax

(1) **Etiology.** Spontaneous pneumothorax may be an idiopathic occurrence in a previously healthy person, or it may be a complication of underlying pulmonary disease.

(2) **Evaluation and diagnosis**

(a) **History.** A high index of suspicion is present whenever a patient with known lung disease experiences the **acute onset** of severe respiratory distress.

(b) **Physical examination.** Decreased fremitus, decreased breath sounds, and hyperresonance are present on the affected side. Asymmetric chest movement and displaced point of maximal impulse may be noted. Percussion over the clavicles on opposite sides reveals minor differences in percussion tones. In the infant and in patients with severe cystic fibrosis lung disease, the physical findings may be minimal, even in the face of extensive collapse.

(c) **Chest roentgenogram.** Sometimes, an expired posteroanterior view will aid diagnosis when the pneumothorax is small.

(d) **Classification.** Generally, a pneumothorax is well tolerated after an initial period of distress because of an adjustment of perfusion to ventilation. (**Pneumothorax can enlarge during reduced inflight cabin pressure,** which can be a problem when transporting sick infants.)

   (i) **Minor to moderate.** Less than 30% collapse

   (ii) **Major.** 30–70% collapse

   (iii) If **complete collapse** occurs, the possibility of tension pneumothorax should be suspected.

(3) **Treatment.** (For infants, see Chap. 6, pp. 144ff.) The following points should be observed:

(a) **If the clinical condition is critical, immediate lifesaving maneuvers become more important than diagnostic procedures.**

(b) If the leak is in visceral pleura, **positive-pressure breathing** can aggravate the situation. If there is a leak in the **parietal pleura** (flail chest), on the other hand, positive pressure may be lifesaving.

(c) **Simple observation** will suffice if the patient can be watched, the clinical condition is stable, there is no evidence of an "open" leak, and the radiologic diagnosis is "minor."

(d) **Cough suppression.** If necessary, dextromethorphan, codeine, or morphine should be used to suppress coughing. The use of respiratory depressants is dangerous and necessitates frequent arterial blood gas measurements.

(e) **Thoracentesis.** Needle aspiration of air at the 2nd anterior intercostal space, midclavicular line may be lifesaving whenever tension pneumothorax is present. Later, a closed thoracostomy drainage system will be in order.

(f) Thoracostomy. Tube thoracostomy is indicated when the pneumothorax is likely to reaccumulate. The term *closed thoracostomy* is used to designate a thoracostomy tube connected to a water-seal bottle. With the water seal (which can be improvised by placing the end of the tube under the surface of some sterile normal saline contained in anything with an air vent), air (and also fluid) drain from the chest, but air cannot reenter the submerged tube tip **if the end of the tube and water seal are below the level of the patient's chest.** It is customary to place the "bottle" on the floor. If the system is functioning well, the fluid will be lifted a few centimeters up the tube as the patient breathes and produces negative (subatmospheric) inspiratory pressure. Later, when the visceral and parietal pleura are adherent, this will not be seen.

(g) Recurrent pneumothoraces require parietal pleural stripping when possible or quinacrine instillation if an operation is precluded by the severity of the underlying lung disease.

f. Exacerbations of chronic pulmonary disease

(1) Bronchopulmonary dysplasia (BPD) is a chronic pulmonary disorder characterized by squamous metaplasia and hypertrophy of small airways with subsequent alveolar collapse and air trapping.

(a) The **etiology** is related to the prolonged mechanical ventilation of premature infants and its high oxygen tensions.

(b) Clinical manifestations and management will depend on the severity of BPD. Multiple systems are secondarily affected, including the respiratory, cardiovascular, and immunologic systems, as well as growth and development. A child with BPD requires very careful handling, since respiratory reserve is minimal in this condition. Hospitalization is often required for an illness that might be relatively benign in other children.

(i) Chronic respiratory insufficiency may be severe and require home use of continuous oxygen therapy. ABGs may show moderate hypoxia or compensated hypercarbia. Acute deterioration of the respiratory status is not uncommon.

(ii) Reactive airway disease similar to that in bronchiolitis is often seen, with wheezing, hyperexpansion, and respiratory failure. Theophylline preparations are often effective.

(iii) Right-sided congestive heart failure secondary to pulmonary hypertension may be severe. Acute weight gain may indicate significant fluid retention. Digitalization and diuretic therapy are often required.

(iv) Lower respiratory infections caused by usually benign viral agents may cause severe respiratory distress. The child should be isolated from others with viral illnesses.

(v) The incidence of **pneumothorax** is increased.

(vi) Sudden infant death syndrome is more common in infants with BPD (see sec. **VII.A.**).

(vii) Nonspecific findings, including lethargy and poor feeding, may indicate worsening respiratory status.

(viii) Radiographic chest abnormalities are common. Areas of hyperaeration and atelectasis may be chronic, making the diagnosis of new infiltrate difficult. Comparison with previous films is usually helpful in revealing acute changes.

(ix) Sepsis in BPD. Fever or a probable bacterial process (new infiltrate on the chest film) may require management similar to that in a febrile neonate (see Chap. 6).

(2) Cystic fibrosis. See also Chap. 10.

(a) Clinical manifestations and management

(i) Reactive airway disease similar to bronchiolitis may cause severe respiratory distress in infants. Respiratory support and bronchodilator therapy may be required.

(ii) **Subacute respiratory deterioration** with decreasing exercise tolerance and increasing respiratory distress is a common problem. Chest x-rays usually reveal increased infiltrative changes. Hospitalization for chest physiotherapy, oxygen, and antibiotics is usually required. *Pseudomonas aeruginosa* and *Staphylococcus aureas* are frequently isolated from sputum cultures.

(iii) **Pneumothorax** is common and should always be considered whenever acute chest pain or respiratory deterioration occurs.

IV. **Cardiac failure.** See also Chap. 9, pp. 248ff.
  A. **Congestive heart failure**
  1. High output failure is seen with severe anemia, hyperthyroid storm, and sepsis. Low output failure is caused by either **myocardial disease** (ischemia, infection, congenital heart disease, metabolic imbalances, arrhythmias) or **obstructive disease** (coarctation of the aorta, critical aortic stenosis, malignant hypertension).
  2. **Evaluation**
    a. **Common symptoms**
      (1) Poor weight gain
      (2) Difficulty in feeding, anorexia
      (3) Chronic unproductive cough unrelated to other upper respiratory symptoms
      (4) Increased perspiration
      (5) Fatigue and poor exercise tolerance
    b. **Physical examination.** Attention is given to the following:
      (1) Chronic malnutrition
      (2) Cardiovascular findings include jugular venous distention, poor perfusion, tachycardia, an S_4 gallop, rales, and tender hepatomegaly. The quality of femoral pulses and presence of murmurs must be evaluated to diagnose anatomic heart disease.
      (3) Respiratory distress
      (4) Evidence of infection, hyperthyroidism, or severe anemia
    c. **Laboratory studies**
      (1) Chest x-ray
      (2) ECG and echocardiogram
      (3) ABGs, CBC, electrolytes, blood sugar, calcium, toxic screen, and thyroid function test if indicated. Measurement of cardiac enzymes (CPK, SGOT, LDH) may be helpful.
  3. **Treatment**
    a. The patient is positioned upright in bed to facilitate breathing; infants are placed in a chalasia chair.
    b. Supplemental oxygen is given. Intubation and mechanical ventilation with positive end-expiratory pressure when indicated.
    c. Patients with severe anemia should be carefully transfused (see Chap. 17, p. 458; see also Chap. 6, pp. 160ff).
    d. Arrhythmias should be treated (see Chap. 9, pp. 235ff).
    e. Diuretics such as furosemide (Lasix), 1 mg/kg/dose, should be given only if the electrolytes are within normal limits.
    f. Morphine (0.05–0.10 mg/kg/dose) is given to allay anxiety and hence decrease the demands on the heart.
    g. Aminophylline is used as a bronchodilator.
    h. Positive inotropic agents (isoproterenol, dopamine, digoxin) can be used to support the myocardium. **Doses** are as follows:
      (1) **Dopamine,** 5–15 µg/kg/min
      (2) **Isoproterenol,** 0.1–0.5 µg/kg/min
      (3) **Digoxin.** A total digitalizing dose is given over the first 24 hr as

follows: 40 µg/kg (use two-thirds of this dose if given parenterally). Give one-half immediately; one-fourth at 8 hr, and one-fourth at 16 hours. The maintenance dose is one-fourth of the total digitalizing dose in divided doses bid. The total digitalizing dose for adults is 1 mg IV, and the adult maintenance dose is 0.125–0.250 mg/kg in divided doses bid.

B. Pericardial tamponade
  1. **Definition:** an accumulation of a large amount of fluid in the pericardial cavity, producing cardiac compression and inadequate diastolic filling and leading to a small, fixed stroke volume and low output heart failure
  2. **Etiology**
    a. **Primary pericardial disease**
        (1) Viral pericarditis
        (2) Bacterial pericarditis
        (3) Rheumatic pericarditis
    b. **Systemic disease that can cause secondary pericardial tamponade**
        (1) Congestive heart failure
        (2) Uremia
        (3) Tumor (usually metastatic)
        (4) Collagen vascular disease
  3. **Evaluation**
    a. **Vital signs** demonstrate tachycardia, tachypnea, and hypotension.
    b. **Physical examination**
        (1) Evidence of low output cardiac failure includes cool extremities, mottled gray skin, and oliguria.
        (2) **Cardiac examination** reveals:
            (a) Muffled heart sound
            (b) Pericardial friction rub
            (c) Jugular venous distension
            (d) Passive hepatic congestion
    c. **Diagnostic studies**
        (1) The chest x-ray shows an increased bulbous cardiac silhouette.
        (2) The ECG shows S–T segment elevation, low voltage, and T wave inversion.
        (3) An echocardiogram shows the effusion.
  4. **Therapy.** Emergency decompression by pericardiocentesis and/or surgery (pericardial window or pericardial stripping) is lifesaving. Pericardiocentesis should be performed by the most experienced person available.
    a. The patient's ECG should be continuously monitored.
    b. **Equipment.** A 10-ml syringe and a 1½-inch 20-gauge needle are adequate for an infant or toddler, whereas a 3-inch spinal needle (20-gauge) can be used in the adult.
    c. Prepare the subxyphoid area with a povidone-iodine (Betadine) and alcohol wash.
    d. Using sterile technique, insert the needle in the subxyphoid area at a 30-degree angle, aiming for the midclavicular to lateral clavicular line. Slight negative pressure should be maintained on the syringe. When the pericardium is entered, fluid will appear in the hub of the syringe; this fluid should be evacuated.
    e. ECG monitoring
    f. **Complications** include pneumothorax, arrhythmias, and myocardial puncture.

C. Tetralogy of Fallot spells
  1. **Etiology.** Caused by an acute increase in pulmonary resistance, leading to an increase in the intracardiac right-to-left shunt. Such spells can last minutes to hours, resolving spontaneously or leading to progressive hypoxia, acidosis, and death.
  2. **Evaluation**
    a. **Clinical findings** include acute cyanosis, restlessness, and agitation.

b. Cardiac and respiratory

(1) A regular rhythm with good pulses is usually present. The murmur of a ventricular septal defect will be heard frequently; the murmur of pulmonary stenosis may decrease during an acute spell.

(2) Examination of the chest is remarkable for the absence of rales and wheezes.

3. Treatment

a. Oxygen is administered.

b. The child should be comforted and quieted.

c. The child should be positioned or held in the knee-to-chest position to increase the systemic resistance.

d. Morphine sulfate (0.1 mg/kg IM or IV) is given for sedation and subpulmonic relaxation.

e. Propranolol (0.02–0.1 mg/kg/IV) is given.

f. Metabolic acidosis should be corrected.

4. The best treatment of tetralogy of Fallot spells is prevention.

a. Treat all hypovolemic states early with volume expansion.

b. During procedures on a child with tetralogy of Fallot, have the parent available to comfort and reassure the child.

V. Central nervous system emergencies

A. Seizures. While seizures carry the risk of hypoxic CNS damage, significant morbidity may also result from injudicious medical intervention.

1. Etiology. See Chap. 20, p. 502.

2. Evaluation and diagnosis

a. The history should identify any underlying disease process. Careful attention should be paid to:

(1) The quality and length of the seizure

(2) The presence of fever or other symptoms (headache, stiff neck, poor feeding, irritability)

(3) History of recent trauma

(4) Past and family history of seizure or other chronic conditions

(5) Prescribed medications and compliance

(6) Possibility of ingestion

b. Physical examination should assess the extent of impairment of cardiorespiratory status and illuminate a direct cause for the seizure activity. Include the following:

(1) Vital signs

(2) Air movement and chest wall excursion

(3) Skin color (perfusion, cyanosis, hypopigmented areas)

(4) Evidence of trauma (bruises, laceration, swelling)

(5) Evidence of sepsis (purpura, petechiae)

(6) Pupil size and reaction

(7) Disk margins and retinal field (papilledema, hemorrhage)

(8) Quality of the fontanelle and transillumination of the skull in children under 18 months of age

(9) Muscle tone, reflexes

(10) Observation of seizure activity

c. Laboratory tests

(1) Blood for immediate bedside glucose determination (Dextrostix); CBC; electrolytes; BUN; glucose; calcium; magnesium toxic screen (including lead); pH and TCO_2; anticonvulsant levels when appropriate; and ABGs when indicated

(2) Urine for urinalysis, and an immediate pregnancy test when appropriate

(3) Lumbar puncture when signs of meningeal irritation are present or for seizures without clear diagnosis once increased intracranial pressure (ICP) has been ruled out (see **B.2;** see also Chap. 20, pp. 494ff).

(4) Roentgenographic studies

(a) Skull films are indicated only with evidence of trauma or when metabolic disease associated with bony abnormalities is suspected.

    (b) A CT scan is indicated when head trauma, increased ICP or a mass lesion is suspected.

3. Therapy is based on assuring adequate **ventilation and oxygenation** and terminating seizure activity.

  a. Airway management is of paramount importance. The vast majority of deaths from seizures are due to the inadequacy of air exchange, either from seizure activity or administered medications.

    (1) Maximize the natural airway by loosening clothing about the neck, removing food particles, etc.

    (2) Suction vomitus or secretions.

    (3) An oral airway should be placed if the tongue is obstructing respirations.

    (4) Administer oxygen **whether or not cyanosis is present.**

    (5) If air movement is inadequate despite the preceding steps, artificial ventilation by bag and mask with 100% O_2 is indicated until spontaneous respirations improve. Intubation may be required when bag-and-mask ventilation is insufficient or when long-term ventilation seems probable.

  b. An IV line should be started if a seizure is ongoing or if signs of other serious conditions are evident (e.g., trauma, shock, sepsis).

    (1) Infusion of 5% dextrose with 0.25 NS is generally begun. When hypoglycemia is suspected, a 10% dextrose solution after a 50% dextrose bolus (1 mg/kg IV) may be given.

    (2) When increased ICP is suspected, fluid administration should be minimized.

  c. Anticonvulsant therapy

    (1) Diazepam (Valium) is useful for terminating seizures quickly but has a short anticonvulsant half-life and can be relied on only for a transient effect.

      (a) The initial dose is 0.1–0.25 mg/kg, given not faster than 1 mg/min with a maximum dose of 10 mg. If there is no response to the initial dose in 15 min, a second dose of 0.25–0.4 mg/kg with a maximum dose of 15 mg can be given.

      (b) Diazepam is supplied as 5 mg/ml and should be slowly pushed close to the IV site until the seizure has terminated. Since the IV tubing volume may be greater than 2 ml, the line should be flushed after each 0.2 ml of diazepam is administered. An alternative is diluting 2 ml (10 mg) of diazepam with 8 ml of NS pushed slowly until the seizure has terminated.

      (c) Diazepam is capable of causing significant respiratory depression and should never be given until equipment and staff for assisted ventilation are available.

      (d) Diazepam used in conjunction with phenobarbital holds a significantly greater risk of respiratory arrest than with each drug alone.

    (2) Phenytoin is effective, and its relatively long duration of action makes it a useful adjunct to diazepam administration. However, the onset of action is usually in 20–40 min. Therefore, it should not be used as a primary drug if immediate cessation of the seizure is paramount.

      (a) Phenytoin should be infused as soon as the diazepam has been given. The dosage is 15–20 mg/kg IV in normal saline over 20 min (not faster than 1 mg/kg/min).

      (b) Cardiac arrhythmias and hypotension are the most important complications. Take care that infusion is not too rapid. Cardiac monitoring is essential.

    (3) Paraldehyde can be used as an adjunct to diazepam and phenytoin if

further therapy is required. In addition, since paraldehyde is administered rectally, it can be used when no IV line can be started. The
dosage is 0.3–0.4 ml/kg (maximum 8 ml) mixed in peanut or corn oil
at a 10:1 (oil-paraldehyde) ratio and administered per rectum via
rectal tube.

(4) Phenobarbital can be used when the preceding therapy has not terminated seizure activity.

  (a) The dosage is 10 mg/kg IV given slowly over 10–15 min. If no
  effect is evident after 20–30 min, this dose can be repeated
  twice.

  (b) Once phenobarbital has been administered, great care should be
  exercised in using diazepam [see **(1)**].

d. With prolonged or refractory seizures, underlying conditions must be
ruled out. The possibility of trauma, intracranial infection, increased ICP
bleeding vascular anomalies, or ingestion of toxic substances or medication should always be reconsidered.

4. Specific disorders

a. Febrile seizures are the most common form of convulsive disorders in
children. They are associated with fever but without CNS infection, a
metabolic abnormality, or any other direct cause and usually occur from 6
months up to 5 years of age. Seizures with fever in children who have
suffered previous **nonfebrile** seizures are excluded.

(1) Evaluation and diagnosis

  (a) The **history** should describe fever and a seizure that is usually
  brief, self-limited (approximately 4–5 min, never longer than 15
  min), generalized, tonic-clonic, and generally with rapid recovery.
  It should include past and family history of seizures, both febrile
  and nonfebrile, and any underlying neurologic or metabolic abnormality (see Chap. 20, p. 503).

  (b) The **physical examination** should be directed to uncovering the
  cause of the fever and ruling out a CNS infection or other abnormality. Great care should be exercised in ruling out the presence
  of meningeal or residual neurologic signs.

  (c) Laboratory investigations should be determined by the child's
  age, history, and physical findings. In children under 20 months
  of age, meningeal signs are unreliable in detecting meningeal
  irritation due to infection. Febrile seizures lasting **more than 15
  min, focal** in nature or associated with transient or permanent
  neurologic abnormalities, have a higher probability of being associated with an underlying infection or metabolic or traumatic
  disorder. These "complex" febrile seizures therefore require more
  aggressive diagnostic testing.

(2) Therapy

  (a) For an ongoing seizure, anticonvulsant therapy is that for seizures in general (see **A.3.C**). "Make haste slowly" in stopping a
  febrile seizure. Note the time anticonvulsant therapy is given to
  evaluate the length of seizures.

  (b) Administer antipyretics and tepid sponge.

  (c) Prophylaxis. See Chap. 20, p. 506.

b. Hypoglycemia (see also Chap. 11) Hypoglycemic seizures are a medical
emergency.

(1) Provide general supportive measures as outlined in **3.**

(2) Look for Medic-Alert bracelet or other evidence of insulin use.

(3) After withdrawing an aliquot of blood for glucose and other determinations, give 1 ml/kg IV of 50% dextrose stat. For **infants,** a 25%
dextrose dilution at the same dose is preferable.

(4) Begin an IV infusion of 10% D/W at the maintenance rate (see Chap.
11, p. 313; see also Chap. 6, p. 164ff).

(5) Investigate the cause of the hypoglycemia.

c. Hypertension
   (1) Provide the general supportive measures outlined previously.
   (2) Rapid therapy for hypertension is required (see Chap. 8, p. 218).
   (3) Ongoing seizures can be treated acutely as outlined in **3** for general seizure disorders. Investigate the cause of the hypertension.
d. Meningitis or encephalitis
   (1) Provide the general supportive measures outlined previously.
   (2) Anticonvulsant therapy is that outlined for a general seizure disorder (see **3.c**).
   (3) Rapid institution of antibiotic therapy is critical.
   (4) To minimize any possible associated cerebral edema, fluid administration should be carefully monitored and kept at the minimum rate required to maintain cardiovascular stability (usually at 75% of maintenance) (see Chap. 7, p. 197).

B. Increased intracranial pressure (ICP)
 1. The **etiology** includes:
   a. Cerebral edema due to hypoxia and ischemia, Reye syndrome, or toxins (i.e., lead)
   b. Increased cerebrospinal fluid (CSF) volume due to hydrocephalus or an obstructed ventricular shunt
   c. Increased intracranial blood volume due to infection (meningitis and encephalitis), trauma, (intraparenchymal bleeding, subdural hematoma), or arteriovenous malformations
   d. Space-occupying lesions due to tumor or abscess
 2. Evaluation
   a. A complete **history** should include any evidence of infection, trauma, hypoxic events, previous seizures, CNS insults, and medications. Neurologic symptoms should be carefully documented, with detailed accounts of the duration and progression.
   b. Physical examination
      (1) Vital signs should be taken and recorded frequently. The Cushing reflex (bradycardia, hypertension, slow and irregular respirations) may be present.
      (2) In the neurologic examination, look for focality and intracranial bruits. In the infant and toddler, be certain to measure the head circumference, feel for split sutures, and transilluminate the head. The Glasgow Coma Scale (Table 3-5) is used if coma is present. Table 3-6 will assist in identifying possible herniation.
      (3) The remainder of the physical examination should attempt to be directed toward finding the causes of the ICP, e.g., evidence of trauma, infection, hepatic disease, cyanotic heart disease, or systemic hemangiomas.
   c. Laboratory studies include:
      (1) A CT scan, once the patient's condition has stabilized
      (2) Skull x-rays are helpful for eliciting splitting of the sutures, calcification, or bone erosion secondary to prolonged increased pressure.
      (3) A lumbar puncture is done **after** the CT scan, to rule out a mass lesion, for pressure measurement, and to aid in the diagnosis of infection or hemorrhage. A lumbar puncture carries a risk of central herniation in the patient with ICP. At times, however, examination of the CSF is essential, and the benefits outweigh the risks of the procedure. In these situations, great care should be taken to have
         (a) Another person available to monitor the patient
         (b) The smallest spinal needle
         (c) An IV in place
         (d) Mannitol at the bedside
 3. Therapy. The goal of therapy is to decrease the ICP by decreasing one or more of the component volumes.

Table 3-5. Glasgow Coma Scale[a]

Response	Score
Eyes	
Open	
Spontaneously	4
To verbal command	3
To pain	2
No response	1
Best motor response	
To verbal command	
Obeys	6
To painful stimulus[b]	
Localizes pain	5
Flexion withdrawal	4
Flexion abnormal	
(decorticate rigidity)	3
Extension (decerebrate rigidity)	2
No response	1
Best verbal response[c]	
Oriented and converses	5
Disoriented and converses	4
Inappropriate words	3
Incomprehensible sounds	2
No response	1
Total	3–15

[a]The Glasgow Coma Scale, based on eye opening and verbal and motor responses, is a practical means of monitoring changes in the level of consciousness. If the response on the scale is given a number, the responsiveness of the patient can be expressed by summation of the figures. The **lowest** score is 3; the **highest** is 15.
[b]Apply knuckles to sternum; observe arms.
[c]Arouse patient with painful stimulus if necessary.

  a. All correctable lesions are treated.
  b. The initial therapy includes:
    (1) Position. To avoid venous obstruction the patient's head should be kept midline, with the head of the bed at a 30-degree upward slant.
    (2) Oxygen and airway. The PaO_2 should be maintained above 100 mm Hg by whatever means required.
    (3) Hypocapnia. Endotracheal intubation and hyperventilation to a $PaCO_2$ of approximately 24 mm Hg will cause vasoconstriction and hence a decrease in the intracranial blood volume. Some patients will hyperventilate spontaneously and do not require mechanical ventilation.
    (4) Osmotherapy. Attempt to achieve an osmolarity of 300–320 mOsm/L, as follows:
      (a) Limit the amount of fluid intake (PO and IV).
      (b) Give mannitol, 0.25–0.50 gm/kg, as a bolus q2–4h.
      (c) Give glycerol as a PG bolus, q6h.
      (d) Give furosemide (Lasix), 1 mg/kg q6–8h.
      (e) Calculate osmolarity if direct laboratory measurement is not available (mOsm = mEq Na + BUN/2.8 + blood glucose/18). The calculated value will be falsely low if other osmotic agents are present in the blood (i.e., mannitol, glycerol) (see also Chap. 7, p. 189).
      (f) During osmotherapy, an accurate record should be kept of intake and output; urine output should not fall below 0.25–0.5 ml/kg/hr.

Table 3-6. CNS Herniation

Level of dysfunction	Respiratory pattern	Pupil size	Extraocular movements	Motor pattern
Diencephalon (central herniation, bilateral)	Cheyne-Stokes	Small	Paresis of upgaze	Decortication
Midbrain (lateral herniation, unilateral, central, or bilateral)	Central neurogenic hyperventilation	Dilated	Preserved abduction (loss of function of cranial nerves III, IV)	Decerebration
Pons	Cluster	Midposition	Absent doll's caloric response	Flaccid
Medulla	Ataxic	Midposition	Absent doll's caloric response	Flaccid

(5) Seizure control is important to avoid a sudden, massive increase i cerebral metabolism.

(6) Normothermia must be maintained to avoid increased blood flow an volume.

(7) Corticosteroids are effective in reducing the edema that surround brain tumors, but their benefit in intracranial hypertension from other causes has not been demonstrated. Dexamethasone (Decadron 1 mg/kg/day in 3 divided doses. Corticosteroids are contraindicated i the treatment of Reye syndrome because of their catabolic qualities

c. Maximum increased therapy. If the preceding maneuvers fail to contro the ICP, more invasive monitoring in the form of a CVP line and an IC monitoring device is required. The following therapeutic maneuvers ma then be tried.

(1) Sedation and muscle relaxation. Muscle relaxants (pancuroniun [Pavulon], 0.1 mg/kg q1–2h) will prevent intracranial hypertensio associated with movement and muscle strain. Sedation with mor phine (0.1 mg/kg/q2–6h) or diazepam (0.1 mg/kg/q2–6h) is used t control the increase of pressure that occurs with noxious stimuli.

(2) Barbiturates. The use of barbiturates for increased ICP is controver sial. They usually lower it, but whether or not they alter the outcom is debatable. The usual preparation is:

   (a) Nembutal, 3–5 mg/kg/bolus, followed by a bolus or infusion of 1– 2 mg/kg/hr, to achieve a blood level of 20–40 mg/L.

   (b) The main complication of barbiturate therapy is the associated myocardial depression. Thus, drug level and cardiac function should be closely monitored.

(3) Hypothermia to 30°C has been used, but it carries many risks, includ ing cardiac arrhythmias, pancreatitis, hyperglycemia, and decreased hepatic drug metabolism (especially a problem if the patient is also receiving barbiturates). It is not recommended.

(4) The duration of maximum increased ICP therapy can extend to weeks. The process of weaning the patient from therapy is started when the ICP is consistently in a normal range. The patient is first weaned from barbiturates and then from pancuronium and mechani cal hyperventilation; osmotherapy is the last to be discontinued. The pace of weaning is dictated by the ICP response.

C. Spinal cord lesions. The patient usually presents with neurologic dysfunction below the level of the lesion. The most common lesions will be discussed here.

1. Trauma, usually as the result of hyperextension, hyperflexion, or vertical crush injuries. The fractures or dislocations most commonly occur at the level of T12–L1, C5–C6, and C1–C2.

   a. Evaluation. Patients may experience a *total loss* of function distal to the lesion (as in cord transections), or **temporary and completely reversible** loss (as seen in localized edema).

   (1) The **history** of the injury should be documented, with meticulous details of the progression and degree of neurologic loss.

   (2) The **physical examination** should include:

      (a) The adequacy of ventilation and cardiovascular status

      (b) Examination for associated injuries

      (c) The neurologic examination will usually demonstrate:

         (i) Loss of **motor and sensory function** below the level of the lesion.

         (ii) **Arreflexia** for 2–6 weeks, often with a return to some reflex activity at a later date.

         (iii) Total **flaccidity** is initially present; **spasticity** follows weeks after the insult.

         (iv) Urinary retention can also be a feature.

   (3) Laboratory studies include:

      (a) Radiographs of the spine

      (b) CT scan of the affected region

      (c) A myelogram may be indicated.

  b. Treatment

    (1) Locate the lesion and attempt to minimize any further damage.

    (2) The neck should be immobilized in a neutral position.

    (3) Respiratory function must be supported as required. Patients with a lesion at C1–C2 will require mechanical assistance.

    (4) The **cardiovascular system** must be supported as required; hypovolemia can result from associated autonomic dysfunction.

    (5) A Foley catheter is placed to avoid bladder distension.

    (6) Traction and/or surgical decompression are usually attempted in an effort to minimize any further damage.

2. Epidural abscess. See also Chap. 15.

  a. Etiology. Usually *S. aureus.* The anatomy of the dura localizes the infection to the dorsal compartment.

  b. Evaluation may reveal exquisite back pain and a preference for the back to be held rigid. There may be distal muscle weakness and radicular pain. The **laboratory examination** includes:

    (1) Plain radiographs

    (2) A CT scan

    (3) Sedimentation rate, CBC, and blood cultures

    (4) If a lumbar puncture is performed, it will reveal a pleocytosis and increased CSF protein.

  c. Therapy includes:

    (1) Surgical drainage

    (2) Antibiotics (see Chap. 15)

3. Transverse myelitis. Transverse myelitis presents as a usually rapidly progressive segmental spinal cord dysfunction.

  a. The **etiology** includes viral disease and vascular and demyelinating disease.

  b. The **evaluation** of this lesion is the same as outlined in **2.b.** All other spinal cord lesions must be ruled out.

  c. The **therapy** is controversial, with very equivocal results.

    (1) Supportive therapy is the mainstay, and is determined by the level of the lesion.

    (2) A trial of corticosteroid (dexamethasone, 1 mg/kg/day in divided doses tid), is often made.

    (3) Plasmaphoresis is currently under consideration as a possible therapeutic maneuver.

D. Hydrocephalus is an increase in the CSF component of the intracranial volume, caused by a blockage in normal CSF flow and resorption (rarely, overproduction of CSF can also cause hydrocephalus).

  1. The **etiology** includes:

    a. Hemorrhage. Intraventricular, traumatic, and secondary to arteriovenous malformation

    b. Tumor. Particularly a posterior fossa tumor that directly blocks the third and fourth ventricle

    c. Infection, including:

      (1) Congenital TORCH infections (toxoplasmosis, rubella, cytomegalic inclusion virus, herpes)

      (2) Ventriculitis

      (3) Tuberculous meningitis

    d. Anatomic abnormality

  2. Evaluation. Signs and symptoms of ICP vary with the age of the patient.

    a. History

      (1) Children under 2 years of age usually demonstrate the following:

        (a) Lethargy with poor sucking and poor feeding

        (b) Apnea

        (c) Spasticity

  (d) High-pitched cry
  (e) Vomiting
 (2) Children over age 2 usually present with
  (a) Headache that is worse in the early morning hours
  (b) Vomiting
  (c) Lethargy
 b. Physical findings
  (1) Children under a few years of age
   (a) Increased head circumference, with split sutures, dilated scalp veins, and bulging fontanelle
   (b) Lower extremity spasticity with opisthotonos
   (c) Optic atrophy
   (d) Pseudobulbar palsy
  (2) Children over a few years of age
   (a) Lower extremity spasticity
   (b) Papilledema
   (c) Gait disturbance
 c. Laboratory examination
  (a) Plain skull radiographs may demonstrate split sutures, intracranial calcifications, and bony erosions.
  (2) A **CT scan** is the best diagnostic tool. With it, ventricular size can be directly evaluated.
  (3) Ultrasound of the head can be used in children under the age of 1 year.
 3. The therapy must be tailored to each clinical situation, but usually will include:
  a. Decompression of the spinal fluid compartment either by an external or an internalized shunt
  b. Tumor removal or irradiation
  c. Systemic corticosteroids are used to decrease tumor-related edema (dexamethasone, 1 mg/kg/day in divided doses tid).
E. Complications of intraventricular shunts
 1. Etiology and evaluation. Ventricular shunts are placed for decompression of the ventricles. Two types of internalized, long-term shunts are used: the first is the ventriculoperitoneal (VP) shunt and the second is the ventriculoatrial (VA) shunt. The most common medical emergencies associated with these shunts are:
  a. Mechanical obstruction presents with the symptoms and signs of ICP (see **B**). When obstruction occurs, the shunt should be tapped acutely, followed by surgical manipulation, or replacement, or both.
  b. Infection. The shunt is a foreign body and as such serves as a nidus for infection. **Treatment** includes antibiotics and very often surgical removal of the shunt. If the shunt must be removed, emergency and perhaps temporary ventricular decompression can be effected by an indwelling ventricular catheter externalized through a burr hole.

VI. Acute abdomen
A. Appendicitis
 1. Evaluation and diagnosis
  a. History. Establish the time of onset. The appendix commonly perforates within 36 hr after pain begins. The pain is periumbilical and is almost always the first symptom. Vomiting is present and always follows the onset of pain. After several hours, pain usually shifts to the right lower quadrant. In the infant, decreased appetite, fever, and vomiting are usually present.
  b. Physical examination, when right lower quadrant pain is present, will usually reveal tenderness, guarding, and rebound. Rectal examination is imperative to elicit tenderness. Diarrhea will be present, especially in retrocecal appendicitis.

c. Laboratory data
  (1) Urinalysis, urine culture and Gram stain
  (2) The WBC usually is elevated, but rarely above 20,000 in a child with a nonperforated appendix.
  (3) Abdominal x-rays will show curvature of the spine to the right due to the spasm of right-sided abdominal musculature. An air-fluid level may be seen in the cecum. A fecalith may be seen and increases the likelihood of a perforation. With perforation, decreased bowel gas in the right lower quadrant and free peritoneal fluids can be seen, especially in children under 2 years of age. A chest film may be helpful, since lower lobe pneumonia may occasionally mimic appendicitis.

2. Therapy
  a. Appendectomy
  b. In suspected perforated appendix, a triple antibiotic regimen (ampicillin, gentamicin, and clindamycin or cephoxitin) is usually given.

B. Obstruction
1. Intussusception
  a. Etiology. Intussusception is usually found in children from 1 month to 2 years of age and occurs when a segment of intestine protrudes into the lumen of an adjacent portion of intestine, causing intermittent and possibly permanent obstruction and necrosis. The majority of cases are idiopathic, but of the identifiable causes, a Meckel's diverticulum is the most common. Henoch-Schönlein purpura is also common.
  b. Evaluation and diagnosis
    (1) History
      (a) Intermittent abdominal pain, vomiting, and bloody ("currant-jelly") stools
      (b) Violent episodes of colicky, severe abdominal pain, causing the child to cry out and draw the legs into flexed position
    (2) Physical examination
      (a) The child may be quiet, listless, or normal appearing between episodes of pain. Irritability or restlessness may also be noted.
      (b) When the process presents later in the course, the child may show signs of prostration, pallor, and altered mental status. Careful vital sign measurement is essential in this setting.
      (c) A vague, sausage-shaped mass is palpable, either abdominally or rectally, in the vast majority.
      (d) Stools should be tested for occult blood.
      (e) Fever is common, particularly in infants.
    (3) Laboratory data
      (a) A characteristic filling defect extending from the cecum to distal parts of the colon is observed in the barium enema.
      (b) Hematocrit
      (c) Electrolytes should be monitored.
      (d) Urine output and the urinalyses should be monitored.
  c. Therapy
    (1) IV fluids
    (2) Barium enema. Most intussusceptions can be reduced by the hydrostatic pressure of the barium during the diagnostic enema. When done in a controlled manner, with close collaboration between the surgeon and radiologist, this procedure is safe and may obviate the need for surgery.
    (3) When hydrostatic reduction is unsuccessful, **laparotomy and direct reduction** is required. If reduction is not possible or if necrotic bowel is present, resection and anastomosis will be necessary.

2. Malrotation and volvulus
  a. Etiology. Congenitally abnormal position of the small bowel and associated abnormal posterior fixation of the mesentery of the small bowel. The most common age of presentation is under 1 month of age.

b. Evaluation and diagnosis

(1) The **history** almost always includes vomiting, usually bile stained. In older children, a past history of attacks that are often misdiagnosed as "cyclic vomiting" may be elicited.

(2) **Physical examination** may reveal abdominal distension, jaundice, blood-stained vomitus or stools, and shock.

(3) **Laboratory data**

(a) Abdominal films may reveal gas in the stomach with a paucity of air in the small intestine.

(b) An upper GI series and small bowel follow-through will confirm the diagnosis, defining the position of the ligament of Treitz and the cecum. Electrolytes and CBC should be carefully followed. Stool testing positive for blood is a poor prognostic sign, indicating significant bowel ischemia.

c. Therapy

(1) Nasogastric tube

(2) **Operative relief** of the obstruction should be attempted as rapidly as controlled conditions allow.

(3) **IV fluids** (see Chap. 7).

3. Pyloric stenosis is a cause of obstruction in the first 8 weeks of life, with a peak in 2–4 weeks. Males are affected 4:1 over females, and it occurs more frequently in infants with a family history of the condition.

a. The **history** reveals the onset of vomiting of feedings.

(1) The vomitus is usually not bile stained.

(2) As the obstruction increases, so, too, does the vomiting.

b. Physical examination. The findings will vary with the severity of the obstructive process.

(1) Dehydration and weight loss (at times, emaciation) are common.

(2) The classic palpation of an olive-sized muscular tumor occurs in the majority of cases.

(3) Gastric peristaltic waves are also common.

c. Laboratory data

(1) **Roentgenographic studies** after a barium meal often reveal stenosis ("railroad-track sign").

(2) Electrolytes, BUN, glucose, pH, and TCO_2 should be followed, since significant abnormalities may accompany the vomiting.

d. Therapy

(1) Nasogastric tube

(2) Correction of the dehydration, alkalosis, and electrolyte abnormalities is a critical aspect of initial therapy (see Chap. 7, p. 196).

(3) Surgical correction should take place as soon as the metabolic abnormalities have been satisfactorily corrected, but certainly within 48 hr after diagnosis.

C. Blunt trauma to the abdomen can be a serious injury, yet may present with subtle symptoms and signs that may mimic other causes of abdominal pain. A careful history of trauma, from even seemingly minor events, should raise this possibility. Abdominal tenderness, particularly in the liver, pancreatic, or splenic area, abdominal bruises, or hematuria are also suggestive. A child with significant internal abdominal injury might present many hours or even days after the traumatic event.

1. Evaluation usually requires surgical consultation.

a. Initially, careful observation for deterioration of vital signs or increasing abdominal tenderness or distension is imperative.

b. Laboratory studies should include: CBC, prothrombin time, partial thromboplastin time, platelet count, and clot for type and crossmatch in case blood loss is significant or surgical intervention is required.

2. Initial therapy should be directed at maintaining adequate blood volume.

3. Surgical intervention may be required if ongoing blood loss is suspected.

D. Ectopic pregnancy has become an important diagnostic consideration in evaluating the acute abdomen in adolescent females.

  1. Etiology. An ectopic pregnancy is one in which the fertilized ovum is implanted at a site other than the endometrium; 98% of ectopic pregnancies occur in the fallopian tube.

  2. Diagnosis. Ectopic pregnancy in an adolescent may present as an abdominal catastrophe or, more subtly, with colicky pain and mild vaginal bleeding. Ectopic pregnancy must be considered in all children who have experienced menarche and present with abdominal pain.

  a. A catastrophic presentation demands a rapid yet careful evaluation.

  (1) The patient usually is in shock, with signs of peritoneal irritation, including tenderness and rigidity but rarely fever.

  (2) Intraperitoneal blood may be palpated as a doughy mass in the cul-de-sac.

  (3) Culdocentesis can be performed to confirm hemoperitoneum.

  (4) Laboratory tests should include preoperative studies and type and crossmatching for at least 4 units of blood.

  b. Nonacute presentation

  (1) Classically, this involves vaginal bleeding after a missed period, lower abdominal pain, and palpation of an adnexal mass.

  (2) Extreme sensitivity to cervical motion is an important finding.

  (3) Blood should be drawn for a CBC.

  (4) An elevated WBC and erythrocyte sedimentation rate may suggest an infectious cause.

  (5) The hematocrit should be followed.

  (6) A urinalysis should help rule out alternative diagnoses, including urinary tract infection and renal calculi. A urine pregnancy test is positive in only half of ectopic pregnancies. Serum human chorionic gonadotropin determinations are more reliable indicators of pregnancy.

  3. Therapy

  a. The catastrophic presentation, with the patient in shock, requires rapid stabilization and transfer to the operating room for definitive surgery.

  b. The differential diagnosis in a nonacute presentation may be difficult, and surgery is performed when there is a high index of suspicion of ectopic pregnancy based on procedures that may include culdocentesis, pelvic ultrasound, examination under anesthesia, and laparoscopy.

E. Pelvic inflammatory disease is an important cause of abdominal pain in female adolescents. Its clinical presentation may be similar to that of appendicitis, ectopic pregnancy, and menstrual cramps. For a discussion of evaluation and therapy, see Chap. 15, p. 399.

VII. Special problems in the emergency room

  A. Sudden infant death syndrome (SIDS) is the leading cause of death in infants between 1 week and 1 year of age. In the United States the incidence is 2–3 deaths/1000 live births. The mortality is similar in rural and urban areas. Although typical cases have been reported in infants under 1 week and over 1 year of age, the peak incidence is between 2–4 months.

  1. Clinical findings. Most cases of SIDS occur during sleep times. Typically, a well-cared for infant is placed in a crib at night and is found dead in the morning. In a study of over 400 infants, 74% died quietly during the early morning hours. In none of these infants was there an agonal outcry, and the dying event went unobserved in all. In this study, one-third of the deaths occurred while **another person was sleeping in the same room.** The quiet nature of the death has been further substantiated by reports of deaths that occurred in car seats while the infant was sleeping and a parent was driving. There have been some infants, however, who have been found in a corner of the crib or grasping blankets, which may indicate a silent terminal motor turmoil. This circumstance, when it has occurred, has not been helpful in determining the pathogenesis.

2. Epidemiology. Epidemiologic studies have provided some data on SIDS that are suggestive.

   a. There is a higher incidence of SIDS in the winter months. This observation is **independent of temperature** and holds true even for cities where there is little seasonal temperature variation.

   b. Although SIDS has a slightly higher incidence in the lower socioeconomic groups, victims come from all social classes.

   c. The incidence is higher in males than in females, and in low-birth-weight infants. Approximately 20% of the infants in two studies had a birth weight below 2,500 gm.

   d. It occurs in both breast-fed and bottle-fed infants, and victims who have been fed only breast milk have been recorded. The incidence is slightly higher in siblings, but there is no predictable genetic pattern.

   e. The least susceptible populations are Orientals (0.51/1,000 live births), followed by whites (1.32), then Mexican-Americans (1.74), and blacks (2.92). Most vulnerable are American Indians (5.93).

   f. Twins are more susceptible than nontwins (3.87/1,000 live births), and triplets are probably at greatest risk (8.33).

   g. In some American cities, a recent decrease in the incidence of SIDS has been seen.

3. Mechanism

   a. Almost all hypotheses proposed to explain the ultimate mechanism of death in SIDS have been disproved. Refuted theories include spinal hemorrhage, aspiration, hypogammaglobulinemia, and allergy to cow's milk. There has been insufficient evidence for rickets, renal dysfunction, tracheal collapse, enlarged thymus, bacterial sepsis, and overwhelming viremia. Studies on diving reflexes, cardiac arrhythmias, and vagal reflexes have been inconclusive. Hypotheses must sufficiently account for

   (1) The age and racial distribution

   (2) Predisposition to occur during sleeping hours

   (3) Incidence in the winter months

   (4) Lack of premonitory signs

   (5) Failure to find a cause of death on autopsy examination

   (6) The rapidity and apparent serenity of the death

   b. New findings have shifted attention from the immediate events of death toward a search for chronic abnormalities. If high-risk profiles can be developed, some deaths may be preventable.

   (1) Currently, most investigative interest is focused on apnea. In several studies of children with documented apnea who died suddenly, autopsies revealed no demonstrable cause of death. Since these initial studies, respiratory physiologists have published additional data about apnea and its possible relationship to SIDS.

   (2) Histologic evidence of the effect of chronic hypoxia has been demonstrated in some infants who have died of SIDS. It has been theorized that chronic underventilation of the lungs occurs during sleep, and many of the infants have chronic hypoxemia prior to death. Hypertrophied pulmonary arteries have been found among infants who have died of SIDS. The investigators considered this evidence of chronic hypoxemia and are now investigating other possible hypoxemic markers, such as extramedullary hematopoiesis, abnormal retention of periadrenal brown fat, abnormal proliferation of astroglial fibers in the brainstem, and postnatal growth slowdown.

   (3) Neonatal abnormalities have been cited that may suggest evidence of prenatal problems. These abnormalities include:

   (a) Feeding patterns

   (b) Temperature regulation

   (c) Motor tone

   (d) Underactivity

    (e) Abnormal cry

    (f) Breathlessness and periods of exhaustion during feeding

4. Reaction to sudden infant death

  a. Parents. The loss of a well-cared for, healthy child, who in the first year of life is the focus of family enthusiasm, evokes the most painful type of grief reaction. Parents turn inward and blame themselves for the death of their child. Typically, they recreate in their own minds the few hours before the death of their child to search for evidence that, in some way, they could have prevented the terminal event.

Although the immediate effect on parents is overpowering, the initial shock gives way to guilt, which often persists in spite of rational explanations. In the usual grief process, an early stage is internal bargaining. When sudden death is due to a known cause, the concrete character of the event can be incorporated into the normal rationalization of mourning. When, however, death is due to an unknown mechanism, as in SIDS, feelings of self-condemnation and inadequacy of parenting are reinforced. This type of death denies parents the prior mourning process that in other terminal illnesses may begin at the time of diagnosis. For young parents this loss may be their first experience with death of a family member. They may often suffer further remorse because of innuendos in the remarks of poorly informed relatives and friends that the parents are at fault.

  b. Surviving children are often the most neglected family members in cases of SIDS. Parents sometimes forget that children have both feelings and fantasies about death. Children may be excluded from the mourning by being separated from immediate family members, which effectively prohibits them from discussing the death.

Children under the age of 5 years view death as a temporary and reversible situation, akin to sleep or short absences. Children 5–10 years of age may look at death in terms of responsibility—something or someone was responsible. By the time most children are 10 years old they are able to understand that death is inevitable, irreversible, and final. Surviving older children appear to be able to resolve the problem of loss, and they do substantially better when they are included in the grief process. For this reason, parents are advised to be as honest as possible with their explanations and their own emotional reactions.

In the course of normal sibling rivalry, children might wish an infant brother or sister to die. Small children indulge in magical thinking, which entails the belief that one can cause events by wishing for them to occur. Or a child may have lightly touched the infant on the night of the death or taken away a blanket or bottle and, because of an immature understanding of death, may implicate himself or herself in the cause. For this reason, siblings need to be assured that the death was unrelated to their feelings or actions.

5. Role of the physician. The physician has the difficult responsibility of explaining SIDS to grieving parents and thus should have some understanding of how the death of a child affects parents. Without this understanding there is a risk of reinforcing the parents' preconceived notions and adding to their guilt feelings.

It should be emphasized that the parents were in no way responsible for the death, that SIDS is unrelated to suffocation, feedings, and sleeping position. In reviewing the few hours before the death, parents often search for minor omissions for which to blame themselves. These should be discussed patiently and gently refuted. Parents may also blame relatives or baby-sitters tending the child at the time of death. This also should be discussed openly. Parents need guidance in future family planning with surviving siblings.

In such circumstances, explaining a death requires compassion and, particularly, sensitivity, since any insinuation of parental neglect is distorted and misinterpreted. By such an approach the physician provides some comfort to parents who have lost their child suddenly and unexpectedly.

6. **Near-miss SIDS** refers to cases in which a significant apneic or terminal event is interrupted. The evaluation must document such an episode and rule out alternative diagnoses.

   a. In the history, evidence of underlying disease should be obtained and the severity and nature of the observed episode determined. Seizure activity, infection, inappropriate feeding mixture, choking or vomiting, recent trauma, and medication should all be included. All these conditions can result in a presentation similar to that of near-miss SIDS.

   b. The **physical examination** should ensure that the infant is in no imminent danger and should carefully identify the underlying disorders. Vital signs measurement and a respiratory and neurologic examination are mandatory.

   c. **Laboratory tests** should include a CBC with differential, electrolytes, calcium, BUN, creatinine, blood glucose (and Dextrostix), and urinalysis. Evidence of infection or a metabolic abnormality should be reviewed. Other tests should reflect specific concerns raised by the history or physical findings: an electroencephalogram, lumbar puncture, and radiologic studies to evaluate swallowing and gastroesophageal reflux (see Chap. 10, p. 282).

   d. **General management** includes a period of in-hospital observation and monitoring. If sepsis is suspected, antibiotics should be started pending negative cultures (see Chap. 15, p. 362). After initial management is decided, further evaluation, including pneumography, parental education and support, and arrangements for home monitoring when appropriate, should be coordinated with a medical center with an active program for near-miss SIDS infants.

B. Child abuse and neglect

1. **Objectives and problems**

   a. Recognition or suspicion of child abuse should be met by a long-range therapeutic plan, with attention to the establishment of supportive relationships. The goal of the initial process of management is protection of the child while the parents are helped through an acute family crisis.

   b. **Problems** include:

   (1) Parental personalities in which denial and projection serve as the principal modes of ego defense.

   (2) The family's anxious confusion in facing an array of clinical specialty services and social agencies, often working in an uncoordinated manner to protect the child.

   (3) The exigencies of poverty, including mistrust of community institutions, racism, unemployment, and drugs.

   (4) The clinical team may be frustrated by missed appointments, angry parental confrontations, time-consuming contacts with outside agencies, and conflicts among the responsible personnel stemming from the emotions brought forth by prolonged contact with disturbed families.

2. **Diagnosis**

   a. **Clinical findings.** Suspect child abuse or neglect whenever a child presents with **any one or a combination** of the following clinical findings:

   (1) Fractures that a simple fall would be unlikely to produce
      (a) Different stages of healing in multiple fractures
      (b) Metaphyseal fractures
      (c) Epiphyseal separations
      (d) Subperiosteal calcifications

   (2) Subdural hematomas

   (3) Multiple ecchymoses that may resemble purpura

   (4) Intestinal injuries, ruptured viscera

   (5) Burns of any kind, especially in infants

  (6) Poor hygiene
  (7) Inadequate gain in weight or height
  (8) Marked passivity and watchfulness; fearful expression
  (9) Bizarre accidents, multiple ingestions
  (10) Malnutrition
  (11) Developmental retardation
 b. **Some frequent behavior patterns of abusive or negligent parents.**
    They may:
    (1) Use severe punishments
    (2) Give a past history of abuse in their own upbringing
    (3) Display suspicion and antagonism toward others
    (4) Lead isolated lives
    (5) Make pleas for help in indirect ways, such as
        (a) Bringing the child to the clinician or emergency room for no
             specific reason or for repeated minor medical complaints
        (b) Insisting that the child be admitted to the hospital for a minor
             illness and expressing anxiety if he or she is not
    (6) Lean on their children for support, comfort, and reassurance
    (7) Sample a variety of health care facilities without establishing a
         relationship with any particular one
    (8) Display poor impulse control or an openly hostile attitude toward
         the child
    (9) Be unable to carry out consistent discipline, yet threaten or punish
         the child if he or she does not live up to an expectation or whim
    (10) Understand little about normal child development and seem unable
         to integrate the information offered about it.

3. Axioms of management
 a. Once child abuse or neglect is diagnosed, the child is at great risk of
    reinjury or continued neglect.
 b. Protection of the child must be a principal goal of initial intervention, but
    this protection must go hand in hand with a program to help the family
    through its crisis.
 c. Traditional social casework cannot in itself protect an abused or ne-
    glected child in a dangerous environment. Medical follow-up is also neces-
    sary, and day-to-day contact with a child care center may help
    significantly to encourage the child's healthy development.
 d. If the child is reinjured and medical attention is sought anew, the parents
    are likely to seek care in a facility other than that where the diagnosis
    was originally made or suspected.
 e. Public social service agencies in both urban and rural areas do not have
    sufficient well-trained personnel, and the quality of administration and
    supervision in these agencies often is not high. These factors militate
    against their operating effectively in isolation from other social agencies.
    Simply reporting a case to the public agency mandated to receive child
    abuse case reports may not be sufficient to protect an abused or neglected
    child or to help the family.
 f. Early attempts by the hospital staff to identify the agent of an injury or to
    determine if neglect was "intentional" may be ill advised. There is rarely
    a need to establish **precisely** who it was who injured or neglected a child
    and why. Clinical experience has shown that it is more important to
    establish confidence and trust in the hospital personnel. This may be
    jeopardized by overly aggressive attempts to ferret out the specific cir-
    cumstances of the injury. On the other hand, lack of evidence for parental
    "guilt" is not a criterion for discharge of the patient.
 g. If there is evidence that the child is at major risk, hospitalization to allow
    time for assessment of the home setting is appropriate. Children under
    the age of 3 are frequent victims; infants under 1 year of age with severe
    malnutrition or failure to thrive, fractures, burns, or bruises of any kind

are especially at risk of reinjury or neglect. Prompt and effective intervention is vital to ensure their survival.

4. Assessment of the child and family

   a. An adequate **medical history** and **physical examination** are necessary at the time the child is brought to the clinician. Photographs and a skeletal survey are made when indicated by the child's condition and the clinician's impression.

   b. If a social worker is available, he or she is called promptly at the time of the family's visit. The physician should introduce the social worker as someone interested and able to help them through this difficult period. After the interview, the physician and social worker should confer.

   c. Interviewing the parents

      (1) In the initial interviews and in subsequent contacts, **no direct or indirect attempt to draw out a confession from the parent is made.** Denial is a prominent ego defense in virtually all abusive parents. Their often bizarre stories of how their child was injured should not be taken as intentional falsifications. These odd accounts frequently indicate a parent's profound distress in acknowledging infliction of an injury or failure to protect a child. In the face of such a threatening reality, they repress it and may offer a blatant fabrication—which must be accepted for the moment.

      (2) One should not accuse the parent or he or she may use more primitive defenses than denial; i.e., a desperate resistance to talking about the problem at all, angry outbursts directed at the interviewer or hospital, and threats to take the child home immediately. This in turn may threaten information gathering and continuing helpful professional relationships and may endanger the child.

      (3) A good interview technique allows parent and child to maintain the integrity of ego and family. It is appropriate to emphasize the child's need for hospital care and protection from harm. At this time the clinician should demonstrate concern and the ability to help the **parents'** distress as well.

   d. In explaining the legal obligation to report the case, the clinician's compassion and honesty will go far to allay the family's anxiety.

   e. The opportunity to observe parent-child interaction and the child's physical and psychological milestones, which might lead to insight into the familial causes of a child's injury or neglect, may not be available to a clinician in an ambulatory setting.

C. Rape and sexual abuse of children are now recognized to be extremely common in the United States, with an estimated one out of four adolescent girls victimized before reaching adulthood. Less than half of these incidents are reported to medical and legal personnel (see also Chap. 12, p. 329).

   1. Definitions

      a. *Rape* is a legal conclusion defined by state law. Most states distinguish between statutory rape and common law rape, the latter being penetration without consent. *Rape* as a term is used to refer to a violent act initiated by an assailant in which a victim is subjected to sexual act(s) performed by force or the threat of force without the victim's consent.

      b. *Sexual abuse* refers to sexual activity involving a child that is inappropriate because of the child's age, level of development, or role within the family. Authority and power allow the perpetrator to coerce the child into compliance. Sexual abuse is more chronic than rape and usually involves an acquaintance or a relative of the child.

   2. Evaluation

      a. The **history** should gather information necessary to assess the need for protective care and support services and the nature of medical therapy. A review of the abuse may be traumatic for the child and family, who should be interviewed together and then separately if possible. Great care and sensitivity must be demonstrated, as with other forms of child abuse (see **B**). The assistance of an experienced social worker, rape counselor, or psychiatrist is helpful.

   b. Evaluation should include:

   (1) The time of the abuse and the circumstances surrounding it

   (2) Identification, when possible, of the perpetrator, to assess the risk involved should the child return home

   (3) The nature of the sexual contact—oral, rectal, penile, or vaginal

   (4) Vaginal discharge or perineal complaints

   (5) Nonspecific complaints that may reflect chronic abuse: abdominal pain, enuresis, encopresis, recent school problems.

   c. The **physical examination** is directed at careful observation and recording evidence of abuse, associated injuries, the presence of ongoing medical problems, and the emotional status of child (Table 3-7). In most cases of sexual abuse (especially chronic intrafamily abuse) there are no positive physical findings. Consequently, the likelihood of sexual abuse is best assessed by examining data from the history and psychological data as well as the results of the physical examination. The examination should be done gently and only after careful explanation to the child and the family. Consent forms and standard evidence collection procedures should be explained and utilized in all suspected cases. Some of these cases may well be prosecuted.

   A full pediatric examination is required. In addition, special attention should be paid to:

   (1) The general emotional state of the child (e.g., anxious, apathetic)

   (2) The presence of bruises, abrasions, lacerations, and other cutaneous lesions

   (3) The presence of significant trauma, including fractures and abdominal injuries

   (4) The external genitalia, which should be carefully examined for ecchymoses, edema, lacerations, and erythema

   (5) An internal vaginal examination must be performed whenever

       (a) A history of vaginal or rectal penetration by a penis, finger, or foreign object is elicited or suspected.

       (b) The history reveals symptoms relating to the vaginal or perineal area (e.g., discharge, dysuria).

       (c) Abnormalities (even minor) are observed on the external genital examination.

       (d) There are questions as to the veracity or completeness of the history regarding the nature and scope of abuse.

   Note. Rape is a crime of violence. More than 80% of rape victims suffer from associated injuries. Great care must be taken to rule out vaginal and internal trauma.

3. Therapy consists of management of acute medical conditions, venereal disease prophylaxis, pregnancy prophylaxis when appropriate, psychiatric support, social service management, and medical follow-up.

   a. The therapy of acute medical conditions should be directed by the history and physical findings. Abdominal and vaginal trauma are common in violent assaults.

   b. Venereal disease prophylaxis is recommended for all patients who have had contact with the assailant's genitals. It is often best administered PO, particularly in young children, in the hope of minimizing the pain and emotional upset (injections are often seen by the child as punitive) associated with the assault.

   (1) Oral prophylaxis. Amoxicillin, 50 mg/kg (maximum 3.0 gm) is given in 1 dose with probenicid, 25 mg/kg (maximum 1.0 gm). **Contraindications** to oral therapy are

       (a) Rectal or oral penetration, since oral medication is ineffective with pharyngeal or rectal gonorrhea.

Table 3-7. Collection of evidence during the rape examination

Study	Equipment	Procedure	Comments
Photograph clothing	Camera	Photograph patient in clothing worn during assault	Not required if not wearing same clothing or if there are psychological contraindications
Collect clothing	Paper bags	Place each article in separate bag	Use of plastic bags may alter evidence
Photograph cutaneous lesions	Camera	Photograph complete view of body and close-ups of sites of injury	Omit if psychological contraindications
Urine for urinalysis, pregnancy test, and toxic screen	Three collection cups	Routine	Urinalysis may reveal urologic injuries or inflammation; pregnancy must be ruled out at time of examination
Wood's light examination of skin	Wood's light	In darkened room, shine light over skin, scalp, and perineum	Fluorescent areas may indicate semen
Sample stains on skin	Saline, cotton swabs, collection tube	Moisten swab with saline, then rub skin; seal in tube	Will be examined for sperm and acid phosphatase
Comb pubic hair	Comb, envelope	Comb pubic hair with envelope or towel underneath	Will be examined for foreign hair
Trim pubic hair	Scissors, forceps, envelope	Trim any hair where suspected seminal fluid is found	Will be examined for sperm and acid phosphatase

Procedure	Equipment	Method	Notes
Aspiration of vaginal fluid	Vaginal speculum, aspiration pipette or eye dropper, collection tube	In adolescents, use water-lubricated speculum for vaginal trauma; in children, use a nasal or otic speculum to aspirate vaginal contents. Make two slides with cover slip, and empty remainder into tube	One slide is examined for motile sperm, the other is saved for laboratory review. The tube fluid is for sperm, blood group, acid phosphatase
Swab vaginal posterior fornix	Cotton swab, saline, collection tube	Moisten swab with saline, and wipe vaginal wall at posterior fornix; place in tube	Will be examined as for aspirated fluids
Vaginal washing	Saline, aspiration pipette, collection tube	Instill 5–10ml saline into vagina, aspirate, and handle as for aspiration of vaginal fluids	Avoid cervix during washings
Pap smear	Two slides, fixative, Pap smear curette	Routine	Sperm may be seen; for general health maintenance
Cervical and rectal gonorrhea culture	Cotton swabs, two Thayer-Martin plates	Routine	Important even for the youngest of children
Rectal washing	Saline, aspiration pipette, collection tube	Instill 5–10ml saline into rectum; aspirate, and handle as for vaginal fluids	Omit if anal penetration not suspected from history or physical examination
Blood sample	Two to four tubes, blood drawing equipment	VDRL, CBC	Required if infection or blood loss suspected
		Blood typing	Identification of patient's and foreign secretions
		Pregnancy test	Confirm urine test

(b) Uncertainty of follow-up VDRL determinations, as oral therapy does not adequately treat incubating syphilis.

(2) Intramuscular prophylaxis. Give procaine penicillin, 100,000 units/kg (maximum 4.8 million units), half in each buttock. Just before injection, give probenicid PO, 25 mg/kg (maximum 1 gm).

c. Pregnancy prophylaxis

(1) Indications. Pregnancy prophylaxis should be considered when the following conditions are met:

(a) There is documentation or strong suspicion that intercourse has occurred.

(b) The patient has experienced menarche and is not presently menstruating.

(c) The time of unprotected intercourse is less than 72 hrs prior to treatment.

(d) The patient would have an abortion if already pregnant from previous intercourse (because of the risk to the fetus of high-dose estrogens).

(2) Prophylaxis consists of **conjugated estrogens** (Premarin), 25 mg PO bid for 4 days. This regimen is almost universally associated with nausea and vomiting. Therefore, prochlorperazine, 5–10 mg PO, given 2 hr prior to estrogen, is usually helpful.

d. Psychiatric evaluation and support are essential, both for child and family. Victims of sexual abuse may suffer from deep emotional disturbances, even those who initially display seeming tranquility or aloofness. Rape counselors provide critical support, and many cities maintain excellent rape counseling services that should be utilized.

e. Social service evaluation is helpful in assessing the circumstances surrounding the abuse and the relative safety of the child if he or she returns home. As in other forms of child abuse, when the safety of the home is uncertain, admission to the hospital or alternative placement is indicated. Sexual abuse is considered a form of child abuse, and state reporting laws will thus apply.

f. Medical follow-up. While the follow-up care is multidisciplinary, it is usually most helpful when one health provider is identified to the child and family and has the responsibility for coordinating the various services and explaining the medical data to the child and family. Medical follow-up should be carefully arranged to encompass the following:

(1) Follow-up examination and assessment of healing injuries

(2) Check of cultures and other laboratory data

(3) Management of adverse effects of prophylactic therapy

(4) Emotional and social service support

D. Psychiatric emergencies

1. Acute psychosis encompasses a group of conditions in which there is a gross impairment in reality testing such that an individual incorrectly evaluates thoughts or perceptions. Direct evidence includes delusions or hallucinations or behavior so grossly disorganized that disturbed reality testing can be implied. Among other concerns are suicidal or homicidal intentions, medication or hospitalization, and social support services. The assistance of an experienced psychiatrist is usually required.

a. Etiology

(1) Nonorganic psychosis includes the schizophrenic, paranoid, and major affective disorders. Specific organic causes have not been identified.

(2) Organic psychosis includes metabolic, infectious, neoplastic, cardiovascular, and traumatic conditions, as well as drug ingestion (see Table 4-4).

b. Diagnosis

(1) An organic cause should be ruled out first. Clues to an organic cause include:

Table 3-8. Medications for the acutely agitated child

Drug	Under 12 years (mg)*	Over 12 years (mg)*
Chlorpromazine	10–25 IM	25–50 IM
Thioridazine	10–25 PO	25–50 PO
Haloperidol	0.5–1.0 PO	2–5 PO
Perphenazine (Trilafon)		4–8 PO

*Medication can be repeated after 1 hr if no improvement is seen.

- **(a)** Clouding of consciousness
- **(b)** Visual hallucination
- **(c)** An acute mental status change
- **(d)** A family history of nonorganic psychosis
- **(2)** A psychiatric evaluation is necessary to assess the nature and course of the disease.
- **c. Therapy**
  - **(1) Indications for hospitalization** include:
    - **(a)** Suicidal or homicidal ideation
    - **(b)** Confusion severe enough to impair daily self-care or family attempts to provide care
    - **(c)** When familial support or understanding of the patient's condition is judged inadequate
    - **(d)** When the cause or nature of psychosis remains unclear
  - **(2) Medication.** Emergency medication (Table 3-8) is indicated when aggression or agitation is severe and unresponsive to supportive reassurance. Ingestion of an anticholinergic agent should be ruled out before antipsychotic medication is administered that it may mimic psychotic agitation.
- **2. Suicide.** In the United States, suicide represents the third leading cause of death in adolescents. Females attempt suicide more commonly than males, but males' attempts are more often successful.
  - **a. Precipitating factors.** Suicide attempts are most commonly related to family problems, depression, school problems, relationship discord, and pregnancy.
  - **b. Evaluation. All suicide attempts should be taken seriously.** Although varying in intent and severity, all suicide attempts imply a significant breakdown of social communication and relationships. The following are relevant to the assessment of suicide risk:
    - **(1) Depression.** Severe guilt, hopelessness, and vegetative signs reflect a serious disturbance and an increased risk of subsequent suicidal behavior.
    - **(2) Previous thoughts, attempts, and careful planning of attempts** usually imply an increased risk of subsequent attempts and a greater requisite intervention.
    - **(3) Social and family dynamics** that precipitated the attempt and show little evidence of potential for rapid amelioration
    - **(4) Psychosis.** Suicidal attempts or ideation secondary to delusions or hallucinations are extremely serious and require hospitalization.
  - **c. Management**
    - **(1) Hospitalization** is indicated if the risk of suicide seems imminent, particularly if the conditions outlined in **b.(1)–(4)** are evident or suspected.
    - **(2) Home management** should be undertaken only after careful psychiatric evaluation and when a sustained follow-up plan can be assured.
      - **(a)** The crucial goal must be to modify the home environment sufficiently to make it tolerable for the child.

(b) Access to immediate telephone or other personal support or counseling can be an important way to defuse a situation that is potentially intolerable for the patient.

3. The violent patient

a. Acute and subacute violence. Aggression is common in children, and usually takes developmentally appropriate and controllable forms. However, occasionally the clinician is confronted by an acutely violent or threatening patient.

To prevent harm to the patient and others, rapid and purposeful control of the patient is imperative. There are generally two types of situations that require intervention.

(1) Acute. An actively combative, dangerous, violent patient whose cooperation is not obtainable

(2) Subacute. A severely agitated, threatening patient in whom violence appears imminent and whose cooperation is questionable

b. Management

(1) Verbal intervention may be useful in younger children in whom violent behavior is part of stereotyped tantrums or rage displays.

(2) Physical restraint should be instituted as quickly and humanely as possible.

(3) Medications should be used judiciously. In the actively violent patient, they should be prepared before the patient is restrained.

(a) Antipsychotics are useful to control agitation or combative behavior. They may enhance the effects of anticholinergic and narcotic agents and may produce hypotension, extrapyramidal reactions, tachycardia, and laryngospasm. **Chlorpromazine** ($10-15$ mg/M^2 q4–6h) can be used.

(b) Benzodiazepines are most effective given IV or PO to patients who are severely anxious rather than actively violent. Respiratory depression with large doses and enhancement of the depressant effects of alcohol, monoamine oxidase inhibitors, phenothiazines, tricyclic antidepressants, and barbiturates may occur. Give **diazepam**, 0.1 mg/kg IV or PO (maximum 10 mg).

(4) Continuing care involves appropriate psychiatric placement, social service, and psychiatric evaluation (see Chap. 21).

(5) Ethical considerations. It is **imperative** that the use of restraints or medication meet the needs of patients and not the needs of the treating facility. In addition, it is often difficult to determine which patients are violent because of primary psychiatric conditions or those who come to violence in response to oppressive social inequities. The potential for the "medicalization" of what are in fact social problems is significant. Strong efforts must be made to prevent the use of psychiatric or medical therapy to subvert the civil rights of patients or undermine the redress of social grievances.

Note: State laws regarding the medicating of patients against their wishes vary. Clinicians should be acquainted with local provisions.

E. Evaluation of a child under 2 years of age with fever. Elevated temperature in a child under 2 signifies the presence of a recognizable or localized febrile illness. However, silent (occult) bacterial illness, including pneumonia, meningitis, and bacteremia, may present with few clinical findings other than fever. The evaluation and management of these children remains controversial.

1. Etiology. The cause depends on age. Children under 3 months old are at risk of bacterial disease from gram-negative organisms and group B beta-hemolytic streptococci. In children age 3–24 months, blood and deep tissue invasion is primarily caused by *Streptococcus pneumoniae* (pneumococcus) and *H. influenzae* type B.

2. The history should include a review of nonspecific responses to infection, e.g., lethargy, poor feeding, and irritability. The onset and height of the fever should be documented. Other specific symptoms, such as cough, congestion, rash, limping, or swelling, will help identify the focus of infection. The medication history should be noted.

3. Physical examination

   a. General appearance. Lethargy, weak cry, poor posture, and decreased eye movements may be important indications of serious illness.

   b. Vital signs. The height of the temperature is related to the likelihood of deep tissue infection. The respiratory rate may reflect the presence of fever, but may also indicate pneumonia. Hypotension may reflect sepsis. The pulse is elevated in a fever, but persistent and extreme tachycardia or bradycardia signifies cardiovascular compromise.

4. Laboratory data

   a. The following are associated with a serious increased risk of bacterial infection:

   (1) An elevated white blood cell count ($\geq 15,000/m^3$), particularly with an elevated erythrocyte sedimentation rate (ESR) (≥ 30).

   (2) A differential count with band forms of $500/m^3$ or a neutrophil count of $10,000/m^3$.

   b. When the temperature shows a significant elevation (39.5°C rectal), no source is identified, and the white count and ESR are elevated, blood for culture should be drawn. In children under 3 months of age a rectal temperature of 39.5°C is reason enough for a blood culture.

   c. Obtain a urinalysis and a urine culture.

   d. If the count listed in **a.(1)** or **a.(2)** is present, a chest film is indicated irrespective of chest examination findings when high fever (39.5°C rectal) is present and no source is apparent.

   e. Lumbar puncture should be performed on all febrile children with meningeal or systemic signs of meningitis (see Meningitis, Chap. 15, p. 392). In infants, meningitis may not be appreciated on initial physical exam. A period of close observation of the child in a comfortable setting (e.g., parent's lap, waiting room) for evidence of irritability, lethargy, toxicity, and other subjective findings will help the clinician assess the need for lumbar puncture. The height of fever, elevation of the WBC, ESR, and band count, and findings during "optimal observation" should determine the need for lumbar puncture.

5. Therapy should be based on the specific illness identified (see Chap. 15, pp. 381ff). With high fever, elevated WBC, ESR, and band count, and **no apparent source** of localized infection (despite a chest x-ray and lumbar puncture when appropriate), a diagnosis of **possible bacteremia** may be entertained. Therapy remains controversial. For a discussion of this, see K. B. Roberts, *Manual of Clinical Problems in Pediatrics,* Little, Brown, 1979. Pp. 5–9.

F. Near-drowning can be divided into two general categories:

   1. Cold versus warm water drowning. Cold water near-drownings are associated with hypothermia, which protects against CNS hypoxic damage by decreasing CNS oxygen consumption. Warm water near-drownings are not associated with any protective mechanisms.

   2. Freshwater versus saltwater drownings

   a. Freshwater near-drowning with aspiration can cause surfactant washout resulting in atelectasis, intrapulmonary right-to-left shunting, and hypoxia; if a large amount of fresh water is aspirated, hypervolemia and water intoxication can also result.

   b. Saltwater near-drowning causes massive pulmonary edema, with intrapulmonary right-to-left shunting, and hypoxia. If a large volume of salt water is aspirated, hypovolemia, hemoconcentration, and hypernatremia can ocur.

   3. Evaluation of near-drowning victims

   a. A **precise history** of the event should be obtained, including:

   (1) The **type of water,** whether cold or warm, fresh or salt

   (2) Associated injuries

   (3) Estimation of the time submerged

(4) Clinical status when rescued. Note if there were any spontaneous respirations or heartbeat.

(5) Type of CPR required and when it was begun

b. A **complete physical examination** should be done, with particular attention given to the following:

    (1) Vital signs: Blood pressure, pulse, respirations, and temperature

    (2) Associated injuries

    (3) The cardiovascular, respiratory, and neurologic systems

c. Laboratory evaluation includes a general screen for hypoxic and hypotensive injury.

    (1) Blood studies: ABGs, electrolytes, blood sugar, calcium, CBC, prothrombin time, partial thromboplastin time, liver function tests. A toxic screen may also be indicated.

    (2) Chest x-ray and other radiographs as required to rule out associated injury

    (3) ECG

    (4) Urinalysis, with a flow chart showing the hourly output

4. Treatment

a. All patients who are victims of near-drowning should be admitted for observation. This includes patients who revive spontaneously at the site of the accident.

b. Initial therapy

    (1) Respiratory support may require CPR and management of the airway and ventilation, with a very low threshold for endotracheal intubation. In both freshwater and saltwater drowning, atelectasis and hypoxia are major problems, and the addition of positive end-expiratory pressure can decrease atelectasis and hence improve oxygenation.

    (2) Temperature resuscitation must begin immediately (see **G**).

c. Subsequent therapy. When initial CPR is successfully completed, the following treatment plan is started:

    (1) Cardiovascular support is given as required (see sec. **II**).

    (2) Recognition and treatment of increased ICP if it occurs (see sec. **V.B**).

    (3) The use of corticosteroids is controversial, but it appears that they do not cause any detrimental effects. The dose used is 1 mg/kg of **dexamethasone**/day in divided doses tid.

    (4) All associated injuries must be treated.

    (5) Antibiotics are used if there is any indication for their use, but blind treatment of all near-drownings with antibiotics is not indicated.

    (6) Early and intense social service intervention is necessary for the family of the victims.

G. Cold-related injury

1. Hypothermia

a. Definition. Hypothermia, or a core temperature less than 35°C, can result from any cold exposure, but in pediatrics is commonly an emergency situation in the near-drowning patient. Hypothermia causes marked depression of all organ systems, but is critical in the cardiovascular system in that it results in a marked decrease in cardiac output with a propensity for malignant arrhythmias. Atrial flutter and atrial fibrillation are noted above 30°C, followed by ventricular ectopy and fibrillation at less than 30°C, and asystole at approximately 26°C.

b. Evaluation

    (1) A **full history** is important, documenting the patient's symptoms, the duration and type of exposure, and any medical therapy that was attempted.

    (2) Physical examination

        (a) The general physical examination will show **profound peripheral vasoconstriction.** The patient should be examined closely for localized tissue damage (frostbite) (see **G.2**) and associated injuries.

(b) **Vital signs.** Temperature must be obtained rectally or by esophageal catheter with a special "cold" thermometer. **Oral and axillary temperature measurements are inadequate.**

(c) The **cardiovascular system** should be assessed for perfusion and any evidence of arrhythmias.

(d) The **neurologic examination** is important. The following guidelines may be helpful:

    (i) **Above 35°C.** Alert, conscious, shivering

    (ii) **35–30°C.** Clouded mentation, dilated pupils with lower temperatures, decreased shivering, atrial arrhythmia

    (iii) **Below 30°C.** Unconscious, diminished deep tendon reflexes, diminished respirations, and ventricular ectopy and fibrillation

    (iv) **26°C and below.** The patient appears dead. Respiration is barely detectable. The heart is in ventricular fibrillation, or the pulses are barely detectable; asystole may be present.

(3) **Laboratory studies.** The requirements for laboratory testing increase with the severity of the hypothermia.

(a) Acutely, ABGs should be obtained.

(b) Later, the following studies are important: electrolytes, BUN, creatinine, CBC, clotting variables, liver function, and a toxic screen if there is any question of a toxic ingestion.

(c) A chest x-ray should be obtained to ascertain if there was any aspiration during the acute event or resuscitation.

c. **Treatment**

(1) **Rewarming should be started immediately.** Various methods are available, but for patients with a temperature below 32°C, core rewarming is necessary. The **methods for rewarming** are as follows:

(a) **External rewarming** has the advantage of ease but the disadvantages of inefficiency and increased complications of afterdrop and rewarming shock.

    (i) **Passive external rewarming.** Remove all clothing, and place the patient in a warm room under warmed blankets. **This method should be used only if the core temperature is greater than 35°C.**

    (ii) **Active external rewarming** is accomplished by applying heat to the body surfaces: warming blankets, water baths (temperature 37–40°C), and hot water bottles over the femoral and axillary areas. **This method should not be used if the temperature is less than 32°C.**

(b) **Core rewarming.** These methods as a group are more effective and efficient than external rewarming methods. Specific methods include:

    (i) Heating all parenteral infusions in a blood warmer to 37–40°C

    (ii) Nasogastric lavage with warmed (38°C) saline

    (iii) Colonic irrigation with warmed (38°C) saline

    (iv) **Airway rewarming.** Inspired gases can be warmed to 42–46°C.

    (v) **Peritoneal dialysis.** The dialysate going into the patient should be warmed to 45°C. This may require bathing the dialysate bottles in a 54°C bath.

    (vi) Cardiac bypass when available

(2) **Cardiac resuscitation must accompany rewarming.** Routine CPR is started, noting the following:

(a) **A patient cannot be pronounced dead until he or she remains asystolic after rewarming to a core temperature of 30°C or the**

patient cannot be rewarmed to 30°C even with invasive measures.

   (b) If the patient presents with an effective cardiac rhythm, try to minimize manipulation. Stimulation can precipitate a malignant arrhythmia.

   (c) If the patient has asystole or ventricular fibrillation, continue CPR while rewarming.

      (i) **Medications** and **countershock** are very ineffective when the temperature is below 30°C.

      (ii) Avoid giving too much $NaHCO_3$; alkalosis can precipitate ventricular fibrillation in these patients. Therefore, ABGs must be monitored.

2. Frostbite and other cold injuries

  a. Etiology. Tissue damage from cold exposure is caused by vascular injury. Cold exposures can cause both

   (1) Freezing injuries (frostbite) that result from exposure to freezing temperatures that cause crystallization of the tissue water.

   (2) Nonfreezing injury (chilblain, immersion foot, trench foot). These usually occur after long exposure to temperatures above freezing, usually with very high humidity.

  b. Evaluation and diagnosis requires the following:

   (1) The **core temperature must be obtained,** and if hypothermia is present, rewarming should be started immediately (see **1**).

   (2) The **level of tissue damage** should be assessed by using the following classification system:

     (a) First-degree injury presents with hyperemia and edema and is quite painful.

     (b) Second-degree injury also presents with hyperemia, but has clear vesicle formation. It also is painful.

     (c) In **third-degree injury,** necrosis of the cutaneous tissue with dark vesicle formation develops.

     (d) Fourth-degree injury demonstrates complete necrosis and loss of tissue extending into and below the subcutaneous level. This is a painless lesion.

  c. Therapy. The goals of therapy are to stop the cold injury and minimize further tissue damage and loss.

   (1) The skin should be rewarmed by

     (a) Removal from the cold

     (b) Removal of any restrictive clothing

     (c) Topical ointments should be avoided.

     (d) The patient should not be allowed to smoke cigarettes or drink alcohol, in order to avoid any vascular reactivity.

     (e) If the area is still frozen when the patient presents (i.e., no sensation, white, hard, brittle skin), the involved skin should be warmed in a water bath of 40°C. **Warm only until the area is unfrozen. The water bath temperature should not exceed 42°C**

   (2) Local care should include only loose, dry dressings. The skin should **not** be rubbed; vesicles and blisters should **not** be broken.

   (3) Tetanus toxoid, 0.5 ml IM, is given unless the patient has received tetanus in the 10 years preceding the cold injury.

   (4) Pain medication may be required: morphine, 0.1 mg/kg/q4–6h is adequate.

   (5) Antibiotics should be given if there is any evidence of infection.

   (6) Physical therapy is required in the convalescent period if there is any tissue damage over a joint.

   (7) Amputation should be delayed until optimal healing has occurred; this may require 2–3 weeks.

H. Heat-related injury
  1. Burns
    a. Severe burn injuries require immediate management with a a team approach.
    b. Evaluation of the burn patient
      (1) The **history** must include:
        (a) The **type of heat** the patient was exposed to (e.g., an open flame, scald burn, electrical burn, explosion)
        (b) How or why the patient was exposed. Try to assess for inadequate supervision or evidence of child abuse.
        (c) Note if there is any **evidence of associated injuries.**
        (d) Assess for the possibility of an inhalation burn. Note if there was an explosion, or if the heat injury occurred inside a closed space. In both cases the possibility of pulmonary burns is increased.
      (2) The **physical examination** must be complete.
        (a) All clothing must be removed and the patient weighed.
        (b) Vital signs should be obtained quickly in order to guide appropriate resuscitation.
        (c) Immediately note if the patient is cyanotic or **shows evidence of an inhalation burn**—singed nasal hairs, pharyngeal edema, or stridor. If any of these is present, intubation should be performed before further physical assessment is completed.
        (d) The surface burn must be assessed for
          (i) Its **surface area.** Charts are available to help estimate the size of the involved area. In children over 12 years of age, the "rule of nines" can be used; in younger patients, burn charts must be used.
          (ii) The **depth of the burn** or level of tissue injury must be evaluated. **First-degree burns** involve the epithelium only. There is vasodilation and little edema. **Second-degree burns** involve destruction of the epithelium and part of the corium, with sparing of the dermal appendages. Capillary damage presents with blister formation. **Third-degree burns** cause destruction of the entire dermis with loss of sensation. Clinically, these burn areas appear white, with no blister formation.
          (iii) The **presence of circumferential burns must be noted** and **distal blood flow assessed.**
        (e) The remainder of the examination should be devoted to an evaluation of neurologic and cardiovascular status and a search for evidence of associated injuries.
      (3) The laboratory examination of the burn victim includes:
        (a) Blood studies: CBC, electrolytes, blood sugar, BUN, creatinine, calcium, prothrombin time, partial thromboplastin time, total protein, carboxyhemoglobin, and—if it is an electrical burn—a CPK
        (b) Chest x-ray
        (c) Urinalysis
        (d) Radiographs to rule out associated injuries
    c. Therapy. The general goals of therapy are to support the cardiovascular system in the face of massive volume loss, to maintain adequate ventilation and oxygenation, and to minimize tissue loss with local care and infection control.
      (1) Check the adequacy of the airway. If there is evidence of a pulmonary burn, the patient should be intubated. Increased ambient oxygen should be administered as required.

(2) Apply cold sterile saline soaks to the burn to stop any remaining thermal damage.

(3) Establish IV access. If the burn is extensive, a CVP line should be placed.

(4) Volume replacement should be started if there are second-degree or third-degree burns involving more than 10% of the body surface area (BSA). Volume replacement can be calculated as follows:

Volume replacement = %BSA burn $\times$ 2 ml/kg + 1,500 ml/M^2/24 hr

This volume is given as lactated Ringer's. One-half is given over the first 8 hr and the remainder over the next 16 hr. For this calculation 50% BSA is the maximum percentage that can be used. While calculations can serve as guidelines, the volume status should be assessed with hourly urine output and CVP measurements.

(5) A **Foley catheter** is placed to monitor urine output.

(6) Sedation is given for pain control: morphine, 0.1 mg/kg/q3–4h.

(7) Tetanus toxoid (0.5 ml IM) is given if the patient has not had a tetanus booster in the past 5 years.

(8) Antibiotic coverage is started. Penicillin, 200,000–400,000 units/kg in divided doses qid, or cephalothin (Keflin), 40–80 mg/kg/day in divided doses qid.

(9) Topical care. Silvadene cream can be used over the entire burn area. Silver nitrate can be used on all surface areas except the face and the hands because of staining of the skin. Sterile, bulky, dry dressings should then be applied.

(10) Early escharotomies and/or fasciotomies should be performed in all circumferential burns if there is any distal circulatory impairment.

d. **Electrical burns: approach and treatment**

(1) The patient should be **examined carefully for an entrance as well as an exit wound.**

(2) The patient should also be **examined for any associated injuries.**

(3) Laboratory evaluation includes CPK and urine for hemoglobin and myoglobin, and an ECG.

(4) A very common burn injury in pediatrics is an electrical burn to the mouth. These patients must be followed closely for a minimum of weeks because of the complications of hemorrhage at the site of the lesion. If the patient presents with active bleeding from the lip, apply pressure acutely. Surgical intervention is often required.

2. **Heat stroke** is a life-threatening syndrome.

a. **Characteristic triad in heat stroke**

(1) Severe CNS disturbances manifested by coma, seizures, headache, or confusion

(2) Hyperpyrexia, or a rectal temperature greater than 41°C

(3) Dry skin with no evidence of sweating

b. **Other clinical symptoms and findings** include:

(1) Tachycardia and hypotension

(2) Oliguria or anuria with acute tubular necrosis

(3) There can be acute changes in the hepatic function, reflected in a slight elevation of the liver function tests.

(4) Rhabdomyolysis, which can complicate and compound renal injury

c. **Evaluation**

(1) The **history** may reveal the following predisposing factors: alcoholism, obesity, heart disease, or fever. A careful history must include the duration of the temperature elevation, the therapeutic maneuver attempted at home, and a history of oral intake and urine output.

(2) The physical examination will reveal the findings enumerated in **2.a** and **b.** A flow sheet should be started to monitor the clinical course

(3) Laboratory evaluation
  (a) Blood studies: electrolytes, blood sugar, serum osmolarity, BUN, creatinine, liver function tests, prothrombin time, partial thromboplastin time, CBC, and CPK
  (b) Urinalysis, urine for myoglobin
d. Therapy
  (1) Cooling. The patient should be cooled by:
    (a) Removing **all clothing**
    (b) Placing the patient in **an ice bath** until the rectal temperature is less than 38.5°C
    (c) Phenothiazines can be given to decrease shivering (which is a heat-producing process), but **be aware that phenothiazines may cause hypotension.**
  (2) The **cardiovascular system** usually requires support with volume replacement; a CVP line is placed as required (see sec. **II**).
  (3) The **renal status** is monitored and an accurate record of the intake and output kept. The patient who is oliguric or anuric should be treated as any other patient with renal failure.
  (4) If **seizures** are present, the patient should receive a loading dose of phenytoin, 10 mg/kg IV, or phenobarbital, 10 mg/kg IV (see sec. **V.A.3.C**).
3. Heat "cramps" are muscle cramps secondary to an acute loss of electrolytes. Treatment includes cooling, and fluid and electrolyte replacement.
4. Heat exhaustion or prostration is a hypovolemic state that presents with progressive lassitude, headache, nausea and vomiting, tachycardia, and hypotension. Treatment includes volume resuscitation with close electrolyte monitoring.

VIII. Intensive care procedures
A. Intubation
1. Indications for tracheal intubation include:
  a. Airway management
  b. Pulmonary toilet
  c. Administration of CPAP (continuous positive airway pressure)
  d. Starting mechanical ventilation
2. Equipment required
  a. Respiratory equipment. Laryngoscopes and blades; positive pressure and anesthesia bags; appropriate-sized masks, oral airways, suctioning equipment, and endotracheal tubes. To estimate the correct endotracheal tube size, the following equation can be used

  ETT size = (16 + age in years) divided by 4
  For example: if a child is 4 years old:
  ETT size = (16 + 4)/4 = 20/4 = 5

  Always have one size larger and one size smaller immediately available.
  b. Medications. Atropine, methohexital (Brevital), succinylcholine, diazepam (Valium), morphine, cocaine, lidocaine (Xylocaine), Cetacaine
3. General instructions for an intubation
  a. Assemble all the necessary equipment.
  b. Pretreat the child with atropine, 0.03 mg/kg IV or IM, to avoid a vagally induced bradycardia.
  c. Hyperoxygenate the child with 100% oxygen by face mask. This will provide a larger margin of error if the intubation proves to be difficult and requires more time than anticipated.
  d. Positioning. The child's head should be in the midline; this position should be maintained by an assistant. Because the child's larynx is more anterior and cephalad than the adult's, head positioning is slightly different. The child should be put in the "sniffing position," which can be

accomplished by placing a small blanket, diaper, or towel under the occiput. Placing a roll under the shoulders may, in fact, obscure the airway.

e. **Laryngoscopy.** The laryngoscope is held in the left hand, while the mouth is opened with the right. The blade of the laryngoscope is placed in the right side of the mouth and advanced to the midline, sweeping the tongue to the left side of the mouth and out of the way. The larynx is then visualized. At this time, further positioning of the head, such as hyperextension, may help bring the larynx into better view. If suctioning is necessary, this is the time to do it.

f. **Intubation.** The endotracheal tube is brought in from the right side of the mouth and placed between the cords under direct visualization. The position of the tube is checked by listening for breath sounds. The tube is then secured into place.

g. **Sedation** and **restraints.** The pediatric patient will often make gallant attempts to remove the tube; therefore, every precaution should be made to protect the airway. This may require sedation (chloral hydrate, 30–50 mg/kg/q6h) or morphine (0.1 mg/kg/q2–4h) and restraints that can be applied as arm/elbow splints. The feet should also be secured.

4. **Sedation and relaxation techniques:**

   a. **Methohexital (Brevital)** and **succinylcholine.** The patient is given methohexital (1.0–1.5 mg/kg IV), after which the adequacy of the airway is assessed with bag-and-mask ventilation. If the airway can be maintained easily, succinylcholine (1 mg/kg IV) is given for muscle relaxation. When the child is fully relaxed, the intubation is completed. The following **limitations of this technique** must be considered:

      (1) **A muscle relaxant should only be given by a person who is competent with intubations,** usually an anesthesiologist.

      (2) **A child with an airway obstruction should not receive a muscle relaxant until an endotracheal tube is in place** (see below).

      (3) **A child with hypotension and any evidence of myocardial compromise should not receive a barbiturate** because it can cause further myocardial decompensation. This child can receive diazepam (Valium) instead of methohexital.

      (4) **Any child with an acute major denervation or burn injury should not receive succinylcholine.** In these conditions, succinylcholine may cause profound hyperkalemia. Children who have renal failure and difficulty with high serum potassium levels should not receive succinylcholine.

      (5) **Any child who has a full stomach should receive cricoid pressure to prevent aspiration before any relaxants are administered.** The cricoid pressure should be maintained until the endotracheal tube is in place.

   b. **Diazepam and narcotics.** Children can be treated with large doses of diazepam (0.5 mg/kg IV) and morphine (0.1–0.5 mg/kg IV) followed by oropharynx and nasopharynx spraying with lidocaine, Cetacaine, or cocaine. This method usually requires some patient cooperation.

   c. Children with obstructed airways can, as a rule, maintain their own airway better than the physician can with bag-and-mask ventilation. **Children with obstructions are most safely intubated in the operating room,** where immediate rigid bronchoscopy and tracheostomy are available. In the operating room, these children are given deep halothane anesthesia prior to the intubation.

   d. **Blind nasotracheal intubations.** In young children, blind nasotracheal intubation is exceedingly difficult but in the older child and adolescent, this technique is a possibility. The nasal-oral airway is sprayed with Cetacaine, lidocaine, or cocaine for local anesthesia. Then, with the child in a sitting position with the head forward, the tube is advanced in the usual manner for nasal intubation.

B. Ventilators
  1. **Definition of terms used in mechanical ventilation**
      a. **Controlled ventilation** is complete mechanical ventilation in which the patient does no spontaneous breathing.
      b. In **assisted ventilation** the patient initiates a breath that the ventilator completes. This is usually combined with an occasional mandatory breath. This mode is not routinely used in children under the age of 12 years because the ventilator does not have an adequate response time to their normally high respiratory rate.
      c. In **intermittent mandatory ventilation (IMV)** the patient receives breaths at a preset rate but can spontaneously generate his or her own respirations at any rate.
      d. In **continuous positive airway pressure (CPAP),** no preset breaths are given, and the patient breathes against a constant distending pressure.
  2. The **types of ventilators** available are outlined below and compared in Table 3-9. Ventilators are classified by the event that terminates ventilation in each machine.
      a. **Pressure-cycled ventilators.** Inspiration continues until the preset pressure is reached.
      b. **Time-cycled ventilator.** Inspiration continues for a preset time.
      c. **Volume-cycled ventilator.** Inspiration continues until the preset volume is delivered.
      In both time-cycled and volume-cycled ventilators, pressure limits can be set to avoid the problems of overdistension and barotrauma.
  3. **Indications for ventilation therapy.** Mechanical ventilation is used to treat or to prevent respiratory failure, indicated by hypoxia, hypercapnia, and respiratory acidosis. Specific clinical situations include:
      a. Apnea
      b. Fatigue from increased work of breathing caused by dynamic airway disease or parenchymal disease. In these cases it is important both to assist ventilation and to decrease or prevent atelectasis.
      c. Neuromuscular disease
      d. Skeletal problems producing restrictive lung disease or an unstable thorax
      e. Mechanical obstruction inhibiting diaphragmatic movement, e.g., massive abdominal distention
  4. **How to use the ventilator:**
      a. **CPAP** prevents or reverses small airway closure and alveolar collapse, decreasing the work of breathing as well as the oxygen requirement. The complications and limitations of CPAP include:
          (1) Overdistention of the alveoli and CO_2 retention.
          (2) Decreased systemic venous return, producing a decrease in the cardiac output. This effect is exaggerated if the patient is hypovolemic.
      b. **Mechanical ventilation** (IMV, assisted, controlled) is used when the patient cannot generate an adequate minute ventilation. Ventilator therapy must be tailored to accommodate each clinical situation.
          (1) If complete mechanical ventilation is the therapy selected, controlled ventilation or IMV at a rate of 15-25 breaths/min is required. In these situations, the patient will need heavy sedation and/or muscle relaxants in order to tolerate the ventilator.
          (2) If intermittent or assisted ventilation is selected, the mechanical rate is set and the patient allowed to generate as much spontaneous ventilation as possible.
          (3) **When a patient is started on mechanical ventilation, it is imperative to evaluate adequacy of oxygenation and ventilation with ABGs.**
C. Central venous pressure (CVP) monitors
  1. **Definition.** CVP lines are intrathoracic catheters used for the assessment of preload or intravascular volume status.

Table 3-9. Ventilators*

	Pressure cycled	Time cycled	Volume cycled
Examples	BIRD	Baby Bird, Healthdyne, Seachrist, Biomed, BP200	MAI, MAII, Emerson
Operation	Very portable, Pneumatically operated, No electrical requirement	Portability and electrical requirements vary with the specific ventilator	Not portable, requires electricity to operate
Modes	Assist or control Not for CPAP, IMV	CPAP, IMV, control Cannot assist	CPAP, IMV, assist, control
Physiology	Tidal volume will change drastically with a change in lung compliance or airway resistance	Tidal volume will change with compliance changes	In patients weighing over 10 kg, tidal volume is relatively stable despite changes in airway resistance and compliance. In smaller children the compressible volume of the tubing is relatively large in comparison with the set tidal volume, so that with changes in airway resistance or compliance, delivered tidal volume is not accurately predictable
Patients	Best used in short-term therapy in patients with normal lungs	Best used in patients weighing less than 10–15 kg; in larger patients it is difficult to maintain a high enough flow rate to deliver an adequate tidal volume	For the reasons enumerated above, best used in patients weighing more than 10 kg
How to start	Child is ventilated by hand with a manometer in line to predict the pressures necessary for adequate chest movement	The same maneuver as with the pressure-cycled ventilator	Tidal volume is estimated to be 15–20ml/kg, and a rate is selected between 10–20 cycles/min

*Whenever a patient is started on mechanical ventilation, it is imperative to evaluate the adequacy of oxygenation and ventilation with ABGs

2. Placement is indicated in
  a. Any situation in which a CVP measurement will help to guide therapy, i.e.,
   (1) Shock
   (2) Anuria or oliguria
   (3) During vasoactive drug therapy
   (4) During therapeutic osmotherapy
   (5) Congestive heart failure
   (6) Situations in which massive fluid shifts are anticipated, i.e. sepsis, burns, major trauma, surgery
  b. Any situation in which secure vascular access is necessary:
   (1) During cardiac arrest
   (2) During chemotherapy
   (3) For hyperalimentation
3. Required equipment includes:
  a. Sterile preparations. Betadine, alcohol, gloves, masks, sterile drapes
  b. Tourniquet, arm board
  c. Long angiocatheters or other catheter
  d. Cutdown tray
  e. Lidocaine 0.5%, without epinephrine
4. How to place the line
  a. Technical line placement is similar in the adult and pediatric patient; but the degree of difficulty is usually inversely related to the size of the patient.
  b. Access sites include:
   (1) The internal jugular vein is a preferred site, but access to this vein can be difficult in infants because of their short, squat necks.
   (2) The external jugular vein is another excellent access site, but it can be difficult to thread the catheter over the clavicle and into the chest. In this situation, a J wire used as a guide can be helpful.
   (3) The subclavian vein is easier to cannulate in the older child than in the infant.
   (4) The brachial vein is another preferred site. In an older child, percutaneous cannulation can be done, whereas a cutdown is often required in an infant.
   (5) Femoral veins offer fast cannulation approaches, but they are associated with a high risk of infection. These lines should not be used if there is any evidence of intraabdominal trauma.
   (6) The umbilical vein offers an easy access route in infants, but it can be difficult to thread the catheter through the liver and into the chest.
  c. All lines should be placed with sterile procedure.
  d. Before beginning the cannulation, estimate the length of catheter that will be required to reach the right atrium.
  e. Once the vein is entered, the catheter should be advanced until the tip is, ideally, in the right atrium, but any intrathoracic placement is acceptable. The position can be evaluated during the procedure by the transducer wave forms. A chest x-ray should be obtained to ascertain the specific location of the catheter.
  f. Once the line is placed, CVP is most accurately measured with an electrical transducer. A water column can be used, but the normal tachycardia of younger children tends to produce a falsely high CVP reading.
5. Complications of CVP placement include:
  a. Infection. The line should be handled with sterile procedure at all times.
  b. Air embolism can occur. The system should be closed to air at all times.
  c. Arrhythmias can occur if the catheter advances into the right ventricle. If a right ventricular tracing is present on the monitor, the line should be pulled back into the correct position.
  d. Pneumothorax or hemothorax can result from line placement. A chest

x-ray should be obtained immediately after line placement to determine whether this complication is present.

D. Swan-Ganz catheters (pulmonary artery lines)

1. **Definition.** The Swan-Ganz is a catheter specifically designed to provide the following information:
   a. CVP, which is obtained from the proximal port
   b. Pulmonary artery pressure, which is measured at the distal port
   c. Pulmonary capillary wedge pressure (PCWP), which is a reflection of the left atrial pressure, is measured at the distal port when the catheter is wedged with the distal balloon inflated.
   d. Cardiac output is obtained by thermodilution techniques. This measurement requires a thermodilution cardiac output computer. The cardiac index can then be calculated by dividing the cardiac output by the patient's surface area in meters squared.

2. **Indications for a Swan-Ganz insertion**
   a. For **cardiac output measurements** in patients suffering cardiogenic shock
   b. For the **measurement of right and left filling pressures** (intravascular volume assessment) in patients in whom right-sided filling pressure does not reflect the left side of the heart. These clinical conditions include:
      (1) Severe pulmonary disease
      (2) Cor pulmonale
      (3) Anatomic heart disease
      (4) Asymmetrical myocardial damage from a vascular or infectious insult.

3. **Equipment required for line placement** includes:
   a. A catheter and introducer of appropriate size
      (1) If the patient is less than 12 years old, a 5F catheter should be used.
      (2) If the patient is over 12 years of age, a 7F catheter is appropriate.
   b. Sterile drapes, gloves, masks, alcohol, and Betadine
   c. A 1-ml syringe for distal balloon inflation
   d. A two-channel pressure recorder
   e. A cardiac output computer
   f. Iced 5% D/W for thermodilution cardiac output

4. **Placement** can be performed on the ward, but occasionally requires fluoroscopy.
   a. Strict sterile procedure is essential.
   b. The catheter is preferably placed through the right internal jugular or the right basilic vein, but any central venous access is acceptable.
   c. During the insertion, the progress of the catheter can be assessed by fluoroscopy or by watching the pressure trace of the distal pulmonary artery port as the catheter is advanced from the right atrium to the right ventricle and eventually into the pulmonary artery, where it can be wedged. The balloon is inflated when the catheter is in the right ventricle. This allows the blood flow to direct the catheter into the pulmonary artery.
   d. When the catheter is in position, a chest x-ray should be obtained and the line securely taped into place.

5. **Complications**
   a. **Arrhythmias** can occur from ventricular irritation during insertion or from an indwelling catheter. These arrhythmias should be anticipated with a continuous ECG monitor during the entire time the pulmonary artery line is in place. Lidocaine should be at the bedside.
   b. The **catheter may permanently wedge** and cause distal ischemia; permanent wedge position can be diagnosed from the pressure tracing and can be remedied by withdrawing the catheter a small distance.
   c. The occurrence of **infection** can be minimized by maintaining sterile procedures and by line removal as soon as possible.

    d. Air embolism can occur. To prevent it, extreme care should be exercised during any infusions or boluses.

    e. Platelet consumption occurs in some patients. The **only way to treat this complication is to remove the catheter.**

    f. The **catheter can knot** on itself during placement, which makes removal difficult and increases the possibility of damaging the vessels.

    g. Vessel perforation can also occur. This complication can result in a critical loss of intravascular volume and/or a pneumothorax.

E. Arterial lines

  1. Definition. An arterial line is a direct cannulation of a peripheral artery for the purpose of ongoing pressure monitoring and/or frequent arterial blood sampling.

  2. Indications for placement

    a. Blood pressure monitoring for any clinical situation characterized by blood pressure lability, e.g., shock, any patient taking cardiotonic or vasoactive drugs

    b. Frequent ABG monitoring (e.g., respiratory failure, therapeutic hyperventilation)

    c. Vascular access for frequent **blood sampling**

  3. Equipment. The general equipment requirements are:

    a. Short Medicuts or angiocatheters (20- or 22-gauge)

    b. Sterile preparations. Betadine, alcohol, gloves

    c. Tape, arm board, tincture of benzoin

    d. A 10-ml syringe with a flush solution of heparinized saline (1 unit heparin/ml)

    e. Pressure monitoring equipment with high pressure tubing

  4. How to place the arterial line:

    a. Any of the peripheral arteries can be used, but preferred sites include

      (1) Use the **radial** artery only after the Allen test is performed to document good ulnar flow.

      (2) Posterior tibial or dorsalis pedis. Both these arteries can be used, but a modified Allen test must be performed to evaluate the adequacy of the artery not being used.

      (3) Temporal artery. The use of **this site is more controversial than the others because of possible ischemic complications.**

    b. The extremity should be securely taped to an arm or foot board. Be certain that the distal toes or fingers are visible, so that distal blood flow can be constantly evaluated.

    c. Cannulation should be performed with a sterile technique.

    d. Percutaneous cannulation or cutdown procedures are acceptable. If the temporal artery is selected, a vascular cutdown is usually easier because of the tortuous route of the temporal artery.

    e. After the line is placed, it should be secured with tape and tincture of benzoin. The patient should be under constant visual supervision while the line is in place.

    f. Normal saline with 1 unit of heparin/ml is infused at a rate of 1–2 ml/hr. This line is **not** a medication line.

  5. Complications of arterial lines

    a. The main complication is vascular compromise distal to the site of insertion, either from spasm or from thromboembolism. In an effort to minimize these complications:

      (1) If there is any evidence of vascular compromise, the line should be removed.

      (2) The line is used only for monitoring and blood sampling, **not** as a medication line.

    b. Massive blood loss can occur if the line becomes disconnected. To prevent this, all lines should be taped securely and kept under visual observation at all times.

    c. Infection, although uncommon, is possible.

F. ICP monitoring
1. **Monitoring devices.** ICP can be measured with one of the following moni toring systems:
    a. The **intraventricular catheter** is advanced through a burr hole into the ventricular system. The main advantage of this method is that CSF can be therapeutically drained, thus effecting a decompression of the ven tricular system.
    b. **Subarachnoid transducers** (Richmond screw, Becker bolt) are mounted on metal screw bolts that are placed through a burr hole into the sub arachnoid space.
    c. **Subdural transducers** (Ladd, Wilkinson) are pressure monitors placed in the subdural space.
2. **Indications and limitations of ICP monitoring devices.** The decision to mon itor the ICP invasively must be made by the primary physician in conjunc tion with the neurologist and the neurosurgeon. There are no absolute crite ria for ICP monitoring, but general groups of patients that **we** monitor include:
    a. **Head trauma** victims with a Glasgow Coma Scale score less than 6 (see Table 3-5).
    b. **Reye syndrome** patients demonstrating a Lovejoy stage three or less and/or a Glasgow Coma Scale score less than 6.
    c. **Patients who experience ischemic or hypoxic events that result in a score of less than 6.** A CT scan can sometimes be helpful in the decision of whether or not to place a monitoring device.
    d. The **technical limitations** of the monitoring devices include the following patient groups:
        (1) Patients with anatomic or surgically created fontanelles have a natural pressure release. Measured ICP is difficult to interpret in these patients.
        (2) Children under 9–12 months of age have very thin calvariums. Place ment of a subarachnoid bolt or screw is very difficult and can be dangerous.
3. **Equipment required**
    a. A neurosurgical drill for burr holes
    b. A catheter or pressure transducer and pressure tubing
    c. **Sterile preparations.** Betadine, alcohol, sterile sheets, gloves, and masks
    d. Lidocaine 1%
    e. Gentamicin is used as a catheter flush solution
4. **Placement should be done by a neurosurgeon under strict sterile pro cedure.**
5. The **complications** of invasive ICP monitoring include:
    a. **Infection** can occur but can be minimized if monitoring is maintained as a closed system and handled with sterile procedures at all times.
    b. **Local trauma** from hemorrhage and/or direct injury to brain tissue can result from the insertion of these monitors. The incidence of these compli cations can be decreased if all coagulopathies are corrected before the procedure is started.

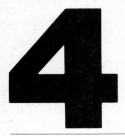

Poisoning

Ingestion of toxic products by children is a common occurrence. It is estimated that annually about 6,000,000 children will ingest a potentially toxic substance. Children under 5 years of age account for 80% of recorded cases of poison ingestion. Fortunately, the majority of these poisonings result in a low morbidity and mortality. Over-the-counter medications, household products, plants, and cosmetics are the toxic agents most frequently encountered in children less than 5 years old. Although an intoxication in a child less than 5 is the result of an accidental ingestion, in adolescents and young adults it is frequently the result of a suicide gesture or attempt. Prescription and nonprescription drugs are those most frequently involved in these cases.

I. **Emergency management**

A. **Identification of the poison.** Usually, the ingested material can be identified by a careful history.

1. The **initial history** should include the identification of the product ingested (containers or bottles should be brought to assist identification), the amount taken (a swallow for a 3-year-old child is approximately 5 ml; for a 10-year-old, 10 ml; and for an adolescent, 15 ml), the time of ingestion, and the child's present condition.

2. The physician should accept the **largest estimated amount** ingested in determining therapy.

3. **Physical examination** will often reveal supporting evidence for a particular ingestion. When the nature of the substance ingested is unknown, the list of common signs or symptoms presented in Table 4-1 may be useful.

4. The specific substance causing a poisoning should be confirmed by **qualitative** analysis performed on blood, urine, or a gastric specimen. When possible, a **quantitative** analysis should be performed on blood.

B. **Removal of the poison.** Removal **prior to** absorption and onset of symptoms is the primary aim. Enhancement of excretion and various methods of dialysis may be useful in more severe ingestions.

1. **Chemical methods. Ipecac syrup** and **apomorphine** are the most effective methods of gastric emptying.

   a. **Ipecac syrup** is now the method of choice because it induces emesis in 15–20 min in 85% of patients with 1 dose and in 30–40 min in 96% of patients with 2 doses. It removes approximately 40–50% of an ingested product when administered within 1 hr of ingestion. It is available without prescription and has a long shelf life, which allows for storage at home for emergency use. It is safe when taken in the recommended dosage.

      (1) For the child 1–10 years old, 15 ml (1 tbs) of ipecac syrup is given, followed by liberal quantities of clear fluid. If vomiting does not occur within 20 min, the same dose may be repeated once.

      (2) For the patient 10 years of age and older, 30 ml of ipecac syrup is given along with clear fluids. If vomiting does not occur in 20 min, the dose may be repeated once.

      (3) For children age 6–12 months, 10 ml is given once only, followed by clear fluids. **It should be administered under medical supervision.**

      (4) Ipecac is **contraindicated** in patients who have ingested caustic agents or hydrocarbons (relative contraindication) or in those who are comatose or having seizures.

Table 4-1. Common signs and symptoms of toxic exposures

Systems involved	Substances involved
Central nervous system	
Depression and coma	Sedative-hypnotics, narcotics, anticonvulsants, tranquilizers, tricyclic antidepressants, phenothiazines, antimuscarinic agents, hypoglycemic agents, alcohols, aromatic hydrocarbons, carbon monoxide, lead, mercury, lithium cyanide, gases, solvents
Stimulation and/or convulsions	Amphetamines, xanthines, sympathomimetic agents, psychotropic drugs (PCP, mescaline), cocaine, nicotine, salicylates, ergot, camphor, lead, strychnine, organophosphate and carbamate, chlorinated insecticides
Hallucinations	Psychotropic drugs, amphetamines, alcohol withdrawal, antihistamines, antimuscarinic agents, cocaine, camphor, tricyclic antidepressants
Hyperpyrexia	Salicylates, atropine
Cardiovascular system	
Arrhythmias	Digitalis, quinidine, tricyclic antidepressants
Tachycardia	Amphetamines and sympathomimetic agents, xanthines, cocaine, tricyclic antidepressants
Bradycardia	Beta blockers, cardioglycosides, quinidine
Hypotension	Narcotics, phenothiazines, antihypertensive agents, tricyclic antidepressants
Hypertension	Cocaine, amphetamines, psychotropic drugs
Gastrointestinal system	
Nausea, vomiting, and diarrhea	Almost any toxic substances can produce these signs or symptoms
Increased salivation	Organophosphate insecticides, mushrooms
Decreased salivation	Antimuscarinic agents, antihistamines
Respiratory system	
Hypoventilation	CNS depressant substances
Hyperventilation	Salicylates, cocaine, nicotine, carbon dioxide
Abnormal odors on breath:	
Alcohol	Alcohols, phenols, chloral hydrate
Acetone	Alcohol, acetone, lacquer
Wintergreen	Methyl salicylate
Garlic	Phosphorus and arsenic
Bitter almonds	Cyanide
Pears	Chloral hydrate
Others	Turpentine, camphor
Ocular system	
Mydriasis	Antimuscarinic agents, sympathomimetic agents, psychotropic drugs, cocaine, amphetamines
Miosis	Narcotics, organophosphate insecticides, parasympathomimetic drugs
Blurred vision	Antimuscarinic agents, alcohols
Colored vision	Digitalis, quinine
Scotomas	Quinine, salicylates
Red eye	Marihuana
Auditory system	
Tinnitus	Salicylates, streptomycin, ergot, quinines

Table 4-1 (continued)

Systems involved	Substances involved
Cutaneous system	
Cyanosis	Nitrites, nitrobenzene, aniline dyes
Jaundice	Carbon tetrachloride, benzene, aniline dyes, chromates, phenothiazines, quinacrine
Staining or coloring	Bismuth black; carbon monoxide and cyanide, pink blood; methemoglobinemia, brown blood; atropine, flushed face
Discoloration of gums	Lead, bismuth, arsenic
Alopecia	Thallium, radium, arsenic, hypervitaminosis A
Abnormal color of urine	
Dark green	Phenol, resorcinal
Yellow	Picric acid

    b. Apomorphine causes emesis in 100% of patients within 2–5 min of its use. However, the patient must come to the hospital or to the physician's office for its administration. The recommended dosage is 0.07 mg/kg/dose SQ. A respiratory depressant, its effect may be reversed with naloxone (Narcan), 0.01 mg/kg/dose IV.

  2. Mechanical methods. The use of blunt objects to induce emesis or lavage is less effective in emptying the stomach than are chemical emetics.

    a. The **disadvantages** of the use of lavage include emotional and physical trauma, ineffectiveness in removing tablets, and the delay involved in bringing the patient to the hospital.

    b. For the comatose patient, a cuffed lavage tube or prior intubation with a cuffed endotracheal tube followed by passage of a lavage tube may be indicated.

    c. Gastric lavage procedure

      (1) Equipment. Catheter, 8–12F, 4-oz Asepto syringe; lavage with 1/2 NS

      (2) For lavage, place the patient on the left side, with the head hanging over the table.

      (3) Cool the tube with ice. Use jelly to facilitate insertion.

      (4) Measure the distance to the stomach, and ensure entrance into the stomach by checking for bubbles under water or injecting air with auscultation over the stomach.

      (5) Aspirate the gastric contents prior to lavage.

      (6) Perform lavage until the return is clear.

      (7) Leave activated charcoal in the stomach on completion, or, if indicated, a specific antidote (e.g., Mucomyst).

      (8) Pinch the tube on removal to prevent aspiration.

  3. Enhanced excretion. Methods of enhancing excretion should be used only in serious poisoning, since they involve some risk. Most cases are handled conservatively, allowing the patient to excrete or metabolize the ingested drug. Only a small percentage will require the more radical forms of therapy that follow.

    a. Fluid diuresis enhances excretion by increasing the rate of glomerular filtration, so that the resorptive sites in the distal tubules have a shorter exposure to the ingested drug. Fluid diuresis will enhance excretion of drugs mainly excreted by the kidneys. A sustained diuresis of 2–3 times normal is recommended.

    b. Ionized diuresis is based on the principle that excretion is favored when a drug is maintained in its ionized state. Excretion of acidic compounds, such as salicylates and long-acting barbiturates, is enhanced by sustained **alkalinization** of the urine. The more acidic the ingested drug, the more effective is alkalinization in enhancing excretion.

c. **Osmotic diuresis** is based on the principle of an osmotic load preventing resorption of an ingested drug in the proximal tubules, Henle's loop, and the distal tubules.

    (1) A diuresis of 2–3 times the normal excretion is recommended.

    (2) Mannitol, 0.5 gm/kg/dose IV of a 25% solution q4–6h, may be used.

    (3) Close monitoring of serum and urinary electrolytes, body weight, and central venous pressure (CVP) is indicated.

    (4) **Contraindications** to the procedure are cardiac disease, oliguria or anuria, hypotension, and pulmonary edema.

d. **Diuretics.** An output 2–3 times normal in a child is sought. Furosemide (Lasix), 2 mg/kg/dose IM or IV, can be used. Urinary and blood electrolytes should be closely monitored.

4. **Dialysis.** Exchange transfusions, peritoneal dialysis, hemodialysis, and hemoperfusion are not part of the usual emergency management of poisoning. Their use is reserved for the most severe cases, with the decision based on the patient's ability to maintain adequate cardiorespiratory function, adequate urinary output, and the inherent toxicity of the ingested drug, but principally on the **effectiveness** of these methods in removing the toxic substances.

    a. **Hemodialysis** and **hemoperfusion** are the most effective techniques. Only substances with a small volume of distribution (<1 L/kg), low protein binding, a low molecular weight, and a low total body clearance will benefit from these methods (Table 4-2). However, only hemodialysis can correct a concomitant electrolyte or acid-base disturbance.

    b. **Peritoneal dialysis** is less effective and should be used only when hemodialysis or hemoperfusion can not be performed (see Chap. 8, pp. 216ff).

    c. **Exchange transfusion** is usually reserved for young children who cannot undergo hemodialysis or hemoperfusion (see Chap. 6, p. 157ff).

C. **Catharsis, dilution, and neutralization**

1. **Catharsis. Cathartics** may hasten transit through the GI tract, thus decreasing absorption of poisons not removed by emesis. Only ionic cathartics, such as magnesium sulfate (250 mg/kg) or magnesium citrate (5 ml/kg) should be used. Enemas may be used to remove overdoses given PR.

2. **Dilution** is a relatively ineffective method, its greatest benefit being its calming influence.

3. **Neutralization** of ingested bases with acids and ingested acids with bases **is no longer advised.** It is generally instituted too late to be effective, and the resultant exothermic reaction may cause secondary tissue damage.

D. **Supportive therapy.** While allowing normal renal and hepatic processes to rid the body of the ingested drug, the principles of supportive therapy must be observed. These principles include the following:

1. **Respiratory support.** Assure adequate respiratory exchange by clearing secretions, supplying sufficient O_2 and humidity, and turning the patient often to prevent pneumonia. Rarely, intubation and mechanical respiration will be required.

2. **Cardiac support.** Correction of shock and arrhythmias

3. **Fluid homeostasis.** Replacement of previous and ongoing losses, as well as correction of electrolyte derangements. In renal failure, dialysis may be needed.

4. **Hematologic.** Correction of hemolytic anemias with packed cell transfusions or whole blood transfusions for external losses of blood

5. **Central nervous system** involvement may require control of seizures with
    a. IV diazepam, phenytoin, or phenobarbital
    b. Supportive measures for prolonged coma
    c. Preventive measures against self-injury

6. **Antibiotic therapy** for bacterial superinfection. Prophylactic antibiotics are discouraged.

7. **General supportive measures** include the monitoring of vital signs, the avoidance of CNS stimulants, and the use of analgesics as indicated.

Table 4.2. Clinical usefulness of dialysis and hemoperfusion

Toxic agent	Peritoneal dialysis	Hemodialysis	Hemoperfusion
Acetaminophen	0	+ +	+ +
Amanita phalloides		+ +	+ +
Aminophylline	+	+ +	+ + +
Amphetamine	+	+	
Arsenic	+	+ +	
Atropine		0	
Barbiturates			
short- and inter-mediate-acting	+	+	+
long-acting	+ +	+ + +	+ + +
Camphor		+ +	
Chloral hydrate (TCE)		+ +	
Chlordiazepoxide		0	
Chloroquine	0	0	
Chlorpromazine	0	0	
Diazepam		0	0
Digoxin	0	0	0
Diphenhydramine			
Ethchlorovynol	0	+	+
Ethyl alcohol	+ +	+ + +	+ + +
Ethylene glycol	+ +	+ + +	
Fluoride	+	+ +	
Glutethimide	0	+	+
Heroin		+	
Iron (free)	0	0	0
Isoniazid	+	+ +	
Isopropyl alcohol	+ +	+ + +	
Lithium	+	+ +	
Meprobamate	+	+ +	+ +
Methaqualone	0	+	+
Methyl alcohol	+ +	+ + +	+ + +
Methyldopa	+	+ +	
Methyprylon	0	+	+
Monoamine oxidase inhibitors			
Paraldehyde			
Paraquat	+	+ +	+ +
Phenytoin	0	+	+
Primidone		+	
Propoxyphene	0	0	
Salicylates	+ +	+ + +	+ + +
Theophylline	+	+ +	+ + +
Tricyclic anti-depressants	0	0	0

Symbols: 0 = ineffective; + = not very effective; + + = moderately effective; + + + = highly effective; no symbol = effectiveness unknown.
Source: Adapted from L. Chicoine, et al. *Emergency Treatment of Poisoning.* Ministry of National Health and Welfare, Canada, 1982.

E. Antidotes
   1. Local antidotes
      a. Activated charcoal, an odorless, tasteless black powder, is the residue from the distillation of wood pulp. It forms a stable complex with the ingested toxin, thus preventing absorption.
         (1) It should not be given before ipecac syrup, since it will bind the syrup and make it ineffective. Its effectiveness depends on its small particle size and large surface area. It should be used for drugs against which it is known to be effective (Table 4-3). **It is not effective against metals, ethyl, isopropyl, and methyl alcohol, alkali, or acid.**
         (2) The dose is 1 gm/kg PO in 8 oz of water or with an ionic cathartic (see **C**). It may be given following induced emesis (1 hr after the last vomiting) or via the nasogastric tube after lavage.
      b. The universal antidote (a mixture of charcoal, magnesium hydroxide, and tannic acid) is **ineffective** and in fact is **hepatotoxic. It should not be used.**
   2. Specific antidotes. The number of ingestions for which there is a specific antidote are few. The following list includes the drugs or substances for which an antidote is available:
      a. Dimercaprol (British antilewisite [BAL]), for arsenic, bismuth, chromium, cobalt, copper, iron, lead, magnesium, radium, selenium, and uranium. The dose is 3–4 mg/kg/dose IM at intervals of 4–8 hr for 5 days and then 3 mg/kg/dose q12h (see sec. **III.D.**).
      b. Ethylenediaminetetraacetate (EDTA), for lead, iron, mercury, copper, nickel, zinc, cobalt, beryllium, and manganese. The dose is 50–75 mg/kg/day IM or IV in 2–3 divided doses for 5–7 days. Add procaine for IM use.
      c. Penicillamine, for lead, copper, and mercury. The dose is 25–50 mg/kg/day PO in divided doses. The maximum daily dose is 1 gm (see sec. **III**).
      d. Amyl or sodium nitrite and thiosulfate, for cyanide. The **dosage** is as follows: amyl or sodium nitrite, 0.33 ml/kg of a 3% solution IV at a rate of 2.5–5.0 ml/min, followed in 15 min by sodium thiosulfate, 1.65 ml/kg of a 25% solution IV at a rate of 2.5–5.0 ml/min.
      e. Naloxone hydrochloride (Narcan), for narcotics and propoxyphene. Give 0.01 mg/kg/dose IV. If there is no response after 2 min, give 0.03 mg/kg IV. Continue this therapy until a narcotic effect is no longer present.
      f. Vitamin K$_1$, for warfarin and bishydroxycoumarin. The dose is 2–5 mg/kg IM or IV.
      g. Deferoxamine, for iron. The dose is 50 mg/kg IM q4h (maximum 1 gm q4h). For severe intoxication, give IV at a rate **not to exceed** 15 mg/kg/hr. Do not exceed 6 gm in 24 hr.
      h. Ethanol, for methanol and ethylene glycol. The loading dose is 1 gm/kg IV (10% solution) or PO (50% solution), followed by 0.5 gm/kg q4h, to maintain the blood ethanol level between 100–150 mg/100 ml.
      i. Atropine sulfate and/or **pralidoxime chloride** (protopam), for organophosphate insecticides (cholinesterase inhibitors). The dose of atropine is 1–4 mg or 0.05 mg/kg IV, with repeat doses of 2 mg at intervals of 2–5 min to reverse muscarinic effects until full atropinization is achieved and then as necessary to maintain atropinization. The dose of pralidoxime is 10–25 mg/kg given slowly IV to reactivate phosphorylated acetylcholinesterase and repeated in 12 hr as needed.
      j. Methylene blue, for methemoglobinemia induced by nitrites, aniline dyes, chlorates, phenacetin, nitrobenzene, sulfonamides, and quinones. The dose of methylene blue is 1–2 mg/kg IV as a 1% solution and is repeated in 4 hr if needed.
      k. Chlorpromazine, for amphetamines. The dose is 1 mg/kg IM or IV q6h. Titrate subsequent doses to the clinical response.
      l. Diphenhydramine (Benadryl), for phenothiazine extrapyramidal reactions. The dose is 1–2 mg/kg IV q6h for 4 doses (maximum single dose is 50 mg IV).

Table 4-3. Drugs and chemicals adsorbed by activated charcoal

Analgesic and antiinflammatory agents
    Acetaminophen
    Aspirin
    Indomethacin
    Mefenamic acid
    Morphine
    Opium
    Propoxyphene
    Phenylbutazone

Anticonvulsants and hypnosedatives
    Barbiturates
    Carbamazepine
    Chlordiazepoxide
    Diazepam
    Glutethimide
    Ethchlorvynol
    Phenytoin
    Sodium valproate

Other drugs and chemicals
    Amphetamines
    Atropine
    Camphor
    Chlorpheniramine
    Cocaine
    Colchicine
    Digitalis glycosides
    Iodine
    Ipecac
    Mercuric chloride
    Methylene blue
    Muscarine
    N-Acetylcysteine (Mucomyst)
    Nicotine
    Oxalates
    Paraquat
    Parathion
    Penicillin
    Phenol
    Phenolphthalein
    Phenylpropanolamine
    Promazine
    Propantheline
    Quinine
    Strychnine
    Tetracycline
    Theophylline
    Tolbutamide
    Tricyclic antidepressants

Table 4-4. Common ingestions of low toxicity

No treatment required	Removal necessary if large amounts ingested
Ballpoint inks	Aftershave lotion
Bar soap	Body conditioners
Bathtub floating toys	Colognes
Battery (dry cell)	Deodorants
Bubble bath soap	Fabric softeners
Candles	Hair dyes
Chalk	Hair sprays
Clay (modeling)	Hair tonic
Crayons with A.P., C.P., or C.S. 130–46 designation	Indelible markers
Dehumidifying packets	Matches (more than 20 wooden matches or 2 books of paper matches)
Detergents (anionic)	Nodoz
Eye makeup	Oral contraceptives
Fishbowl additives	Perfumes
Golf balls	Suntan preparations
Hand lotion and cream	Toilet water
Ink (blue, black, red)	
Lipstick	
Newspaper	
Pencils (lead and coloring)	
Putty and Silly Putty	
Sachets	
Shampoo	
Shaving cream and shaving lotions	
Shoe polish (occasionally, aniline dyes are present)	
Striking surface materials of matchboxes	
Sweetening agents (saccharin, cyclamate)	
Teething rings	
Thermometers	
Toothpaste	

   m. Oxygen for carbon monoxide (100% O_2 for 30 min–4 hr)
   n. N-acetylcysteine, for acetaminophen. Give 140 mg/kg PO as a loading dose and then 70 mg/kg q4h for 17 doses.
   F. Prevention. No course of therapy, no matter how trivial the ingestion, is complete without a discussion about why the poisoning occurred and a review of ways to ensure that the incident will not be repeated. Recognition that the agent, an unpredictable child, and an emotionally or socially unstable milieu may play a part in poisoning is essential in such discussions.
II. Specific ingestions. Table 4-4 lists certain common substances of low toxicity that either require no treatment when ingested or require only emesis when ingested in large quantities. The specific ingestions listed in this section are chosen because their management remains complex and difficult.
   A. Caustics
      1. Etiology. The severity of the caustic burn is related to the concentration and duration of contact. Following ingestion, a **burn** ensues during the first week, **granulation tissue** during the second week, and **fibrosis** during the third week. Typical **acids** ingested are toilet-bowl cleaners, metal-cleaning fluids, and industrial bleaching products. Typical **alkalis** ingested are powerful detergents, toilet-bowl cleaners, and dishwasher and laundry granules.

Table 4-5. Petroleum products: Estimation of aspiration hazard versus systemic toxicity

Product	Source(s)	Systemic toxicity	Aspiration hazard*
Toluene, xylene, benzene, or ether	Industrial or rubber solvents	+ + +	+
Gasoline	Fuel	+	+ + +
Naphtha	Solvent, lighter fluid, dry cleaner, thinner	+	+ + +
Kerosene	Fuel, charcoal lighter fluid, thinner, pesticide solvent	+	+ + +
Mineral seal oil	Furniture polish	+	+ + +
Diesel oil	Fuel	+	+ +
Mineral oil		−	+
Lubricating oil	Motor oil, cutting oil, transmission fluid	−	−

+ = low risk; + + = moderate risk; + + + = high risk; − = no risk.
*Formulations with increased viscosity have decreased aspiration hazard.

2. Evaluation and diagnosis
    a. Pain in the mouth and retrosternal area may be experienced. **Oropharyngeal burns** may develop. **The absence of oral burns and symptoms is not sure evidence against esophageal involvement.** Other symptoms include nausea, vomiting, abdominal pain, and bloody diarrhea.
    b. Esophageal perforation with mediastinitis and **gastric perforation** with peritonitis may occur. **Aspiration** may lead to pulmonary necrosis or glottic edema. Bacterial **superinfection** may occur during the first and second weeks and **esophageal stricture** formation in later weeks.
    c. If a skilled surgeon is available, **esophagoscopy** is the best way to determine the presence and extent of esophageal injury. If not, a **barium swallow** can sometimes be informative of esophageal mucosal injury.

3. Treatment
    a. Emesis and lavage are contraindicated.
    b. Neutralization with acids or alkalis is contraindicated. The caustic should be washed off the esophagus with water or milk.
    c. If esophageal burns are present, **corticosteroids** should be begun within 48 hr (prednisone, 2 mg/kg/day) and continued for 3–4 weeks. A barium swallow is indicated following corticosteroid therapy to confirm the presence or absence of stricture formation; if present, subsequent dilations will be necessary.
    d. Liquids and soft foods may be given when the patient can swallow.
    e. Perforations, volume losses, and infection should be treated accordingly.
    f. Prophylactic antibiotics are not indicated.

B. Hydrocarbons
  1. Etiology
    a. Aromatic hydrocarbons (benzene, toluene, xylene, styrene) affect mainly the CNS and pulmonary systems. The liver, kidney, myocardium, and bone marrow may also be involved. Organ toxicity results from **absorption** (Table 4-5).
    b. Aliphatic hydrocarbons (gasoline, naphtha, kerosene, lighter fluid) produce mainly pulmonary damage. Pulmonary involvement is caused by

aspiration during ingestion or subsequent vomiting (see Table 4-5). CNS and myocardial involvement are primarily due to hypoxia.

2. **Evaluation**
   a. Ingestion of hydrocarbons may induce **mucous membrane irritation**, nausea, vomiting, diarrhea, and perianal excoriation.
   b. **Pulmonary involvement** may be subclinical or evidenced by coughing, dyspnea, cyanosis, and rales.
      (1) **Pneumatocele, pneumothorax, pleural effusion,** and **pneumonia** may complicate the pulmonary picture.
      (2) **Fever** and **leukocytosis** with pulmonary involvement are frequently present in the first 48 hr.
      (3) **Radiologic findings do not correlate with the clinical picture.**
   c. **CNS** manifestations include restlessness, confusion, drowsiness, and coma.

3. **Treatment**
   a. Removal of **aromatic hydrocarbons** is indicated if an amount greater than 1 ml/kg has been ingested.
   b. For **aliphatic hydrocarbons,** the danger from aspiration is greater than the risk from GI absorption. Removal is indicated only if large amounts (>5 ml/kg) have been ingested, or if a more toxic substance is ingested along with the hydrocarbon (metals, pesticides).
   c. In the **alert** patient, emesis with ipecac syrup is a safer method of removal than lavage. In the **obtunded** patient, protection of the lungs with a cuffed endotracheal tube and subsequent lavage constitute the therapy of choice.
   d. **The use of activated charcoal and olive oil may lead to spontaneous vomiting.**
   e. For pulmonary involvement, O_2, humidity, and bronchodilators may be necessary. Antibiotics should be reserved for superinfection.
   f. Present evidence does not support the use of corticosteroids.
   g. Infiltrates may take weeks to resolve fully.
   h. Management of CNS, liver, and renal involvement is supportive.
   i. Due to myocardial irritability, **sympathomimetic drugs should be avoided.**

C. **Iron**
1. **Etiology.** Because iron tablets and vitamins with iron are ubiquitous in homes, iron ingestion is common.
2. **Evaluation and diagnosis**
   a. Symptoms generally occur 30 min–2 hr following ingestion. Early symptoms include vomiting, bloody diarrhea, abdominal cramps, and drowsiness.
   b. After the initial phase (6–24 hr after ingestion), fever, metabolic acidosis, hepatic impairment, restlessness, convulsions, shock, and coma may appear.
   c. **Stricture** of the GI tract is an infrequent and late complication, occurring 3–4 weeks after ingestion.
   d. Initial laboratory studies should include a CBC, glucose, serum electrolytes, serum iron, total iron-binding capacity, and an x-ray film of the GI tract to detect the presence of radiopaque iron tablets.
3. **Treatment**
   a. Early **emesis** with ipecac syrup is indicated if 20 mg/kg or more of elemental iron has been taken.
      (1) A flat plate of the abdomen should be obtained after emesis, to see if all iron tablets have been removed.
      (2) Activated charcoal is not indicated.
      (3) Deferoxamine (5–10 gm in 50 ml H_2O) or sodium bicarbonate (50–100 ml of a 1% solution) by mouth may decrease absorption of iron.
   b. IV fluids, sodium bicarbonate, and volume expanders should be used to correct acidosis and fluid loss.

c. Deferoxamine
   (1) Chelation test
      (a) Indications include:
         (i) History of a large amount ingested, with symptoms other than minimal vomiting and diarrhea *or*
         (ii) Serum iron level exceeding the total iron-binding capacity *or*
         (iii) A symptomatic patient, with a WBC count greater than 15,000 or glycemia greater than 150 mg/100 ml.
      (b) Administration. Deforoxamine, 50 mg/kg (maximum 1 gm), is given IM. The urine turns burgundy red when the serum iron level exceeds the total iron binding capacity (TIBC) (serum iron >500 mg/100 ml).
   (2) Deferoxamine therapy
      (a) Indications include:
         (i) Coma or shock
         (ii) Serum iron level exceeding the total iron-binding capacity
         (iii) Positive provocative chelation
      (b) Administration
         (i) The parenteral route, whether IM or IV, will depend on the clinical state of the patient and the serum concentration. The IM dose is 50 mg/kg (maximum 1 gm) q4h.
         (ii) In case of coma, hypotension, or acidosis, the IV route should be used. Give 50 mg/kg over 4 hr by slow infusion at a rate not exceeding 15 mg/kg/hr.
         (iii) Cessation of therapy is dictated by improvement in the patient's clinical condition, a serum iron concentration within normal range, and the disappearance of the color in the urine.
   (3) Dialysis. Ferrous sulfate is not dialyzable except when bound to deferoxamine. Dialysis is indicated only in the presence of oliguria or anuria.
D. Salicylates are the most frequent drug encountered in poisoning in children less than 5 years of age.
   1. Etiology. Accidental ingestion or excess salicylate used at therapeutic doses
   2. Evaluation
      a. Salicylates produce an initial respiratory alkalosis due to hyperventilation secondary to central stimulation. The body compensates by excreting base via the kidneys. A state of metabolic acidosis, especially in young children, is quickly superimposed. Dehydration and worsening acidosis occur due to hyperventilation, renal solute loss, an increased metabolic rate, and vomiting. Presenting symptoms in the younger child generally include metabolic acidosis and respiratory alkalosis. The adolescent presents with respiratory alkalosis alone.
      b. The first symptoms seen in both alkalosis and acidosis are deep, rapid respiration, thirst, vomiting, and profuse sweating. In severe intoxication, confusion, delirium, coma, convulsions, circulatory collapse, and oliguria may ensue.
      c. Salicylates increase body metabolism, prolong prothrombin times, cause platelet dysfunction, and may induce either hyperglycemia or hypoglycemia. They are first excreted in the urine within ½ hr after ingestion, and peak serum levels occur 2 hr after ingestion. Of an ingested load of aspirin, 75% is excreted through the kidneys, and 25% is handled by oxidation.
      d. Initial laboratory studies include a CBC, electrolytes, blood gases, serum ketones, blood glucose, prothrombin time, serum salicylate level, and urine acetone, pH, protein, and ferric chloride.
   3. Diagnosis. Ingestion of 150 mg/kg will cause symptoms. A salicylate level of 50 mg/100 ml causes mild symptoms; 50–80 mg/100 ml produces symptoms of moderate severity; and 80–100 mg/100 ml produces severe symptoms. The

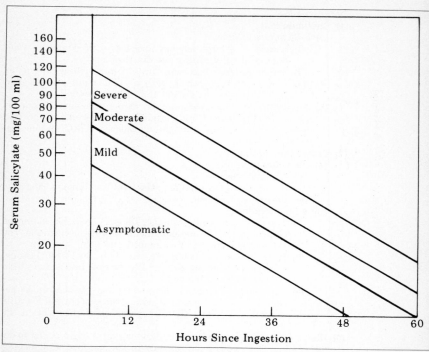

Fig. 4-1. Nomogram relating serum salicylate levels to expected clinical severity of intoxications following a single dose of salicylate. (From A. K. Done, *Pediatrics* 26:800, 1960. Copyright © 1960 by the American Academy of Pediatrics.)

nomogram in Fig. 4-1 will be of assistance in determining the expected severity of clinical illness following a single-dose ingestion of aspirin. A level of 50 mg/100 ml or any symptoms (except mild hyperventilation) generally indicate that hospitalization is necessary.

4. **Treatment**
   a. Induction of emesis with ipecac syrup is required when a toxic dose (greater than 150 mg/kg) has been ingested.
   b. IV fluids to replace fluid losses (see Chap. 7, pp. 197) and adequate glucose to correct hypoglycemia.
   c. Lowering of temperature elevation with tepid sponging.
   d. Vitamin K to combat bleeding due to hypoprothrombinemia.
   e. Alkalinization of the urine (2–3 mEq/kg of $NaHCO_3$ q4–6h) and monitoring of the urinary pH (keeping it above 7.5) will result in enhanced excretion of salicylates with serum half-lives being lowered from 24–36 to 6–8 hr. Generous amounts of potassium (3–5 mEq/kg/day) are necessary to replace potassium loss and *allow alkalinization of the urine.*
   f. Potentially fatal serum levels (100–150 mg/100 ml), oliguria or anuria, and cardiac disease are all indications for dialysis. A poor response to $NaHCO_3$, coma, and seizures are *relative* indications for dialysis.

E. **Acetaminophen**
   1. **Etiology.** At present, acetaminophen is used more than aspirin as an analgesic and antipyretic. It is consequently widely available in homes and is thus one of the drugs most frequently ingested by children and adolescents.

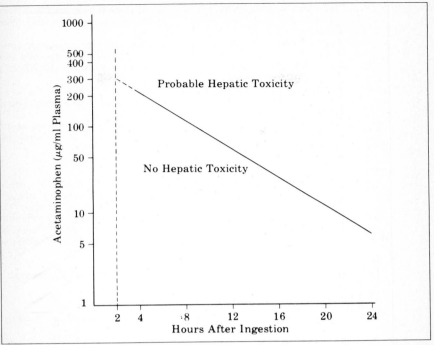

Fig. 4-2. Semilogarithmic plot of plasma acetaminophen concentration versus time based on data from adult patients. Patients with concentrations above the line at the corresponding times after ingestion may develop hepatotoxicity. Patients with concentrations below the line have a low probability of developing hepatotoxicity. (From B. H. Rumack and H. Mathews, *Pediatrics* 55:871, 1975. Copyright © 1975 by the American Academy of Pediatrics.)

2. **Evaluation**
   a. The major target organ of acetaminophen overdose is the liver.
   b. Signs and symptoms within the first 12–24 hr of ingestion include nausea, vomiting, and diaphoresis. Evidence of hepatotoxicity appears 24–36 hr after ingestion and includes hepatic enlargement with tenderness and jaundice, hyperbilirubinemia, hyperammonemia, and prolongation of the prothrombin time. Liver biopsy shows focal hepatocyte cytolysis and centrizonal necrosis. Serum transaminase activity peaks by 3–4 days following ingestion and returns to normal within a week in those who recover.
   c. Metabolites of acetaminophen, rather than the parent compound, are hepatotoxic. In overdose, normal metabolic pathways are saturated, and reactive intermediates are consequently formed that bind to liver macromolecules, causing liver necrosis.
   d. The consequences of acetaminophen ingestion cannot be anticipated from the initial nonspecific signs. Although the history is often unreliable, a single ingested dose of 3 gm in a 2- or 3-year-old (approximately 150 mg/kg) and a dose greater than 8 gm in the adolescent may result in hepatic damage.
   e. *An acetaminophen blood level drawn 4 hr following ingestion is the best predictor of subsequent hepatotoxicity.* When interpreted on the Rumack-Mathews nomogram (Fig. 4-2), a plasma concentration greater than 200

μg/ml at 4 hr or 50 μg/ml at 12 hr after ingestion is associated with liver damage. A half-life that exceeds 4 hr is indicative of possible liver damage.

    f. Acetaminophen overdose must be distinguished from Reye syndrome, amino acid disorders, and alpha$_1$-antitrypsin deficiency in the child and from drug abuse (alcohol, heroin, volatile hydrocarbons) and Wilson's disease in the adolescent.

  3. Treatment

    a. Removal of the ingested dose with ipecac syrup or gastric lavage when the patient is seen within 4 hr of ingestion.

    b. Activated charcoal will bind acetaminophen. **Its use should be deferred if N-acetylcysteine (Mucomyst) is to be used,** since it will bind the antidote, thereby reducing its effectiveness.

    c. Avoid enzyme inducers such as phenobarbital and alcohol.

    d. Avoid forcing fluids or ionized diuresis.

    e. When acetaminophen has been taken in high doses, or when acetaminophen levels are in the range likely to cause hepatotoxicity, N-acetylcysteine should be administered. The loading dose is 140 mg/kg PO. Maintenance doses of 70 mg/kg q4h should be administered thereafter for 17 doses. N-acetylcysteine should be diluted to a 5% solution before it is administered and repeated if vomiting occurs within 1 hr of administration.

F. Theophylline

  1. Etiology. Theophylline is a xanthine bronchodilator widely used in the treatment of obstructive lung disease.

  2. Evaluation

    a. Signs and symptoms

      (1) Gastrointestinal symptoms are the most frequent and include nausea, vomiting, and hematemesis.

      (2) CNS toxicity includes agitation, restlessness, irritability, or mild obtundation. **Seizures** may occur in severe poisonings.

      (3) Mild supraventricular tachycardia is frequent, but life-threatening arrhythmias are less frequent than in adults.

    b. Therapeutic serum concentrations range between 10–20 μg/ml. The severity of the toxicity increases with increasing serum concentrations. Life-threatening arrhythmias and seizures usually occur with serum concentrations greater than 80–100 μg/ml after acute overdose.

    c. Prolonged absorption may occur after an overdose, especially with slow-release preparations.

  3. Treatment

    a. Remove theophylline by inducing emesis with ipecac syrup or, if necessary, by gastric lavage.

    b. Activated charcoal and ionic cathartics are indicated (see secs. **I.C** and **E**).

    c. Theophylline serum concentrations should be obtained and followed q4h to evaluate the effectiveness of treatment.

    d. Do not induce fluid diuresis.

    e. Diazepam, phenytoin, and/or phenobarbital should be used in the treatment of seizures (see Chap. 3, pp. 58ff).

    f. Monitor for cardiac arrhythmias.

    g. Hemodialysis or hemoperfusion should be considered in patients unresponsive to adequate supportive care and/or serum concentration above 80–100 μg/ml.

G. Tricyclic antidepressants

  1. Etiology. These drugs are widely prescribed for mood disorders. Overdoses are frequently intentional. Other drugs may be ingested concomitantly.

  2. Evaluation

    a. Signs or symptoms usually develop within 4 hr of ingestion. Anticholinergic signs—**mydriasis, dry mucous membranes, tachycardia, decreased peristalsis**—are usually the first to appear.

    b. Confusion, agitation, and hallucinations or various stages of coma may be present. Seizures may also occur.

    c. Sinus tachycardia is present in virtually every intoxication, but serious cardiac arrhythmias occur in patients with serum concentrations greater than 1000 ng/ml and/or a prolongation of the QRS complex greater than 100 msec. Ventricular arrhythmias, conduction blocks, and hypotension may occur.

  3. Treatment

    a. Gastric emptying by induced emesis or gastric lavage is indicated.

    b. Activated charcoal and ionic cathartics should be administered and repeated q4–6h for 24 hr in severe intoxication.

    c. Fluid diuresis, dialysis, or hemoperfusion are **ineffective.**

    d. Seizures should be treated with diazepam, followed if necessary by phenytoin or phenobarbital (see Chap. 20, p. 504).

    e. Cardiac arrhythmias should be treated with appropriate agents (see Table 9-1).

    f. Hypotension should be treated with fluid followed by vasopressors (dopamine or dobutamine) if necessary.

    g. Physostigmine, 0.5 mg in children, 1 mg in adolescents, given slowly IV, should be reserved for the treatment of severe agitation or hallucination or refractory seizures or arrhythmias.

    h. Continuous cardiac monitoring may be ended when the patient has been completely asymptomatic and the ECG normal for 24 hr.

H. Substances of abuse

  1. Etiology. Drugs and chemicals abused by adolescents and young adults depend on age, sex, race, socioeconomic group, and geographic location.

  2. CNS depressants include narcotics, hypnotic-sedative agents (barbiturates and nonbarbiturates), benzodiazepines (e.g., diazepam, chlordiazepoxide), and alcohols.

    a. Evaluation

      (1) Following an acute overdose, all induce CNS depression (see Table 3-5) and cardiorespiratory depression as well.

      (2) Pupils are usually small, or constricted in the case of narcotics.

      (3) Reflexes are diminished. Seizures are more frequent with propoxyphene, meperidine, and methaqualone.

      (4) In ethanol intoxication there is a correlation between ethanol serum concentration and CNS effects:

        (a) Blood concentrations above 100–150 mg/100 ml: ataxia and incoordination

        (b) Blood concentrations 150–300 mg/100 ml: dysarthria, visual disturbances, and somnolence

        (c) Blood concentrations 300–500 mg/100 ml: coma

        (d) Above 500 mg/100 ml: potentially lethal

      (5) Hypoglycemia is associated with alcohol intoxication in young children.

      (6) All these substances can produce physical and psychological dependence. Withdrawal symptoms can be expected with their abrupt cessation. However, severe manifestations, such as **seizures, delirium, cardiovascular collapse** and **possibly death,** are seen only in the case of alcohol and barbiturate withdrawal.

    b. Therapy

      (1) If the patient is comatose, administer naloxone, 0.01 mg/kg IV. If there is no response within 1 min, administer 0.03 mg/kg IV. If there is still no response, narcotic overdose is **ruled out.** If naloxone is successful in reducing coma, continue to administer it as needed.

      (2) Gastrointestinal decontamination should be instituted (see sec. I). Adequate supportive care (e.g., of respiration, circulation) should be provided.

       (3) Hemodialysis should be considered for patients with severe ethanol intoxication unresponsive to adequate supportive care and/or with serum ethanol concentrations above 500 mg/100 ml.

3. CNS stimulants include amphetamines and amphetaminelike drugs, caffeine, and cocaine.

    a. Evaluation

       (1) Increased CNS excitation may culminate in seizures.

       (2) Pulse rate and blood pressure are increased.

       (3) The pupils are dilated and the reflexes hyperactive.

       (4) These substances can induce psychological and physical dependence. The withdrawal syndrome is characterized by lack of energy, prolonged periods of sleep, increased appetite, and psychological depression.

    b. Therapy

       (1) Following acute intoxication, GI decontamination measures (see sec. I) should be instituted.

       (2) Hypertension is usually of short duration and rarely necessitates treatment. If necessary, phentolamine may be used.

       (3) Amphetamine psychotic reaction may be treated with chlorpromazine or haloperidol. Diazepam is the drug of choice for the treatment of **hyperactivity** and **seizures.**

       (4) Acidification of the urine with ammonium chloride and ascorbic acid can enhance amphetamine elimination.

4. Substances modifying CNS perception include the hallucinogens phencyclidine, lysergic acid diethylamide, and mescaline; the cannabis group including marihuana and hashish; and volatile inhalants, namely, butyl nitrites and hydrocarbon (sniffing).

    a. Evaluation

       (1) Hallucinogens induce euphoria, anxiety, or panic. The affect is inappropriate; the patient experiences time and visual distortion and visual hallucinations.

       (2) PCP overdose produces extreme hyperactivity or cyclic coma, nystagmus, muscle rigidity, seizures, and hypertension. The pupils are small. Flashbacks may occur.

       (3) The cannabis group usually induces a state of euphoria and feeling of well-being. Hallucinations are rare. The pupils are unchanged but the conjunctivae are injected.

       (4) Transient euphoria can be experienced by volatile inhalant users. Cardiac arrhythmias are the major acute complication. Lead intoxication can occur with gasoline sniffing. Butyl nitrite can produce methemoglobinemia.

       (5) Physical dependence on substances modifying CNS perception does not develop. Psychological dependence is possible. No withdrawal syndrome is seen.

    b. Therapy

       (1) The patient presenting with hallucinations or distorted perceptions should be provided a quiet and safe environment.

       (2) Physical or chemical restraints should be avoided. If necessary, diazepam may be used (0.03 mg/kg PO or IV [maximum 10–20 mg]).

       (3) GI decontamination measures should be reserved for the severely intoxicated patient (i.e., comatose patient).

       (4) Acidification of the urine may enhance PCP elimination.

III. Lead poisoning

  A. Etiology. Lead poisoning in childhood results mainly from the ingestion of lead-based paint or plaster or other materials or objects saturated or coated with lead-based paint (lead content > 0.06%) and from ingesting lead-containing soil and household dust. Airborne lead contributes to increased lead absorption by ingestion of fallout on soil or dust rather than by inhalation.

Recent studies indicate that blacks have a greater incidence of lead poisoning than whites, irrespective of socioeconomic status, but the reason is obscure. Malnutrition enhances lead toxicity. The National Health and Nutrition Examination Survey II data (1976–1980) indicate that 4% of all American children under age 6 have elevated lead levels (2% of whites; 12% of blacks). The incidence is highest among the urban poor, but cases can be readily found among suburban, middle-class children. Predisposing factors include iron, calcium and zinc deficiency, conditions of poor housing, low socioeconomic status, and pica.

B. Evaluation

    1. The **history** should emphasize the location, age, and condition of the home or other frequented areas. Although common, the presence of pica is not a sine qua non in lead poisoning. Questions should be asked about the child's appetite, bowel habits, general behavior, and nutrition, as well as about signs of irritability and lethargy.

    2. A **complete physical examination** should include a thorough neurologic examination and, if possible, a developmental assessment and psychometric examination.

    3. **Laboratory studies**

        a. Blood lead levels should be determined by **venous samples** whenever possible, to avoid the problem of skin contamination by lead-laden soil. If a fingerstick sample is used, the finger should be carefully washed and rinsed.

        b. Erythrocyte protoporphyrin (EP) is widely accepted as reflecting lead toxicity. Since the interpretation of values is complicated by the effect of iron deficiency on EP, **absolute criteria for lead poisoning are difficult to establish.** Normal mean EP levels are $\cong 20$ μg/100 ml of whole blood. Up to 35 μg/100 ml of whole blood is considered acceptable. In the presence of iron deficiency, EP values of 50–125 μg/100 ml of whole blood are common. **However, levels of this kind can be due to moderate lead poisoning as well.** In general, values of EP above 100 μg/100 ml of whole blood usually reflect an effect of lead exposure. Rare exceptions occur, including erythrocytic protoporphyria.

        Because 1–3 weeks of lead exposure is required to elevate protoporphyrin levels, it is possible for lead levels to be elevated in the presence of normal EP.

        For a complete discussion, see the Centers for Disease Control's pamphlet, *Preventing Lead Poisoning in Young Children.*

        c. **Other blood tests.** Blood tests in any child with elevated blood lead, EP, or both should include a CBC, with attention to basophilic stippling of the erythrocyte, iron and iron-binding capacity, serum ferritin, BUN, and serum creatinine. Even in the **absence** of clinical anemia, elevated levels of EP can be due to lead, iron deficiency, or both. Similarly, because EP reflects events at the cellular level, serum iron and iron-binding capacity can be normal when EP is not.

        d. **X-ray films** of the knees are helpful in detecting widening and increased density of the zones of provisional calcification in the distal femur, proximal tibia, and proximal fibula (chronic ingestion). Anteroposterior views of the abdomen should be obtained for radiopacities (acute ingestion). Knee films in children 18–30 months of age should be interpreted cautiously, since a wide range of normal changes during rapid growth can mimic "lead lines." However, when widening and increased density of the zone of provisional calcification include the proximal fibulas as well as the proximal tibia and distal femur, the likelihood is increased that chronic exposure to a heavy metal, most probably lead, is responsible for the findings.

        e. *If encephalopathy is suspected, a CT scan of the skull should be obtained immediately to evaluate the possibility of cerebral edema.*

        f. **Lumbar puncture is contraindicated** unless it is certain that cerebrospinal fluid (CSF) pressure is not increased. Lumbar puncture adds little to the evaluation, and the findings do not affect therapy.

g. Lead mobilization test (provocative chelation)

(1) **Indications.** In children with only moderate elevations of blood lead in whom the results of the preceding tests are conflicting or who have already undergone chelation therapy, the lead mobilization test can clarify the size of the **mobilizable** pool of lead. Since this pool has been correlated with indicators of toxicity, a positive lead mobilization test should be considered an indication for therapy.

(2) **Procedure.** 500–1000 mg/M^2/24 h of calcium disodium EDTA is administered IM or by IV drip. The dose may be divided or given in toto in a single dose. Urine is collected quantitatively for up to 24 hr. The test is positive if the 24-hr collection yields more than 1 μg of lead/mg of EDTA injected.

Alternatively, on an outpatient basis, a shorter urine collection (6–8 hr) may be used, with a concomitant reduction in the yield of lead. In this case the dose of EDTA is given in toto at the beginning of collection. Because the large bulk of lead is excreted within 6–12 hr following the EDTA dose, an excretion of ≥ 0.6 μg of lead/mg of EDTA injected is considered positive. Under some conditions, a smaller "yield" could still be considered an indication for chelation therapy, particularly in a very young child or in a child with lingering elevated lead levels.

Note that determinations of the urinary **concentration** of lead are **not** helpful. It is the **absolute** excretion of lead per time interval per chelation dose that is measured, requiring quantitative urine collections and good hydration during the test, which is no mean feat in the toddler who is not yet toilet trained.

Indications for the lead mobilization test are as follows:

(a) Venous blood lead ≥ 25–49 μg/100 ml and EP ≥ 35 μg/100 ml.

(b) To assess need for further chelation in patient under therapy.

h. Nerve conduction times may be abnormal in chronic lead poisoning, reflecting segmental demyelination. This is seen particularly in children with sickle cell disease but has little clinical value.

i. Routine urinalysis may show pyuria, casts, glucosuria, or aminoaciduria, particularly when lead levels exceed 100 gm/100 ml. A Fanconi-type tubular acidosis characterized by aminoaciduria, glucosuria, and hypophosphatemia may be found in such patients.

C. Diagnosis. See Table 4-6.

D. Therapy. At all costs, the source of lead must be removed despite the existence of other problems.

1. **Commonly used chelating agents** are EDTA, BAL, and D-penicillamine. (For a complete discussion of the use of chelating agents, see *J. Pediatr.* 73:1, 1968, and *Pediatrics* 53:441, 1974.)

a. EDTA

(1) **Mechanism of action.** Urinary lead excretion is increased 20-fold–50-fold. Lead is removed from the soft tissues and CNS, but **not** from red blood cells. Bone pools of lead are reduced after multiple chelations with EDTA. EDTA enhances removal of other metals, notably zinc.

(2) **Route of administration.** EDTA may be given IV or IM. When it is given IV, a slow drip gives the best results. In IM administration, EDTA should be given with procaine (0.5–2.0 %) in deep injection. Oral preparations of EDTA have been shown to enhance absorption of lead from the GI tract. Thus, **oral EDTA is contraindicated.**

(3) **Dosage.** Under most circumstances, a total daily dose of 1000 mg/M^2 will provide sufficient lead diuresis. This dose is administered up to 5 days sequentially and then discontinued for at least 48 hr to permit clearance of the lead-EDTA complexes and permit some reequilibra-

Table 4-6. Clinical and laboratory evidence of lead intoxication

Mild	Moderate	Severe
Clinical		
Lead exposure, usually to soil or dust	Probably paint exposure	Pica for paint
Asymptomatic	Predisposing iron deficiency	Secondary iron deficiency
May be predisposing iron deficiency	Positive family history	Abdominal pain, irritability, lethargy, fever, hepatosplenomegaly
Cognitive sequelae	Usually asymptomatic	Ataxia, seizures, coma, increased intracranial pressure, neurologic sequelae
	Loss of appetite and behavior changes	
	Behavioral and cognitive sequelae	
Laboratory		
Lead levels in whole blood 25–49 μg/100 ml	Lead levels 49–70 μg/100 ml	Lead levels > 70 μg/ml
EP in whole blood 35–125 μg/100 ml	EP in whole blood 125–250 μg/100 ml	EP levels > 250 μg/100 ml
KUB and knee x-rays usually negative	KUB x-rays negative	KUB x-rays positive
Serum iron/iron-binding capacity ≤ 16%	Knee x-rays positive	Knee films positive
Serum ferritin < 40 μg/ml	Serum iron/iron-binding capacity ≤ 16%	Serum iron/iron-binding capacity ≤ 16%
CBC normal	Ferritin < 20 μg/100 ml	Ferritin < 10 μg/100 ml
Lead mobilization test: ≤ or ≅ 1 μg Pb/mg EDTA/24 hr	CBC shows mild anemia	CBC shows basophilic stippling, anemia
	Lead mobilization test: ≅1 μg Pb/mg EDTA/24 hr	Decreased nerve conduction time
		CT scan shows increased intracranial pressure
		Aminoaciduria, glycosuria
		Lead mobilization test: > 1 μg Pb/mg EDTA/24 hr

tion of lead stores. Under these conditions, as many 5-day courses of EDTA as indicated can be administered. As a rule, the longer the hiatus between courses of EDTA, the lower the risk of toxicity. In severe lead poisoning (blood lead ≥ 100 μg/100 ml or symptoms present) the dose can be increased to 1500 mg/M^2, **although the risk of renal toxicity is thereby also increased.**

  (4) Toxicity. The kidney is the principal site of toxicity, with renal effects seen at doses as low as 65 mg/kg/24 hr. The risk of toxicity is increased in patients with very high lead burdens. During chelation, daily urinalyses and careful monitoring of BUN, creatinine, and calcium should be done. Although hypocalcemia is avoided by the use of the calcium salt of EDTA, **hyper**calcemia, usually mild, can be seen with prolonged therapy. **Other toxic effects** include removal of zinc and other metals. When chelation therapy is completed, replacement of iron and, if indicated, zinc should be undertaken.

 b. BAL

  (1) Mechanism of action. Two molecules of BAL combine with one of heavy metal to form a stable complex. Fecal as well as urinary excretion of lead is enhanced. In addition, BAL diffuses well into erythrocytes. It can be administered in the presence of renal impairment because it is predominantly excreted in bile.

  (2) Route of administration. BAL is available only for IM administration in oil.

(3) Dosage. The usual dosage is 300 mg/M^2/day (up to 600 mg/M^2/day in severe cases) in 3–6 divided doses. Since BAL is mainly used to lower the blood lead rapidly, it need not be given for a full 5 days with EDTA (see **E.2.d**); 48–72 hr may suffice, **provided EDTA is continued.**

(4) Toxicity. Toxic reactions may occur in as many as 50% of patients. A febrile reaction peculiar to children occurs in 30%, which may lead to the erroneous conclusion that infection is present. The presence of a transient granulocytopenia may further confuse the observer. In both adults and children, other reactions include transient hypertension, nausea, headache, burning sensation of the oropharynx, conjunctivitis, rhinorrhea and excessive salivation, paresthesias, a burning sensation in the penis, sweating, abdominal pain, and occasional sterile abscesses. Such reactions are most likely with the inappropriate use of BAL, i.e., when heavy metal concentration is relatively low.

c. D-**Penicillamine** is the only available oral chelating agent. The D-isomer has relatively low toxicity and can be given over a long period. Side effects can be minimized by beginning with a lower dose and gradually increasing to the full dose [see **(4)**].

(1) Mechanism of action. D-Penicillamine enhances the urinary excretion of lead, although not as effectively per mole as EDTA. Lead is not removed from erythrocytes. Excreted lead is not necessarily in the form of chelated complexes, and the specific mechanism is not well understood.

(2) Route of administration. The D-isomer is administered PO. It is currently available as both 125-mg and 250-mg tablets and capsules. The capsules may be opened or the tablets crushed and suspended in liquid, if necessary.

(3) The usual **oral dose** is 20–40 mg/kg (600–1200 mg/M^2). Side effects can be minimized by initiating therapy with small doses; e.g., 25% of the expected dose and increasing after 1 week to 50% and again after 1 week to the full dose, as well as by monitoring for toxicity.

(4) Toxicity and side effects. The D-isomer of penicillamine is relatively nontoxic. However, as many as 20% of patients receiving the drug will experience some form of mild toxicity, usually reactions resembling those of penicillin sensitivity, including fevers, rashes, leukopenia, thrombocytopenia, and eosinophilia. Anorexia, nausea, and vomiting are infrequent. Of most concern, however, are isolated reports of nephrotoxicity, possibly from hypersensitivity reactions. Toxicity may be reduced by concurrent administration of pyridoxine, although no controlled studies of this effect are available. D-**Penicillamine should not be administered to patients with known penicillin allergy.**

2. Monitoring chelation therapy. Urinary lead excretion may be used to monitor the effectiveness of chelation therapy, since the blood lead can be misleading in the presence of chelating agents.

a. During chelation therapy, serum calcium, BUN, and lead in the blood and urine, as well as urinalyses, are monitored for evidence of hypocalcemia or renal toxicity due to EDTA. If such evidence is present, EDTA can be reduced or discontinued, and renal function usually returns to normal.

b. Occasionally, symptoms may worsen during therapy. Removal of lead should continue, with attention to CNS changes suggestive of cerebral edema (see **E.3**).

c. EDTA is administered for up to 5 days at a time. In general, urinary lead excretion tends to fall off after the fourth day regardless of the lead burden, while the risk of EDTA nephrotoxicity increases after the fifth day. For this reason, EDTA chelation is interrupted after 5 days, and a

Table 4-7. Indications for chelation therapy

1. Venous blood lead $\geq$ 50 μg/100 ml on two successive occasions, *or*
2. Venous blood lead $\geq$ 25–49 μg/100 ml and EP $\geq$ 125 μg/100 ml *or*
3. Positive lead mobilization test

Factors contributing to indications
    Age, degree of exposure, underlying developmental level, iron deficiency

"rest period" of at least 48–72 hr is initiated. If the lead burden, indicated by initial blood lead and urine lead excretion, is very high, chelation is again begun after 48–72 hr, and a new 24-hr urine lead is obtained for comparison. In this manner, as many chelations as are indicated by the lead burden can be undertaken without significant risk until such time as the initial 24-hr urine lead excretion fails to yield $\geq$ 1 μg lead/mg EDTA. Therapy is then discontinued and long-term follow-up begun. Subsequent chelation may well be necessary, but a longer hiatus between chelations can now ensue.

    d. Because of the "rebound" phenomenon during reequilibration of body lead stores, blood lead and EP levels immediately following chelation tend to be misleading and are best obtained 2–3 weeks following therapy.

    e. The goal of therapy is to reduce body lead burden to safe levels (i.e., blood lead < 25 μg/100 ml) and EP to normal (i.e., < 35 μg/100 ml). Because chelation therapy tends to be less efficient as the body burden is lowered, the clinician must exercise judgment to decide when enough therapy has been administered. Such factors as the child's age, degree of exposure, likelihood of continued exposure, discomfort, and side effects of parenteral chelation must be weighed. In general, the most complete therapy should be applied to children under 3 years of age.

E. Management of plumbism. The criteria for chelation therapy proposed in Table 4-7 are intended as guidelines. Each child is different. Important variables include age, duration of exposure, risk factors such as iron deficiency, sickle cell disease, and metabolic acidosis, and developmental levels.

  1. Mild lead poisoning

    a. Identify and remove the **lead source.** Parents can help by vacuuming and wet-mopping the home to reduce lead dust.

    b. Administer **oral iron** (6 mg/kg elemental iron/24 hr) to correct iron deficiency and reduce further lead absorption.

    c. Repeat lead and EP determination monthly or more frequently. If values remain elevated longer than 2 months, consider a **lead mobilization test.**

    d. If the lead mobilization test is **negative,** or the child is over 3 years old, D-penicillamine (900 mg/M^2/24 hr in 2 divided doses PO) may be useful in reducing lead and concomitant EP values. The possibility of continued lead exposure, although not desirable, is not a contraindication to the use of D-penicillamine.

    e. If the lead mobilization test is **positive,** begin chelation therapy by administration of calcium disodium EDTA (Versenate) for 5 consecutive days, giving 1000 mg/M^2/day IM in single doses with procaine. Hospitalization is not necessary unless daily clinic or office visits are not feasible.

    f. Daily urinalyses, BUN, creatinine, and lead and iron studies should be obtained on the first and fifth days of treatment.

    g. If further chelation therapy is warranted, provide a hiatus of at least 48–72 hr between courses of treatment.

    h. After chelation therapy is completed, restart iron therapy until both lead and EP values have returned to normal.

  2. Moderate lead poisoning

    a. Identify and remove the **lead source.** If "deleading" is undertaken, remove the child **completely** from the home during the process and until a thor-

ough cleanup is completed. **Permitting children to return home at night during the deleading of a home risks further serious exposure.**
   b. Administer oral iron (see **1.b.** preceding) for 1 month or until EP stabilizes.
   c. Administer a lead mobilization test and proceed as described in **l.d.** and **e.**
   d. It is likely that more than one course of chelation therapy will be needed. Parents should be informed of this as early as possible to enlist their cooperation in the treatment process.
   e. Mild, transient elevations of blood lead following chelation therapy are commonly due to "rebound" (reequilibration of residual body stores of lead) rather than reexposure. However, reexposure can and does occur and is usually accompanied by significant increases in EP values shortly afterward.
   f. As in **l.h.,** iron therapy should begin following completion of chelation and continued until the EP either stabilizes or returns to normal.
3. **Severe lead poisoning without encephalopathy**
   a. **Identify and remove the lead source.**
   b. **Hospitalize** the child.
   c. Give 1.5 times the usual **maintenance fluids** (see Chap. 7, p. 197).
   d. Administer EDTA IV if possible or IM if necessary (1000 mg/M^2 daily in 3 divided doses). If the IM route is chosen, the dose can be given bid or even in a single injection.
   e. If the lead burden appears high on the basis of urinary excretion, add BAL IM in 3 divided doses of $300 \text{ mg/M}^2/24 \text{ hr}$ for 48–72 hr.
   f. Monitor BUN, blood, 24-hr urine lead, and the urinalyses.
   g. After chelation is completed, administer iron (see **1.b** preceding).
4. **Severe lead intoxication with encephalopathy**
   a. **This is a medical emergency.**
   b. Give maintenance fluids.
   c. Begin EDTA IV, $1500 \text{ mg/M}^2/\text{day}$ in 3 divided doses by slow drip.
   d. Begin BAL IM, $600 \text{ mg/M}^2/\text{day}$ in 3–6 divided doses.
   e. Treat cerebral edema with mannitol and dexamethasone (Decadron) (see Chap. 3, p. 62).
   f. **Continue chelation therapy at all costs, since cerebral edema will not respond to therapy until the lead burden is reduced.**
   g. Treat seizures with anticonvulsants (see Table 20-3).
   h. After 5 days, discontinue therapy for 48 hr and restart.
   i. Monitor BUN, calcium, electroencephalograms, urinalysis findings, and blood and 24-hr urine lead.
   j. Continue with a close monthly follow-up as long as the child is at risk.
5. **Sequelae.** Both symptomatic **and** asymptomatic lead poisoning produce sequelae. Gross screening tests are generally not sensitive enough to distinguish subtle deficits and are frequently performed in children too young to provide reproducible results.
   All children with histories of increased lead burden should undergo thorough neuropsychological evaluation prior to entering school, ideally at ages 5–6. At a minimum, this should include evaluation of visual-motor skills, expressive and receptive language skills, visual and auditory perceptual skills, and fine and gross motor skills. I.Q. testing may be misleading because it fails to reflect specific functional deficits. With these results in hand, the clinician can alert the school to a child's difficulties and recommend remedial or special education where deficits exist. Conversely, when none is found, the family and school authorities can be appropriately reassured. Behavior problems related to lead poisoning, such as hyperactivity, may respond to pharmacologic therapy.
F. **Prevention. Lead poisoning is a preventable disease.** Strong laws are in effect in some states requiring removal of lead paint from the market and strong

penalties for nonremoval from houses in cases of plumbism. **Proper precautions are needed during deleading and renovation of old housing lest incidental exposure occur. Children should be removed completely from such homes while such work is going on. Heating and sanding of lead paint are particularly dangerous** and should be avoided and scraping or chemical stripping used. Continued reduction of leaded gasoline consumption is necessary to reduce lead "fallout" in soil and household dust, particularly near heavily trafficked areas. Intensive screening of children to identify those at risk, widespread inspection of housing, and stringent enforcement of sanitary and housing codes can reduce morbidity in this disease.

Management of the Newborn, I

I. General principles of the newborn evaluation and care

A. Prenatal care

1. **Antenatal care of the high-risk fetus.** The factors making a pregnancy high risk are listed in Table 5-1. The important information to obtain in a high risk pregnancy is gestational age, maturity of specific organ systems, fetal size and rate of growth, and evidence of fetal/placental health.

    a. **Gestational age is determined by**

    (1) The date of the last menstrual period
    (2) The date of quickening
    (3) The time of appearance of fetal heart sounds
    (4) Pregnancy tests
    (5) Size of the uterus
    (6) Early ultrasonographic findings
    (7) **Amniotic fluid (AF) measurements.**

        (a) **An AF creatinine concentration of over 2 mg/100 ml indicates a full-term fetus with a 94% confidence level.**
        (b) **An AF bilirubin concentration** approaches zero at term in infants without hemolytic disease.
        (c) **Greater than 50% of fetal cells staining positive for fat globules,** using Nile blue sulfate stain, indicates a full-term fetus.

    b. **Maturity of specific organ systems.** Pulmonary maturation is determined by measurement of AF phospholipids (see Chap. 6, p. 141).

    c. **Fetal size and rate of growth** are determined by uterine size and by ultrasonography.

    d. **Placental function and fetal well-being**

    (1) Human chorionic gonadotropin
    (2) Human placental lactogen
    (3) Estriols in maternal blood and urine
    (4) Nonstress monitoring
    (5) Oxytocin challenge test
    (6) Fetal breathing patterns
    (7) Amniocentesis for meconium or evidence of infection (white cells or bacteria)

    e. **Real-time ultrasonography for the diagnosis of**

    (1) Malformations such as anencephaly, meningocele, cardiac defects, renal malformation, GI malformation
    (2) Disorders of fetal activity as in neurologic or muscular disorders and placental insufficiency
    (3) Ascites and hydrops in hematologic disease of the newborn
    (4) Assessing fetal growth for calculating gestational age and in such disorders as maternal diabetes and hypertension
    (5) An aid for procedures such as amniocentesis and fetal surgery

    f. **Intrapartum tests of fetal well-being include:**

    (1) Fetal heart rate monitoring
    (2) Fetal scalp pH
    (3) Fetal scalp transcutaneous oxygen tension

Table 5-1. Perinatal risk factors associated with an increased risk to the newborn

Condition	Risk to newborn
Maternal condition	
Maternal age over 35	Chromosomal abnormalities, SGA
Maternal age under 16	Prematurity
Poverty	Prematurity, infection, SGA
Infertility	Low birth weight, congenital anomalies, increased prenatal mortality
Smoking	SGA, increased perinatal mortality
Drug or alcohol abuse	SGA, fetal alcohol syndrome, withdrawal syndrome, sudden infant death
Diabetes	Stillbirth, hyaline membrane disease, congenital anomalies
Thyroid disease	Goiter, hypothyroidism, hyperthyroidism
Renal disease	SGA, stillbirth
Heart or lung disease	SGA, stillbirth, prematurity
Hypertension, chronic or preeclampsia	SGA, asphyxia, stillbirth
Anemia	SGA, asphyxia, stillbirth
Isoimmunization (red cell antigens)	Stillbirth, anemia, jaundice
Isoimmunization (platelets)	Stillbirth, bleeding
Thrombocytopenia	Stillbirth, bleeding
Polyhydramnios	Anomalies (anencephaly, GI obstruction, renal disease, goiter)
Low urinary estriols	SGA, stillbirth
Bleeding in early pregnancy	Prematurity, stillbirth
Bleeding in third trimester	Anemia, stillbirth
Premature rupture of membranes, fever, infection	Infection
TORCH infections	See TORCH infections, p. 168
Past history of infant with jaundice, respiratory distress syndrome, or anomalies	Increased risk of recurrence in neonate
Maternal medications, corticosteroids, antimetabolites, antithyroid medications, reserpine, salicylates, etc.	See individual package inserts. See also J. P. Cloherty and A. R. Stark (Eds.), *Manual of Neonatal Care.* Boston: Little, Brown, 1980.
Fetal conditions	
Multiple birth	Prematurity, twin transfusion syndrome, asphyxia
Poor fetal growth	Asphyxia, stillbirth, congenital anomalies
Abnormal fetal position	Trauma, hemorrhage, deformities
Abnormality of fetal heart rate or rhythm	Asphyxia, heart failure, heart block
Acidosis	Asphyxia, respiratory distress syndrome
Condition of labor or delivery	
Premature labor	Respiratory distress, asphyxia
Labor occurring 2 weeks or more after term	Stillbirth, asphyxia, meconium aspiration
Long labor	Asphyxia, stillbirth
Meconium-stained amniotic fluid	Asphyxia, meconium aspiration syndrome, stillbirth

Table 5-1 (continued)

Condition	Risk to newborn
Prolapsed cord	Asphyxia
Maternal hypotension	Asphyxia, stillbirth
Rapid labor	Trauma
Analgesia and anesthesia	Respiratory depression, hypotension
Neonatal condition	
Low Apgar score	Intracranial hemorrhage, respiratory distress, anoxic–ischemic encephalopathy
Foul smell of baby, amniotic fluid, or membranes	Infection
Placental anomalies	
Small placenta	SGA
Large placenta	Hydrops, heart failure
Torn placenta	Blood loss
Vasa previa	Blood loss

SGA = small for gestational age; TORCH = Toxoplasmosis, rubella, cytomegalic inclusion disease, and herpes simplex.

    (4) Fetal scalp platelet counts
    (5) Tests of vaginal blood for fetal red blood cells
2. Prenatal diagnosis of specific diseases
  a. Amniocentesis is done to obtain fluid and cells for specific studies such as:
    (1) AF alpha fetoprotein (AF-AFP) is elevated in the presence of open neural tube defects. About 10% of neural tube defects may be closed, and the levels of AF-AFP may be normal. AF-AFP is best measured at 16–18 weeks. Elevated AF-AFP unrelated to a neural tube defect may be found in:
      (a) Fetal or placental bleeding caused by amniocentesis
      (b) Omphalocele
      (c) Cystic hygromas
      (d) Fetal nephrosis
      (e) Fetal death
      When AF-AFP levels are abnormal, an acetylcholinesterase assay should be done, the morphology of AF cells should be examined, and the percentage of rapidly adherent cells should be estimated. These tests may help confirm the presence of neural tube defects. Anatomic studies by **ultrasonography** should be carried out in all instances of elevated AF-AFP. **Amniography** or **fetoscopy** should be considered when the diagnosis is uncertain.
    (2) **Chemical analysis** of AF may be done for AF **bilirubin** in cases of hemolytic disease of the newborn. Organic acids may be measured in cases of suspected organic acidemias, such as methymalonic acidemia. Hexosaminidase A activity may be measured in patients at risk for Tay-Sachs disease, and 17 α-hydroxyprogesterone may be measured in cases of suspected 21-hydroxylase deficiency.
    (3) **AF cells** may be obtained for culture between the fourteenth and sixteenth week of pregnancy to determine:
      (a) **Abnormal chromosomes.** A karyotype is obtained to rule out chromosomal abnormalities such as Down syndrome and other trisomies in pregnancies where a positive family history of

chromosomal abnormalities is present and in pregnant women over 35 years of age.

- (b) **Sex chromosome karyotype.** This identifies fetal sex in cases of X-linked inherited diseases.
- (c) **Enzyme or substrate concentrations indicating inborn errors of metabolism.** The list of those disorders that can be diagnosed by this method is long and includes such diverse conditions as gangliosidoses type I, Hurler syndrome type I, galactosemia, maple syrup urine disease, and the adrenogenital syndrome. In general, disorders that are expressed in skin fibroblasts will also be expressed in cultured AF cells.

b. **Fetoscopy** may be used for the diagnosis of malformations and to assist in fetal tissue sampling.

c. **Fetal tissue sampling.** Fetal skin, blood, or tissue may be obtained for diagnosis of hemoglobinopathies, chronic granulomatous disease, hemophilia, or congenital ichthyosis.

B. General assessment of the newborn

1. **Physical examination of the newborn.** At no other time than at birth is more information obtained from the general overall visual and auditory appraisal of a naked infant and less information obtained from an exhaustive system-by-system examination. Three categories are of utmost importance: **cardiorespiratory status,** the **presence of congenital anomalies,** and the **effects of gestation, labor, delivery, anesthetics, and signs of infection or other disease.**

   a. **Initial examination.** A fretful infant should be quieted with a nipple. The usual order of examination is as follows:

      (1) **Respiratory.** Evaluation of respiratory status includes color, presence of acrocyanosis, and respiratory rate (normal 40–60 and often periodic), including the presence of apnea. Rales and questionable breath sounds are usually insignificant if the infant is otherwise well. On the other hand, retractions, nasal flaring, and respiratory grunting are significant in the absence of crying. Percussion has little value.

      (2) **Cardiac.** Evaluation of the heart includes the position of maximal impulse, palpation of femoral and brachial pulses, and auscultation of the heart for rate, rhythm, and presence of murmurs. Because of rapid alterations in systemic and pulmonary pressures, murmurs do not always reflect the presence of significant heart disease.

      (3) **Abdomen.** Observation for asymmetry, including the musculature, masses, and fullness, is critical. Palpation with gentle pressure from lower to upper quadrants is most useful. Bowel sounds may or may not be present initially. The normal liver may be as much as 2.5 cm below the right costal margin. Palpate for both kidneys.

      (4) **Genitalia and rectum.** Observe for symmetry, presence of both testicles, and normal placement and patency of the urethral orifice and anus.

      (5) **Extremities, spine, and joints.** Observe for anomalies of the digits, structural abnormalities, hip dislocation, and positional anomalies.

      (6) **Head, neck, and mouth.** Inspect for cuts, bruises, caput, cephalohematoma, mobility of suture lines, and skull molding. Measure the head circumference from occiput to midbrow. Observe for neck flexibility and asymmetry and cleft palate and lip.

      (7) **Neurologic examination.** Observations for neurologic status can usually be made concurrently while handling the baby for the preceding examinations. Observe for tone, activity, symmetry of the extremities and facial movements, alertness, consolability, and reflexes, including the Moro, suck, root, grasp, and plantar reflexes.

      (8) **Eye examination.** (Periorbital edema from silver nitrate may interfere.) Usually, the presence of cataracts and tumors can be evaluated

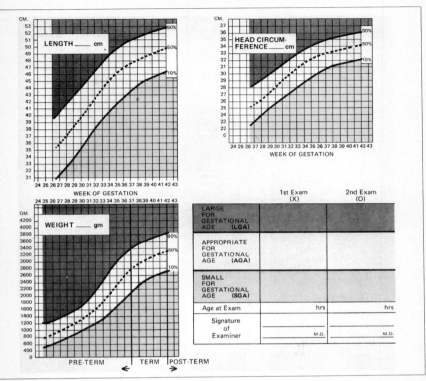

Fig. 5-1. Classification of newborns based on maturity and intrauterine growth. (Adapted from L. C. Lubchenco, C. Hansman, and E. Boyd, *Pediatrics* 37:403, 1966; and F. C. Battaglia and L. C. Lubchenco, *J. Pediatr.* 71:159, 1967. Copyright © 1978, Mead Johnson & Co., Evansville, Ind.)

by elicitation of the red reflex. Scleral hemorrhage and pupillary size can be assessed.

   b. The **discharge examination** should include attention to cardiac status (congestive heart failure or new murmur), abdomen (masses), stools, urine, skin (jaundice, infection), cord (infection), feeding (amount), maternal competence, and follow-up.

   2. Assessment of gestational age. Gestational age is estimated by using modifications of the Dubowitz examination shown in Figures 5-1 and 5-2. These forms were developed by Jacob L. Kay, M.D., Seton Hall Medical Center, Austin, Tex., with Mead Johnson, Evansville, Ind.

C. Nursery care

   1. Feeding and nutrition. Requirements for full-term neonates are between 110–130 kcal/kg/day. The protein requirement is 2–3 gm/kg/day. Fat intake makes up 55–65 kcal/kg/day, and the balance is carbohydrate.

   a. Breast-feeding

   (1) Breast milk is of proved nutritional and emotional value for the feeding of the full-term infant and should be encouraged for all full-term infants and most premature infants.

   (2) Whether or not breast milk is nutritionally adequate for the premature infant is disputed. The protein in breast milk is 60% whey (β-

NEUROMUSCULAR MATURITY

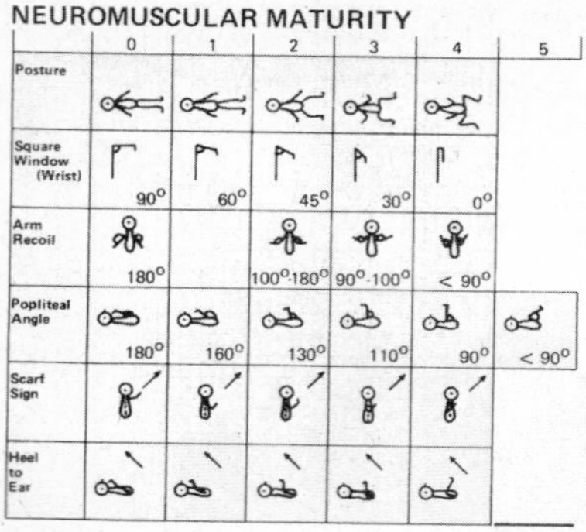

PHYSICAL MATURITY

	0	1	2	3	4	5
SKIN	gelatinous red, transparent	smooth pink, visible veins	superficial peeling &/or rash, few veins	cracking pale area, rare veins	parchment, deep cracking, no vessels	leathery, cracked, wrinkled
LANUGO	none	abundant	thinning	bald areas	mostly bald	
PLANTAR CREASES	no crease	faint red marks	anterior transverse crease only	creases ant. 2/3	creases cover entire sole	
BREAST	barely percept.	flat areola, no bud	stippled areola, 1–2 mm bud	raised areola, 3–4 mm bud	full areola, 5–10 mm bud	
EAR	pinna flat, stays folded	sl. curved pinna, soft with slow recoil	well-curv. pinna, soft but ready recoil	formed & firm with instant recoil	thick cartilage, ear stiff	
GENITALS Male	scrotum empty, no rugae		testes descending, few rugae	testes down, good rugae	testes pendulous, deep rugae	
GENITALS Female	prominent clitoris & labia minora		majora & minora equally prominent	majora large, minora small	clitoris & minora completely covered	

Gestation by Dates ______________ wks

Birth Date ____________ Hour ____________ am pm

APGAR ____________ 1 min ____________ 5 min

MATURITY RATING

Score	Wks
5	26
10	28
15	30
20	32
25	34
30	36
35	38
40	40
45	42
50	44

SCORING SECTION

	1st Exam=X	2nd Exam=O
Estimating Gest Age by Maturity Rating	______ Weeks	______ Weeks
Time of Exam	Date ______ Hour ______ am pm	Date ______ Hour ______ am pm
Age at Exam	______ Hours	______ Hours
Signature of Examiner	______ M.D.	______ M.D.

Fig. 5-2. Newborn maturity rating and classification: Estimation of gestational age by maturity rating. (Adapted from A. Y. Sweet. Classification of Low-Birth-Weight Infants. In M. H. Klaus and A. A. Fanaroff (Eds.), *Care of the High-Risk Infant.* Philadelphia: Saunders, 1977. P. 47; and J. L. Ballard et al., A simplified assessment of gestational age. *Pediatr. Res.* 11:374, 1977. Copyright © 1978, Mead Johnson & Co., Evansville, Ind.)

lactoglobulin and lactalbumin) and 40% casein and relatively digestible by the premature. However, the low total protein content of breast milk may be inadequate to support optimal growth in premature infants. Prematures not growing adequately on breast milk may therefore require protein supplementation (up to 2 gm/day) (see Table 5-2). Some prematures may also have a transient lactase deficiency that requires lactose-free formula.

(3) Human milk contains a number of antimicrobial components not found in infant formulas: immunoglobulins, leukocytes, lactoferrin, the third component of complement in colostrum, and lysozymes. In areas where sanitation is poor, the use of nonhuman milk formulas has been clearly associated with increased infant mortality from infection.

(4) Fostering successful breast-feeding

(a) Both the obstetrician and the pediatrician should discuss nursing prenatally with the mother.

Table 5-2. Commonly used supplements to increase calorie content of formula

Product	Cal/gm	Cal	CHO (gm)	Protein (gm)	Fat (gm)	Na (mg)	Food sources
Casec (MJ)	4	17		4		7.1	Calcium caseinate (88%, milk fat)
Glucose	4	35	8.75				
Karo Syrup	4	60	15			22	Corn syrup/tbsp: 4 gm glucose, 1 gm sucrose, 2 gm maltose, 2 gm trisaccharides, 5.5 gm polysaccharides
Lipomul-Oral (Upjohn)	9	90			10		Corn oil
MCT oil (MJ)	9	115			13.8		Coconut oil, MCTs easily absorbed; need no bile salts or lipase for absorption
EMF	4	60		15			Predigested collagen
Polycose (Ross)	4	30	7.5			10	Hydrolyzed cornstarch, glucose polymer

   (b) Experienced nursing mothers should be available to discuss the satisfactions and techniques of breast-feeding with expectant mothers.
   (c) Obstetric ward and neonatal unit practices should be altered to foster successful nursing. Some of these changes include:
      (i) Decreasing the amount of sedation or anesthesia given to mothers
      (ii) Allowing the mother to nurse the infant immediately after delivery, if possible
      (iii) Encouraging "rooming in" to avoid separation of mother and infant
      (iv) Having infants fed on demand rather than on a rigid schedule
      (v) Seeing that the personnel caring for new mothers are actively supportive of breast-feeding
   (5) For a discussion of contraindications to breast-feeding, see J. Cloherty and A. Stark (Eds.), *Manual of Neonatal Care,* Boston, Little, Brown, 1980.
b. Formula feeding. A number of commercially available formulas are adequate (Table 5-3). Those based on cow's milk (e.g., Similac, Enfamil) are the usual formulas for full-term infants.
   (1) Modified formulas (e.g., Special Care or Enfamil Premature) are best for premature infants in the first weeks of life because of the whey-casein and calcium-phosphorus ratios.
   (2) Soy-based formulas and formulas whose caloric density is greater than 20 cal/oz are for special situations.
   (3) Protein, medium-chain triglycerides (MCTs), and glucose-polymer caloric supplements (see Table 5-2) should be used only for babies who require caloric supplementation. These supplements may increase the likelihood of late metabolic acidosis and prevent absorption of Ca^{2+} and other minerals. They are also expensive.

Table 5-3. Composition of formulas per liter

	Human milk*	Special Care 20	Special Care 24	Enfamil Premature 20	Enfamil Premature 24	"Preemie" SMA	PM60/40	SMA
kcal/L	510–700	680.3	800	680	800	680	680	680
Protein (gm)	11	18.3	22	20	24	20	15.8	15
Source	Casein, lactalbumin	Nonfat milk, whey	Nonfat milk, whey	Nonfat milk, whey	Nonfat milk, whey	Nonfat milk, whey	Nonfat milk, whey	Nonfat milk, whey
Fat (gm)	45	36.7	44	34	41	44	37.6	36
Source		MCT oil (50%), corn oil (30%), coconut oil (20%)		Corn oil (40%), MCT oil (40%), coconut oil (20%)		Oleo, coconut, soy, safflower oils (87.5%), MCT oil (12.5%)	Coconut and corn oil	Coconut, safflower, soy, oleo oils
CHO (gm)	68	71.7	86	74	89	86	68.8	72
Source	Lactose	Glucose polymers (50%), lactose (50%)		Corn syrup (60%), lactose (40%)		Lactose (50%), glucose polymers (50%)	Lactose	Lactose
CA (mg)	250	1,200	1,440	790	950	750	400	447
P (mg)	159	600	720	400	400	400	200	332
Ca/P ratio		2:1	2:1	2:1	2:1	1.9:1	2:1	1.3:1
Na (mg)	194	310	380	260	320	320	160	149
K (mg)	590	940	1,120	750	900	750	580	562
Cl (mg)	460	640	710	570	690	530	400	372
Mg (mg)	40	83	100	71	85	70	42	53
Fe (mg)	0.1	2.5	3.0	1.0	1.2	3	1.5	12
I (μg)	30	130	150	54	64	83	42	69
Zn (mg)	0.4	10	12	6.7	8.1	5.0	5.0	3.7
Cu (mg)	0.4	1.7	2.0	0.6	0.8	0.7	0.6	0.5
Mn (mg)	0.07	0.08	0.1	0.2	0.2	0.2	0.3	0.16
Vitamin A (IU)	1,900	4,580	5,500	2,100	2,300	3,200	2,500	2,647
Vitamin D (IU)	22	1,000	1,200	420	510	510	400	423
Vitamin E (IU)	2.7	25	30	13	16	15	20	9.5
Vitamin K (μg)	15	83	100	66	76	70	30	58
Vitamin C (mg)	43	250	300	57	69	70	55	58
Vitamin B_1 (thiamine) (mg)	0.16	1.7	2.0	0.5	0.6	0.8	0.65	0.7
B_2 (riboflavin) (mg)	0.38	0.4	0.5	0.6	0.7	1.3	0.7	0.7
B_6 (mg)	0.1	0.3	0.3	0.4	0.5	0.5	0.4	0.4
B_{12} (μg)	0.3	3.7	4.5	2.0	2.5	2.0	1.5	1.0
Niacin (mg)	1.5	34	40	8.4	10.0	6.3	7.3	10.2
Folic acid (mg)	0.05	0.25	0.3	0.2	0.24	0.1	0.1	.05
Panthothenic acid (mg)	1.8	12.5	15.0	3.0	3.8	3.6	3.0	2.1
Biotin (μg)	0.002	25	30	15.8	19.0	18	30	15
Osmolality (mOsm/kg H_2O)	288	250	300	244	300	268	260	296
Renal solute load (mOsm/L)	230	128	154	170	210	175.2	96	91

*Human milk data from S. J. Fomon, *Infant Nutrition* (2nd ed.). Philadelphia: Saunders, 1974. P. 362.
Sources: Wyeth Laboratories, Philadelphia, Pa., 1982; Mead Johnson Laboratories, Evansville, Ind., 1983; Ross Laboratories, Columbus, Ohio, 1982; table prepared by Patricia M. Queen, M.M.Sc., R.D., Assistant Director of Clinical Nutrition, Department of Nutrition and Food Service, Children's Hospital, Boston.

Prosobee	Isomil	Isomil SF	Portagen	Pregestimil	Nutramigen	Similac	Similac with whey	Enfamil
680	680	680	670	670	680	680	680	680
20	20	20	24	19	22	15	15	15
Soy	Soy	Soy	Sodium caseinate	Casein hydrolysate	Casein hydrolysate	Nonfat milk	Nonfat milk, whey	Nonfat milk
36	36	36	32	27	26	36.3	36.3	38
Coconut, soy oils	Coconut, soy oils	Soy, coconut oil	MCT oil (83%), corn oil, soy oil	MCT oil (40%), corn oil (60%)	Corn oil	Coconut, soy oil	Coconut, soy oil	Coconut, soy oil
69	68	68	78	91	88	72.3	72.3	69
Corn syrup	Corn syrup, sucrose	Glucose polymers	Corn syrup, sucrose	Corn syrup, tapioca starch	Sucrose, tapioca starch	Lactose	Lactose	Lactose
630	700	700	630	630	630	510	400	460
500	500	500	480	420	480	390	300	320
1.3:1	1.4:1	1.4:1	1.3:1	1.5:1	1.3:1	1.3:1	1.3:1	1.4:1
290	320	320	320	320	320	230	230	210
780	770	770	850	740	690	800	750	690
550	590	590	580	580	480	500	430	420
74	50	50	137	74	74	41	50	53
12.7	12	12	12.7	12.7	12.7	1.5	12	1.1
69	100	100	48	48	48	100	100	69
5.3	5.0	5.0	6.3	4.2	4.2	5.0	5.0	5.3
0.6	0.5	0.5	1.0	0.6	0.6	0.6	0.6	0.6
0.2	0.2	0.2	0.8	0.2	0.2	0.03	0.3	1.0
2,100	2,000	2,000	5,300	2,100	1,690	2,000	2,000	2,100
420	400	400	530	420	420	400	400	420
21	20	20	21	15.8	10.6	17	20	21
106	100	100	106	106	106	55	55	58
55	55	55	55	55	55	55	55	55
0.5	0.4	0.4	1.1	0.5	0.5	0.65	0.65	0.5
0.6	0.6	0.6	1.3	0.6	0.6	1.0	0.65	1.1
0.4	0.4	0.4	1.4	0.4	0.4	0.4	0.4	0.4
2.0	3.0	3.0	4.2	2.1	2.0	1.5	1.5	2.0
8.5	9.0	9.0	14.0	8.4	8.4	7.0	7.0	8.5
0.1	0.1	0.1	0.1	0.1	0.1	0.1	0.1	0.1
3.0	5.0	5.0	7.0	3.1	3.1	3.0	3.0	3.0
53	30	30	53	53	50	10	10	15.8
200	250	150	220	350	480	290	300	300
130	131	131	150	180	132	105	101	100

c. Supplements (vitamins, iron, and calcium)

(1) Breast-feeding

(a) Breast-fed infants need supplementation with 400 IU/day of vita-min D. Although vitamins A and C are not necessary, they will not be harmful in the doses provided in commercially available vitamin preparations (vitamin A, 1500 IU; vitamin D, 400 IU, vitamin C, 50 mg).

(b) The use of iron supplements in breast-fed infants is controversial (see *Pediatrics* 63:52, 1979). Some have suggested a dose of 2 mg/kg/day of elemental iron.

(c) If infants are fully breast-fed they should receive fluoride sup-plementation as in **(2)(b)** even if the mother drinks fluoridated water.

(2) Formulas

(a) Formulas usually contain adequate vitamins (1 quart formula/day), though iron supplementation after 4–8 weeks of age may be necessary (2 mg/kg/day elemental iron).

(b) Fluoride should be supplemented if babies are not receiving fluoridated water (0.25 mg/day up to age 2, 0.50 mg/day age 2–3 years, 1.0 mg/day 3–16 years).

(c) Small prematures should be given vitamin E (25–50 IU/day) for prevention of hemolysis.

(d) Vitamin K, 0.5 mg IM weekly, should be given to infants not being fed orally or taking antibiotics.

(e) Supplemental calcium (150 mg/kg/day elemental Ca^{2+} is the rec-ommended total daily consumption) may be necessary, since for-mulas contain approximately 1 mg Ca^{2+}/cal.

d. Special nutritional needs of the low-birth-weight infant

(1) Fluid intake of the low-birth-weight infant should increase from 75 ml/kg/day on day 1 to approximately 150 ml/kg/day after day 5. Daily caloric requirements are 50–100 kcal/kg by 3 days of age and 110–150 kcal/kg during later growth.

Low-birth-weight infants usually tolerate feeding q2–3h better than larger feedings q4h.

(a) If the infant is under 1,250–1,500 gm, start an IV with 10% D/W at about 100 ml/kg/day. Continue IV until PO feedings are 100 ml/kg/day.

(b) Follow Dextrostix at ½, 1, and 2 hr of age, then q4h prn. The Somogyi effect can occur if the IV infiltrates.

(2) See Table 5-4 for recommended schedule of gavage feeding.

(3) Close monitoring of urine and specific gravity, skin turgor, body weight, serum and urine osmolarity, and electrolyte concentrations is necessary.

(4) **Supplements** as needed for oral supplementation to increase caloric concentrations of formula should never be over 25 cal/oz (see Table 5-2).

(a) **Carbohydrates.** Glucose polymer (Polycose), 4 cal/gm

(b) **Fat.** MCT oil, 8.3 cal/gm, 9 cal/gm

(c) **After 1 week**

(i) 25–50 IU vitamin E (Aquasol E) qd PO

(ii) 1 ml multivitamins qd PO (including vitamin D, 400 IU; vitamin A, 1,500 IU; vitamin C, 25–50 mg)

(iii) 0.25–1.0 mg folate qd PO

(iv) Vitamin K_1, 0.5 mg weekly, if the patient is on long-term antibiotics or total parenteral nutrition

(v) Calcium gluconate 10% (9 mg Ca^{2+}/ml) added to the formula for a calcium dose of 150 mg/kg (this should be done gradu-ally over 1 week)

Table 5-4. Schedule of gavage feeding

Weight (gm)	Age (hrs)	Size of feeding (ml)	Interval	Content of feeding
Less than 1,200 (expected gastric residual* is 1–2 ml)	4–12	1–2	q2h	Sterile water, then 5% D/W
	12–24	2–4	q2h	5% D/W
	24–48	3–6	q2h	Equal parts of formula and 5% D/W
	48–72	4–8	q2h	Equal parts of formula and 5% D/W
	>72	5–10	q2h	Full-strength formula
1,200–1,500 (expected gastric residual* is 2 ml)	4–12	2–3	q2–3h	Sterile water, then 5% D/W
	12–24	4–6	q2–3h	Equal parts of 5% D/W and formula
	24–48	6–9	q2–3h	Equal parts of 5% D/W and formula
	48–72	8–12	q2–3h	Equal parts of 5% D/W and formula or full-strength formula
	>72	10–15	q2–3h	Full-strength formula
1,500–2,000 (expected gastric residual* is 3 ml)	4–12	5–15	q3–4h	Sterile water, then 5% D/W
	12–24	5–15	q3–4h	Equal parts of 5% D/W and formula
	24–48	10–25	q3–4h	Equal parts of 5% D/W and formula or full-strength formula
	48–72	15–35	q3–4h	Full-strength formula
	>72	20–45	q3–4h	Full-strength formula

*For intermittent gavage feeding, if the prefeeding residual is more than 25% of the amount of the feeding, the volume of the feeding should be reduced or alternative feeding methods considered.

Note: After 72 hr, the amount of each feeding should be increased each day by 1–2 ml in babies weighing less than 1,200 gm, 2–3 ml in babies weighing 1,200 to 1,500 gm, and 5–15 ml in babies weighing 1,500 to 2,000 gm, up to a volume of 150–175 ml/kg/24 hr.

Source: J. P. Cloherty and A. R. Stark (Eds.), *Manual of Neonatal Care.* Boston: Little, Brown, 1980.

(5) Keep gastric intake *below* 200 ml/kg/day to avoid aspiration. Infants who need to suck in excess of their appetite can be appeased with pacifiers.

(6) On discharge, discontinue vitamin E and begin iron (2 mg elemental iron/kg/day).

(7) Infants who are unable to tolerate oral gavage feedings need parenteral nutrition (see Chap. 10, pp. 257ff).

(a) Fluid needs are as described in Table 7-8, but they may vary, depending on the need to restrict fluid (e.g., as in hyaline membrane disease) or the need to give extra fluid (e.g., small prematures with large insensible water losses, who may have fluid requirements up to 200 ml/kg/day or more).

Table 5-5. Neutral thermal environmental temperatures

Birth weight		Incubator air temperature (°C)	First 24 hours (°F)
kg	lb		
	2	35.0	95.0
1		34.9	94.9
	3	34.2	93.6
1.5		34.0	93.2
	4	33.7	92.7
2		33.5	92.3
	5	33.3	92.0
2.5		33.2	91.8
	6	33.1	91.6
3		33.0	91.4

   (b) On day 2, 3 mEq/kg/day of sodium and 2 mEq/kg/day of potassium are required.
   (c) Caloric requirements are initially provided as **dextrose** 8–10% (4 kcal/gm) as tolerated and as **protein** (4 kcal/gm) as protein hydrolysates or free amino acids in gradually increasing dosage from 1 gm/kg/day on day 2 to 2.5 gm/kg/day on days 4–7.
   (d) Fat (9 kcal/gm) is given as 10% soybean emulsion. *Intralipid* may be used to provide additional calories without excessive fluid intake if the infant is receiving inadequate calories *after* the first week of life (see Chap. 10, p. 262) or when bilirubin is under 8 mg/100 ml (5 mg/100 ml for small prematures).
2. **Temperature control.** Heat loss may be minimized by placing an infant in a neutral thermal environment, or the thermal condition at which heat production is minimal yet core temperature is within normal range (Table 5-5).
   a. **Healthy infant.** The skin should be dried and the infant wrapped. Examination in the delivery room should be performed under a radiant warmer with a skin probe, keeping the skin temperature at 36.5°C.
   b. **Sick infant.** The skin should be dried and the infant wrapped and transported in a heated incubator. A radiant warmer with a servocontrol is used for procedures. Very sick neonates, to whom access is important, may be kept in an open radiant warmer with servocontrol of skin temperature; a small, clear-plastic heat shield will prevent loss by convection and radiation and may be used when observation is less important.
3. **Premature infants** (under 37 weeks gestation)
   a. **Delivery.** If possible, infants under 30 weeks gestation should be delivered in a hospital with an intensive care nursery. The need for infant transport adds to the mortality and morbidity of this group.
   b. **Respiration.** Hyaline membrane disease may be prevented by the measurement of the lecithin-sphingomyelin (L/S) ratio in amniotic fluid and prenatal treatment of the mother with corticosteroids when indicated. Perinatal hypoxia and apnea should be anticipated and treated.
   c. **Cardiovascular.** Fluid overloading should be avoided. Patent ductus arteriosus is common.
   d. **Hematologic.** Blood component therapy (packed cells, plasma, platelets) may be necessary for anemia, hypovolemia, or bleeding.
   e. **Hyperbilirubinemia,** hypoglycemia, hypocalcemia, hyponatremia, temperature control problems, and special nutritional needs must be anticipated.
4. **Small for gestational age (SGA) infants** (birth weight below the 10th percentile for gestational age). Conditions associated with SGA infants are listed in Table 5-6.

Table 5-6. Disparities with gestational age

Infants large for gestational age	Infants small for gestational age	
Constitutionally large infants	Advanced maternal age	Chronic hypertension
Infants of diabetic mothers	Multiparity	Sickle cell disease
Postmaturity	Race	Chronic disease
Transposition of the great vessels	Infertility	Smoking
Erythroblastosis fetalis	Previous spontaneous abortions	Multiple fetuses
Beckwith syndrome	Unwed state	Placental lesions
Parabiotic syndrome	Drug abuse	Congenital anomaly
	Maternal heart or renal disease	Chromosomal anomaly
	Toxemia	Congenital infections

   a. **During pregnancy,** monitor fetal well-being by urinary measurements and ultrasonographic measurements of the fetus.
   b. **At delivery,** anticipate fetal distress, meconium aspiration, hypoxia, and heat loss. In the **newborn,** monitor for polycythemia, hypoglycemia, and hypocalcemia. Evaluate for fetal causes of poor growth, including anomalies and congenital infection. Examination of the placenta is frequently useful.
5. **Large for gestational age** (LGA) (birth weight over the 90th percentile for gestational age). Conditions associated with LGA infants are listed in Table 5-6.
   These infants are at high risk of obstetric trauma, including dystocia, leading to fractures, brachial plexus injuries, or central nervous system injury. Polycythemia and hypoglycemia may be present.
6. **Postmature infants** (gestation over 42 weeks). The etiology is usually unknown, but postmaturity is associated with anencephaly, trisomy 18, and Seckel's dwarfism.
   a. **Management** during pregnancy includes careful estimation of fetal gestational age by dates, ultrasound, and monitoring of fetal well-being.
   b. **Delivery** may be elective depending on lung maturity or fetal distress. Intrapartum asphyxia, meconium aspiration, neonatal hypoglycemia and polycythemia are seen in postmature infants.

Management of the Newborn, II

I. Care of the newborn in the delivery room

A. Preparation

1. A thorough knowledge of the maternal and fetal history is essential.
2. The factors associated with increased risk to the newborn are listed in Table 5-1. A physician and nurse skilled in the resuscitation of the newborn should be present at the delivery of a high-risk infant.
3. Prior to the delivery of a high-risk infant, the pediatrician and pediatric nurse should discuss with the parents their plans for the care of the infant in the delivery room and nursery.
4. **Equipment**
   a. Radiant warmer bed, blankets (prewarmed)
   b. Infant suction bulb
   c. A flow-through anesthesia bag capable of delivering 100% oxygen. The bag should have an adjustable "pop-off" control and be fitted with an in-line manometer for observing airway pressure should assisted ventilation be required.
   d. Infant face masks of various sizes
   e. Stethoscope
   f. Larynogscope with No. 0 and No. 1 blades, batteries, and bulbs
   g. Cole orotracheal tubes with 2.5-, 3.0-, and 3.5-mm internal diameters, two of each
   h. **Drugs.** $NaHCO_3$, 0.5 mg/ml; epinephrine, 1:10,000; dextrose, 25 or 50%; calcium gluconate 10%; atropine; naloxone (Narcan), 0.2 mg/ml; saline; and albumin
   i. Umbilical catheterization tray with 3.5 and 5F catheters
   j. A prewarmed transport isolette with a portable oxygen supply

B. Delivery

1. Place the infant on a warming table.
2. Suction the nares and mouth with a suction bulb. **Gastric aspiration and deep suctioning in the first 5 min of life may produce bradycardia and should not be done routinely.**
3. If thick meconium is present, suction the oropharynx before the shoulders are delivered, and intubate and suction the trachea before the onset of breathing.
4. Dry the infant.
5. Evaluate the condition of the infant by the Apgar Score (Table 6-1).
   a. **Apgar 8–10.** No intervention required. Keep the infant warm. Avoid unnecessary invasive measures.
   b. **Apgar 5–7.** Stimulate the infant by gently slapping the feet or rubbing the back, and provide an oxygen-rich atmosphere to breathe by placing the mask over the baby's face.
   c. **Apgar 3–4.** If the heart rate is below 100, clear the airway and ventilate with bag and mask with pressures of 20–25 cm H_2O at 30 breaths/min. Higher pressures may be required to open collapsed alveoli.
   d. **Apgar 0–2.** For treatment of infants whose Apgar scores are 0–2, see Fig. 6-1.
6. All infants should have a brief general examination for anomalies.

Table 6-1. Apgar score*

Sign	0	1	2
Heart rate	Absent	Slow, less than 100/min	Over 100/min
Respiratory effort	Absent	Weak cry, hypoventilation	Crying lustily
Muscle tone	Limp	Some flexion of extremities	Well flexed
Reflex irritability	No response	Some motion	Cry
Color	Blue, pale	Pink body, blue extremities	Entirely pink

*Score infant at 1 and 5 minutes of age.

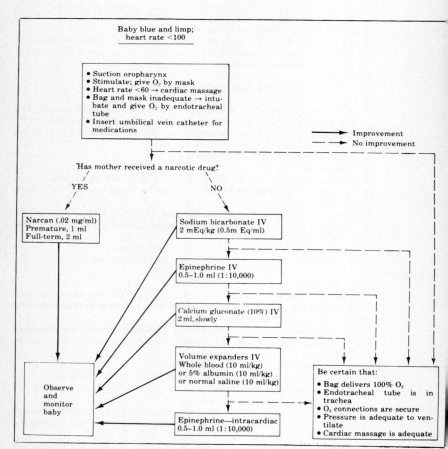

Fig. 6-1. Treatment in an infant with an Apgar score of 0–2. (Adapted from J. Kattwinckel, Continuing Education Program, University of Virginia.)

7. If the mother is awake and the infant appears well, encourage her to hold the infant as soon as she wishes.

II. Intensive care of the newborn

A. Procedures for respiratory complications

1. Remove foreign material, such as meconium and vomitus, by suction.
2. Establish patency of the airway using an oral airway (size 00 or 1) as necessary. The infant can usually be adequately ventilated by a bag and mask until preparations are made for intubation.
3. **Intubation**
   a. **Equipment.** In the delivery room or in an emergency, oral intubation is quickest and easiest with Cole tubes. Cole tube sizes are Nos. 14, 16, and 18 for a full-term infant and Nos. 10 and 12 for a premature infant. When the infant's condition is stabilized, Cole tubes are changed to a soft, cuffless nasotracheal tube (e.g., Portex) for chronic intubation. Portex tube sizes are as follows:

Infant weight (gm)	Portex tube size (internal diameter in mm)
Under 1,250	2.5
1,250 to 2,000	3.0
Over 2,000	3.5

   Additional equipment includes a laryngoscope with size 0 and size 1 blades, tincture of benzoin, adhesive tape, and Magill forceps. If possible, a clinician experienced in the intubation of infants should be in attendance.

   b. **Method**
   (1) Suction the mouth and upper airway.
   (2) If the intubation is elective, empty the infant's stomach, attach a cardiac monitor and a transcutaneous PO_2 monitor to the baby.
   (3) For nasotracheal intubation, measure for proper tube length **prior to intubation** (Fig. 6-2).
   (4) The baby should be ventilated with a bag and mask just prior to intubation.
   (5) The infant's head should be in the neutral position, avoiding excessive extension of the neck. The laryngoscope is held between the thumb and first finger of the left hand, with the second and third fingers holding the chin and stabilizing the head. Pushing down on the larynx with the fifth finger of the left hand (or having an assistant do it) and keeping the infant's head straight may help to visualize the vocal cords (trachea). The laryngoscope is passed into the right side of the mouth and then to the midline, swinging the tongue out of the way.
   (6) The endotracheal tube is held with the right hand and inserted between the vocal cords to about 2 cm below the glottis. During nasotracheal intubation, Magill forceps can be useful to guide the tube between the cords. If the fifth finger is pressing on the trachea, the tube can be felt as it slips into place.
   (7) Check the tube position by auscultation to ensure equal aeration of both lungs. If air entry is poor over the left chest, pull back the tube until aeration is improved.
   (8) During the procedure, one person should continually observe the infant and monitor the heart rate. The infant should not be allowed to become hypoxic or have bradycardia during intubation. If bradycardia occurs, stop the procedure and ventilate the infant with a bag and mask. Attaching an anesthesia bag on one side to 100% oxygen and on the other to the intubation tube adapter will deliver 100% oxygen to the pharynx during the intubation procedure. (An in-line pop-off valve should be present so that pressures do not exceed 25 cm H_2O.)
   (9) Intubation in the delivery room is usually temporary, and the tube can be held in place by hand. If prolonged ventilation is required, the

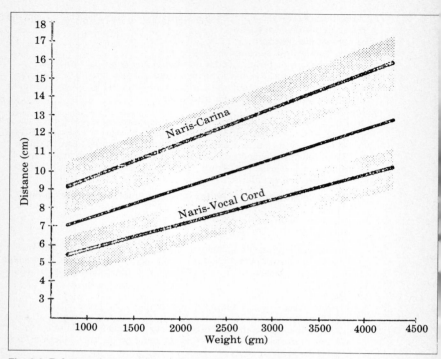

Fig. 6-2. Relation of naris-carina and naris-glottis distance to body weight. (From J. Coldiron, *Pediatrics* 41:823, 1968. Copyright © 1968 by the American Academy of Pediatrics.)

tube should be secured by tape, and an x-ray obtained to check its position.

4. Ventilation

   a. Principles

   (1) Delivery room

   (a) Artificial ventilation is used to oxygenate the infant and, when necessary, to initiate spontaneous ventilation. First, the airway is cleared and ventilation is established with a mask and an anesthesia bag capable of delivering an FIO_2 of 1.0.

   (b) A maximal inspiratory pressure of 25 cm H_2O with a rate of 30–40 breaths/min is usually adequate. However, higher pressures may be required to open collapsed alveoli, e.g., when initiating the first breath or in ventilating an infant with hyaline membrane disease (HMD). Pressure should always be monitored with an in-line manometer.

   (c) The adequacy of ventilation is assessed by listening for equal breath sounds over both hemithoraces and by observing chest wall motion. Pressure should be increased if the chest wall is not moving in spite of a tightly fitting face mask. A good response is shown by a rise in heart rate, good skin color, and an increase in the baby's activity. If these signs are not observed, the baby should be promptly intubated and ventilated.

   (d) After intubation, ventilation should be performed and the adequacy of ventilation reassessed as described in **(a)** and **(b)**. If ventilation is still not adequate, do the following:

   (i) Recheck the position of orotracheal tube to be sure it is not in the esophagus and, if in the trachea, is not advanced too far.

   (ii) Evaluate the infant for possible pneumothorax by auscultation, transillumination, or portable chest x-ray (see sec. **III.C**).

   (iii) If the tube is in a good position, there is no pneumothorax, and adequate ventilatory pressure is being used, anatomic or developmental abnormalities should be considered and ruled out by appropriate clinical or x-ray examinations (e.g., diaphragmatic hernia, hypoplastic lungs, severe lung immaturity).

(2) Nursery

(a) Continuous distending airway pressure (CDAP) is indicated:

   (i) In hyaline membrane disease (HMD), when an FIO_2 greater than 0.4–0.6 is required to maintain a PaO_2 of 50–70 mm Hg, or when there is significant clinical worsening during the 1st day of life. Application of CDAP early in the course of HMD decreases the time spent in high oxygen concentrations and lessens the need for mechanical ventilation.

   (ii) Apnea unresponsive to other forms of therapy (see sec. **III.D**)

   (iii) Contraindications to CDAP without positive-pressure ventilation are increasing $PaCO_2$, persistent acidosis, and diseases not associated with decreased pulmonary compliance.

(b) Intermittent positive-pressure ventilation (IPPV) is indicated:

   (i) In HMD, when the PaO_2 is less than 50 mm Hg at an FIO_2 of 0.6 in adequate CDAP.

   (ii) When PCO_2 is over 60–70 mm Hg from any cause

   (iii) In persistent respiratory acidosis

   The actual levels of PaO_2 and $PaCO_2$ selected for intervention depend on the disease course. Respiratory support is adjusted so that PaO_2 = 50–70 mm Hg, $PaCO_2$ = 35–50 mm Hg, and pH = 7.30–7.40. These values are optimal in HMD and differ for certain diseases (e.g., persistent pulmonary hypertension).

b. Methods. For a detailed discussion of the methods used in providing CDAP or IPPV and recommendations for ventilation and care of the infant on the respirator, consult J. P. Cloherty and A. R. Stark (Eds.), *Manual of Neonatal Care*, Boston, Little, Brown, 1980.

c. Long-term complications of respirator therapy

(1) Bronchopulmonary dysplasia (BPD). Chronic lung disease in the form of bronchopulmonary dysplasia occurs in 5–30% of survivors of respirator therapy for HMD. These infants often require prolonged treatment with oxygen and respiratory therapy because of severe disease. Most recover slowly, although some may die of infection or cor pulmonale during the first year of life.

(2) Retrolental fibroplasia (RLF). Premature infants receiving oxygen therapy are at risk of retrolental fibroplasia. (To avoid visual impairment, close attention must be paid to PaO_2.) All premature infants treated with oxygen should have an ophthalmologic examination prior to discharge. In very small prematures (weighing < 1,000 gm) RLF may occur even if the PO_2 did not exceed 100. Some studies have shown that the use of Vitamin E may prevent severe RLF.

(3) Neurologic impairment is estimated to occur in 10–15% of the survivors of respirator therapy for HMD. Infants with less severe disease are presumably less affected.

(4) Familial psychopathology. Little is known about the long-term effects of HMD and its management on parent-infant interaction. The

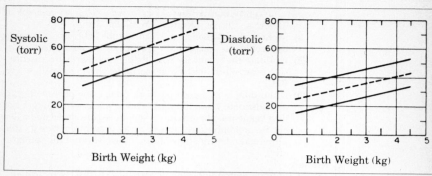

Fig. 6-3. Linear regressions (*broken lines*) and 95% confidence limits (*solid lines*) of systolic (*left*) and diastolic (*right*) aortic blood pressures on birth weight in 61 healthy newborn infants during the first 12 hours after birth. (From H. T. Versmold et al., *Pediatrics* 67:607, 1981. Copyright © 1981 by the American Academy of Pediatrics.)

incidence of child abuse may be high in infants who have significant medical problems at birth.

B. Shock. See Chap. 3, pp. 42ff, for a discussion of the causes and therapy of shock in the newborn. Figure 6-3 shows the normal blood pressure in healthy newborn infants of various birth weights during the first 12 hr of life.

C. Other emergency procedures

1. **Blood gases.** Samples may be obtained from a warmed heel in a heparinized Natelson tube by heel stick or by direct puncture of the radial, temporal, or posterior tibial artery. Brachial and femoral arterial punctures should be avoided. If the infant's condition is unstable, cannulation of the umbilical, radial, or posterior tibial arteries may be necessary.

2. **Umbilical artery catheters** aid greatly in parenteral therapy, monitoring blood gases, and withdrawing blood samples. However, **indwelling arterial catheters carry great potential dangers, including life-threatening infection and thromboembolism.**

   a. **Indications.** Umbilical artery catheters should not be used unless the infants under care are considered to have a high risk of death from their primary disease (e.g., gross prematurity, birth weight < 1,000 gm, HMD, severe aspiration pneumonia, shock).

   b. **Methods**

      (1) Complete sterility is required, including gloves, gown, and mask.

      (2) The cord and the surrounding area are washed carefully with povidone-iodine (Betadine) and alcohol, and the infant's abdomen is draped with sterile towels.

      (3) Cut the cord 1.0–1.5 cm from the skin. Tie the base with a cord tie.

      (4) Identify the arteries. Gently insert the tip of an iris forceps into the lumen of one artery. Allow the forceps to expand and dilate the artery while the cord stump is held between the thumb and forefinger.

      (5) Insert a saline-filled catheter (5F for infants weighing over 1,250 gm and 3.5F for infants weighing under 1,250 gm) into the artery for the appropriate distance (Fig. 6-4).

      (6) X-ray films should be taken after placement of all umbilical catheters. The tip should be either at or below the level of L3–L4 or just above the diaphragm (T6–T10).

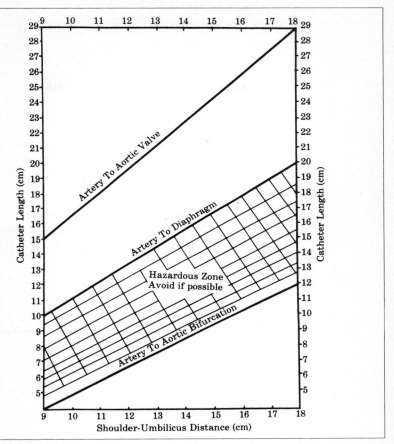

Fig. 6-4. Shoulder-umbilicus distance measured above lateral end of clavicle to umbilicus versus length of umbilical artery catheter needed to reach designated level. (From P. M. Dunn, *Arch. Dis. Child.* 41:69, 1966.)

   (7) When adequate placement is assured, the catheter should be secured by a suture as well as by adhesive tape. The umbilical stump should be covered with an antimicrobial agent (e.g., Betadine ointment) and left open to air.
   (8) The infusion solution should contain 1 U of heparin/ml of infusate.
   (9) Arterial catheters should be removed as soon as possible. Use of the transcutaneous PO_2 monitor and heel-stick blood gas determinations will permit this.
3. **Umbilical vein catheters**
   a. **Indications.** Umbilical vein catheters are used for emergency access to the circulation and for exchange transfusion. Because of the risks of thrombosis and infection they are not used for chronic care. Small prematures ($\approx$ 750 gm) may have to be managed with umbilical vein catheters.

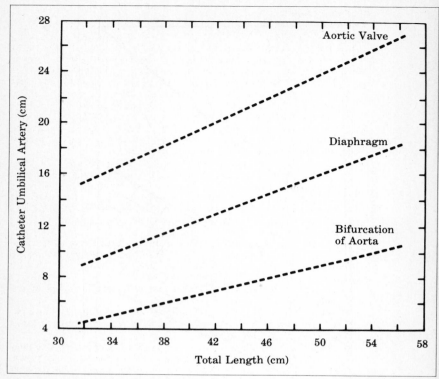

Fig. 6-5. Length from shoulder to umbilicus versus length of umbilical vein catheter. (From P. M. Dunn, *Arch. Dis. Child.* 41:69, 1966.)

In the latter case, it must be verified by x-ray that the catheter is in the vena cava or right atrium before hypertonic infusions are begun.

   b. Methods

     (1) Prepare as for umbilical artery catheterization.

     (2) Identify the vein, remove visible clots, and dilate with an iris forceps.

     (3) Insert a saline-filled, 5F (< 1,250 gm) or 8F (> 1,250 gm) catheter. A multiholed catheter is used for exchange transfusions, a single-holed catheter for long-term replacement (see Fig. 6-5 for position).

     (4) When free blood flow is achieved (usually at a distance of 5–7 cm), the catheter is adequately placed for exchange transfusion.

     (5) Keep the catheter and surrounding area sterile during exchange transfusion. In general, conditions as close to sterile as possible should be maintained in long-term placement as well.

     (6) Following exchange, place a purse-string silk suture around the vein before removing the catheter. For subsequent exchanges the cord should be soaked with warm saline until it is soft. The suture will assist in identification of the vein and reinsertion of the catheter.

III. Respiratory diseases

  A. Hyaline membrane disease (HMD)

    1. Etiology. The cause of HMD is an absence or deficiency of surfactant, a phospholipid that normally lines alveoli. The disease is associated with prematurity and factors that affect lung maturation and surfactant production.

2. **Prenatal evaluation**
   a. Measurement of the lecithin-sphingomyelin (L/S) ratio and disaturated phosphotidyl choline (DSPC) concentration in amniotic fluid is a reliable index of fetal lung development in pregnancies that are not complicated by maternal diabetes or Rh sensitization. The incidence of HMD is under 5% if the L/S ratio is greater than or equal to 2:1. The incidence is 1% if the DSPC is greater than or equal to 500 µg/100 ml. The L/S ratio must be greater than 3.5 to 1 and DSPC greater than or equal to 1,000 to predict pulmonary maturity in infants of diabetic mothers.
   b. **Use of maternal corticosteroids.** If an infant of less than 33 weeks' gestation with evidence of pulmonary immaturity (L/S < 2:1) must be delivered, alleviation of pulmonary immaturity may be accomplished by the administration of glucocorticoids to the mother.
      (1) A full course of **dexamethasone,** 4 mg IM q8h for 48 hr, or beta-methasone, 12 mg IM q24h for 48 hr, must be given to ensure a beneficial effect.
      (2) If the infant remains undelivered for more than 7 days after the course of glucocorticoids, the AF should be retested and if the L/S and DSPC are still immature a repeat course should be given.
3. **Postnatal evaluation**
   a. Signs and symptoms of HMD include grunting respirations, retractions, tachypnea, and hypoxia starting shortly after birth. The infant is usually premature.
   b. **Laboratory studies**
      (1) Gastric aspirate should be obtained during the first hour of life for the following:
         (a) A gram stain for neutrophils and bacteria (5 neutrophils/high-power field or the presence of bacteria in the first hour of life is associated with infection)
         (b) A gastric aspirate shake test to assess the amount of pulmonary surfactant in the newborn's lungs if the L/S ratio is not known. This test has an approximately 10% false-negative rate, but only 1% false-positive. The gastric aspirate must be uncontaminated with blood or meconium to give a reliable result. It is performed as follows:
            (i) Absolute alcohol, 0.5 ml, is added to 0.5 ml of gastric aspirate in a 4-ml glass tube, 82.0 by 10.25 mm (No. 4852 Red Stopper Tube, Becton, Dickinson & Co.) (as supplied new from the manufacturer). The test tube, capped by the thumb, is vigorously shaken for 15 sec and allowed to stand for 15 min.
            (ii) The test is then **read** as follows:

Negative	No bubbles
1 +	Very small bubbles in meniscus extending one-third or less of the distance around the test tube (a magnifying glass is usually required to determine that these small bubbles are indeed bubbles as opposed to particles)
2 +	A single rim of bubbles extending one-third to all around the test tube (a magnifying glass is not necessary)
3 +	A rim of bubbles all the way around the test tube

            (iii) The test is **interpreted** as follows:

Negative	High risk of HMD
1 + or 2 +	Intermediate risk of HMD
3 +	Little chance of HMD

      (2) **Chest x-ray.** Classically, this shows generalized reticulogranular pattern with air bronchograms.

(3) Arterial blood gas (ABG) should be obtained and $TcPO_2$ monitoring (if available) begun.

(4) An ECG and several blood pressure measurements should be taken.

(5) Cultures should be made of the skin (nose, throat, ear canal, umbilicus, and rectum), gastric aspirate, urine, and blood. Spinal fluid should be included if the infant's condition allows.

(6) A CBC, including a platelet count, should be obtained. Hematocrit, electrolytes, glucose, calcium, and bilirubin should be determined initially and followed every 6–12 hr thereafter, depending on the clinical status of the infant and the observed rate of change of the individual variables. Smaller low-birth weight infants, in whom rapid changes in fluid and metabolic balance are more likely, should be monitored more frequently.

4. **Treatment**
   a. **Oxygen**
      (1) **Dosage.** Sufficient oxygen should be used to maintain the PaO_2 at about 60–70 mm Hg. Care must be taken to administer the lowest oxygen concentration required to maintain adequate arterial saturation. Oxygen should be fully, but not excessively, warmed and humidified and the humidity chamber changed daily to avoid bacterial growth. Oxygen should be administered via oxygen-air blenders that allow precise control over the concentration of administered oxygen. The oxygen concentrations being administered should be checked at least every hour. If an infant requires intermittent assisted ventilation with a Mapleson bag, the oxygen concentration administered via the bag should be similar to that usually required by the infant. When supplemental oxygen is used, PaO_2 should be checked no less than q4–6h—more frequently if the status of the infant is changing rapidly. Blood gases should be obtained 15–20 min after a change in respiratory therapy. The use of a transcutaneous PO_2 ($TcPO_2$) monitor allows the continuous assessment of the infant's oxygenation and decreases the need for frequent arterial or capillary blood gas monitoring.

      (2) **Toxicity. Arterial oxygen concentration (PaO_2) over 100 mm Hg may be hazardous to the retina.**

      (3) **Delivery of oxygen.** If the infant's oxygen requirement exceeds that which can be delivered by hood (PaO_2 is less than 50 mm Hg and FIO_2 is greater than 0.6), or if hypercapnia ($PaCO_2 > 60$ mm Hg) or apnea uncontrolled by other therapies is present, the use of CDAP or mechanical ventilation is indicated (see sec. II.A.4).

   b. Careful attention should be paid to **temperature control**, especially in the low-birth-weight infant (see Chap. 5, p. 130).

   c. Normal **fluid and electrolyte requirements** should be provided (see sec. VIII). Careful monitoring of electrolytes, calcium, glucose, bilirubin, and hydration status is essential, especially in the low-birth-weight infant, who is particularly susceptible to rapid fluid and metabolic changes.

   d. Severe metabolic acidosis should be corrected with bicarbonate infusion. In profound metabolic acidosis, treat by infusing a solution of 0.25–0.5 mg $NaHCO_3$/ml to correct the calculated base deficit (mEq = 0.3 × kg × base deficit) at a rate no faster than 1 mEq/kg/min. If the acidosis is less severe (pH < 7.25 but > 7.10), correct by slow infusion over several hours of a $NaHCO_3$-dextrose solution to replace the calculated deficit. A solution of 15 mEq of $NaHCO_3$/100 ml of 5 or 10% D/W will provide adequate treatment of the acidosis while avoiding the use of hyperosmolar solutions, which have been associated with intraventricular hemorrhage in the premature neonate. **Always be sure that the infant is adequately ventilated before administrating $NaHCO_3$.**

   e. Follow the **blood pressure** carefully (see Fig. 6-3). If the infant is hypovolemic, maintain intravascular volume with slow transfusions of packed RBC or fresh frozen plasma (FFP) as appropriate, depending on the infant's hematocrit and clinical status.

    f. Maintain adequate **blood volume** and **oxygen-carrying capacity** by transfusion with packed RBCs if the hematocrit is less than 40–45% or blood loss from blood sampling is greater than 7–10% of estimated blood volume. Monitor blood glucose with Dextrostix frequently during transfusions to avoid hypoglycemia secondary to the interruption of the IV dextrose infusion.

    g. Because pneumonia can mimic the symptoms and x-ray picture of HMD, antibiotic coverage (e.g., ampicillin and an aminoglycoside) should be started after appropriate cultures have been obtained. If clinical and laboratory evaluation make infection unlikely and cultures are negative, antibiotics may be discontinued after 72 hr.

    h. Hypocalcemia and hyperbilirubinemia should be corrected as described in secs. **VI.D.3** and **V.A.3.**

    i. **Nutritional requirements** should be provided. If the course of the illness is relatively mild, feedings may often be begun by the third or fourth day. In more severe illnesses, however, this may not be possible, and IV hyperalimentation can be used to provide additional calories (see Chap. 10, pp. 257ff).

    j. The infant should be observed closely for the development of complications such as intraventricular hemorrhage, patent ductus arteriosus, pneumothorax, retrolental fibroplasia, and bronchopulmonary dysplasia.

B. Meconium aspiration before or during birth can obstruct airways, interfere with gas exchange, increase pulmonary vascular resistance, and cause severe respiratory distress.

    1. Etiology. One-half of infants with meconium-stained amniotic fluid have meconium in the trachea on suction. Such infants frequently are postmature or have suffered intrapartum asphyxia.

        a. Prevention of passage of meconium in utero. Tests of fetal well-being, such as nonstress testing with fetal monitoring and scalp pH sampling, may be done in pregnancies with evidence of uteroplacental insufficiency. High-risk pregnancies include those in women with toxemia or hypertension, in heavy smokers, in chronic maternal disease, with poor fetal growth, and in postmaturity.

        b. Prevention of meconium aspiration

            (1) When thick particulate or "pea-soup" meconium is present, the obstetrician should attempt to clear the infant's nose and oropharynx before the chest is born. This can be done with a bulb syringe followed by the passage of a de Lee catheter through the nose to the oropharynx.

            (2) When the birth is completed, the infant should then be passed to the anesthesiologist or pediatrician, who should suction the trachea with the largest orotracheal tube that will fit. The tube should be introduced **into the trachea** under direct laryngoscopy and sucked by mouth as it is being withdrawn. Two to four intubations are usually sufficient.

            (3) Oxygen by mask should be administered after the trachea has been cleared.

            (4) To the extent possible the airway should be cleared and ventilation initiated *before* significant bradycardia occurs. Once the child has had a few breaths, meconium in the airway has moved from the trachea to the smaller bronchi, so exhaustive attempts to remove it at that point are unwise. Similarly, *no* positive pressure should be used until *after* the trachea is sucked out.

            (5) The trachea should also be suctioned in infants with thin meconium and Apgar scores of 6 or less.

    2. Evaluation and diagnosis

        a. The severity of the disease is directly related to the amount and thickness of the meconium.

b. If tachypnea or respiratory distress increases, evaluation should include:

   (1) Arterial blood gas (ABG) determination. Unlike infants with HMD, in meconium aspiration arterial desaturation due to right-to-left shunting is likely to be more of a problem than is carbon dioxide retention.

   (2) Chest x-rays of infants with meconium aspiration show coarse, irregular pulmonary densities. Also, 10–20% of infants may have associated pneumothorax or pneumomediastinum.

   (3) A CBC and calcium and glucose determination should be done.

   (4) If an infiltrate is seen on the chest x-ray, cultures of the blood, skin, and trachea are indicated, because meconium enhances the growth of bacteria, and differentiating pneumonia from meconium aspiration is difficult.

3. Therapy

   a. Infants with significant aspiration often have severe problems. Following diagnosis:

   (1) Respiratory physiotherapy and **oropharyngeal suction** should be done every 30 min for the first 2 hr and every hour for the next 8 hr. The trachea should be suctioned if a tube is in place.

   (2) Hypoxia should be eliminated by increasing the inspired oxygen concentration, and severe metabolic acidosis should be corrected with a bicarbonate infusion (see sec. **A.4.d**). Careful monitoring of blood gases is essential, and the placement of an indwelling arterial catheter for blood sampling and infusion is usually required. For persistent hypoxia ($PaO_2 < 50$ mm Hg) or for severe hypercapnia ($PaCO_2 > 60$ mm Hg), intubation and mechanical ventilation are indicated (see sec. **I.B.2** and **3**).

   (3) Maintenance fluid and electrolyte requirements should be provided. Hematocrit, electrolytes, calcium, and glucose should be monitored carefully. Transfuse with packed RBCs if the hematocrit is less then 40–45%.

   (4) The use of **antibiotics** is individualized, but, in general, if an infiltrate is seen on chest x-ray, broad-spectrum antibiotics are used after cultures have been obtained.

   (5) Hypoxia and acidosis may contribute to persistent pulmonary artery hypertension with continued severe hypoxia and right-to-left shunting of blood via the patent ductus arteriosus or foramen ovale. (For a full discussion of the evaluation and management of persistent pulmonary hypertension see J. P. Cloherty and A. R. Stark (Eds.), *Manual of Neonatal Care*, Boston, Little, Brown, 1980).

   (6) Pneumothorax or pneumomediastinum develops in approximately 10–20% of infants with meconium aspiration. Therefore, close observation for the development of this complication is indicated. (See **C** for a discussion of air leaks and their management.)

C. Air leak

   1. Etiology. Air leak in the newborn infant results from alveolar rupture or dissection of air into the pulmonary parenchyma outside the bronchial tree. Infants who have HMD or pneumonia, or who have required resuscitation, or who have sustained meconium aspiration are at increased risk of pneumothorax.

   2. Evaluation and diagnosis

   a. Clinical signs of **pneumothorax** develop rapidly and include moderate to severe respiratory distress, cyanosis, a shift of the apex beat, a change in breath sounds, a drop in blood pressure and perfusion.

   b. Pneumomediastinum may be manifested by subcutaneous emphysema. A dramatic change in blood pressure or perfusion may indicate a shift of the mediastinum or dissection of air along the aorta.

   c. Pneumopericardium will cause an immediate deterioration in blood pressure, heart rate, and arterial oxygen. This problem should be consid-

ered in the presence of pneumomediastinum and pneumothorax. It will
lead to death unless diagnosed and treated quickly.

  d. Anteroposterior and cross-table lateral x-rays will help differentiate
pneumothorax and pneumomediastinum from other causes of respiratory
distress.

  e. For acute evaluation of an infant who deteriorates dramatically, the
fiberoptic transilluminator may be used to diagnose pneumothorax.

3. Treatment

  a. Pneumothorax

    (1) Uncomplicated pneumothorax. In infants with no underlying pul-
monary disease or complicating therapy (respirator or positive end-
expiratory pressure [PEEP]) and who are not in distress from
pneumothorax or pneumomediastinum, there may be no continuing
air leak. Under these conditions, conservative therapy may be adequate. This consists of observation in an incubator, frequent small
feedings to minimize crying, and a follow-up x-ray. The extrapulmonary air will usually resolve in 24–48hr.

The use of 100% oxygen, while effective in speeding the resolution of
pneumothorax, **is not recommended** because of the danger of retrolental fibroplasia.

    (2) Needle aspiration. The occasional infant who has no underlying pul-
monary problem or continuing air leak, but **who is in distress** from
the pneumothorax, may be treated by **needle aspiration.**

      (a) Place the infant in a sitting position if possible.

      (b) Attach a 25-gauge needle to a 50-ml syringe via a three-way
stopcock. Place a hemostat about 1 cm from the needle tip to
prevent deep penetration.

      (c) The needle should enter through the second intercostal space in
the anterior axillary line lateral to the pectoralis major muscle.
Hit the rib with the needle and slide it over the top to minimize
the chance of bleeding from the intercostal artery.

      (d) If air continues to leak, a chest tube must be inserted. If the infant
is breathing or crying after the visceral pleura opposes the
parietal pleura, the needle tip may cause a bronchopleural fistula.
This is not a common occurrence, but it is prudent to remove the
needle as soon as possible.

    (3) Chest tube placement. Infants with a continuing air leak, underly-
ing pulmonary disease causing continued distress, or on respirator
therapy or PEEP require **chest tube placement** and suction for drainage of pneumothorax. This should be performed or supervised by experienced nursery personnel.

  b. Pneumomediastinum. Chest tubes are not placed in infants with
pneumomediastinum alone.

  c. Pneumopericardium

    (1) Symptomatic pneumopericardium may be drained using a 20-gauge,
1½-inch needle attached via a three-way stopcock to a 10–20-ml syringe.

      (a) Following surgical preparation, insert a needle at the subxyphoid
region, aiming for the posterior left shoulder, and, with suction on
the syringe, advance the needle until air appears.

      (b) When the air stops flowing, withdraw the needle.

    (2) Often, a single aspiration results in clinical improvement. About 25–
40% of patients will have a recurrent symptomatic pneumoperi-
dium, which may be treated as just described.

    (3) Infrequently, the pneumopericardium will act as if constant air drain-
age into the pericardial space has occurred. Placement of a 16-gauge
Intracath into the pericardial space is appropriate in this situation.

D. Apnea. In *apnea spells,* breathing is absent for a defined period of time (i.e., 15–

30 sec) or ineffective, after which such changes as bradycardia, cyanosis, pallor, hypotonia, or metabolic acidosis are seen. *Prolonged apnea* is apnea lasting over 16 sec in a full-term infant and over 20 sec in preterm infants. *Periodic breathing* is defined as pauses in breathing of 3 sec or longer, interrupted by respirations for less than 20 sec. *Disorganized breathing* is irregular breathing with short apnea and bradycardia.

Bradycardia and **cyanosis** are usually present after 20 sec of apnea, although they may occur more rapidly in the small premature infant. After 30–45 sec, **pallor** and hypotonia are seen, and the infant may be unresponsive to tactile stimulation. The majority of very small premature infants (under 30 weeks' gestational age) have occasional apneic spells. As many as 25% of all premature infants weighing under 1,800 gm (about 34 weeks) will have at least one apneic episode. These spells generally begin at 1–2 days of age and may recur for 2–3 weeks postnatally, although most occur within the first 10 days of life.

1. **Etiology**
   a. **Hypoxemia** from congenital heart disease, respiratory disease (HMD, pneumonia), anemia, or hypovolemia
   b. **Respiratory center depression** due to hypoglycemia, hypocalcemia, electrolyte disorders, sepsis, drugs, or intracranial disorders
   c. **Abnormal or hyperactive reflexes** due to suction or stimulation of the pharynx, fluid in the airway or pharynx from feeding or gastroesophageal reflux, and paradoxical apnea after lung inflation
   d. **Airway obstruction** due to passive neck flexion, pressure on the lower rim of a face mask, submental pressure, and supine position are all encountered during nursery procedures. Spontaneously occurring airway obstruction, which tends to occur when preterm infants assume a position of neck flexion, may contribute to the **prolongation** of apneic spells.
   e. **Temperature.** Apnea is more frequent in the absence of a skin-core temperature gradient. Infants in Isolettes servocontrolled to maintain skin temperatures at 36.8°C have more frequent spells than do those maintained at 36.0°C. Sudden increases in incubator temperature increase the frequency of apneic spells.
   f. *Apnea of prematurity* is prolonged apnea in the absence of any of the preceding conditions. It may be related to decreased CO_2 sensitivity or to decreased afferent stimulation from peripheral receptors.

2. **Monitoring and evaluation**
   a. All infants of less than 34 weeks' gestational age or weighing under 1,800 gm should be placed on heart rate monitors for at least 10 days. Since impedance apnea monitors may not distinguish respiratory efforts during airway obstruction from normal breaths, the **heart rate** should be monitored.
   b. When a monitor alarm sounds, the clinician should respond to the **infant,** not the monitor. Check for bradycardia, cyanosis, and airway obstruction.
   c. Following the first apneic spell, the infant should be evaluated for a possible underlying cause, and specific treatment should be initiated. A precipitating cause is more likely in infants of more than 33–34 weeks' gestational age. Treatable causes should be considered first.
   d. A bag and mask should be available near every infant being monitored for apnea. The oxygen concentration should be similar to that which the infant has been breathing. Equipment for intubation and full resuscitation should be present.

3. **Treatment**
   a. Individual spells are treated with diffuse tactile stimulation. Infants who fail to respond should be ventilated during the spell with bag and mask, generally with an FiO_2 of under 0.40 or equal to the FiO_2 prior to the spell, to avoid marked elevations in arterial PO_2.
   b. For repeated prolonged spells, i.e., more than two to three/hr or spells requiring frequent bagging, treatment should be initiated in the order of

increasing invasiveness and risk. The number of spells may be reduced by:

(1) Increasing afferent stimulation by rocker beds, oscillating water beds, or recurrent cutaneous stimulation

(2) A blood transfusion to elevate the hematocrit slightly (i.e., to about 45%), despite the absence of significant anemia

(3) Decreasing environmental temperature to the low end of the neutral thermal-environment range. Placing a heat shield around a small premature infant may prevent swings in temperature.

(4) It is important to avoid stimuli that may trigger apnea. These may be suctioning, nipple feeding, and cold or warm stimulation of the trigeminal area of the face.

(5) **Theophylline** PO or aminophylline IV in divided doses of 5–7 mg/kg/day q4–6h should be started if the preceding measures fail.

    (a) If the neonate has severe apneic spells and more rapid action is desired, a loading dose of aminophylline, 5–7 mg/kg IV over 1 hr, can be given. The usual maintenance doses can be given after 6 hr.

    (b) Serum levels should be obtained during therapy, and the dosage should be adjusted to maintain the theophylline concentration in the range of 7–13 μg/ml. The dosage should be reduced if tachycardia or GI toxicity becomes evident.

    (c) Clinical responses may be seen at levels from 3–14 μg/ml. The maximum response may take from 3–4 days.

(6) Caffeine citrate may decrease the frequency of apneic spells. As with theophylline, the acute and long-term toxicity of caffeine in newborn infants is not well established, although no significant heart rate changes are noted with caffeine. A suggested **dosage schedule** for caffeine citrate is a loading dose of 10–20 mg/kg PO or IV, followed by a maintenance dose of 5–10 mg/kg qd–bid for 3 days. The drug is then stopped for 24 hr and resumed if apnea recurs.

(7) Small increases in FIO_2 (0.25–0.26) may reduce the frequency of apneic spells. However, without a continuously reading oxygen electrode to monitor arterial oxygenation, the **risk of retrolental fibroplasia** makes this intervention relatively hazardous.

(8) In some infants, CPAP at low pressures (3–4 cm H_2O) is effective.

(9) If all these interventions fail, **mechanical ventilation** may be required until the infant matures.

(10) Most neonates with apnea of prematurity will not require therapy or monitoring by the time they are ready for discharge from the hospital. If infants are free of apnea for 2 weeks while being monitored in the hospital, their medication can be stopped. If they are free of apnea, off medication, for 2 weeks while being monitored in the hospital, it is usually safe to discharge them.

(11) If there is any concern about the possibility of recurrence of apnea, a pneumogram to assess breathing patterns, obstructive apnea, and bradycardia may be useful (the use of the pneumogram to predict apnea is controversial). If there is a documented need for medication (abnormal pneumogram or clinical apnea off medication), the pneumogram must be repeated with the infant on medication. If the infant is normal, he or she may be discharged on the same daily dose per kilogram and the blood level that was associated with a normal pneumogram.

(12) Monthly follow-up pneumograms with the infant off medication while being monitored are done to assess the need for continued medication.

(13) If pneumograms are abnormal or clinical apnea occurs at theophylline levels of 12–15 μg/ml, home monitoring may be required.

Each hospital should have its own guidelines for both hospital and home management of apnea of prematurity.

IV. Cardiac disease in the newborn. Severe congenital cardiac disease occurs in approximately 1 out of 400 infants.

A. Congestive heart failure

1. Etiology. Patent ductus arteriosus (PDA) in premature infants is the most common cause of congestive heart failure (CHF) in the newborn period. Other causes are hypoplastic left heart syndrome, complex congenital heart disease, myocarditis, arteriovenous fistula in the brain or liver, and idiopathic paroxysmal tachycardia.

2. Evaluation

    a. Common signs of heart failure in the newborn are tachycardia, tachypnea, hepatomegaly, cardiomegaly, and diaphoresis.

    b. ABGs, chest x-rays, ECG, echocardiography, radionuclide angiography, and cardiac catheterization are all useful in evaluation.

3. Diagnosis

    a. PDA. Most premature infants with PDA do not require cardiac catheterization, since a PDA is usually evident by clinical examination, and its hemodynamic significance can be quantitated by noninvasive tests.

        (1) For signs and symptoms see Table 6-2.

        (2) The diagnosis of a PDA can be confirmed and the amount of the left-to-right shunt quantitated by 2-dimension echocardiography.

    b. The diagnoses of other causes of CHF are also given in Table 6-2.

4. Treatment

    a. General medical treatment is directed toward decreasing the work load on the heart.

        (1) Although digoxin has been the mainstay of treatment in all age groups for many years, recent work suggests that **digoxin may be of little benefit to the very immature preterm infant with CHF secondary to PDA** (see Chap. 9, pp. 248ff).

        (2) Other therapeutic measures include diuretics, fluid restriction to under 120–150 ml/kg/day, use of a low-solute formula (e.g., Similac PM 60/40 or breast milk), maintenance of a neutral thermal environment (see Chap. 5, p. 130), and decreasing the work of feeding, e.g., gavage rather than nipple feedings.

        (3) For adequate myocardial oxygenation,

            (a) Maintain the hematocrit at over 40% (use packed red blood cells, 5 ml/kg, given over 2–4 hr and repeated as necessary) and

            (b) Increase FiO_2 as necessary to maintain the PaO_2 at 60–80 mm Hg.

    b. Cardiotonic drugs are the cornerstone of CHF treatment.

        (1) For specific recommendations regarding **digitalis** and **diuretics**, see Chap. 9, pp. 235, 250.

        (2) Isoproterenol (Isuprel). Isoproterenol can be used in severe CHF when other means fail to maintain adequate cardiac output (see Chaps. 3 and 9).

        (3) Dopamine has been used in the newborn for the treatment of severe hypotension. It has also been used to reverse the hypotensive effects of tolazoline (Priscoline) when it is used in the treatment of persistent fetal circulation.

    c. If the cardiac failure caused by the PDA is not adequately controlled by other medical treatments, a trial of indomethacin is warranted. (See J. P. Cloherty and A. R. Stark (Eds.), *Manual of Neonatal Care,* Boston, Little, Brown, 1980, p. 184, for a discussion of evaluation, dosage, potential side effects, and contraindications to the use of indomethacin.) If it is contraindicated, or it fails to be effective, surgical ligation of the ductus is indicated.

B. Cyanosis can indicate life-threatening illness.

1. **Etiology**
   a. The major cardiac causes of cyanosis in the newborn are transposition of the great arteries, critical pulmonary stenosis, or atresia, or both, tetralogy of Fallot, tricuspid atresia, anomalous pulmonary veins, and Ebstein's anomaly.
   b. Major pulmonary causes are HMD, meconium aspiration, pneumothorax, and persistent fetal circulation.

2. **Evaluation**
   a. These infants must be evaluated rapidly by ECG, chest x-ray, right radial ABGs in room air and 100% oxygen, and an echocardiogram. If available, a cardiologist should be promptly consulted.
   b. Early measurement of PaO_2 in 100% oxygen in a child with developing pulmonary disease can be helpful when cyanotic congenital heart disease is being considered later in the infant's course. Many infants with HMD may have a PaO_2 greater than 100 mm Hg in 100% oxygen early in their disease, but not by day 2 or 3. A PaO_2 over 150 in an adequately ventilated infant virtually excludes significant cyanotic heart disease.

3. **Treatment** of cardiac causes of cyanosis in the newborn is a **medical emergency.** The infant must be given enough oxygen to keep the PaO_2 over 60 mm Hg. Therapy for CHF as outlined in **A.4** must be given. Surgery is frequently required.

C. **Rhythm disturbances.** See also Chap. 9, p. 235.

1. **Bradycardia.** Both sinus bradycardia and that due to congenital heart block are rare.
   a. **Etiology.** Elevated intracranial pressure, hypertension, potassium intoxication, hypothyroidism, and congenital heart disease. Congenital heart block may be secondary to maternal collagen vascular disease.
   b. **Treatment**
      (1) Treat the underlying cause if possible. If the low heart rate persists after treatment but there is no evidence of cardiovascular compromise, observation without treatment is a wise course. In general, infants with a heart rate between 50–70 beats/min may be asymptomatic and need no treatment if they remain well for over 72 hr with a normal QRS complex on the ECG.
      (2) In infants with a heart rate under 50, respiratory distress, cyanosis, and CHF are frequent. Treatment consists in the use of a chronotropic agent such as isoproterenol to raise the heart rate acutely (see **A.4.b**). If asymptomatic bradycardia persists when medication is withdrawn, insertion of a pacemaker may be necessary.
      (3) When fetal heart rate monitoring indicates a pesistent fetal bradycardia, arrangements for a cardiologic consultation should be made prior to delivery.

2. **Paroxysmal atrial tachycardia (PAT)** is relatively common.
   a. **Etiology.** Congenital PAT may be associated with Wolff-Parkinson-White syndrome, structural congenital heart disease, or no evident cardiac abnormality.
   b. **Evaluation**
      (1) The heart rate is 200–300/min; P waves are rarely seen, and the QRS may be normal or abnormal.
      (2) If PAT is present prenatally, it carries a risk of CHF in utero, with a possibility of fetal hydrops, or stillbirth, or both. Treatment of the mother with digoxin should be instituted and early delivery planned in conjunction with determination of pulmonary maturity (L/S ratio).
   c. **Treatment** consists of attempts to convert to sinus rhythm. Infants in good condition at delivery can usually tolerate up to 24 hr of tachycardia without CHF.
      (1) Occasionally, infants respond to vagal stimulation (rectal examination) or pressure applied to the fontanelle.

Table 6-2. Presenting signs and findings in congenital heart disease

Diagnosis	Age	Presenting signs	Auscultation	X-ray findings	ECG
Transposition of the arteries					
Intact ventricular septum	First hours or days	Cyanosis	Unremarkable	Cardiac enlargement Pulmonary vasculature $\uparrow$	Right ventricular hypertrophy
Ventricular septal defect	First weeks	Congestive heart failure	Pansystolic murmur	Cardiac enlargement Pulmonary vasculature $\uparrow\uparrow$	Combined ventricular hypertrophy
Ventricular septal defect and pulmonic stenosis	First days or weeks	Cyanosis	Pansystolic and stenotic murmurs	Cardiac enlargement Pulmonary vasculature $\rightarrow$	Combined ventricular hypertrophy
Tetralogy of Fallot	First days or weeks	Cyanosis	Early stenotic murmur, single S_2 at upper left sternal border	Cardiac enlargement 0 Pulmonary vasculature $\downarrow$	Right ventricular hypertrophy
Pure pulmonary stenosis	First weeks or months, occasionally days	Cyanosis	Late stenotic murmur, widely split S_2, faint P_2	Cardiac enlargement + Pulmonary vasculature $\downarrow$	Right ventricular hypertrophy marked

Hypoplastic left heart	First days	Cyanosis and congestive heart failure, with all pulses ↓	Late systolic murmur; single S_2	Cardiac enlargement ++ Pulmonary vasculature ↑ ↑	Right ventricular hypertrophy marked
Ventricular septal defect	First weeks	Congestive heart failure	Pansystolic murmur, narrowly split S_2, loud P_2	Cardiac enlargement+ Pulmonary vasculature ↑	Combined ventricular hypertrophy
Coarctation of the aorta	First weeks	Congestive heart failure with hypertension, ↓ femoral pulses	Stenotic murmur across back	Cardiac enlargement+ Pulmonary vasculature (passive) ↑	Right ventricular hypertrophy
Patent ductus arteriosus with pulmonary artery hypertension	First weeks	Congestive heart failure Bounding pulses	Crescendic systolic murmur, ± early diastolic murmur, split S_2, loud P_2	Cardiac enlargement+ Pulmonary vasculature ↑	Combined ventricular hypertrophy

  (2) Infants with PAT should be rapidly digitalized whether or not the are responsive to vagal stimulation.

  (3) Verapamil, a calcium channel–blocking agent, has been used success fully in the treatment of supraventricular tachycardias in the new born. This drug should be used under guidance of a pediatric car diologist experienced in the use of this medication.

  (4) If the infant's clinical state deteriorates, cardioversion may be neces sary. Begin at 10 watt-sec and increase by 10 watt-sec until successfu reversion to sinus rhythm occurs. After normal sinus rhythm is estab lished, digoxin therapy is usually maintained for 6–12 months.

V. Hematologic problems

A. Jaundice (including erythroblastosis)

1. Etiology

 a. *Physiologic hyperbilirubinemia* in full-term infants is defined as uncon jugated hyperbilirubinemia (total serum bilirubin < 12 mg/100 ml, di rect fraction < 15% of the total) that appears on or after the third day o life and resolves prior to 10 days. It is caused by an increased biliru bin load and poor hepatic uptake conjugation and excretion of bilirubin The same factors in the premature infant may cause the bilirubi to go higher. The term *physiologic* does not imply that the bilirubin i nontoxic.

 b. *Nonphysiologic jaundice* is jaundice due to an abnormality of bilirubi production, metabolism, or excretion. It is manifested by clinical jaundic (bilirubin > 7) in the first 36 hr of life, a total bilirubin over 12 in a full term infant or over 15 in a premature infant, and by direct bilirubin ove 1.5–2.0 or clinical jaundice over 10 days in a full-term infant or over : weeks in a premature infant.

  (1) Indirect hyperbilirubinemia. Direct bilirubin is less than 15% of the total bilirubin. The causes of nonphysiologic hyperbilirubinemia i the neonate are as follows:

   (a) Excess bilirubin production due to

    (i) Maternal-fetal blood group incompatibility

    (ii) Hereditary spherocytosis

    (iii) Hemolytic anemia

    (iv) Extravascular extravasation of blood

    (v) Polycythemia

    (vi) Swallowed blood

    (vii) Increased enterohepatic circulation of bilirubin as in pylori stenosis, delayed emptying of the intestine, and poor flui intake

    (viii) Genetic and ethnic factors

   (b) Decreased clearance of bilirubin due to

    (i) Errors of metabolism, including familial nonhemolyti jaundice type I and II (Crigler-Najjar syndrome), Gilber syndrome, Dubin-Johnson syndrome, Rotor syndrome galactosemia, tyrosinosis, and hypermethionemia

    (ii) Prematurity

    (iii) Endocrine abnormalities of hypothyroidism and hy popituitarism, breast-feeding infants of diabetic mother.

    (iv) Poor perfusion of the liver

  (2) Direct hyperbilirubinemia (direct bilirubin > 15% of the total biliru bin). Causes of direct hyperbilirubinemia are sepsis; intrauterine vi ral infections; neonatal hepatitis, intrahepatic biliary atresia syn drome, extrahepatic biliary atresia, choledocal cyst, biliary trac obstruction by an abdominal mass or annular pancreas; trisomy 18 galactosemia; tyrosinemia; Rotor syndrome; Dubin-Johnson syn drome; hypermethionemia; alpha$_1$-antitrypsin deficiency; cysti fibrosis; posthemolytic disease of the newborn syndrome (inspissate bile syndrome); and prolonged total parenteral nutrition.

2. Evaluation and diagnosis

  a. Infants who appear jaundiced have serum bilirubin levels greater than 6 mg/100 ml. A full-term infant whose bilirubin is over 5 mg/100 ml within the first 24 hr of life, over 10 mg/100 ml within the first 48 hr, or over 13 mg/100 ml after 72 hr requires investigation. Premature or sick infants should have daily serum bilirubin measurements until they are past the danger of hyperbilirubinemia. In infants known to be at risk of hyperbilirubinemia, such as infants born to Rh-sensitized mothers, cord blood bilirubin should be measured.

  Other tests to evaluate jaundice and place the infant in the correct diagnostic group include direct and indirect bilirubin; the blood groups of mother and infant; a direct Coombs test and identification of the antibody if it is positive; a CBC, blood smear for red cell morphologic study, and a reticulocyte count. In persistent jaundice or direct hyperbilirubinemia liver function tests are indicated.

  b. While tests to assess bilirubin binding may help predict whether the infant is at increased or decreased risk, none is reliable enough to predict the absolute safety of any bilirubin level.

  c. *Kernicterus* is a toxic effect of non-albumin-bound, unconjugated bilirubin on the CNS. Susceptibility to kernicterus is increased by factors that decrease albumin binding (hypoalbuminemia; elevated free fatty acids; lipid infusion or sepsis with catecholamine-stimulated lipolysis; acidosis; hypoglycemia; sulfonamides; organic anions) and factors that increase diffusion of free bilirubin into the brain (increased concentration of bilirubin and/or increased duration of exposure to elevated levels of bilirubin; anoxic-ischemic encephalopathy).

  d. Sublethal bilirubin encephalopathy results in mild CNS developmental deficits.

3. Treatment

  a. The goal of evaluation is to decide at what serum bilirubin level treatment should be instituted to avoid kernicterus or sublethal bilirubin encephalopathy.

   (1) In full-term infants, kernicterus is unlikely to occur if indirect bilirubin concentrations are kept under 20 mg/100 ml, provided there are no factors disturbing the blood-brain barrier or interfering with the binding of bilirubin to albumin. As far as is known at present, no absolute level exists below which there is no risk of bilirubin encephalopathy.

   (2) Kernicterus has been described at autopsy in premature infants whose bilirubin levels never exceeded 10 mg/100 ml. However, there is no consistent relationship between subsequent neurologic development and bilirubin levels in low-birth-weight infants if bilirubin levels stay under 20 mg/100 ml. The bilirubin encephalopathy seen in low-birth-weight infants may be related more to alterations in the blood-brain barrier caused by anoxia, ischemia, or hyperosmolarity than to the actual bilirubin level.

  b. The general guidelines used for treatment are in Figs. 6-6 and 6-7. The goal of therapy is to prevent the presence of unconjugated free (unbound) bilirubin in the serum of all infants and to prevent bilirubin encephalopathy.

   (1) Establish that the baby has adequate fluid intake. In breast-fed infants, supplement the diet with 5% D/W or formula if indicated. Give IV fluids if indicated.

   (2) Correct asphyxia, hypotension, hypoxia, hypothermia, and hypoglycemia. Avoid drugs that may interfere with the binding of bilirubin to albumin, and avoid factors that may disturb the blood-brain barrier.

  c. Phototherapy

   (1) Indications

    (a) Phototherapy should be instituted if there is a risk that unconjugated bilirubin will rise to levels that might saturate albumin-binding sites or that would possibly result in the need for an exchange transfusion.

(b) Prophylactic phototherapy may be indicated in special circumstances (i.e., in tiny infants in whom dangerous levels of bilirubin are likely to develop; in severely bruised prematures; in hemolytic disease while waiting for exchange transfusion). In hemolytic disease, phototherapy is used as an adjunct to exchange transfusion.

(c) Effectiveness. The amount of skin exposure and radiant energy impinging on the skin are of primary importance for effective phototherapy. Blue light (wavelength 450–500 nm) is more effective in lowering bilirubin, but cool white light provides better visualization of cyanosis in the infant. We use light banks which have alternating blue and white lights.

(2) Technique of phototherapy

(a) Shield both the infant's eyes. Observe the infant for nasal obstruction from the eye shields.

(b) Be certain all electric outlets are properly grounded.

(c) Use a Plexiglass cover or shield to prevent harm to the infant in case of lamp breakage and to screen out wavelengths below 300 nm, thus protecting the infant from ultraviolet light.

(d) Placing lights over, beside, and under the baby will increase the exposure. Lights can be placed under the baby by using a transparent plastic crib and placing the baby on a plastic air bubble mattress.* The baby should be turned over q4h.

(e) Monitor the temperature q2h to prevent hypothermia or hyperthermia. Use a control alarm if possible and a servocontrolled incubator if necessary.

(f) Weigh the infant daily—or, if the infant is small, twice daily—and provide extra fluid as necessary.

(g) Do not use skin color as a guide to hyperbilirubinemia in infants under phototherapy. Instead, monitor bilirubin at least q12h.

(h) Change the lamps q2,000h of use (alternatively, change them all every 3 months). Monitoring the energy output in the range of 425–475 nm will give more precise information on energy output.

(3) Side effects include:

(a) Increased insensible water loss, which requires a 20–30% increase in fluid intake

(b) Transient rashes

(c) Diarrhea

(d) Bronze baby syndrome, a rare complication usually seen in infants with parenchymal hepatic disease who are treated with phototherapy. Do not use phototherapy in infants with liver disease or obstructive jaundice.

(4) Toxicity. No significant long-term toxicity has been described. However, phototherapy should be used with the same caution as with any other treatment.

d. Exchange transfusion

(1) Indications

(a) Exchange transfusion should be instituted to correct severe anemia or if evaluation of bilirubin levels indicates any potential that free (unbound to albumin) unconjugated bilirubin could be present or that the infant is at risk of bilirubin encephalopathy (see **2**) (see Figs. 6-6 and 6-7). The level of bilirubin at which exchange transfusion is recommended for low-birth-weight infants is controversial. There are no studies which permit recom-

*Thermo-GARD, Tower Products, Inc., 1919 South Butterfield Road, Mundelein, Ill. 60600

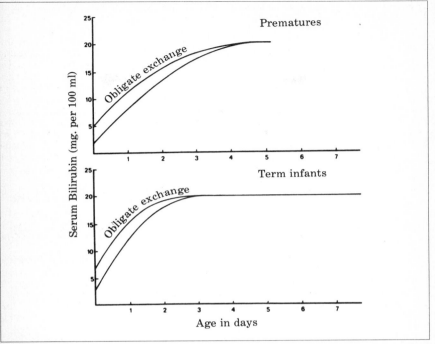

Fig. 6-6. Serum bilirubin levels plotted against age in premature and full-term infants with erythroblastosis. Levels above the top line are predictive of an ultimate bilirubin level of over 20 unless the natural course is altered by treatment. Levels below the bottom line predict that the level will not eventually reach 20. Between the lines is an intermediate zone where the ultimate level could be below or above 20. (Adapted from J. Lucey et al., *Pediatrics* 41:1, 1968.)

mendations to be made for the treatment of low-birth-weight infants with bilirubins under 20 mg/dl. Current recommendations from the American Academy of Pediatrics (*Guidelines for Perinatal Care*, 1983) state:

Many physicians currently use published guidelines and are aggressive in their treatment of jaundice in low-birth-weight neonates, initiating phototherapy early and performing exchange transfusions in certain neonates with very low bilirubin levels (<10 mg/dl). Nevertheless, it must be recognized that this will not prevent kernicterus consistently. Some pediatricians may prefer to adopt a more conservative therapeutic stance and allow serum bilirubin levels to approach 15–20 mg/ dl (257–342 µmol/liter), even in low-birth-weight neonates, before considering exchange transfusion. At present, both of these approaches to treatment must be considered acceptable. In either case, the finding of low bilirubin kernicterus at autopsy in certain low-birth-weight neonates cannot necessarily be interpreted as a therapeutic failure. Like retrolental fibroplasia, kernicterus is a condition that, in certain neonates, is essentially unpreventable.

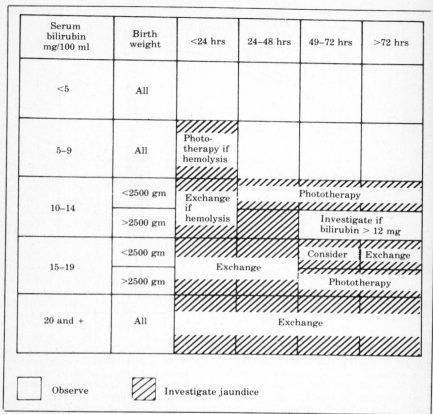

Fig. 6-7. Guidelines for the management of hyperbilirubinemia. Phototherapy should be used after any exchange transfusion. Hyperbilirubinemia should be treated as though it were in the next higher category in the presence of the following: (1) perinatal asphyxia, (2) respiratory distress, (3) metabolic acidosis (pH 7.25 or below), (4) hypothermia (temperature below 35°C), (5) low serum protein (5 gm/100 ml or less) (6) birth weight less than 1,500 gm, and (7) signs of clinical or central nervous system deterioration. (From M. J. Maisels, in G. B. Avery [Ed.], *Neonatology*. Philadelphia: Lippincott, 1972.)

(b) Failure of phototherapy to control bilirubin levels in hemolytic disease is a frequent indication.

(c) Early exchange transfusion is often indicated in the presence of hydrops, in a known sensitized infant, or in an infant with anemia.

(d) The indications for immediate (at birth) exchange transfusion are hydrops or severe anemia. When a hydropic baby is expected, preparation for exchange should begin by alerting blood bank personnel prior to delivery, thus avoiding unnecessary delay.

(e) A cord hemoglobin < 12 mg/100 ml and a cord indirect bilirubin > 3.5 mg/100 ml are usually indications for exchange transfusion, but the rate of rise of the indirect serum bilirubin is the best indication. A bilirubin rise of over 0.5 mg/100 of ml/hr usually signifies a need for exchange transfusion.

   (f) Late exchange transfusion in hemolytic disease is usually indicated when the bilirubin in full-term infants is 10 mg/100 ml at 24 hr and 15 mg/100 ml at 48 hr in spite of phototherapy.

(2) Blood preparations for exchange transfusions

   (a) Fresh (under 24-hr-old) **blood** should be used in sick infants. In other cases, blood under 72 hr old should be used to prevent problems with hyperkalemia and acidosis.

   (b) Irradiated blood should be used if the infant has received intrauterine transfusions.

   (c) Heparinized blood (usually 25 mg of heparin/500 ml) has the advantage of causing little effect on the ionized calcium, electrolytes, and acid-base balance in recipient infants. The disadvantages are as follows: It must be used within 24 hr of drawing; it may have a low glucose level, resulting in hypoglycemia during an exchange transfusion; and heparin causes a rise in nonesterified free fatty acids, which may interfere with binding of bilirubin to albumin. Heparin may also interfere with coagulation of the infant's blood. Heparinized blood bags are not available in most centers.

   (d) Citrate-phosphate-dextrose (CPD) blood has the advantage that it can be used up to 72 hr after drawing and that there is no rise in nonesterified free fatty acids in recipients. The disadvantages are as follows: low pH (6.9–7.0), which may not be tolerated by sick infants; hypernatremia; high glucose content, which may cause late hypoglycemia in hyperinsulinemic infants with erythroblastosis; and binding of calcium and magnesium. Sodium, potassium and the pH of blood should be checked if the blood is over 48 hr old.

   (e) Fresh (<24 hr old) heparinized or CPD blood should be used in hydropic or otherwise compromised newborns. Blood should be compatible with the mother's, with a low titer of anti-A and anti-B. Subsequent transfusions should be done with blood compatible with that of the mother and infant.

   (f) Acid-base problems, hyperkalemia, and hypernatremia can be avoided by using centrifuged packed red cells under 72 hr old resuspended in thawed fresh frozen AB plasma just prior to exchange.

   (g) In all blood over 4 hr old there are defects in platelet function.

(3) Technique of exchange transfusion. Asphyxia, hypoglycemia, acidosis, and temperature problems should all be corrected before exchange transfusion.

   (a) General. In all infants, exchange should be done under a radiant heater, servocontrolled to the infant. A cardiac monitor should be in place, as should a reliable peripheral IV line to improve glucose control during and after the exchange.

   (b) The umbilical vein should be used if possible. If the umbilical vein cannot be entered, the safest route is through a central venous pressure (CVP) line placed through the antecubital fossa (see Chap. 3, p. 91) This line can be left in for future exchanges.

   (c) In sick, hydropic infants, exchange is best performed through umbilical arterial and venous catheters, so that blood may be removed and replaced simultaneously.

   (d) In sick infants who are anemic (hematocrit under 35%) a partial exchange transfusion can be given with packed red blood cells (25–80 ml/kg) to raise the hematocrit to 40%. After stabilization, more exchange transfusions can be given for hyperbilirubinemia.

The blood for these exchanges should be set up prior to deliver and packed with the plasma separated into a side bag, so that i can be remixed if a packed cell exchange is unnecessary.

(e) Albumin (salt-poor albumin, 1 gm/kg 1–2 hr prior to exhange increases the amount of bilirubin removed by the exchange. A bumin is contraindicated in CHF or severe anemia and is nc usually used in early exchanges in which the goal is to remov sensitized red cells rather than bilirubin.

(f) An infant's blood volume is usually about 80 mg/kg, and ex change transfusion should be done using double the infant's bloo volume (160 ml/kg), in aliquots of 10–20 ml, depending on th infant's tolerance for the procedure. (An aliquot should neve exceed 10% of the infant's estimated blood volume.) A usefu approach is to start with 10-ml aliquots, increasing to 20-ml ali quots in infants weighing over 2 kg if all goes well. A two-volum exchange removes 87% of the infant's red blood cells.

(g) The rate of exchange has little effect on the amount of bilirubi removed; however, small aliquots and a slower rate reduce th stress on cardiovascular adaptation. The recommended time fo an exchange in a full-term infant is 1 hr.

(h) Blood should be kept at 37°C by a temperature-controlled wate bath that has an alarm to signal overheating.

(i) Blood should be gently shaken often, since the RBCs will settl rapidly, and the settling can lead to an exchange with relativel anemic blood at the end of the exchange.

(j) If heparinized blood is used, a Dextrostix blood sugar should b obtained from the blood and from the baby during the exchange 10 ml of 5% dextrose can be given as an umbilical vein push afte each 100 ml of blood if necessary. If the catheter tip rests abov the liver, a more concentrated sugar solution may be used. Whe citrated blood is used, the infant's blood sugar should be checkec for several hours after the exchange, and oral feedings or par enteral glucose should be given.

(k) When using CPD, most infants will not require additional cal cium; following cessation of exchange transfusion, the Ca^{2+} leve rapidly returns to normal. If needed, 0.5–2.0 ml of 10% calciun gluconate may be given following each 100 ml of exchange blood However, this measure increases the ionized Ca fraction only temporarily. There is a risk of severe bradycardia unless calciun is given very slowly.

(l) Heparinized blood usually contains 25 mg of heparin/500 ml o blood. **Protamine** is administered following the exchange to neu tralize the heparin estimated to be remaining in the baby (1 m protamine/mg of heparin left in the baby—usually 10 mg in a 3 kg baby).

(m) When the transfusion is finished, place a silk purse string sutur around the vein and leave a "tail" so that it will be easy to find th vein for the next exchange.

(n) When the catheter is removed, the cord tie is "snugged up" for ar hour. If it is not removed, skin necrosis may occur.

(o) The venous catheter should be removed by pulling all the way ou quickly.

(p) Although their use is controversial, prophylactic antibiotics are recommended if a catheter was passed through an old, dirty cord if there is great difficulty in passing the catheter, or if there are multiple exchanges.

(q) Subsequent exchange is indicated at bilirubin levels suggesting that unbound bilirubin is potentially present (Figs. 6-6 and 6-7)

(4) Complications of exchange transfusions
  (a) Vascular. Embolization with air or clots, and thrombosis
  (b) Cardiac. Arrhythmias, volume overload, and arrest
  (c) Electrolytes. Hyperkalemia, hypernatremia, hypocalcemia, and acidosis
  (d) Clotting. Overheparinization and thrombocytopenia
  (e) Infections. Bacteremia, hepatitis, cytomegalovirus
  (f) Miscellaneous. Mechanical injury to donor cells, perforation of vessels, hypothermia, hypoglycemia, and possibly necrotizing enterocolitis
e. Phenobarbital, 5–8 mg/kg/day, will increase bilirubin conjugation and excretion. It may take 3–7 days to be effective. It is most useful in Crigler-Najjar syndrome type II and many cases of direct hyperbilirubinemia.

B. Anemia
  1. The **causes** of anemia include blood loss, hemolysis, decreased production, and physiologic decreased erythropoiesis.
  a. Blood loss
    (1) Etiology. The causes of blood loss are hemorrhage from the fetal to the maternal circulation; twin-twin transfusion; placenta previa; placental absorption; umbilical cord rupture or hematoma; incision of the placenta or cord; traumatic amniocentesis; rupture of anomalous placental vessels; intracranial bleeding; rupture of the liver or spleen; and GI bleeding due to ulcer, enterocolitis, or thrombosis. Iatrogenic anemia due to inadequate replacement of blood drawn for studies is a frequent cause of anemia in the neonate.
    (2) Evaluation. If blood loss is **acute,** the **manifestations** are shock, tachypnea, tachycardia, low venous pressure, weak pulses, and pallor. The hematocrit may initially be normal. **Chronic** blood loss is manifested by extreme pallor and a low hematocrit, with less distress than one would expect given the low hematocrit. These infants may be **normovolemic.** They may have CHF or hydrops.
    (3) Laboratory evaluation
      (a) A Kleihauer-Betke smear of maternal blood to detect fetal red cells in the maternal circulation
      (b) The APT test for fetal hemoglobin in gastric aspirate or stool
      (c) Intracranial and abdominal ultrasound
      (d) Peritoneal aspiration in cases of suspected liver or splenic rupture
      (e) Careful examination of the placenta and its vessels
  b. Hemolysis
    (1) Etiology. The causes of hemolysis include:
      (a) The isoimmune anemias: RH incompatibility, ABO incompatibility, minor blood group incompatibility (e.g., Kell, "e", "c", "E")
      (b) The acquired hemolytic anemias: infection, disseminated intravascular coagulation (DIC), vitamin E deficiency, and drug reactions
      (c) The hereditary hemolytic anemias: red cell membrane defects (spherocytosis); enzyme defects (pyruvate kinase [PK] and glucose 6-phosphate deficiency [G-6-PD])
      (d) The thalassemia syndromes
    (2) Evaluation. Manifestations may include jaundice, hepatosplenomegaly, pallor, hydrops, a positive Coombs test, an elevated reticulocyte count, and an abnormal red cell morphology on smear.
    (3) Laboratory evaluations include hematocrit, serum bilirubin, and reticulocyte count; examination of a peripheral blood smear for red blood cell morphology; direct Coombs test on an infant's red cells, with identification of the antibody if positive; antibody screen of maternal serum; enzyme screen of infant's or parents' red cells (G-6-PD or PK deficiency); and screening for infection.

   c. **Decreased production.** The causes of decreased production include Blackfan-Diamond syndrome; Fanconi's anemia; hemoglobinopathies such as thalassemia; reactions to drugs; infections and infiltrative diseases such as leukemia, neuroblastoma and storage diseases.

   d. **Physiologic anemia of full-term and premature infants** is due to physiologic decreased erythropoiesis.

     (1) Full-term infants have a nadir of the hemoglobin level at 9.5–11.0 gm/100 ml at 6–12 weeks; prematures (body weight 1,200–1,400 gm) have a nadir of 8–10 gm/100 ml at 5–10 weeks; and prematures (body weight under 1,200 gm) have a nadir of 6.5–9.0 gm/100 ml at 4–8 weeks.

     (2) The laboratory manifestations of physiologic anemia are a decreased hematocrit and a low reticulocyte count. When the infant's oxygen demand increases, erythropoietin will increase, and if iron stores are adequate, the reticulocyte count will increase, and the hemoglobin level will rise.

2. Therapy

  a. Transfusion

     (1) If an infant appears to have had acute blood loss at birth, a catheter should be placed into the umbilical vein. Venous pressure should be measured and blood drawn for studies and crossmatching.

     (2) If hypovolemic shock is present (decreased venous pressure, pallor, tachycardia), 20 ml/kg of a volume expander should be given. Unmatched type O, Rh-negative blood should be kept available for this purpose. Albumin (5%), plasma, or normal saline are secondary choices, in that order.

     (3) If blood loss was acute and not continuing, as in a fetal-maternal hemorrhage, there will be immediate dramatic improvement. If there is continuing internal hemorrhage, the improvement will be less. Infants in shock from asphyxia will have little response.

     (4) A repeat transfusion of 10–20 mg/kg may be given if there are signs that the first transfusion was inadequate (decreased venous pressure, tachypnea, tachycardia, and shock). If plasma or albumin was given initially, packed red cells are given in the second transfusion.

     (5) In chronic fetal blood loss (low hematocrit without evidence of hypovolemia), packed red cells (10 ml/kg) are given if the hematocrit is under 30. If the hematocrit is under 25 in a normovolemic or hypervolemic infant who may be in failure, a partial exchange transfusion with packed RBCs is indicated.

     (6) Premature infants may be comfortable with hemoglobin (Hgb) in the range of 6.5–8.0 gm/100 ml. The level itself is **not** an indication for transfusion. However, if any other condition (e.g., sepsis, apnea, pneumonia, bronchopulmonary dysplasia) requires increased oxygen-carrying capacity, transfusion is indicated.

     (7) When multiple samples are being drawn from sick infants, a careful record must be kept of the amount drawn. Blood should be replaced as whole blood when 5% of the volume has been removed. (Average blood volume in a neonate is 80 ml/kg.)

     (8) The hematocrit in infants with cardiac or respiratory diseases should be kept above 40 with transfusions of packed red blood cells (10 ml/kg).

     (9) Transfusion to replace red blood cells is calculated with the formula

$$\text{Volume transfusion} = \frac{\begin{array}{c}\text{weight (in kg)} \times \text{blood volume/kg} \\ \times \text{(Hgb desired} - \text{Hgb observed)}\end{array}}{\text{Hgb of blood to be given}}$$

(The average hemoglobin of packed red cells is 23 gm/100 ml.)

(10) These transfusions are usually given as 10 ml/kg of packed red cells. Infants should be monitored during transfusion.

3. Prevention or amelioration of the anemia of prematurity

   a. Premature infants are given 25 IU of water-soluble vitamin E daily until they are 8 weeks of age.

   b. Formulas similar to mother's milk in that they are low in linoleic acid are used to maintain a low content of red blood cell polyunsaturated fatty acids.

   c. Iron is not used for the first 2 months, since therapeutic doses (6 mg/kg/ day) enhance lipid peroxidation of red blood cell membranes.

   d. After 8 weeks, iron supplements (2 mg/kg/day) as fortified formula or therapeutic iron are used to decrease the late anemia of prematurity.

C. Bleeding disorders

   1. Etiology. See Chap. 17, pp. 447ff.

   2. Evaluation and diagnosis. See Chap. 17, pp. 447ff.

   3. Treatment. Also see **B.**

   a. Any underlying disease, such as shock, asphyxia, or infection, must be treated.

   b. A reliable IV line must be placed.

   c. After blood is drawn for studies. 1.0–2.0 mg of vitamin K_1 (AquaMEPHYTON) or vitamin K_1 oxide (Konakion) should be given IV over 2–3 min. The onset of action may be 2–3 hr. If liver disease is present, the onset of action may be longer.

   d. Fresh frozen plasma, 10 ml/kg IV q12h, provides immediate replacement of clotting factors.

   e. If thrombocytopenia or thrombocytopathia is present, give 1 unit of platelets (platelets from 1 pint of blood)/3 kg IV. **Platelets must not be given through an arterial line.** This should elevate the platelet count to 100,000 unless platelet destruction is continuing. In isoimmune thrombocytopenia, platelets from the mother or compatible with the mother are given if there is bleeding.

   f. Packed red cells, plasma, and platelets are usually used. However, fresh whole blood will replace platelets and clotting factors and provide red blood cells. The amount used is initially 10 ml/kg. This is repeated as needed to replace blood lost.

   g. Clotting factor concentrates are used if there is a known factor deficiency.

   h. Disseminated intravascular coagulation (DIC) should be treated by treating the underlying cause (sepsis, necrotizing enterocolitis) and giving fresh frozen plasma and platelets to keep the platelet count about 50,000. If bleeding continues, an exchange transfusion with fresh citrated blood may be helpful. If DIC is associated with gangrenous thrombosis of the skin, toes, or fingers, an exchange transfusion with fresh heparinized blood, followed by heparin, 50 μ/kg q4h for 2–3 days, may be useful. If fresh heparinized blood is not available, heparin, fresh frozen plasma, platelets, and red cells may be used.

4. Prevention

   a. Infants should be given vitamin K_1, 1 mg IM, at birth.

   b. Mothers taking phenytoin should be given 10 mg of vitamin K_1 IM 24 hr prior to delivery. These newborns should have cord blood prothrombin time and partial thromboplastin time measured. If these levels are prolonged, the infants should be given fresh frozen plasma, 20 ml/kg.

   c. Mothers should refrain from taking aspirin for 1 week prior to delivery.

D. Polycythemia

   1. Etiology

   a. Placental overtransfusion

   b. Placental insufficiency

   c. Other causes include maternal diabetes, congenital adrenal hyperplasia, Beckwith syndrome, neonatal thyrotoxicosis, Down syndrome, and trisomy D.

2. Evaluation and diagnosis
   a. Most infants with polycythemia are asymptomatic.
   b. Suggestive symptoms include cyanosis (due to unsaturated hemoglobin) priapism, hypoglycemia, and jaundice (bilirubin load to the liver: 1 gm of hemoglobin produces 34 gm of bilirubin).
   c. Central hematocrits should be checked to diagnose or rule out polycythemia.

3. Treatment
   a. Any **central hematocrit** above 60 is of concern.
   b. Any symptomatic child should have a partial exchange transfusion if the central hematocrit is **above 65.**
   c. Asymptomatic infants with a central hematocrit of 60–70 can usually be managed by pushing fluids.
   d. Exchange transfusion is probably indicated with a central hematocrit more than 70 in the absence of symptoms.
   Exchange is done with fresh frozen plasma if available, or 5% albumin to bring hematocrit to 60 by the following calculation:

$$\text{Volume of exchange (ml)} = \frac{\text{Blood volume} \times (\text{observed Hct} - \text{desired Hct})}{\text{Observed Hct}}$$

VI. Metabolic problems
A. Metabolic disorders. Genetically determined metabolic disorders are seen in 1 of every 200 infants (see Chap. 14).
   1. Etiology See Chap. 14.
   2. Evaluation and Diagnosis (also see Chap. 14).
      a. These disorders should be suspected in the following **clinical situations:**
         (1) A positive family history of any such disorder
         (2) A history of unexplained neonatal deaths in the family
         (3) Neonatal symptoms and signs, such as poor feeding, lethargy, hypotonia, coma, seizures, vomiting, diarrhea, tachypnea, rashes, coarse facial features, hepatomegaly, jaundice, cataracts, dehydration, constipation, temperature instability, unusual odor of urine or sweat, failure to thrive, and poor progression of development
         (4) Onset of symptoms in an infant who was well at birth
         (5) Onset of symptoms after a change in diet
         (6) Onset and progression of symptoms without evidence of asphyxia, infection, CNS hemorrhage, or other congenital defects.
      b. Laboratory signs of these disorders include: hypoglycemia; metabolic acidosis; lactic acidosis; ketosis; hyperammonemia; hyperbilirubinemia; abnormal amino acid pattern in the blood; ketonuria; positive ferric chloride test of the urine; and reducing substance in the urine. For purposes of genetic counseling, it is important to make an accurate diagnosis even if the affected infant dies. Infants who die with symptoms that may be caused by a metabolic disorder should be photographed, have full body x-rays, and an autopsy. Blood should be saved for chromosomes and blood and serum saved for analysis. Skin should be saved for fibroblast culture, and rapidly frozen liver and brain tissue should also be saved.
   3. Treatment
      a. If a metabolic disorder is suspected, a metabolic disease center should be contacted. Rapid transfer to a newborn unit with access to a laboratory capable of performing sophisticated tests should be considered, since many of these disorders are rapidly fatal unless properly treated.
      b. Exchange transfusion or peritoneal dialysis should be considered for stabilization while awaiting a specific diagnosis.
      c. An attempt must be made to prevent protein catabolism with possible accumulation of toxic by-products. The infant should be given oral or parenteral glucose. Dextrose polymers (Polycose, [Ross Laboratories, Co-

lumbus, Ohio], medium-chain triglycerides, Nil-Priote [product 80056, Mead Johnson]), glucose, emulsifiable fat, minerals, vitamins, and Intralipid should be considered for use. When a diagnosis is made, specific dietary or vitamin therapy should be started if possible.

4. Some specific disorders which are lethal in the newborn will be outlined here:
   a. **Galactosemia**
      (1) **Symptoms:**
         (a) Jaundice
         (b) Hepatomegaly
         (c) Lethargy
         (d) Weight loss
         (e) Sepsis
         (f) Cataracts
         (g) Hypoglycemia
      (2) **Diagnosis.** Reducing substance in the urine (positive Clinitest) with negative urine for glucose (negative glucose oxidase dipstick test); assay of blood for galactase 1-phosphate-uridytransferase (Bentlen test); assay of urine for galactose
      (3) **Treatment.** Elimination of galactose from the diet.
   b. **Organic acidemias.** Methylmalonic acidemia, propionic acidemia, and isovaleric acidemia
      (1) **Signs and symptoms.** Poor feeding, vomiting, lethargy, tachypnea, coma, hypotoxicity, spasticity, and seizures
      (2) **Diagnosis.** Metabolic acidosis, ketoacidosis, hyperammonemia, hypoglycemia, ammonia odor from sweat or urine, bacterial inhibition assay for specific amino acid, gas layer chromatography, and high-voltage electrophoresis
      (3) **Treatment.** Reversal of metabolic acidosis, dietary therapy, and vitamins
   c. **Hyperammonemic syndromes.** These syndromes include urea cycle disorders; carbamylphosphate synthetase deficiency; ornithine transcarbamylase deficiency; citrullinemia; arginosuccinic acidemia; argininemia; ornithine transaminase deficiency; oroticacidurias; hyperornithinemia; and hyperlysinemia.
      (1) **Symptoms and signs.** Feeding problems, lethargy, irritability, hypertonicity, hypotonicity, tachypnea, coma, and convulsions
      (2) **Diagnosis.** Metabolic acidosis, hyperammonemia, bacterial inhibition assay, gas layer chromatography, and high-voltage electrophoresis
      (3) **Treatment** is dietary. Limit protein intake; avoid constipation; acidify colonic contents with lactulose to decrease ammonia absorption; and give antibiotics to decrease colonic flora. Peritoneal dialysis and exchange transfusion have been tried. Some disorders may respond to specific treatment; e.g., oroticaciduria may be treated with uridine.

B. **Infants of diabetic mothers**
   1. **Pregnancy.** Management during the diabetic pregnancy should include:
      a. Close cooperation between obstetrician, pediatrician, and internist
      b. Frequent prenatal visits
      c. Accurate dating of time of conception by menstrual history, early examination, and early ultrasound
      d. Maintenance of a maternal normoglycemia by diet, insulin, or both. Maternal blood sugar should be monitored by frequent blood glucose determinations, by measurement of the daily amount of glycosuria (keep under 20 gm/day), and by measurement of hemoglobin A_1c. There is evidence that the maintenance of normoglycemia in early pregnancy may be associated with a decreased incidence of major congenital anomalies, and the maintenance of normoglycemia in late pregnancy may be associated with a decrease in macrosomia and neonatal hypoglycemia. **Oral**

hypoglycemic agents should not be used because they cross the placenta and are associated with severe and prolonged neonatal hypoglycemia.

   e. Fetal ultrasonography should be done in early pregnancy for the detection of congenital anomalies such as anencephaly. Maternal alpha fetoprotein should be measured.

   f. As pregnancy progresses into the third trimester, frequent determinations of fetal well-being should be made by ultrasonography, estriols, and nonstress tests (see Chap 5, p. 119).

   g. When delivery is being considered, amniotic fluid should be obtained for assessment of fetal pulmonary maturity (lecithin-sphingomyelin [L/S] ratio, disaturated lecithin, and phosphatidyl glycerol).

   h. The decision on the timing of delivery is made by a balancing of risks to fetus, mother, and newborn. The risks to the fetus are intrauterine death and growth retardation. The risks to the mother are hypertension, renal failure, retinal hemorrhage and unmanageable hyperglycemia. The risks to the newborn from early delivery are prematurity and respiratory distress.

2. **Evaluation of the newborn.** Infants of diabetic mothers are subject to the following: perinatal asphyxia, birth trauma, congenital anomalies, hypoglycemia, hypocalcemia, hyperbilirubinemia, RDS, polycythemia, feeding problems, and renal vein thrombosis.

3. **Diagnosis**
   a. At delivery, a sample of amniotic fluid can be obtained for a shake test, L/S ratio, disaturated lecithin, phosphatidyl glycerol, and Gram stain.
   b. Gastric aspirate should be obtained for shake test and Gram stain.
   c. **Laboratory data.** Determine the following:
      (1) **Blood sugar** at birth and at 1, 2, 3, 6, 12, 24, and 48 hr (Dextrostix reading)
      (2) Calcium at 6, 12, 24, and 48 hr
      (3) Hematocrit at 1 and 24 hr
      (4) Bilirubin as needed
      (5) Chest x-ray and ABGs as indicated for evaluation of respiratory distress or cyanosis
      (6) ECG and cardiac ultrasound for evaluation of cardiac disease as indicated.

4. **Therapy**
   a. See treatment of RDS, sec. **III,** cardiac problems, sec. **IV,** hypoglycemia, sec. **VI.C,** hypocalcemia, sec. **VI.D,** polycythemia, sec. **V.D,** and hyperbilirubinemia, sec. **V.A.1.a.**
   b. These infants are given 10% D/W by mouth or gavage hourly starting at 1 hr of age until the blood glucose is stabilized. If this is not tolerated, parenteral glucose is given.
   c. If the infant is hypoglycemic, glucagon (300 µg/kg SQ, to a maximum dose of 1.0 mg) may be used to raise the blood sugar while an IV infusion is being started. Rapid infusions of concentrated dextrose solutions may stimulate insulin release in these hyperinsulinemic infants. If an IV line is suddenly lost, there may be rebound hypoglycemia.

C. *Hypoglycemia* in the neonate is defined as any blood sugar less than 40 mg/100 ml with hypoglycemic symptoms that disappear after IV glucose. Thus, any blood glucose less than 40 mg/100 ml should be a cause for concern, and a blood glucose under 30 mg/100 ml requires treatment.

   1. **Etiology.** See Table 6-3.
   2. **Evaluation and diagnosis**
      a. **Symptoms** include lethargy, apathy, limpness, tremors, apnea, hypothermia, cyanosis, seizures, weak or high-pitched cry, and poor feeding.
      b. **Laboratory data.** In the newborn, glucose oxidase methods that measure true glucose should be used rather than those that measure total reducing substances. Dextrostix and the Ames Eyetone Instrument can be

Table 6-3. Etiology of neonatal hypoglycemia

Decreased hepatic glucose stores, production, or release

Prematurity
Intrauterine growth retardation
Hypoxia
Asphyxia
Hypothermia
Sepsis
Congenital heart disease
Glucagon deficiency
Glycogen storage disease (type I)
Galactosemia
Fructose intolerance
Adrenal insufficiency

Increased utilization of glucose (hyperinsulinism)

Infant of diabetic mother
Erythroblastosis fetalis
Exchange transfusions (intraexchange hypoglycemia if heparinized
   blood is used, postexchange phyoglycemia if citrated blood is used)
Beckwith-Wiedemann syndrome
Nesidioblastosis
Islet cell adenoma
Leucine sensitivity
Maternal chlorpropamide therapy
Maternal benzothiadiazide therapy

Other causes

Maternal therapy with beta-sympathomimetics
Maternal or neonatal salicylate therapy

---

useful. Plasma insulin levels should be measured in certain cases of prolonged hypoglycemia.
3. **Treatment.** The lower level of blood glucose at which CNS damage occurs in
the neonate is not known. We try to keep the blood glucose level over 40 mg/
100 ml.
   a. Anticipation and **prevention** is more important than treatment.
      (1) The blood sugar of well infants who are at high risk of hypoglycemia
          should be measured at 3, 6, 12, and 24 hr of age, and they should be
          given early oral or gavage feedings with 10% glucose and water q2h
          until the sugar level is stable. At this point, they can be weaned to
          milk, with continuing attention to their blood sugars for the first 2
          days of life.
      (2) Asphyxiated infants, infants with seizures and any infant with symp-
          toms that could be due to hypoglycemia should be given parenteral
          glucose. Parenteral glucose should also usually be given during and
          after exchange transfusions.
      (3) Infants at high risk of hypoglycemia should often be given parenteral
          glucose at a rate of 4–8 mg glucose/kg/min until feedings are estab-
          lished and the risks of hypoglycemia are gone.
   b. **Symptomatic hypoglycemia** is best treated by first drawing blood for
      appropriate studies and then giving the following:
      (1) **Glucose,** 0.2–0.4 gm/kg of body weight by IV push. This is done by
          giving 1 ml of 25% D/W/kg at a rate of 1 ml/min.
      (2) The glucose should be followed by a continuous infusion of dextrose at

a rate of 4–8 mg glucose/kg/min. A constant infusion pump should be used. The glucose concentration of the fluid will depend on the daily fluid requirement. On day 1, the fluid requirement is 65 ml/kg/day, or 0.045 ml/kg/min; 10% D/W provides 4.5 mg of glucose/kg/min, and 15% D/W provides 6.75 mg of glucose/kg/min. Either may be used. For most patients, 10% D/W at daily maintenance rates will provide adequate IV glucose.

(3) The concentration of glucose and the rate of infusion are increased as necessary to maintain a normal blood sugar (e.g., some infants with hyperinsulinism will require 15% D/W).

(4) Glucagon at a dose of 30 μg/kg IM can be administered to mobilize glucose in infants with adequate glycogen stores. Infants of diabetic mothers will require 300 μg/kg IM (maximum dose 1 mg). This may be used until an IV line is placed.

(5) Hydrocortisone, 5 mg/kg/day IV or PO, may be used in cases that do not respond to glucose infusions.

(6) Epinephrine, diazoxide, and growth hormone are to be used **only with endocrinologic consultation** in special cases of chronic intractable hypoglycemia.

(7) Phenobarbital should be used with glucose in the treatment of hypoglycemic seizures.

D. *Hypocalcemia* is defined as a serum total calcium concentration less than 7 mg/100 ml or an ionized calcium concentration below 3.0 to 3.5 mg/dl.

1. Etiology. Hypocalcemia usually is related to decreased calcium intake and transient neonatal hypoparathyroidism.

a. First 3 days

(1) **Maternal.** Diabetes, toxemia, or obstetric complications, severe dietary calcium deficiency, or maternal hyperparathyroidism

(2) **Intrapartum.** Asphyxia or prematurity

(3) **Postnatal.** Hypoxia, shock, asphyxia, poor intake, RDS, or sepsis. A normal serum total calcium and a decreased ionized calcium may be seen in alkalosis caused by treatment with bicarbonate or hyperventilation. The same condition may be seen after exchange transfusion with citrated blood.

b. After 3 days (see Chap. 11, p. 309). Any of the preceding causes and also a high-phosphate diet (milk, cereals), magnesium deficiency, intestinal malabsorption, renal disease, hypoparathyroidism, and vitamin D deficiency or metabolic defect

2. Evaluation and diagnosis

a. Signs of hypocalcemia in the newborn are nonspecific, and the classic Chvostek's sign and carpopedal spasm are helpful only **if present.**

b. Irritability, jitteriness, hypotonia, a high-pitched cry, and seizures are the most common presenting symptoms.

c. Calcium levels should be measured frequently in infants with the preceding conditions and substantiated if necessary with ECG measurement of the Q–OTC (Q–onset of T/R–R), or Q–T interval. They should be measured at 6, 12, 24, and 48 hr of age in infants of diabetic mothers; at 1, 3, 6, and 12 hr of age in intrapartum asphyxia; and at 12, 24, and 48 hr of age in premature infants.

d. Ionized calcium, serum phosphorus, magnesium, BUN, creatinine, parathyroid hormone, and calcitonin may be measured in persistent hypocalcemia. Absence of the thymus on chest film may be associated with hypoparathyroidism.

3. Prevention and treatment

a. Preparations. It is preferable to use only one calcium salt (gluconate) for either IV or PO administration; e.g., calcium gluconate 10%, PO or IV (1 ml of 10% calcium gluconate = 100 mg of calcium gluconate = 9 mg of elemental calcium or 0.45 mEq/ml).

b. Indications. Infants who are at risk of hypocalcemia because of poor intake or transient hypoparathyroidism (prematures, infants with RDS) may be monitored carefully and treated if they become hypocalcemic, or they may be given anticipatory calcium supplementation. We usually do the former.

c. Dosage

(1) For asymptomatic hypocalcemia (Ca < 7 mg/100 ml without symptoms), give 5–10 ml/kg/day of 10% calcium gluconate PO or IV. This provides a maintenance calcium (45–90 mg/kg/day of elemental calcium). Start with a low dose and increase the dose as needed. The oral dose is mixed in with the total day's feeding. The IV dose is given by slow continuous infusion over 24 hr. If the cause of the hypocalcemia has resolved, the dose can be gradually decreased over 48 hr.

(2) Acute symptomatic hypocalcemia with significant symptoms such as seizures or cardiac arrhythmias

(a) Give 2 mg/kg of 10% calcium gluconate IV stat.

(b) The maximum dose is 5 ml for prematures and 10 ml for full-term infants. This amount can be given slowly IV (1 ml/min), with careful observation of the heart rate—and the vein if a peripheral vein is being used. This dose is conservative and can be repeated in 15 min if there is no clinical response.

d. Maintenance

(1) Following the acute dose, maintenance calcium, 45–90 mg/kg/day of elemental Ca, should be given parenterally or by mouth. A low-phosphate milk (e.g., breast milk or Similac PM 60/40) should be used when oral feeding is started. Calcium can be added directly to the formula if necessary.

(2) Treatment of hypocalcemia is rarely necessary for more than 4–5 days unless other complications are present. During treatment, calcium levels should be monitored q12–24h and the dose gradually tapered as indicated. By 1 week of age, most infants of diabetic mothers remain normocalcemic on a regular formula or breast milk and without supplements.

e. The **risk of treatment** can be minimized by noting the following:

(1) Most hypocalcemia causes no symptoms and does not need rapid correction. Aggressive, rapid therapy of asymptomatic hypocalcemia often causes more problems than it solves.

(a) A rapid push of calcium can cause a sudden elevation of serum calcium, leading to bradycardia or other cardiac arrhythmias. This is especially true if the umbilical vein is being used. The injection rate should be no faster than 1 ml/min. A cardiac monitor should be in place in infants receiving parenteral calcium as a bolus or as maintenance.

(b) Extravasation of calcium solutions into subcutaneous tissues can cause severe tissue necrosis. This occurs most often when an infusion pump is used. However, an infusion pump is best to provide a steady dose of calcium. The only way to minimize this problem is to use a reliable access (IV cannula) and closely observe the vein.

(c) Calcium cannot be mixed with $NaHCO_3^-$, since this may produce $CaCO_3$ precipitation.

(d) Calcium can cause necrosis of the liver if it is administered via an umbilical vein catheter that is in the portal system.

(e) Calcium pushed into the aorta may be a factor in necrotizing enterocolitis. Therefore, it should be given only by slow maintenance drip if an umbilical artery catheter is used for access.

f. Associated hypomagnesemia

(1) Hypocalcemia may be associated with hypomagnesemia and will not respond unless the hypomagnesemia is treated. Normal magnesium levels in newborns are 1.2–1.8 mEq/L, or 2.4–3.6 mg/100 ml. Associated with neonatal hypomagnesemia are maternal magnesium deficiency, maternal hypoparathyroidism, maternal diabetes, small-for-gestational-age infants, intestinal magnesium malabsorption, liver disease, exchange transfusions with citrated blood, and increased phosphate intake.

(2) Seizures caused by acute hypomagnesemia are treated with 0.1–0.2 ml/kg of 50% $MgSO_4$ IV or IM, repeated if necessary q12h, and the addition of 3 mEq/L of magnesium to maintenance IV fluids. If the infant is able, 0.1–0.2 ml/kg/day diluted at least 1 to 10 with water or formula may be given PO. If specific magnesium intestinal malabsorption is present, up to 1.2 ml/kg/day may be needed.

g. Persistent hypocalcemia. If the infant remains hypocalcemic despite adequate calcium supplementation and normal magnesium levels, a search for other causes of hypocalcemia must be started (see Chap. 11, p. 309).

h. For the long-term calcium needs of prematures see Chapter 5, p. 128

VII. Infection. Infection accounts for 10–20% of infant deaths.

A. Congenital and natal infections

1. **Torch** (toxoplasmosis, rubella, cytomegalovirus [CMV], herpesvirus [HSV], syphilis, and others (hepatitis B virus [HBV] and enterovirus)

    a. Evaluation and diagnosis

    (1) **Maternal history.** Most maternal infections with these agents are asymptomatic. Screening should be considered with the following maternal history:

    (a) Known history of congenital infection

    (b) Habitual abortion

    (c) Infertility

    (d) Contact with cats or mice

    (e) Ingestion of raw meat

    (f) Immunosuppressive therapy

    (g) Rash

    (h) Unexplained adenopathy

    (i) Unexplained illness during pregnancy

    (j) Oral or genital lesion

    (k) Occupational exposure to congenital infection (neonatal nurses, dialysis workers)

    (2) **Maternal diagnosis.** All mothers should be screened early in pregnancy for antibody to syphilis and rubella. Serologic testing is available for HSV, CMV, and HBV. Viral cultures are available for HSV, rubella, CMV, and enterovirus. Maternal vaginal cultures are used to diagnose maternal gonorrhea, and group B streptococci.

    (3) **Neonatal manifestations** include prematurity, intrauterine growth retardation, failure to thrive, and hepatomegaly with elevated direct bilirubin. **Disease-specific manifestations** include:

    (a) **Syphilis.** Mucocutaneous lesions (snuffles), periostitis, osteochondritis, hepatomegaly, and rash

    (b) **Toxoplasmosis.** Chorioretinitis, hydrocephalus, and intracranial calcifications

    (c) **CMV.** Microcephaly with periventricular calcifications, thrombocytopenia, and hepatosplenomegaly

    (d) **Rubella.** Retinopathy, cataracts, patent ductus arteriosus, pulmonary artery stenosis, deafness, and thrombocytopenia

    (e) **Group B streptococci.** Neonatal sepsis and pneumonia and late meningitis

    (f) **HSV.** Skin vesicles, hepatitis, pneumonia, encephalitis, and DIC

    (g) **HBV.** Hepatitis between 1 and 6 months of age

    (h) **Enterovirus.** Encephalitis, sepsislike syndrome, hepatitis, and DIC

    (4) **Laboratory examination.** See also Chap. 15.

    (a) Draw sera for a TORCH screen (5–10 ml of blood) (prior **to transfusions**) or cord blood (serum), and pair with a sample from the

mother, drawn at the same time. This should include a search for IGM-specific immunofluorescent antibodies. Convalescent serum from the mother and baby must be sent in 2–8 weeks, depending on the clinical situation. Sera may be required at 3–6 months.
- **(b)** Measure cord blood IgM (normal < 20 mg/ml).
- **(c)** Viral cultures (HSV, rubella, CMV, enterovirus)
- **(d)** Tzanck preparation smear of vesicles from the infant or mother
- **(e)** Urine cytologic study after millipore filtration for CMV
- **(f)** Histologic study of the placenta
- **(g)** Hepatitis B surface antigen (HBsAg), antibody to surface antigen (anti-HBs), hepatitis B core antigen (HBeAg), and antibody to hepatitis B core antigen (anti-HBe).
- **(h)** Liver enzymes, SGOT, and SGPT
- **(i)** Platelet count and clotting studies

b. Treatment. See also Chap. 15, pp. 412ff.
- **(1)** No specific treatment is available for rubella or CMV infection.
- **(2)** HSV has been successfully treated with both Ara-A and acyclovir (see Chap. 15, p. 415). Topical idoxuridine (see Chap. 23, p. 553) eyedrops and large doses of gamma globulin (10–20 mg IM) have been used.
- **(3)** Treatment is available for toxoplasmosis (see Chap. 16, pp. 434ff).
- **(4)** If varicella develops in the mother within 5 days of delivery, there will be insufficient time for transfer of maternal antibody to the fetus. These infants should receive 2 ml of zoster immune globulin (ZIG) or varicella-zoster immune globulin (VZIG). Mothers in whom varicella develops after delivery are also a risk to their nonimmune offspring.

c. Prevention
- **(1)** Congenital **rubella** is prevented by adequate immunization of child-bearing women (see Chap. 2, pp. 19ff).
- **(2)** **Toxoplasmosis** (see Chap. 16, p. 434) may possibly be prevented by avoiding cats and the eating of raw meat during pregnancy.
- **(3)** Since the majority of neonatal HSV infections are acquired at the time of vaginal delivery, the infants of mothers with active genital herpes should be delivered by cesarean section. If the membranes are ruptured, the baby should be delivered by cesarean section as soon as possibe. Postnatal infection can be acquired from mothers with active lesions. Some have treated exposed infants with ISG, 0.6 ml/kg. If the mother has a primary HSV infection with positive cultures at the time of delivery, consideration can be given to treatment of the infant with Ara-A (30 mg/kg/day) for 14 days.
- **(4)** Infants born to mothers in whom hepatitis A develops near term should be given ISG, 0.5 ml. Infants born to mothers in whom HBV infections develop should be treated with hepatitis B immune globulin (HBIG), 0.5 ml, at birth. The dose should be repeated at 3 and 6 months. These infants should also be given hepatitis B vaccine starting at 3 months of age. If the mother is HBsAg positive, HBeAg negative, anti-HBC positive, and has given birth to another unaffected child, one might withhold HBIG and HB vaccine.

2. Syphilis. See also Chap. 15, p. 402.
- **a. Etiology.** Transplacental transmission of *Treponema pallidum*
- **b. Evaluation and diagnosis**
  - **(1) Perinatal** clinical signs include stillbirth, fetal hydrops, and prematurity.
  - **(2) Postnatal** manifestations include failure to thrive, persistent rhinitis, lymphadenopathy, rash, jaundice, anemia, hepatosplenomegaly, nephrosis, and meningitis.
- **c. Laboratory tests**
  - **(1) Mother.** Rapid plasma reagin (RPR) with titers and fluorescent-treponemal antibody absorption test (FTA-ABS) with titers. Test at first antenatal visit and in third trimester.
  - **(2) Infant**

(a) RPR with titer and FTA-ABS with titer

(b) If available, IGM-FTA-ABS is most specific for fetal infection.

(c) X-rays of long bones may provide evidence of metaphyseal demineralization or periosteal new bone formation.

(d) Dark-field examination of any nasal discharge

(e) CSF examination

d. **Treatment.** See also Chap. 15, p. 408.

(1) Pregnant women with primary, secondary, or latent syphilis are treated as follows:

(a) **Benzathine penicillin G.** The dose is 2.4 MU IM (1.2 MU in each buttock initially). Repeat 7 days later. The total dose is 4.8 MU. Alternatively, give **aqueous procaine penicillin G,** 1.2 MU/day IM for 10 days.

(b) If penicillin allergy is present, **erythromycin** (stearate, ethylsuccinate, or base), 500 mg PO qid for 15 days is used. Erythromycin crosses the placenta in an unpredictable manner. **Tetracycline** in the same dose is effective, but it may have teratogenic effects. Cephaloridine in the same dose has been used.

(2) **Mothers with syphilis of more than 1 year's duration** (latent syphilis of indeterminate or more than 1 year's duration, cardiovascular syphilis, late benign syphilis, neurosyphilis)

(a) **Penicillin**

(i) **Benzathine penicillin G,** 7.2 MU total, 2.4 MU IM weekly for 3 successive weeks, *or*

(ii) **Aqueous procaine penicillin G,** 9.0 MU total, 600,000 units IM daily for 15 days

(b) If penicillin allergy is present, give

(i) Erythromycin (stearate, ethylsuccinate, or base), 500 mg qid for 30 days, *or*

(ii) Tetracycline hydrochloride, 500 mg qid for 30 days

(3) **Infant**

(a) If the infant's serologic test results are negative and he or she has no disease, no treatment is necessary.

(b) If the serologic test results are positive, treat the symptomatic infant. Treat the asymptomatic infant when

(i) The titer is 3–4 times higher than the mother's.

(ii) The FTA is 3–4$^+$.

(iii) IGM is elevated (> 20 mg/100 ml).

(iv) The mother was inadequately treated or untreated.

(v) The mother is unreliable, and follow-up is doubtful.

(vi) The mother's infection was treated with a drug other than penicillin.

(c) If the baby has a positive RPR, or FTA, or both, and the history and clinical findings (including x-ray) make infection unlikely, it is safe to await the IGM report and repeat RPR and FTA titers. Any significant rise in titer or any clinical signs require treatment. If the antibodies are transferred maternal antibodies, the baby should have a falling titer.

(d) Give procaine penicillin G in aqueous suspension, 50,000 units/kg IM in 1 daily dose for 10–14 days or aqueous penicillin G, 50,000 units/kg/day q12h IM for 10–14 days (see Table 15-12).

3. Gonorrhea

a. **Etiology.** Intrapartum infection with *Neisseria gonorrhoeae*

b. **Evaluation and diagnosis**

(1) **Gonococcal ophthalmia** usually presents within 3 days of birth. If the eyes are infected before birth in association with premature rupture of the membranes, symptoms may be present at birth. Usually, a watery, then mucopurulent, then bloody conjunctival discharge develops. There is prominent edema of the conjunctiva and lids, followed by

corneal edema and ulceration. There may be perforation of the globe with panophthalmitis. A presumptive diagnosis is made by demonstration of gram-negative diplococci on Gram stain of the exudate. Definitive diagnosis is by culture. Conjunctivitis from silver nitrate, HSV, staphylococci, pneumonococci, *Escherichia coli,* and *Chlamydia* should be considered in the differential diagnosis.

  (2) Other gonococcal infections are rhinitis, anorectal infection, arthritis, sepsis, and meningitis.

  (3) In infants born to mothers with gonococcal infection, eye, nasopharyngeal, ear, gastric, and anorectal Gram stains and cultures should be done.

c. Treatment. See Table 15-11.

  (1) Asymptomatic infants. If a Gram stain or culture from a maternal or neonatal source is positive for *N. gonorrhoeae,* the infant should be treated with one dose of 50,000 units of aqueous crystalline penicillin G IM or IV, even in the absence of clinical infection.

  (2) Symptomatic infections (opthalmia, arthritis, sepsis) should be treated with 100,000 units/kg/day of aqueous crystalline penicillin G for 10 days. (see Table 15-11).

  (3) Gonococcal ophthalmia should also be treated with saline irrigations and instillation of tetracycline or chloramphenicol eyedrops.

  (4) The possibility of penicillin-resistant gonococcus should be considered (see Table 15-11). Sensitivity testing should be done on all positive cultures. Failure of clinical response or demonstration of penicillin resistance requires systemic treatment with chloramphenicol. There is little experience with spectinomycin in neonates.

d. Prevention

  (1) Pregnant women should have endocervical cultures for gonorrhea.

  (2) Application of 1% silver nitrate to the infant's eyes at the time of birth will usually prevent gonococcal ophthalmia.

  (3) Infants born to mothers with positive cultures should be treated as in c.(1).

B. Acquired infections (see also Chap. 15). The incidence of sepsis in the newborn is 2 in 1,000. The meninges will be involved in 25% of the cases of neonatal sepsis.

  1. Sepsis

  a. Predisposing factors include:

  (1) Premature onset of labor

  (2) Prolonged rupture of membranes

  (3) Maternal fever

  (4) Maternal colonization with group B streptococci

  (5) Indwelling catheters

  (6) Tracheal intubation

  b. Etiology. Organisms associated with neonatal infections are listed in Table 6-4.

  c. Evaluation. Sepsis should be suspected in the following situations:

  (1) Any sudden change for the worse

  (2) Temperature control problems, metabolic acidosis, and infant "not doing well"

  (3) Common symptoms include poor feeding, lethargy, apneic spells, spitting, vomiting, and diarrhea.

  (4) Signs include respiratory distress, abdominal distension, cyanosis, ileus, pustules, petechiae, purpura, omphalitis, and seizures.

  (5) Laboratory and radiographic evaluation

  (a) Leukopenia below 5,000 mm^3, a total neutrophil count under 2,500 mm^3, and a ratio of immature to total neutrophils of 0.15 or greater are clues to infection.

  (b) A Gram stain of gastric aspirate is obtained at or shortly after birth for neutrophils and bacteria.

Table 6-4. Organisms associated with newborn infection

Early infection

 Group B streptococci
 Escherichia coli
 Klebsiella-Aerobacter
 Enterococcus
 Listeria monocytogenes
 Streptococcus (Diplococcus) pneumoniae
 Group *A* streptococci
 Haemophilus influenzae
 Neisseria gonorrhoeae
 Anaerobes: *Clostridium, Bacteroides*

Late nursery infection (> 5 days of age)*

Staphylococcus aureus	*Pseudomonas*
E. coli	*Serratia*
Klebsiella-Aerobacter	*Staphylococcus epidermidis*

*The causative organisms vary with the flora of the nursery and with its personnel.

 (c) Isolation of an organism from sites such as gastric aspirate, ear canal, nasopharynx, skin, or rectum reflects colonization with the organism. The ratio of colonization to disease for the major neonatal pathogens (group B streptococci and *E. coli*) is approximately 100:1.
 (d) Examination of the buffy coat of a spun hematocrit tube by Gram stain may reveal bacteria.
 (e) The erythrocyte sedimentation rate may be elevated in infected infants. (Normal values are 1–2 mm/hr at 12 hr of age to 20 mm/hr at 2 weeks of age.)
 (f) A radionuclide bone scan may reveal osteomyelitis.
 (g) Chest x-ray
 (h) Recovery of an organism by culture or Gram stain from such sites as the blood, CSF, bladder-tap urine, abscesses, bone, joints, middle ear space, pleural space, or peritoneal cavities is confirmation of infection.
 (i) Demonstration of polysaccharide bacterial antigen in the blood, urine, or CSF confirms systemic infection.
 d. Treatment of sepsis. See Chap. 15; see also Table 15-1, 15-2.
  (1) When sepsis is suspected, treatment should begin **before** culture results are available.
  (2) IV antibiotics should be initiated in high, frequent doses (see Appendix Table 6-1).
  (3) Infants who become septic in the first 4 days of life (Table 6-4) should be treated for gram-positive cocci infection (group B streptococci) and gram-negative enteric bacteria. In this group, ampicillin and gentamicin are recommended for initial therapy. Ampicillin is used for initial therapy because of its effectiveness against streptococci, *L. monocytogenes*, enterococci, and some gram-negative bacteria. After the fourth day of life, treatment should cover *Staphylococcus aureus*, gram negatives, and other hospital-acquired pathogens. These pathogens will vary with the local experience but will often include *E. coli, Klebsiella-Aerobacter, Pseudomonas, Serratia* and *Staphylococcus epidermidis*. **The pattern of antibiotic susceptibility of the common agents causing nosocomial infections in the nursery should be known.** The initial treatment of late (> 4 days) infections includes a

Table 6-5. Cerebrospinal fluid findings in high-risk neonates without meningitis

Laboratory study	Term	Preterm
WBC count (cells/mm^3)		
No. of infants	87	30
Mean	8.2	9.0
Median	5	6
S.D.	7.1	8.2
Range	0–32	0–29
± 2 S.D.	0–22.4	0–25.4
Percentage neutrophils	61.3%	57.2%
Protein (mg/100 ml)		
No. of infants	35	17
Mean	90	115
Range	20–170	65–150
Glucose (mg/100 ml)		
No. of infants	51	23
Mean	52	50
Range	34–119	24–63
CSF and blood glucose (%)		
No. of infants	51	23
Mean	81	74
Range	44–248	55–105

Source: Modified from L. D. Sariff, et al., *J. Pediatr.* 88(3): 473, 1976.

penicillinase-resistant penicillin, such as oxacillin, and gentamicin. The new aminoglycosides amikacin and tobramycin should not be used routinely in the newborn except for kanamycin-resistant and gentamicin-resistant gram-negative infections. The third generation cephalosporins moxalactam and cefotaxime may be useful in these cases. However, ampicillin should also be used to cover *Listeria* and group B streptococcus infections (see **3.a**).

(4) Careful attention should be paid to temperature, hydration, caloric intake, acid-base balance, and any coagulopathy.

(5) When confirmatory cultures are ready, antibiotics should be "tailored" to the sensitivities of the organism or organisms recovered. Penicillin is used for group B streptococci (200,000–300,000 units/kg/day in 3–4 doses/day) (see **3.d**). Ampicillin (200 mg/kg/day) is used for *L. monocytogenes* and enterococci. An aminoglycoside should be used with ampicillin for enterococcal and gram-negative sepsis. Carbenicillin is used with an aminoglycoside for some gram-negative infections, especially *Pseudomonas* and indole-positive *Proteus* infections. Penicillin is effective against most anaerobic infections but is ineffective against *Bacteroides fragilis,* in which chloramphenicol is effective. Carbenicillin is effective against many strains of *B. fragilis.*

(6) IV therapy is continued for 10–14 days.

(7) Infants who fail to respond to the preceding therapy may benefit from exchange transfusion, fresh frozen plasma, or white cell transfusions.

2. Meningitis

    a. Etiology. Group B streptococci and *E. coli* account for 70% of all cases of neonatal meningitis in North America. *Listeria monocytogenes,* miscellaneous gram-positive and gram-negative organisms, *H. influenzae,* and anaerobes account for the rest.

    b. Evaluation and diagnosis

        (1) Any infant suspected of sepsis should have a lumbar puncture. Normal values are given in Table 6-5.

   (2) Neonatal meningitis is rapidly fatal, and few if any clinical signs may be present up to and including its terminal stages.
   (3) A full fontanelle is a late sign of meningitis.
   (4) Fever may or may not be present.
   (5) Laboratory studies. See **C.5.**
   (6) The diagnosis is confirmed when more than 10 WBC/mm^3 are present (see Table 6-6) and by a positive CSF culture.
 c. Treatment of meningitis. See also Chap. 15, pp. 392ff.
   (1) The initial therapy for meningitis is the same as for sepsis (Appendix 6-1). The higher ranges of doses are used.
   (2) The Gram stain of CSF or recovery of specific bacterial antigens may guide therapy until cultures are ready. Broad-spectrum coverage should not be dropped until an organism is identified.
   (3) Specific therapy is given when the organism and its antibiotic sensitivities are known.
   (4) In meningitis due to group B streptococci, penicillin and gentamicin are given for 14 days, and penicillin alone may be given an additional 7 days (see **3.d.(1)**).
   (5) The morbidity and mortality in gram-negative neonatal meningitis caused by penicillin-resistant organisms remain so high that early, aggressive therapy must be instituted. The poor penetration of systemically administered gentamicin into the cerebrospinal space may result in an inadequate bactericidal activity against gram-negative organisms. If the organism is ampicillin resistant, there will often be poor results. Intrathecal and intraventricular therapy with gentamicin have not been useful. This has led to therapy with chloramphenicol or moxalactam.
   (6) Chloramphenicol in appropriate doses should be considered as an alternative to aminoglycosides, or as an additional treatment in gram-negative meningitis.
     (a) The emergence of chloramphenicol resistance during the treatment of gram-negative infections has been reported.
     (b) Great care must be used if chloramphenicol is given in the presence of hemolytic anemia (due to the drug's toxic effect on bone marrow red cells) and of granulocytopenia. The drug should also be used cautiously in the presence of liver disease.
     (c) Measuring chloramphenicol levels in the blood and CSF is helpful in preventing dose-related chloramphenicol toxicity (bone marrow suppression and "gray baby syndrome"). The assay for chloramphenicol (as well as for all aminoglycosides) can be obtained from as little as 10 μl of serum. The ratio of CSF to serum chloramphenicol levels is 0.65 (range 0.48–0.99).
   (7) To ensure rapid sterilization of the blood and CSF, repeat cultures of blood and CSF should be done in the patient receiving therapy.
   (8) General supportive care of the patient is essential. Attention must be paid to electrolyte balance (inappropriate antidiuretic hormone secretion), clotting factors (DIC), seizures, nutrition, and ventilation.
   (9) Treatment of meningitis is intravenous, for 14–21 days. Gram-negative meningitis requires 21 days of treatment.
   (10) Moxalactam is active against most aminoglycoside-resistant gram-negative bacteria. It is also active against *Bacteroides* species. It has good penetration into the CSF. It is not very effective against group B streptococci. Moxalactam should be considered in cases of gram-negative meningitis.
 3. Group B streptococcal infection. The group B streptococcus is now the major cause of sepsis in most nurseries in the United States. The attack rate of group B sepsis is 2 in 1,000 live births.
  a. Etiology. Group B streptococci are recovered from the vaginal cultures of 25% of American mothers at the time of delivery. Of their infants, 25%

have positive skin or nasopharyngeal cultures, or both. For every 100 colonized infants, one will become ill.

b. Evaluation

(1) The early-onset type may present as mild respiratory distress or "transient tachypnea of the newborn," progressing rapidly to shock and death in an infant with few or no risk factors for infection. If the disease presents within a few hours of birth, the mortality is high, irrespective of therapy.

(2) Late infections may present as meningitis at 2–4 weeks of age.

(3) **Laboratory studies** include CBC, chest x-ray, blood culture, urinalysis and culture, "surface" cultures, lumbar puncture, and gastric aspirate.

c. Diagnosis

(1) The **diagnosis** is confirmed by positive blood, urine, or CSF cultures.

(2) The chest x-ray may show pneumonia, "retained lung fluid," or a pattern not unlike that of HMD.

(3) The gastric aspirate may show gram-positive diplococci with neutrophils.

d. Treatment

(1) Infants suspected of having group B streptococcal pneumonia or sepsis should be treated with aqueous penicillin, 200,000–300,000 units/kg/day in 3–4 doses/day, or ampicillin, 200 mg/kg/day, and gentamicin (see Appendix Table 6-1).

(2) If sepsis or meningitis is proved, treatment should be carried out for 14 days.

(3) The use of exchange transfusion and immune serum globulin has been advocated for very sick infants.

e. Prevention

(1) Polyvalent **group B streptococcus vaccine** is being evaluated for use in nonimmune pregnant women.

(2) Administration of **ampicillin** or **penicillin** to colonized pregnant women prior to labor or IV 6 hr prior to delivery has been advocated.

(3) Administration of **penicillin** to all infants within 1 hr of delivery has been advocated.

4. Pneumonia

a. Etiology

(1) **Congenital pneumonia**

(a) Transplacental agents include TORCH agents, enteroviruses, *Treponema pallidum, L. monocytogenes, Mycobacterium tuberculosis,* and genital *Mycoplasma.*

(2) Pneumonia acquired perinatally is associated with inhalation of infected amniotic fluid (often associated with prolonged rupture of the membranes). These pneumonias are due to maternal vaginal flora and are caused by group B streptococci, *E. coli,* and other gram-negative enteric bacteria, staphylococci, pneumococci, anaerobic organisms, *Chlamydia, Mycoplasma,* and HSV.

(3) Pneumonia acquired after birth may come from nursery personnel, other infants in the nursery, or nursery equipment. Staphylococci, gram-negative enteric bacteria, enteroviruses, respiratory syncytial virus, adenovirus, parainfluenza virus, *Chlamydia,* and HSV are among the common agents.

b. Evaluation

(1) **A history** of maternal fever, premature delivery, prolonged rupture of membranes, excessive obstetric manipulation, or foul-smelling amniotic fluid should increase suspicion of neonatal pneumonia.

(2) **Physical examination.** Fever, lethargy, tachypnea, grunting, flaring of nasal alae, retractions, irregular breathing, rales, and cyanosis may be present.

(3) **Laboratory tests** should include a CBC, a chest x-ray for evidence of

pulmonary infiltrate or pleural fluid, and a gastric aspirate for Gram stain and cultures. The presence of neutrophils is correlated with pneumonia more than is the finding of bacteria. Cultures, and Gram stain of the blood, urine, CSF and tracheal aspirate, should be obtained.

(4) If pleural fluid is present, **a pleural tap** should be done. Direct lung aspiration or lung biopsy is rarely indicated in cases unresponsive to therapy.

c. Diagnosis. The diagnosis of pneumonia is usually made by the presence of physical signs (see **B.2**) and a chest x-ray showing a pulmonary infiltrate.

d. Treatment

(1) General supportive measures include:

(a) Fluid, electrolyte, and acid-base balance

(b) Maintenance of hematocrit, blood volume, and blood pressure

(c) Nutrition

(d) Temperature control

(2) Respiratory support includes:

(a) Respiratory physical therapy; oxygen as needed

(b) Intermittent positive pressure ventilation, if indicated

(c) Drainage of pleural fluid if the fluid is compromising respiration

(3) Antibiotics are used as in the treatment of sepsis, depending on the suspected cause.

5. Omphalitis. The devitalized umbilical cord is an excellent culture medium for many bacteria. In areas where there is poor maternal immunity to tetanus and inadequate aseptic technique, neonatal tetanus due to omphalitis is a major cause of death.

a. Etiology. The cord is colonized shortly after birth with the local flora. Infection with streptococci and staphylococci is common. **Phlebitis** may spread to the liver, causing liver abscess or thrombosis of the hepatic vein. **Arteritis** may interfere with postnatal obliteration of the umbilical vessels and cause bleeding.

b. Evaluation and diagnosis

(1) Infection can cause peritonitis and septic emboli to the lungs, pancreas, kidney, skin, and bone.

(2) If true omphalitis is present, the infant should have a full evaluation for sepsis, including blood, urine, and CSF cultures.

c. Treatment

(1) As in sepsis, IV antibiotics are administered before culture results are available. Because *Staphylococcus* is a common agent, oxacillin and either gentamicin or kanamycin are preferred.

(2) Any catheter in the umbilicus should be removed.

(3) Leaving the cord open to the air to dry may decrease the number of flora.

6. Tuberculosis in the newborn. In the United States, when maternal tuberculosis (TB) is present or suspected at the time of delivery, management of the newborn is a major clinical problem. For a brief discussion see Chap. 15, p. 409. For a complete discussion, see V. P. Cloherty and A. R. Stark, *Manual of Neonatal Care*, Boston, Little, Brown, 1980.

7. Urinary tract infection may be secondary to sepsis or a primary source of infection. The diagnosis is by examination and culture of urine obtained by a bladder tap. Initial systemic treatment with ampicillin and an aminoglycoside is indicated. Medication can be changed after sensitivities are known. Parenteral treatment should be given for 14 days. Ultrasound and contrast studies of the urinary tract are indicated after treatment.

8. Skin pustules may be caused by staphylococci and will show gram-positive cocci on Gram stain. When there are only a few pustules, bathe with hexachlorophene solution, and local application of bacitracin ointment may suffice. If there are multiple pustules or the infant appears sick, a septic workup and systemic treatment with oxacillin is indicated. Erythema

Table 6-6. Body fluid in premature and newborn infants

Gestational age	TBW as percentage of BW*	ECW as percentage of BW*	ICW as percentage of BW*
Premature at 32 weeks	80	52	28
Full-term infant	75	40	35

BW = body weight, TBW = total body water, ICW = intracellular water, ECW = extracellular water.
*There is a 10% loss of BW in the first 7–10 days of life. This is mostly a loss of ECW.
Source: Adapted from H. S. Dweck, *Perinatology* 2:183, 1975; and J. C. Sinclair et al., *Pediatr. Clin. North Am.* 17:863, 1970.

Table 6-7. Fluid losses in infants at basal metabolic rate

Source of loss[a]	ml/kg/24h
Insensible water loss[b]	26–35
Pulmonary	8–10
Skin	18–23
Urine (at 300 mOsm/L)[c]	30–40
Stool	4
Total	60–77[d]

[a]The major variable in infants is the amount of insensible water loss.
[b]Will vary. See Table 6-8.
[c]Will vary with osmolar load plus renal function.
[d]Extra fluid will be required for growth.
Source: Adapted from H. S. Dweck, *Perinatology* 2:183, 1975; and J. C. Sinclair et al., *Pediatr. Clin. North Am.* 17:863, 1970.

toxicum will show eosinophils on Gram stain. Wounds from scalp monitors or abrasions related to delivery may cause both local and systemic infection. Organisms will include the maternal vaginal flora, especially group B streptococci, coliforms, and anaerobic organisms. Local treatment with warm saline soaks and application of Betadine may be adequate therapy. Systemic illness or local spread in spite of local therapy requires the use of systemic parenteral antibiotics and occasionally incision and drainage.

9. **Septic arthritis or osteomyelitis** may result from a bactermia or local trauma (heel sticks). Diagnosis is by clinical examination, aspiration of fluid, and occasionally by bone scan. Treatment involves systemic antibiotics for 4 weeks after local signs are gone. Aspiration or drainage is required in septic arthritis. Usually, gonococcal arthritis requires only 10 days of treatment and no drainage.

VIII. **Fluid and electrolyte management.** The goal of therapy is to provide fluid and electrolytes for maintenance and growth and to replace losses due to pathologic states. The principles are the same as in older children (see Chap. 7). In the newborn, problems can occur because of differences in body composition (Table 6-6), in the type and amounts of losses of fluid and electrolytes (Tables 6-7 and 6-8), and the limitations in the renal function of premature and newborn infants.

A. **Electrolytes**
   1. **Sodium**
      a. The usual maintenance requirement for sodium is 2–3 mEq/kg/day starting on the second or third day. Preterm infants may require 4–8 mEq/kg/day. This amount will gradually decrease after the first few weeks.
      b. Some causes of **hyponatremia** in the newborn are:

Table 6-8. Insensible water loss and body weight

Insensible water loss* (ml/kg/hr)	Body weight (gm)
2.7	< 1,000
2.3	1,000–1,250
1.5	1,250–1,500
1.0	1,500–1,750
0.8	1,750–2,000

*Factors that increase insensible water loss are ambient temperature above neutral thermal environment, fever, activity, radiant warmer, and phototherapy. Factors that decrease insensible water loss are assisted ventilation with warm and humidified air, heat shield, and incubation with high humidity.
Source: Adapted from H. S. Dweck, *Perinatology* 2:183, 1975; and J. C. Sinclair et al., *Pediatr. Clin. North Am.* 17:863, 1970.

   (1) Maternal. Hypotonic fluid overload, diuretics, and oxytocin use in labor, which causes an increase in antidiuretic hormone (ADH) in the mother and fetus
   (2) Neonatal. CNS disease, causing increased ADH; decreased renal readsorption of sodium due to prematurity, adrenal insufficiency, or diuretics; water intoxication from nebulization or excess free water; and low salt intake in premature infants fed breast milk or low-sodium formula.
   c. Hypernatremia is caused by sodium overload, diarrhea and vomiting, failure to provide adequate free water in infants with increased insensible water loss (IWL).
   d. Treatment of hyponatremia and hypernatremia is similar to that used in older children (see Chap. 7, p. 190).
 2. Potassium
   a. The usual maintenance requirement for potassium is 2–3 mEq/kg/24h. This is usually started on the second or third day.
   b. Hyperkalemia in the newborn may be caused by adrenal insufficiency, exchange transfusion with old blood and by iatrogenic means. The ECG may show peaked T waves.
   c. Hypokalemia in the newborn is often seen in adrenal problems, in failure to replace ongoing potassium losses, in association with vomiting as in pyloric stenosis or with use of diuretics. The ECG may show depressed T waves.
   d. For treatment of hypokalemia and hyperkalemia, see Chap. 7, p. 191.
 3. Calcium. See Chap. 7, p. 192.
B. Renal factors in the newborn. As compared with the kidneys of older children, the newborn kidney has a limited ability both to dilute and to concentrate urine; has a decreased glomerular filtration rate, blood flow, and tubular resorption of glucose, sodium, and bicarbonate; and has an inability to excrete an acid and a phosphate load. These limitations of function are more severe with decreasing gestational age.
C. Fluid and electrolyte monitoring in the newborn should include:
 1. A physical examination
 2. Blood. Osmolarity, Na, K, glucose, BUN
 3. Urine. Specific gravity or osmolarity, Na, K, and glucose
 4. An **accurate record of intake and output.** A calibrated infusion pump is necessary for accurate hourly infusions. A pediatric urine collector should be used to measure output. In small male infants, the penis can be inserted in a test tube to facilitate accurate assessment of output. Weighing diapers or pads before and after voiding may be done to avoid the use of tape with consequent breakdown of skin.

    5. Fluid and electrolyte therapy must be adjusted frequently, depending on the size of the infant and the results of the preceding determinations.

D. Fluid and electrolyte requirements

  1. Term infants

    a. Fluid requirements

Fluid requirement	ml/kg/day
Day 1	70
Day 2	80
Day 3	100
Day 4 on	120–150

    IV fluids are usually given as 10% dextrose in water.

    Decrease in renal failure, cardiac failure, decreased IWL, increased ADH

    Increase in excess IWL, low humidity, fever, activity, increased renal loss.

    b. Na. 2–3 mEq/kg/24h starting on day 2

    c. K. 2–3 mEq/kg/day starting on day 2

    d. Ca. 30–45 mg/kg/day (see p. 128)

  2. Premature infants

    a. Fluid requirements (ml/kg/day):

Body weight (gm)	Days 1–2	Day 3	Days 15–20
2,000–1,750	80	110	130
1,750–1,500	80	110	130
1,500–1,250	90	120	130
1,250–1,000	100	130	140
1,000–750	105	140	150

    b. Prematures weighing under 1,000 gm may require up to 200 ml/kg/day because they are often on open beds and under radiant warmers and phototherapy (see Table 6-8). Failure to provide this amount of fluid will lead to significant hypernatremia.

    c. Small prematures may be unable to metabolize the glucose load in 10% D/W and hyperglycemia and glucosuria will develop. Glucose intake must be measured as gm/kg/hr and gradually increased until the infant can tolerate the glucose load. Some useful numbers to help with this calculation are:

Infusion rate		Amount of glucose received	
ml/kg/hr 5% D/W	ml/kg/hr 10% D/W	gm/kg/hr	gm/kg/day
4	2	0.2	4.8
6	3	0.3	7.2
8	4	0.4	9.6
10	5	0.5	12.0

    For example, 2 ml/kg/hr of 10% D/W will provide 0.2 gm/kg/hr or 4.8 gm/kg/day of glucose.

    d. Electrolyte requirements

      (1) Na. Prematures require at least 2–3 mEq/kg/day starting on day 2 or 3. Many require up to 4–8 mEq/kg/day. Serum and urine sodium should be monitored.

      (2) K. 2–3 mEq/kg/day should be started on day 2 or 3 if there is no renal problem.

      (3) Ca. Acute requirements are often 30–45 mg/kg/day. Long-term calcium requirements are 100–150 mg/kg/day (see nutrition, p. 128).

IX. Neurologic problems
  A. Neonatal seizures. See Chap. 20, pp. 506ff.
  B. Intraventricular hemorrhage. Periventricular-intraventricular hemorrhage (PV-IVH) is the most common neonatal intracranial hemorrhage. It has an incidence of 30–40% in infants weighing under 1,500 gm and is associated with prematurity and hypoxia.
    1. Evaluation
        a. The catastrophic syndrome progresses rapidly in minutes to hours with shock, stupor, coma, bradycardia, respiratory irregularity, and apnea There may be tonic seizures, decerebrate posturing, dilated pupils, flaccid quadriparesis, a full fontanelle, a fall in hematocrit, temperature abnormalities, and metabolic acidosis.
        b. The saltatory presentation may progress over hours or days. The signs are a change in level of consciousness, hypotonia, abnormal eye movement, changes in respiration pattern, and an unexplained fall in hematocrit.
        c. The condition should be suspected in premature infants who have any abnormal neurologic signs. If available, a real-time **ultrasound sector scanner** should be used as the initial diagnostic tool. In its absence, a careful **lumbar puncture** is performed. The finding of bloody CSF is an indication for an attempt to make a definitive diagnosis of intracranial hemorrhage by ultrasound or **CT scan.** Xanthochromia, elevated protein and late hypoglycorrhachia are often seen in the CSF. Meningeal irritation from blood may cause a CSF pleocytosis and raise concerns about infection.
        d. A CT scan is the most accurate means of diagnosing intracranial hemorrhage, but because of the requirement to transport small, sick infants, it is difficult to obtain.
    2. **Diagnosis.** Intraventricular hemorrhage is usually classified as follows:

        Grade I   Subependymal bleeding
        Grade II   Intraventricular hemorrhage without ventricular dilation
        Grade III Intraventricular hemorrhage with ventricular dilation
        Grade IV   Intraventricular hemorrhage with parenchymal hemorrhage

    3. **Therapy**
        a. General supportive measures to treat seizures, hypoxia, apnea, hypercapnia, acidosis, hypothermia, and hypoglycemia should be instituted.
        b. Cerebral perfusion should be maintained to prevent hypoxic-ischemic damage to the brain. The blood pressure should be maintained in the normal range and no wide swings permitted. This must be done carefully since excess cerebral perfusion may increase cerebral bleeding. Intracranial pressure may be decreased by performing a lumbar puncture since in the immediate posthemorrhagic period a communication exists between the ventricles and the subarachnoid space.
        c. Avoid arterial hypertension, hypercapnia, infusion of hyperosmolar solutions, or rapid expansion of intravascular volume.
        d. If the infant survives the acute insult, serial assessment of the hemorrhage and ventricular size should be done by ultrasound or CT scan.
        e. Grade I hemorrhages have a good prognosis and usually need only supportive therapy
        f. **In more severe hemorrhages,** serial lumbar punctures are useful to lower intracranial pressure in the period immediately after the hemorrhage but do not appear to decrease the long-term incidence of hydrocephalus. Serial lumbar punctures may stabilize the infant and allow the CSF to clear.
        g. In acute hydrocephalus unresponsive to serial lumbar punctures, a temporary external ventriculostomy may be necessary.
        h. If slow, progressive ventricular dilation occurs, glycerol in an initial dose of 1 gm/kg q6h PO, progressing over 1 week to 2 gm/kg q6h PO, may

be used. The serum osmolarity, sodium, BUN, and glucose must be monitored. If effective, the drug is continued for 3–6 months. Furosemide
(LASIX) and acetazolamide (Diamox) have also been used for this purpose.

  i. A ventriculoperitoneal shunt is used if a shunt is necessary after a ven-
triculostomy has been in place for 5–7 days or in slowly progressive
hydrocephalus if glycerol is ineffective.

  4. Prevention. Most PV-IVHs occur in the first 2–3 days of life in prematures.
Preventing major fluctuations in brain perfusion may prevent PV-IVH.

X. Necrotizing enterocolitis

  A. Etiology is not clearly defined. The primary event is believed to be damage to the
intestinal mucosa that allows invasion of the bowel wall and circulation by
intestinal flora with subsequent sepsis and perforation. Factors suggested to
cause mucosal damage include ischemia, feeding of hypertonic formulas or medications, and bacterial invasion.

  B. Evaluation and diagnosis

    1. Bloody diarrhea in a small premature infant with abdominal distention and
bloody or bile-stained gastric aspirates suggests necrotizing enterocolitis.
Other frequently associated systemic signs include temperature instability,
Clinitest positive stools, apnea, and lethargy.

    2. Clinical and laboratory abnormalities often associated with necrotizing en-
terocolitis (NEC) include shock, DIC, neutropenia, thrombocytopenia,
acidosis, hyponatremia, and hypoglycemia.

    3. Evaluation should include ABGs, CBC, differential, platelet count and
smear, electrolytes, BUN, glucose, creatinine, prothrombin time and partial
thromboplastin time, cultures of blood, stool and CSF, KUB, and cross-table
lateral x-ray.

    4. The presence of pneumatosis intestinalis on abdominal x-ray confirms the
diagnosis. Free peritoneal gas or gas in the portal venous system may be
seen. Both are ominous signs.

  C. Treatment

    1. The infant should receive nothing by mouth.

    2. A nasogastric tube should be placed for drainage.

    3. After appropriate cultures have been obtained, the infant should be started
on broad-spectrum systemic antibiotics, including ampicillin and gentamicin
(unless the nursery has a high incidence of gentamicin-resistant pathogens
or the surveillance stool cultures for the infant with NEC yield gentamicin-
resistant organisms, in which case an alternative aminoglycoside should be
selected based on the known sensitivity).

    4. Correction of shock, acidosis, hyponatremia, thrombocytopenia, or DIC
should be instituted as detailed in the individual sections dealing with these
problems.

    5. Frequent vital signs and clinical examinations are essential; follow serial
abdominal x-rays, CBC with platelet count, electrolytes and pH q6h until the
individual variables are stable and the infant is improving.

    6. Early surgical consultation is essential. The usual indications for surgery
include perforation or the persistent clinical deterioration of the infant on
optimal medical management.

    7. Peripheral or central hyperalimentation should be instituted.

    8. Treatment should be continued for 10–14 days.

    9. Since intestinal strictures are a possible sequelae of NEC, the infant should
be observed closely for symptoms of obstruction.

XI. Drug withdrawal in the newborn

  A. Etiology. Withdrawal symptoms may be seen in infants born to mothers taking
narcotics, methadone, diazepam, phenobarbital, alcohol, ethchlorvynol, pentazocine, chlordiazepoxide, or other drugs that may cause addiction.

  B. Evaluation and diagnosis

    1. Maternal history. Discreet, sensitive history taking is necessary to elicit a
history of drug abuse.

2. The **infant's symptoms** include disturbed patterns of sleeping and waking rhythms; nasal congestion, sneezing, and yawning; high-pitched cry; increased sucking, ravenous appetite; irritability, jitteriness; hypertonicity, hyperreflexia, and clonus; sweating and tachypnea; vomiting, diarrhea, and dehydration; fever; and seizures and tremors.

3. **Infants of methadone-treated mothers** may have severe, prolonged withdrawal. Some have "late" withdrawal that may be of the following two types:
   a. The first group shows symptoms shortly after birth, improves, then relapses at 2–4 weeks.
   b. The second group shows no symptoms at birth, but symptoms develop 2–3 weeks later. These infants may also have a history of a sudden, tremendous increase in appetite.

4. Blood and urine samples from the mother and infant for toxic screen within 24 hr after delivery may help, but drugs given to the mother during labor can sometimes confuse the results. Clinical suspicion and careful history usually lead to the diagnosis.

C. **Treatment.** The goal of treatment is an infant who is not irritable, is not vomiting, has no diarrhea, and can sleep between feedings, yet is not heavily sedated.

1. Swaddling, holding, and rocking may help infants who are not severely affected.

2. **Drugs.** Infants in whom the preceding therapy is inadequate will need medication.
   a. **Phenobarbital,** 5–8 mg/kg/day IM or PO in 4 divided doses, and tapered over 2 weeks, can be given. The side effects are sedation, poor sucking, and no control of diarrhea.
   b. **Chlorpromazine,** 1.5–3.0 mg/kg/24 hr in divided doses q6h, is given initially IM then PO. This dose is maintained for 2–4 days, then tapered as tolerated every 2–4 days. The length of treatment is from 1–6 weeks. Methadone-dependent infants tend to need a longer course of treatment.
   c. **Paregoric,** 0.05/ml/kg (2 drops/kg/dose), is given q4h. The dose is increased by 2 drops (0.05 ml) at the end of a 4-hr period if no improvement is seen. Some babies will need medication more often than q4h. Once the adequate dose is determined, it can be tapered by 10 percent daily. The length of treatment is 1–6 weeks. **Side effects** include sleepiness and constipation. **The effects of oral benzoic acid on bilirubin binding to albumin are not known. Camphor is a CNS stimulant.**
   d. **Tincture of opium, U.S.P.** For the above reasons, if a narcotic is to be used it may be best to use **tincture of opium, U.S.P.,** a 10% solution (equal to 1.0% morphine). Dilute this 25-fold to a concentration equal to that of paregoric (0.4% opium or 0.04% morphine) and give in the same dose as paregoric.
   e. **Diazepam.** The dose is 1–2 mg IM q8h until symptoms are controlled. The dose is then halved, then changed to q12h, then halved again. The length of treatment ranges from 2–7 days, and it seems to be effective in a shorter time than are other medications. **Note that sodium benzoate included in parenteral diazepam interferes with bilirubin binding.**
   f. **Methadone** should not be routinely used until more data on toxicity are available. **Methadone is excreted in breast milk,** and thus methadone-treated mothers should not breast-feed. When administration has been necessary, the doses used have been 0.5–1.0 mg q4–8h.

3. The major problem for these children is proper disposition and follow-up. Most states require reporting of these infants as battered children, and social agencies should be involved in the decision for disposition (see Chap. 3, p. 72). Some risk factors to consider in sending infants home with their mothers are:
   a. **Maternal age.** The risk increases as age decreases.
   b. **Length of drug use.** The risk increases as the length of usage increases.
   c. Availability of a drug program
   d. Drug use while on methadone suggests increased risk.

Table 6-9. Relative incidence of esophageal anomalies

Type	Relative incidence* (%)
EA with distal TEF	88
EA without TEF	8
TEF without EA	2
EA with proximal and distal TEF	0.6
EA with proximal TEF	0.8

EA = esophageal atresia; TEF = tracheoesophageal fistula.
*TEF/EA is often associated with other major malformation; 20% have congenital heart disease, and 10% have imperforate anus. TEF/EA is sometimes associated with Down syndrome or the VATER syndrome of: vertebral and vascular defects, imperforate anus, EA with TEF, radial dysplasia, and renal defects. Of infants with EA, 20% are premature, and another 20% are small for gestational age.

    e. Inability of the mother to make and keep commitments suggests a high risk to the child.
XII. Surgical emergencies
  A. Tracheoesophageal fistula (TEF) **with or without esophageal atresia** (EA)
    1. Etiology. Esophageal anomalies in the newborn are classified as type A–E. Their frequency is given in Table 6-9.
    2. Evaluation. Depending on the presence and location of the fistula and the presence or absence of esophageal atresia, symptoms include excessive salivation, regurgitation of feedings, coughing from aspiration of feedings or gastric contents, abdominal distension, or a schaphoid, airless abdomen.
    3. Diagnosis
      a. EA is diagnosed by the inability to pass a catheter from the nose or mouth into the stomach. Listening over the stomach as air is injected and withdrawn from the stomach by a syringe attached to the catheter confirms the patency of the esophagus. If EA is present, a plain chest film may show a dilated upper esophageal pouch. It will also demonstrate a catheter coiled in the upper pouch.
      b. The absence of abdominal gas on x-ray suggests EA without a distal TEF. A lateral chest film taken after 1 ml of barium is injected into the upper pouch will be diagnostic of EA. The barium should be immediately removed to prevent aspiration.
      c. TEF without EA may be suspected because of recurrent aspiration with feeding and excessive gas in the bowel. Diagnosis may be difficult. A barium swallow in the face-down position or simultaneous esophagoscopy and bronchoscopy with a dye placed in the trachea may be diagnostic. When clinical symptoms make the diagnosis very likely, surgical exploration of the neck should be considered.
    4. Treatment. Once the diagnosis of EA with TEF is made, the pediatrician's role is to prevent aspiration and to provide nutrition and support until definitive surgical therapy is carried out. Measures should include:
      a. Sump catheter drainage of the upper pouch
      b. Provision of a reliable IV line for nutrition and fluids
      c. Keeping the baby in a 30-degree head-up position
      d. Treatment with antibiotics for pneumonia even if it is not clinically or radiologically evident
      e. Provision of adequate respiratory support
      f. If the baby has complications that will delay primary repair, a **gastrostomy** is usually indicated to decompress the abdomen and prevent aspiration of gastric contents. Definitive repair may be early, delayed, or staged.

B. Omphalocele and gastroschisis
  1. Omphalocele
    a. Etiology. An omphalocele is caused by failure of development of part o the abdominal wall. The defect, which is evident at birth, is covered wit a translucent membrane holding the bowel and viscera. This membran may rupture at delivery.
    b. Emergency medical treatment includes:
      (1) Insertion of a nasogastric tube, which is placed to suction.
      (2) Protecting the lesion by
        (a) Covering with gauze soaked in warm saline and surrounding by a "protective wall" of saline-soaked gauze
        (b) Covering the gauze with Saran Wrap to prevent fluid an evaporative heat loss and then wrapping the abdomen with cotton bandage
      (3) Starting IV fluids
      (4) Starting antibiotics (ampicillin and gentamicin) if the sac is rupture
      (5) Monitoring temperature and blood pressure
      (6) Arranging immediate surgical treatment. The sac should not b pushed back into the abdomen, since this may impede venous retur and respiration.
  2. Gastroschisis is managed medically in the same manner as omphaloce until definitive surgical treatment is carried out. Antibiotics are **alway used** because there is no membrane. Infants with omphalocele and gastro chisis should be evaluated for malformation of the colon and intestinal atre sia.

C. Intestinal obstruction
  1. Etiology. The causes are listed in Table 6-10.
  2. Evaluation
    a. The **symptoms** of intestinal obstruction vary with the site of the lesior Lesions below the pylorus present with bile-stained vomiting. Lesion high in the gut such as malrotation with midgut volvulus will preser with little abdominal distention, and lesions low in the bowel such as ilea atresia will show distention. There may be a history of polyhydramnios
    b. Laboratory tests include hematocrit, CBC, ABGs and pH, an x-ray of th abdomen taken with the infant in the upright and flat positions, a bariur enema, and a sweat test in cases of meconium ileus.
  3. The **diagnosis** of some common causes of intestinal obstruction in the new born are:
    a. Pyloric stenosis may present in the newborn period as nonbilious projec tile vomiting. An enlarged pylorus may be palpated. A large gastric ai shadow may be seen on x-ray. A barium swallow is diagnostic.
    b. Duodenal atresia may be associated with other anomalies such as Dow syndrome, cardiovascular malformations, and other gastrointestina malformations. There may be a history of polyhydramnios. Symptom and signs are bilious vomiting and upper abdominal distention. A plair x-ray of the abdomen will show air in the stomach and upper part of th duodenum ("double bubble").
    c. Jejunoileal atresia presents with abdominal distention, bilious vomiting and failure to pass stools. X-ray films show air-fluid levels and a bariur enema shows a microcolon. There may be multiple atretic segments.
    d. Malrotation of colon with midgut volvulus is an extreme emergency. I may present as bile-stained vomiting without much abdominal distensior in an infant who has previously been passing stools. There may be ab dominal tenderness. X-rays may show duodenal obstruction with little ai in the rest of the bowel. A barium enema may show the cecum in th upper right or central abdomen.
    e. Meconium ileus is often associated with meconium peritonitis, a positiv sweat test for cystic fibrosis, and an x-ray showing dilated small bowe filled with a granular appearing material or tiny bubbles. Treatment ma

Table 6-10. Etiology of intestinal obstruction in newborn

Mechanical obstruction

Congenital	*Extrinsic*
Intrinsic	Malrotation with or without midgut vol-
Pyloric stenosis	vulus
Duodenal atresia	Volvulus without malrotation
Jejunoileal atresia or stenosis	Peritoneal bands
Imperforate anus	Incarcerated hernia (premature infants)
Intraluminal cysts	Annular pancreas
Meconium ileus with or without cystic	Duplications
fibrosis	Aberrant vessels
	Hydrometrocolpos
Acquired	
Intussusception	
Adhesion	
Mesenteric artery thrombosis	
Formation of intestinal concretions (lactobezors)	
Stenosis secondary to healed necrotizing enterocolitis	

Functional obstruction

Prematurity	Sepsis
Defective innervation (Hirschsprung's disease)	Enteritis
	CNS disease
Drugs	Necrotizing enterocolitis
Hypermagnesemia	Endocrine disorders such as hypothyroid-
Heroin	ism and adrenal insufficiency
Hexamethonium bromide	

require enemas as in functional obstruction, gastrograffin enemas after adequate and continuous intravenous hydration and occasionally surgery.

   f. Functional obstruction due to disorders such as prematurity, meconium plug syndrome, and hypermagnesemia will often respond to glycerine suppositories, gentle enemas (one-half strength saline in a dose of 5 ml/kg of body weight) given with a soft rubber catheter, or rectal stimulation with a soft rubber catheter. Frequent small feedings and adequate hydration are also helpful. A barium enema, performed in an infant who has functional obstruction due to prematurity, may compound the problem. If contrast enemas are to be done, consideration should be given to using gastrograffin after adequate and ongoing intravenous hydration.

  4. Treatment of most causes of mechanical intestinal obstruction includes:
    a. Nasogastric suction
    b. Fluid and electrolyte therapy; volume replacement (colloid) if indicated
    c. Antibiotics—if there is a question of integrity of the bowel or the infant appears sick
    d. Surgery if indicated

D. Diaphragmatic hernia occurs once in every 3,000 births. Most diaphragmatic hernias of Bochdalek are on the left side.
  1. Evaluation. Mortality in this disease is high due to the hypoplastic lungs and abnormal pulmonary vasculature. There often are severe complications due to the persistence of the fetal circulation pattern and myocardial dysfunction secondary to hypoxia and acidosis. Infants with large diaphragmatic hernias may present at birth with cyanosis, respiratory distress, a scaphoid abdomen,

decreased or absent breath sounds on the side of the hernia, and heart sounds heard best on the side opposite the hernia. Small hernias, right sided hernias, and substernal hernias of Morgagni may have a more subtle onset, manifested by feeding problems and mild respiratory distress.

2. **Diagnosis.** The diagnosis is confirmed by chest x-ray.
3. **Treatment.** When a diaphragmatic hernia is suspected, the following measures should be employed:
   a. A large tube should be placed into the stomach and put to suction to remove air and gastric contents, which, if allowed to accumulate, will increase mediastinal shift and lung compression.
   b. The infant should receive oxygen and respiratory support as needed.
   c. A reliable IV line should be placed.
   d. Hypoxia and acidosis should be treated.
   e. Prompt surgical correction should be carried out.

Appendix Table 6-1. Doses of selected antibiotics for use in newborns

Drug	Dose, route, and schedule	Comments
Amikacin	15 mg/kg/day IM or IV infused over 30 min	
Ampicillin	< 1 week old: 100–150 mg/kg/day IM or IV q12h > 1 week old: 200 mg/kg/day IM or IV q8h	

Carbenicillin	Initial dose 100 mg/kg IV
	Follow by:
	  Newborns weighing < 2,000 gm:
	    < 7 days old: 225 mg/kg/day IV q8h
	    > 7 days old: 400 mg/kg/day IV q6h
	  Newborns weighing > 2,000 gm:
	    < 3 days old: 300 mg/kg/day IV q6h
	    > 3 days old: 400 mg/kg/day IV q6h	

Chloramphenicol	< 2,000 gm: 25 mg/kg/day IV q12h < 1 week old: 25 mg/kg/day IV q12h > 2,000 gm and 1 week old: 50 mg/kg/day IV q12h	IM chloramphenicol is erratically absorbed. **Toxic effects** are seen with serum levels over 50 μg/ml; serum levels should be kept under 25 μg/ml to avoid the "gray baby syndrome." Goal should be 15–20 μg/ml.
Gentamicin sulfate	< 34 weeks' gestational age: 2.5 mg/kg/dose over 30 min IV or IM q18h > 34 weeks' gestational age: 2.5 mg/kg/dose over 30 min IV or IM q12h	Optimal serum level is 4–8 μg/ml 1 hr after IV dose and under 2.0 μg/ml before a dose

Appendix Table 6-1 (continued)

Drug	Dose, route, and schedule	Comments
Kanamycin sulfate	15 mg/kg/day: IM or slow IV over 30 min q12h	Risks of ototoxicity and nephrotoxicity are increased when renal function is poor. Try to keep the total dose under 500 mg/kg, since ototoxicity is related to total dose. Therapeutic serum level is 15–20 μg/ml. The predose level should be under 10 μg/ml
Moxalactam	< 7 days of age: 50–100 mg/kg/day IV q12h > 7 days of age: 100 mg/kg/day IV q12h	
Oxacillin sodium	50 mg/kg dose IM or IV < 2,500 gm, < 2 weeks old: bid–tid < 2,500 gm, > 2 weeks old: tid–qid	Use higher dose more frequently in severe infection
Penicillin G, crystalline	< 7 days of age: 50,000–100,000 units/kg/day IV or IM q12h > 7 days of age: 100,000–300,000 units/kg/day IV or IM q8h *In group B streptococcal infections use 200,000–300,000 units/kg/day even in infants < 7 days of age	
Vancomycin	< 7 days of age: 30 mg/kg/day q12h IM or IV infused over 30–60 min > 7 days of age: 45 mg/kg/day q8h IM or IV infused over 30–60 min	

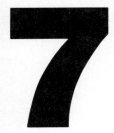

Fluid and Electrolytes

I. General principles

A. Renal function. The glomerular filtration rate (GFR) is relatively depressed in infants and reaches a "normal" adult value (corrected for surface area) only at age 1½–2 years. Other functions similarly depressed include renal plasma flow (RPF), free-water clearance, acid excretion, phosphate excretion, and T_m glucose (Table 7-1).

B. Fluid and volume physiology. At birth the total body water (TBW) constitutes 75–80% of the infant's weight. The TBW falls to 60% in childhood. A rapid diuresis ensues over the first few days of life, during which 7% of TBW is lost.

1. Body fluids

    a. The TBW comprises two major compartments:

        (1) Extracellular fluid (ECF) constitutes 35–45% of body water in infants and 20% in adults (15% interstitial and 5% intravascular).

        (2) Intracellular fluid (ICF) constitutes 40% of body water in both infants and adults.

2. Regulatory mechanisms

    a. The **kidney** regulates (1) water balance, (2) osmolality of fluids by controlling free-water excretion, and (3) distribution of body water through sodium retention and excretion.

    b. Principles

        (1) Tonicity (concentration, osmolality) is conserved in preference to volume.

        (2) The kidneys provide better protection against **dilution** of body fluids than against **dehydration.**

        (3) ECF volume is controlled by **sodium,** and the intracellular compartment (cell volume, ionic content) is dependent on ECF. Hence, sodium control is the key to overall volume control and, indirectly, to ICF regulation.

    c. Osmolality: refers to the number of osmotically active particles per 1,000 gm water in a solution (units = mOsm/kg); whereas osmolarity refers to the number of osmotically active particles per unit volume of solution (units = mOsm/L). The serum osmolality is generally higher than the osmolarity due to the high specific volume of proteins. The terms *osmolality* and *osmolarity* frequently are confused. Osmolality is theoretically more appropriate than osmolarity for the calculation of osmotic relationships.

        (1) ECF osmolality is somewhat higher than that of the ICF because of the contribution by plasma proteins.

        (2) Water flux follows ionic (osmolal) flux to equalize fluid concentrations.

        (3) Osmolality is determined by freezing point depression of the solution. Also, as a rule of thumb:

$$\text{Osmolality} = 2(\text{Na}^+) + \frac{\text{BUN}}{2.8} + \frac{\text{glucose}}{18}$$

Osmolal excretion depends on the concentrating ability of the kidney. To produce a minimal urinary volume requires a maximum osmolal-

Table 7-1. Normal values of renal function*

Measurement	At birth	1–2 Weeks	6 Months– 1 year	1–3 Years	Adult
GFR (ml/min/m^2)	15 ± 11	31 ± 15	45 ± 12	55 ± 13	68 ± 1●
RPF (ml/min/m^2)	51 ± 12	89 ± 20	203 ± 42	310 ± 70	354 ± 5●
T$_m$ PAH (mg/min/m^2)		8 ± 1	30 ± 12	38 ± 11	46 ± 7
T$_m$ glucose (mg/min/m^2)		10 ± 12			196 ± 2●

m^2 = body surface area in square meters.
*Mean ± S.D.

ity: This ranges from 1,200 mOsm/kg in the healthy child (600–700 mOsm/kg in the healthy infant), down to 300 mOsm/kg in the diseased kidney.

d. **Volume** is a sine qua non for organ function. Regulatory factors include cardiac output, peripheral resistance, aldosterone, renin-angiotensin axis, prostaglandins, and catechol levels. Since the body's Na$^+$ content determines ECF distribution, its adjustment is essential to volume regulation. By cation exchange, aldosterone operates in the distal tubule to conserve Na$^+$. Active transport of cation brings about passive water transfer, thereby restoring ECF volume. In addition, ADH release in response to hemoconcentration augments water retention and thereby aids volume repletion.

e. **"Third space"** accumulations occur in many disease states, trapping fluid, electrolytes, and drugs outside their normal boundaries and thus robbing the body of effective volume.

C. Electrolyte physiology

1. **Sodium (Na$^+$).** 1 mEq = 23 mg; 1 gm = 43.5 mEq; plasma concentration = 135–140 mEq/L. **Note:** 1 gm salt (NaCl) = 18 mEq Na$^+$.

   a. Sodium is the principal volume regulator. Normally, Na$^+$ accounts for 90% of extracellular cationic osmolality.

   b. Although Na$^+$ is principally distributed in the ECF, the true Na$^+$ space is the TBW (about 60% of body weight). The serum Na$^+$ concentration is determined by the total body Na$^+$ load and the TBW.

   c. Measurement of Na$^+$ by flame photometer is artifactually depressed in hyperlipemic and hyperglycemic states. **Rule of thumb:** Na$^+$ is depressed 5 mEq/L for every 200 mg/dl of glucose concentration above 100 mg/dl.

   d. Requirements for Na$^+$ vary. A typical daily requirement is 40–60 mEq/M^2, or 1–3 mEq/kg. When excretory capacity is impaired (heart failure, renal compromise) or overwhelmed (salt poisoning), edema formation and expansion of the TBW occurs.

   Symptoms of inadequate sodium include confusion, restlessness, seizures, and eventually coma and death. Hypotension and circulatory failure can result from acute, severe sodium depletion.

   e. The administration of salt (PO, IV, or by clysis) results in uptake by the ECF. One-third enters the plasma space, while two-thirds is taken up by the interstitium.

   f. **In the newborn,** the sodium and volume regulatory mechanisms are functionally limited. Excretory capacity is reduced by a relative concentrating defect (maximal urine osmolality approximately 600–700), and therefore obligatory solute loads require extra free water for their elimination (see Table 5-3 for solute contents of various infant diets). Since infants cannot control their fluid intake, sufficient fluid must be provided to balance needs for solute excretion.

2. **Potassium (K$^+$).** 1 mEq = 39.1 mg; 1 gm = 25.6 mEq; plasma concentration 3.4–5.5 mEq/L (may be higher in neonates).

    a. Potassium is the principal cation of the ICF (which contains 98% of the body potassium) and contributes to the maintenance of intracellular tonicity and cell membrane (ECF) resting potential, permitting electrical "discharge."

    b. The proportion of K$^+$ in the ECF is controlled by multiple factors, including body pH and body Na$^+$ load and K$^+$ load. Thus, measurement of serum K$^+$ provides only an indirect assessment of total body K$^+$ stores and may therefore be misleading (e.g., diabetic ketoacidosis). **No practical estimate of K$^+$ space can be given for therapeutic replacement purposes.**

    c. A typical daily K$^+$ requirement is 30–40 mEq/M^2/24 hr, or 1–3 mEq/kg. There is an obligatory K$^+$ loss via the urine, since tubular resorption cannot lower U$_{K^+}$ below 10 mEq/L.

    d. The limit of tolerance for IV potassium is 250 mEq/M^2/24 hr, or about 8 mEq/M^2/hr. An absolute maximal 1-hr IV dose is 1 mEq/kg, hand administered into a large vein. IV administration of K$^+$ in concentrations greater than 40 mEq/L usually leads to phlebitis.

    e. The danger of **abnormal K$^+$** is exacerbated by abnormalities of Ca^{2+} in the opposite direction.

    f. **Hypokalemia** due to a renal tubular defect, starvation, chronic diarrhea or vomiting, diabetic ketoacidosis, hyperaldosteronism, chronic use of diuretics, or inadequate long-term IV replacement is usually accompanied by chloride depletion with metabolic alkalosis. Recently, carbenicillin has been reported to cause hypokalemia.

        (1) Symptoms include muscle weakness, cramps, paralytic ileus, decreased reflexes, lethargy, and confusion.

        (2) A urine K$^+$ concentration of 10 mEq/L or less suggests severe K$^+$ depletion. Acid urine in the presence of metabolic alkalosis (paradoxical aciduria) also indicates K$^+$ depletion. Hypokalemic metabolic alkalosis is usually accompanied by a K$^+$ deficit of at least 4–5 mEq/kg.

        (3) Cardiac effects seen by ECG are a low-voltage T wave, the presence of a U wave, and a prolonged Q-T interval.

        (4) Chronic explosure to low potassium damages the kidney's concentrating ability, thus producing a vasopressin-resistant **diabetes insipidus.**

    g. **Hyperkalemia** occurs with renal failure, hemolysis, tissue necrosis, Addison's disease, congenital adrenal cortical hyperplasia, certain diuretics, and overdose of K$^+$ supplements. A specific renal tubular defect with hyperkalemia, hypertension, and growth failure has been described.

        (1) Hypocalcemia, hyponatremia, and acidosis all exacerbate the dangerous effects of hyperkalemia.

        (2) The toxic effects are mainly cardiac. Rising K$^+$ interferes with normal nodal and bundle conduction. ECG changes include peaked T wave, increased P-R interval and widened QRS, depressed S-T segment, and atrioventricular or intraventricular heart block. As serum K$^+$ rises beyond 7.5 mEq/L, there is grave danger of heart block, ventricular flutter, and ventricular fibrillation.

3. **Chloride (Cl$^-$).** 1 mEq = 35.5 mg; 1 gm = 28 mEq; 1 gm salt (NaCl) = 18 mEq Cl$^-$; plasma concentration = 99–105 mEq/L.

    a. Chloride is the principal anion of both intravascular fluid and gastric juice. Although chloride may undergo active renal tubular transport, it can be considered to behave passively and in parallel to sodium.

    b. Abnormal losses occur with vomiting, diuretic therapy, and cystic fibrosis (excess sweating) and tend to lead to metabolic alkalosis.

Paradoxical aciduria occurs when Cl^- is in short supply in conjunction with dehydration. Avidity for Na^+ causes preferential retention of Na^+ and rejection of H^+ into the urine; the alkalosis is worsened. Cl^- must be replaced as NaCl.

4. **Calcium (Ca^{2+}).** 1 mEq = 20 mg; 1 gm = 50 mEq; plasma concentration = 9.5–10.5 mg/dl or 4.7–5.2 mEq/L except in the newborn and premature.

   a. Ionized calcium constitutes about 40 percent of total serum calcium; 50 percent is protein bound (principally to albumin), and 10 percent remains complexed. The calcium space is approximately 25% of body weight.

   b. A change in serum albumin of 1 gm/100 ml changes serum calcium concentration, in the same direction, by 0.8 mg/100 ml.

   c. The ionized portion of Ca^{2+} carries out functions in enzyme regulation, stabilizing neuromuscular membranes, coagulation processes, and bone formation. Acidosis increases ionized calcium, while alkalosis decreases it, even to the point of symptomatic tetany. In hypoproteinemic states a lower **total** serum Ca^{2+} is tolerated.

   d. Calcium dynamics are active in the growing child, primarily under the control of vitamin D hormones. Even in states of hypocalcemia, only about 50% of ingested calcium can be absorbed.

   e. **Hypocalcemia** is most commonly seen in rickets, renal compromise, the hypoalbuminemic states of liver disease or nephrosis, and in the neonate who is fed cow's milk formulas. Other conditions producing lowered calcium are discussed in Chap. 11.

      Drugs that cause hypocalcemia include furosemide, glucagon, calcitonin, mithramycin, bicarbonate, and corticosteroids. Exchange transfusion with acid citrate-preserved blood can produce hypocalcemia (see Chap. 17).

      (1) **Symptoms** of depressed ionized Ca^{2+} include the Chvostek and Trousseau signs, carpopedal spasm, ECG changes, and, occasionally, mental confusion. Neonates commonly become jittery and may have seizures with tetany of the newborn (see Chap. 6, p. 166).

      (2) Neonatal tetany occurs because a "relative" hypoparathyroid state in the normal infant is stressed by the excess phosphate found in cow's milk formulas (see Table 5-3).

      (3) In hypocalcemia the ECG shows prolongation of the Q-T interval relative to the rate.

      (4) **Treatment** of hypocalcemia includes IV and PO administration of Ca^{2+}. An IV bolus of calcium will only transiently (for about 1 hr) raise the serum Ca^{2+} level. Continuous IV administration is hazardous (cardiac arrhythmias, phlebitis, subcutaneous calcifications) and should be reserved for critical situations.

   f. **Hypercalcemia** is seen with hyperparathyroidism, vitamin D intoxication, sarcoidosis, cancer, immobilization, thyroid disease, Addison's disease, hypophosphatasia, and the milk-alkali syndrome in those taking antacids. In the Williams syndrome, infantile hypercalcemia is associated with elfin facies and obstructive heart disease (especially supravalvular aortic stenosis). **Symptoms** of excess calcium include nausea, anorexia, vomiting, constipation, polyuria, dehydration, mental confusion, and eventually coma. Chronic elevation of calcium can lead to nephrocalcinosis, extraskeletal calcification, and renal calculi.

5. **Magnesium (Mg^{2+}).** 1 mEq = 12 mg; plasma concentration = 1.9–2.5 mg/dl or 1–2 mEq/L.

   a. Magnesium is located primarily in the intracellular compartment. In the serum, about one-third is protein bound, and the pH of plasma has an effect similar to that on calcium. A magnesium deficiency state may simulate hypocalcemia.

   b. **Hypomagnesemia** occurs in patients on long-term parenteral nutrition, in parathyroid abnormalities and hyperthyroidism, and after mercurial diuretics.

Table 7-2. Values of H^+ with varying pH

pH	$(H^+)(nEq/L)$
6.70	200
6.80	159
6.90	126
7.00	100
7.10	80
7.20	63
7.30	50
7.40	40
7.50	30
7.60	29
7.70	20

    c. Hypermagnesemia may be seen in the newborn following magnesium sulfate administration to the mother with eclampsia. Symptoms are seen when the Mg^{2+} level exceeds 4 mEq/L. Hypotension and diminished responsiveness are early signs; at a level greater than 7 mEq/L, there is a loss of deep tendon reflexes. Coma occurs at levels of 12 mEq/L. Hypermagnesemia has occasionally developed in patients with renal failure who are treated with magnesium-containing antacids to lower phosphate. The ECG shows a prolonged Q-T interval, atrioventricular block, and, with extreme elevations, cardiac arrest.

  6. Bicarbonate (HCO_3). Plasma concentration = 23–25 mEq/L. The bicarbonate ion serves as part of the buffering system employed by the body in its pH regulatory mechanism. The role of bicarbonate is to maintain a normal plasma pH (see **D**).

D. Acid-base physiology

  1. General principles. A shift of 0.1 pH units, at pH 7.40, represents a change of only 10 nanoequivalents (nEq)/L in hydrogen ion concentration (Table 7-2). This delicate regulation comes about through blood buffering, respiratory activity, and renal compensatory mechanisms.

    a. Blood buffers include erythrocyte hemoglobin proteinate, organic and inorganic phosphates, carbonate (from bone), and both plasma and red cell bicarbonate. About half the buffering capacity derives from bicarbonate and roughly one-third from hemoglobin.

    b. Ventilation removes thousands of milliequivalents of carbon dioxide per day, thus preventing buildup of the weak acid H_2CO_3, formed when CO_2 remains dissolved in plasma.

    c. Children ingest 1–2 mEq/kg/day of "fixed" acid in their diet as sulfate from amino acids, nitrate, and phosphate (from phosphoproteins) and produce organic acids from incomplete oxidation of fat and carbohydrate (e.g., lactic acid). Blood chemical buffers provide immediate defense against this tide of acid, but the kidney maintains long-term pH homeostasis through (1) recovery of filtered plasma bicarbonate; (2) excretion of titratable acid (buffered by phosphate); and (3) NH_4^+ production. The proximal tubules reabsorb 85% of filtered bicarbonate by bulk transfer, while the distal tubule H^+ gradient permits recovery of the last 15% of bicarbonate via H^+ excretion.

  2. Determination of acid-base status requires measurement of blood pH and bicarbonate. Bicarbonate, total CO_2 content, and CO_2 combining power pro-

Table 7-3. Normal blood values*

Blood sample	pH	PCO_2	HCO_3^-	TCO_2
Arterial	7.38–7.45	35–45 mm Hg	23–27 mEq/L	24–28 mEq/L
Venous	7.35–7.40	45–50 mm Hg	24–29 mEq/L	25–30 mEq/L

*In infants, the normal range for TCO_2 is 20–24, and pH is lower by approximately 0.05.

vide the same basic information, with total CO_2 (TCO_2) 1–2 mEq/L lower than combining power.

Bicarbonate also can readily be calculated from pH and PCO_2 as follows, a method that is particularly handy for assessing acid-base status, since the apparatus for blood gas determination is now ubiquitous and requires only a few minutes for results.

a. $pH = pK + \log \dfrac{(base)}{(acid)}$, thus

b. $pH = 6.1 + \log \dfrac{(HCO_3^-)}{dissolved\ CO_2}$, thus

c. $pH = 6.1 + \log \dfrac{(HCO_3^-)}{0.03 \times PCO_2}$

This can be rearranged to

d. $(HCO_3^-) = \dfrac{23.9\ (PCO_2)}{(H^+)}$

Thus, knowing PCO_2 and H^+ (from pH) (see Table 7-2), one can calculate bicarbonate. With pH and serum bicarbonate values, the extent of a patient's acid-base imbalance can be measured and the nature of the disturbance determined.

3. **Laboratory values.** Ideally, arterial samples are obtained for the diagnosis of acid-base disturbances. Venous samples may prove inaccurate in patients with impaired peripheral circulation, local tissue damage, or blood stasis caused by a tourniquet. Normal values for arterial and venous blood are given in Table 7-3. A heparinized syringe minimizes collection errors in drawing blood. If a Vacutainer is used, it should either contain an oil film to seal the blood sample and prevent CO_2 diffusion, or it should be a small (3-ml), heparinized tube, completely filled by the blood sample.

4. **Acid-base abnormalities.** By convention, acid-base disorders are divided into the following categories (Fig. 7-1): **respiratory** versus **metabolic, acute** versus **chronic, simple** versus **mixed,** and **pure** versus **compensated** and resulting in either **acidosis** or **alkalosis,** depending on pH. In pure imbalances of pH, the disequilibrium results from a deviation of either PCO_2 (respiratory) or HCO_3^- (metabolic) from the norm. As can be seen from the Henderson-Hasselbalch equation **c** (see I.D.2.a), a rise in PCO_2 increases the denominator and pH falls; this constitutes **respiratory acidosis.** Conversely, a fall in PCO_2 diminishes the denominator and pH rises, leading to **respiratory alkalosis.** Similarly, retention of HCO_3^- causes **metabolic alkalosis,** and a drop in HCO_3^- results in **metabolic acidosis.**

These situations prevail only for brief periods. The change in the internal milieu brings compensatory mechanisms into play. Compensation is rarely sufficient to offset the primary disturbance completely, and the condition is usually only partially corrected, so that the patient has a compensated acid-base disorder (Table 7-4).

a. Respiratory acidosis results from retention of CO_2 and a consequent increase in H_2CO_2. Normally, the rise in PCO_2 stimulates a ventilatory

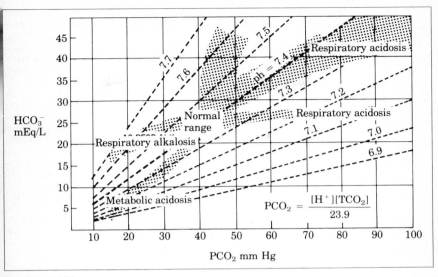

Fig. 7-1. Acid-base nomogram.

Table 7-4. Compensation in acid-base disturbances

Acid-base disturbances	pH	HCO$_3^-$	PCO$_2$	Compensation
Metabolic acidosis	↓	↓		↓ PCO$_2$; acid urine
Respiratory acidosis	↓		↑	Acid urine
Metabolic alkalosis	↑	↑		↑ PCO$_2$; alkaline urine
Respiratory alkalosis	↑		↓	Alkaline urine

effort to eliminate the hypercapnia. In the acute phase of respiratory acidosis, available buffering mechanisms and renal compensation are minimal, and pH falls rapidly as PCO$_2$ exceeds 50 mm Hg (for a discussion of acute respiratory failure, see Chap. 3). Renal compensation functions very effectively in chronic respiratory acidosis via the induction of enzyme systems for ammonium production. By acidifying the urine, the kidney can raise ECF bicarbonate to 40 mEq/L or more to compensate for marked hypercapnia. Usually, neonates are incapable of this adaptation and will remain severely acidotic with respiratory distress syndrome.

b. Respiratory alkalosis is not a common pediatric problem. Hyperventilation (usually due to tachypnea rather than increased tidal volume alone) occurs in patients managed with mechanical ventilators (especially newborn infants with RDS) in the Reye syndrome, in the early phase of salicylate intoxication, in anxious or hysterical states, and in hypermetabolic states. Rapid correction of metabolic acidosis can result in respiratory alkalosis, since correction of the pH in the cerebrospinal fluid lags behind the ECF, and continuing CNS acidosis stimulates the medullary ventilatory drive. Acute respiratory alkalosis can precipitate tetany (see Chap. 11, pp. 308ff.) and makes the patient feel light-headed. In psychogenic cases, symptoms of an acute anxiety state often dominate. Laboratory diagnosis rests on the triad of decreased PCO$_2$, elevated pH, and normal bicarbonate.

    c. Metabolic acidosis results from increased blood H^+ with a concomitant fall in pH. Buffer base (bicarbonate and other blood buffers) is consumed, and TCO_2 falls.

      (1) Accumulation of organic acids is reflected by a rise in the anion gap. The anion gap is an estimation of anionic substances, usually metabolic by-products, that are not measured by the usual laboratory techniques. The anion gap is the difference between serum cations (Na^+) and anions (Cl^- and HCO_3^-) and normally is ~12 mEq/L, but is somewhat higher in newborn infants. If metabolic acidosis results exclusively from bicarbonate loss, the anion gap changes little, since chloride rises proportionately. In lactic acidosis (e.g., secondary to anaerobic metabolism in shock), the large anion gap reflects accumulation of the "unmeasured" anion.

      (2) In response to the acidemic stress, both the kidney and lung undertake corrective measures. There is a prompt increase in minute ventilation, and PCO_2 falls (even more markedly than in primary respiratory alkalosis, in which PCO_2 usually remains above 25 mm Hg), while urinary acidification maximizes over a few days within the limits of both reduced circulation and GFR.

      (3) In children, chronic metabolic acidosis most commonly can be traced to a kidney abnormality, either parenchymal disease, obstruction, or a tubular disorder. Growth failure invariably accompanies chronic acidemia, and corrective therapy is necessary if severe impairment of normal development is to be avoided.

    d. Metabolic alkalosis usually occurs as part of a generalized derangement in fluid and electrolytes. It necessarily involves either gain of a strong base or bicarbonate by the ECF or else a loss of fixed acid, which is analogous. Although the list of causes is long, the source of metabolic alkalosis in the majority of affected children is the GI tract. Most commonly, pyloric stenosis presents with metabolic alkalosis, due to the loss of HCl because of vomiting.

      (1) Potassium plays a central role in both the development and correction of metabolic alkalosis. In acute alkalosis, K^+ moves from the ECF to the ICF to help maintain electroneutrality, since H^+ ion is lost. Although serum K^+ may then be low, total body K^+ remains normal.

      (2) Conditions that produce K^+ depletion also stimulate aldosterone production. The kidney then becomes avid for sodium; as potassium depletion reduces available K^+, the distal tubule exchanges H^+ for sodium as it attempts to replete diminished circulating volume (e.g., due to a GI disturbance) by sodium resorption. The outcome is aciduria, coexisting with systemic alkalosis (paradoxical aciduria), and it tends to perpetuate the derangement.

    e. Mixed disorders of acid-base homeostasis result from disturbances in both respiratory and renal function. Their diagnosis is simplified by reference to Fig. 7-1. Since the shaded areas in Fig. 7-1 represent the 95% confidence bands for each disturbance (including the normal compensatory response), any combination of values of PCO_2 and HCO_3^- that falls outside these areas represents a mixed disturbance.

    f. As a rule, **compensatory mechanisms** modify the acid-base disturbances as shown in Table 7-4 to the following degree:

        Metabolic acidosis: PCO_2 ↓ 1–1.5 × fall HCO_3^-

        Metabolic alkalosis: PCO_2 ↑ 0.5–1.0 × HCO_3^-

        Acute respiratory acidosis: HCO_3^- ↑ to maximum 30 mEq/L

        Chronic respiratory acidosis: HCO_3^- ↑ 4 mEq/L/10 mm ↑ PCO_2

        Acute respiratory alkalosis: HCO_3^- ↓ 2.5 mEq/L/10 mm ↓ PCO_2 (to minimum 18 mEq/L)

        Chronic respiratory alkalosis: HCO_3^- falls to 15 mEq/L

II. Maintenance of normal fluid and electrolyte balance
A. Estimation of fluid requirements

1. **Rationale.** Fluid is continually lost from the body through several mechanisms, both regulated (renal) and unregulated (insensible). *Maintenance fluid requirement* is the amount of fluid required to keep total body fluid in balance. There are several methods of **estimating** the maintenance fluid requirements for an average patient under average conditions; the **actual** maintenance requirements may vary considerably from the usual estimations because of unusual circumstances (see **3**).

2. **Components of maintenance fluid requirements**
   a. **Insensible losses** account for about 50% of the total fluid lost per day. The usual sources of insensible losses (and the usual percentages of the total losses) are:
      (1) **Respiratory** (humidification of exhaled air) = 15%.
      (2) **Skin** (evaporation, not sweat) = 30%.
      (3) **Feces** = 5%.
   b. **Urine losses** account for the other 50% of fluid loss. Actual urine volume depends mainly on the level of hydration, but there is a minimal obligatory urine volume required to dissolve excreted metabolic waste products and electrolytes.
   c. **Intrinsic fluid sources.** The water of oxidation is water gained as a by-product of normal metabolism; it can replace about 15% of the usual fluid losses. This is normally considered when estimating maintenance fluid requirements (i.e., maintenance fluid requirement = insensible losses + urine losses − intrinsic fluid sources).

3. **Methods of estimating maintenance fluids**
   a. **Surface area.** Levels of renal function and body fluid requirements correlate best with body surface area (BSA). Hence, the unit of measurement used is the square meter (M^2), and water needs are expressed as $ml/M^2/24$ hr. The nomogram (Fig. 7-2) correlates weight to surface area in children with normal body proportions. This system works well for children weighing **more than 10 kg** and has the advantage that a single formula can be used for all ages. The normal water requirement is about 1,500 ml/$M^2/24$ hr (Table 7-5).
   b. **Calories expended.** This method computes water requirements from metabolic expenditure. Figure 7-3 depicts energy use as a function of weight. To calculate fluid requirement, one allows 100−150 ml/100 cal metabolized.
   c. **Body weight**
      (1) General rule is
         100 ml/kg for the **first** 10 kg of body weight
         50 ml/kg for the **next** 10 kg of body weight
         20 ml/kg for the weights above 20 kg

         Example: A 25-kg child would require:
         100 ml/kg × 10 kg = 1,000 ml for first 10 kg
         50 ml/kg × 10 kg =   500 ml for next 10 kg
         20 ml/kg × 5 kg =   100 ml for last   5 kg

         Total   1,600   25 kg

      (2) The main advantage of this method is that it is easy to remember and calculate.
   d. **Allowances for unusual maintenance requirements.** Changes in normal maintenance requirements are affected by several conditions, shown in Table 7-6.

4. **The fluid needs of the newborn**
   a. Maintenance needs are 60 ml/kg for the first 24 hr, advancing to 125 ml/kg/24 hr after the first week of life. A low solute load is better tolerated,

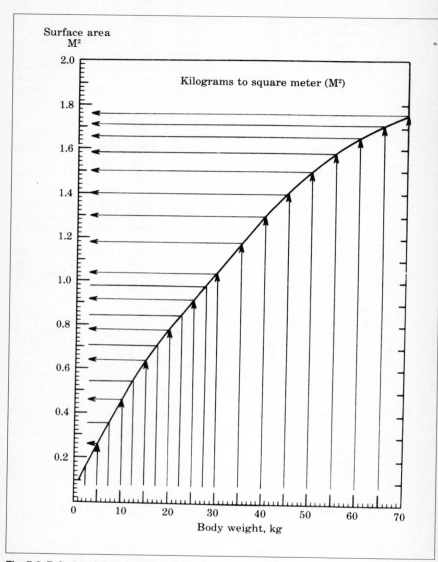

Fig. 7-2. Relations between body weight in kilograms and body surface area. (Adapted from N. B. Talbot, R. R. Richie, and J. D. Crawford. *Metabolic Homeostasis*. Cambridge, Mass.: Harvard University Press, 1959. P. 1.)

Table 7-5. Fluid balance in children

Losses	
Respiratory and skin	775 ml/M^2/24 hr[a]
Gastrointestinal	100 ml/M^2/24 hr
Urine	875 ml/M^2/24 hr[b]
Total	1750
Sources	
Water of oxidation	250 ml/M^2/24 hr
Net maintenance requirement	
Water	1500 ml/M^2/24 hr

[a]Varies with size of child; e.g., 1,200 ml/M^2 in a toddler versus 700 ml/M^2 at age 8–10 years.
[b]Based on excretion of isotonic urine, 300 mOsm/L, and minimal solute intake, e.g., dextrose in water.

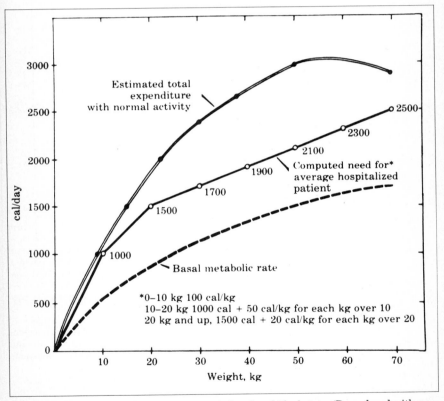

Fig. 7-3. Comparison of energy expenditure in basal and ideal state. (Reproduced with permission from W. E. Segar, Parenteral fluid therapy. *Curr. Probl. Pediatr.* 3(2):4, 1972. Copyright ©1972 by Year Book Medical Publishers, Inc., Chicago.)

Table 7-6. Conditions affecting normal fluid requirements

Condition	Adjustment
Increased metabolic rate	
Fever	Increase H_2O by 12%/°C
Hypermetabolic state	Increase H_2O by 25–75%
Decreased metabolic rate	
Hypothermia	Decrease H_2O by 12%/°C
Hypometabolic state	Decrease H_2O by 10–25%
Unusual insensible losses	
High environmental humidity	Decrease IWL to 0–15 ml/100 cal
Hyperventilation	Increase IWL to 50–60 ml/100 cal
Excessive sweating	Increase H_2O by 10–25 ml/100 cal

Table 7-7. Newborn fluid and electrolyte therapy

Solute	Amount	Age
10% D/W	65 ml/kg/24 hr	Day 1
	80 ml/kg/24 hr	Day 2
	100 ml/kg/24 hr	Day 3
Sodium	Add 2–3 mEq/kg/14 hr	Day 3
Potassium	Add 1–2 mEq/kg/24 hr (if urine output adequate)	Day 2
Calcium	10 mg/kg elemental Ca^{2+} IV push	
	30 mg/kg/24 hr IV maintenance	
Bicarbonate	1 mEq/kg (1 ml of 8% solution) IV	
	(may repeat for persistent acidosis)	

so 0.2% saline in 5 or 10% dextrose, with added bicarbonate and calcium as needed, is a reasonable choice for uncomplicated cases (Table 7-7).

  b. To provide the small volumes that newborns require, IVs should be run with constant infusion pumps. Frequent determination of blood chemistries (electrolytes, BUN, creatinine, calcium, phosphorus, pH, TCO_2, osmolality) is **mandatory**.

  c. Phototherapy increases, and mechanical ventilators with humidified oxygen substantially reduce, insensible water loss.

5. Urine output accurately reflects both circulatory status and adequacy of hydration. Although urine volume varies, about 50 ml/kg/24 hr is typical for the normal child. Infants excrete less urine in the first 24–48 hr of life but excretion increases thereafter. **An output less than 0.5 ml/kg/hr suggests pathologic oliguria and requires attention.**

B. Estimation of electrolyte requirements (see also Tables 7-5 and 7-7). Na^+, K^+, Cl^-, and HCO_3^- requirements vary significantly because of the kidney's ability to conserve them or to excrete any excess. General estimates of Na^+ and K^+ daily maintenance requirements calculated by three methods follow.

1. BSA.	20–50 mEq Na^+/M^2 BSA	20–50 mEq K^+/M^2
2. Caloric requirement.	2–4 mEq Na^+/100 cal	2–3 mEq K^+/100 cal
3. General method.	2–4 mEq Na^+/100 ml fluid	2–4 mEq K^+/100 ml fluid

Table 7-8. Estimation of dehydration

	Degree of dehydration		
Clinical signs	Mild	Moderate	Severe
Weight loss (%)	5	10	15
Behavior	Normal	Irritable	Hyperirritable to lethargic
Thirst	Slight	Moderate	Intense
Mucous membrane	May be normal	Dry	Parched
Tears	Present	+/−	Absent
Anterior fontanelle	Flat	+/−	Sunken
Skin turgor	Normal	+/−	Increased

C. **Estimation of caloric requirements**
   1. To reduce protein catabolism and avoid ketosis, 75–100 gm glucose/M^2/day is required. However, this will **not meet caloric needs.** To do so requires 1200–1500 cal/M^2/24 hr, not allowing for extra requirements imposed by illness.
   2. Dextrose solutions (5–10%) are tolerated peripherally, whereas 15/30% sugar can be administered through a central IV line.
   3. To provide high caloric content, total parenteral nutrition may be needed (see Chap. 10, p. 257).

III. **Assessment of abnormalities of fluid and electrolyte balance**
   A. **General comments**
      1. The most useful way to consider dehydration is based on the amount of **sodium and potassium lost in relation to water.** Hence, we conventionally divide the dehydration states into isotonic (isonatremic), hypotonic (hyponatremic), and hypertonic (hypernatremic) for purposes of management.
         a. **Hypotonic.** Na^+ < 125 mEq/L; ECF depletion with relative sparing of intracellular contents; hence, early vascular compromise
         b. **Isotonic.** Na^+ 130–150 mEq/L; balanced loss of water and ions
         c. **Hypertonic.** Na^+ > 150 mEq/L; ICF depletion; allows more chronic dehydration.
      2. The best indicator of **short-term quantitative fluid loss** is change in body weight. Table 7-8 presents a rough clinical estimate of signs and degree of dehydration.
      3. **Role of solute load.** In understanding dehydration states, it is important to consider the contribution of **intake** in producing a negative balance as well as the role played by **output** via diarrhea or vomiting. Renal solute load hastens dehydration by causing obligatory urinary free-water loss in the infant struggling to excrete an ingested solute load.
         This means that the solute stress of a given feeding is different from the formula's measured osmotic load. Since infants cannot effectively concentrate urine much beyond 600 mOsm/kg, it is apparent that cow's milk causes free-water losses **three times greater** than those of human milk, while boiled skim milk imposes a fourfold free-water loss. Thus, to avoid hypertonic dehydration, renal solute load should be minimized in infants with fluid losses.
      4. **Initial assessment** of the dehydrated child should include the following:
         a. **History.** Urine output, weight change, infectious disease contacts, and estimate of stooling or vomiting frequency
         b. **Clinical.** Urine output, skin turgor, mucous membrane moisture, eye turgor, fullness of fontanelle, and mental state
         c. **Laboratory.** Weight, CBC, serum and urine Na^+, K^+, Cl^-, pH, Co_2,

Table 7-9. Deficits in moderate to severe dehydration

Type of dehydration	Range of Na$^+$ (mEq/L)	Losses			
		Water (ml/kg)	Na$^+$ (mEq/kg)	K$^+$ (mEq/kg)	Cl$^-$ + HCO$_3^-$ (mEq/kg)
Isotonic	130–145	100–150	7–11	7–11	14–22
Hypotonic	< 125	40–80	10–14	10–14	20–28
Hypertonic	> 150	120–170	2–5	2–5	4–10

Source: Modified from R. W. Winters. *Principles of Pediatric Fluid Therapy.* North Chicago: Abbott Laboratories, 1970. P. 56.

BUN, creatinine, osmolality, glucose, and calcium. **Urinalysis.** SG, pH, glucose, ketones, amino acids (ferric chloride), and appropriate cultures.

5. **Urinalysis** is particularly important. The specific gravity should be well above 1.015 **unless intrinsic renal disease** is contributing to the problem. Ketonuria often accompanies dehydration without diabetes. Trace or 1+ protein can be present, along with cellular debris and a few hyaline casts. However, a very active sediment signals underlying primary renal disease. Alkaline urine should raise the question of renal tubular acidosis.

6. **Water and electrolyte losses.** Estimates of deficits in moderate to severe dehydration are given in Table 7-9.

B. **Assessment of Na$^+$ and K$^+$ losses**

1. **General.** There is no practical means of assessing true K$^+$ loss; serum K$^+$ does not accurately reflect total body K$^+$ stores (see sec. **I.C.2.b**). Nonetheless, one may assume in most instances that K$^+$ losses are equivalent to Na$^+$ losses.

2. Estimations of Na$^+$ and K$^+$ deficits in a child who appears severely dehydrated and in whom the serum Na$^+$ is known can be made using Table 7-9.

3. Calculation of Na$^+$ deficit is based on the current (dehydrated) serum Na$^+$ concentration, the desired "normal" serum Na$^+$ concentration (usually 135 mEq/L), and the volume of distribution of Na$^+$, the TBW (see sec. **I.C.1**). The assumption on which the calculations are based is that Na$^+$ is the **sole** cation used for rehydration. This is a prudent assumption, since rehydration preferentially should preserve the ECF (and thus the vascular space) over the ICF. In practice these calculations actually provide the deficits of total cations (Na$^+$ and K$^+$). This should be remembered when both Na$^+$ and K$^+$ are provided in the solutions used for rehydration. The Na$^+$ deficit (Na$_d^+$) is the difference between the normal total body Na$^+$ (Na$_n^+$) and the current (dehydrated) total body Na$^+$ (Na$_c^+$).

$$Na_d^+ = Na_n^+ - Na_c^+$$

Thus, $Na_d^+ = (TBW \times 135) - [(TBW - FL) \times Na^+]$

or $Na_d^+ = TBW (135 - Na^+) + FL (Na^+)$

Where TBW = 0.6 × normal weight and FL is the fluid loss (or equivalent of weight change) and Na$^+$ is the current serum sodium concentration (mEq/L).

C. **Ongoing losses**

1. **General.** *Ongoing losses* are abnormal losses of fluids and/or electrolytes that occur while the patient is under observation. The losses may be continuous or sporadic, and while the changes in renal output can often accommodate small ongoing losses, appropriate management dictates that the losses be replaced in an orderly fashion.

2. **Estimation of ongoing losses**

a. **Fluid.** Abnormal losses (nasogastric suction, surgical drainage, vomitus) usually can be measured directly.

Table 7-10. Composition of body fluids

Source	Na$^+$ (mEq/L)	K$^+$ (mEq/L)	CL$^-$ (mEq/L)	HCO$_3^-$ (mEq/L)	pH	Osm (mOsm/L)
Gastric	50	10–15	150	0	1	300
Pancreas	140	5	50–100	100	9	300
Bile	130	5	100	40	8	300
Ileostomy	130	15–20	120	25–30	8	300
Diarrhea	50	35	40	50	Alk	
Sweat	50	5	55	0		
Blood	140	4–5	100	25	7.4	285–295
Urine	0–100*	20–100*	70–100*	0	4.5–8.5	50–1400

*Varies considerably with intake.

    (1) In the absence of direct measurement, **weight changes** can be used to determine fluid losses. Daily changes in weight can be assumed to reflect losses or gains of TBW.

    (2) Patients receiving maintenance fluids and calories should remain at a constant weight.

    (3) Patients receiving maintenance fluids, but insufficient calories, should lose about 0.5% of their weight per day. This weight loss accounts for the body fat stores metabolized to H$_2$O and other by-products.

    (4) Newborn infants should lose weight over the first 3–5 days of life and subsequently gain weight consistent with the usual growth curves (approximately 30 gm/day for full-term infants) if given sufficient nutrition.

  b. Electrolytes

    (1) The electrolyte content of abnormal body fluid losses frequently can be **measured directly.** This is particularly important for **abnormal** urine losses, since the composition can vary widely.

    (2) The usual composition of body fluids is shown in Table 7-10.

3. Strategy for replacement of ongoing losses

  a. Generally, ongoing losses of fluids and electrolytes are measured or calculated over fixed time periods and replaced evenly over an equivalent period of time.

    (1) If there are large ongoing losses, these periods should be short (e.g., every half-hour or hour).

    (2) If losses are small, adjustment can be made daily.

  b. Patients without deficits at the initiation of the therapy

    (1) The therapy is designed to provide **maintenance** fluid and electrolytes plus replacing the **ongoing** losses.

    (2) If there are unusual urine losses or if the urine output is erratic, therapy is designed to provide **insensible** fluid losses plus urine and ongoing losses.

  c. Patients dehydrated at the initiation of therapy (e.g., vomiting or diarrhea)

    (1) The measured or extenuated ongoing losses are **added to** the calculated replacement of maintenance and deficit fluid and electrolytes. Adjustments should be made frequently. Urine losses are ignored, since they are accounted for in the maintenance calculations.

    (2) It is important **not** to recalculate the overall deficits in rehydrating a dehydrated patient with ongoing losses; this usually leads to an **underestimation** of true deficits. Add ongoing losses to previously estimated deficits.

   d. When providing replacement for large or unusual ongoing losses, periodically monitor and reassess the patient's condition (see sec. **V**).

IV. Correction of abnormalities of fluid and electrolyte balance

A. Acute fluid management and resuscitation: general concepts. See also Chap. 3.

1. Weigh the patient.
2. If shock is present, or if no urine is produced in the first half hour, give 20–30 ml/kg Ringer's lactate, or 5% albumin IV until adequate circulation returns.
3. After the first hour, give 10 ml/kg/hr of Ringer's lactate until shock is alleviated and actual fluid and electrolyte deficits can be accurately calculated.
4. If the patient is asymptomatic and/or dehydration is hyponatremic or isotonic, one-half the fluids calculated for 24 hr should be administered in the first 8 hr. The remaining half should be administered in the remaining 16 hr
5. If hypertonic dehydration is present after correcting shock, correct the deficit slowly and evenly over 48 hr.
6. Temperature will affect total maintenance needs; with fever, add 12% of the maintenance amount per degrees centigrade.
7. In most situations, do **not** add K^+ to the IV solutions until after the patient has voided. If the patient has hemolytic uremic syndrome or acute tubular necrosis, IV K^+ may lead to severe hyperkalemia.
8. In **diabetic ketoacidosis,** however, K^+ may be added to the initial solution, since rapid correction of dehydration, acidosis, and hyperglycemia may precipitate severe hypoglycemia (see Chap. 13, p. 333).
9. **Adequacy of therapy** is indicated by urine output of 40 ml/M^2/hr (1.5 ml/kg/hr), urine $Na^+ \sim 40$ mEq/L, normal circulation, and restoration of weight.

B. Hypotonic dehydration. In this condition the fluid loss comes mainly from the intravascular and interstitial compartments rather than the intracellular reservoir. Hence, circulatory compromise appears early, and there is marked loss of turgor. Patients arrive at this state when enteric losses are replaced with low-solute fluids (e.g., fruit juice, Coca-Cola).

1. **Clinically,** infants present soon after the onset of illness because symptoms become apparent early. For a given weight loss, the clinical signs are more marked than in isotonic or hypertonic dehydration. Thus, estimates of weight loss should follow a 3, 6, 9 percent rule of thumb for mild, moderate, and severe, respectively. Seizures occur infrequently, even with marked hyponatremia, but generalized lethargy is common, and vascular collapse can occur early.
2. **Treatment.** Since loss is mainly ECF, replacement therapy can advance rapidly, with volume and sodium restored by the end of 24–36 hr.
3. **Strategy for replacement of deficits (first day of treatment) after resuscitation**
   a. Calculate or estimate the total deficits of fluid and electrolytes and add the maintenance requirement. Subtract the amount given during the initial resuscitation period. The result is the remaining deficit and maintenance to be provided in the first day.
   b. If the patient is asymptomatic and dehydration is hypotonic or isotonic, one-half of the remaining deficit and maintenance fluids and electrolytes should be administered in the next 8 hr and the other half over the subsequent 16 hr. (Some authors suggest one-half the deficit and one-third the maintenance in the 1st 8 hr, followed by one-half the deficit and two-thirds the maintenance in the next 16 hr. This plan makes little practical difference.)

C. Symptomatic hyponatremia. Regardless of the cause, whether Na^+ loss or water excess, therapy is directed at raising the sodium concentration quickly, to stop symptoms.

1. Use hypertonic saline (3% = 513 mEq Na^+/L) to deliver approximately 5 mEq/kg/hr. The approximate sodium deficit is given in **III.B.3.**

2. Symptomatic hyponatremia may be seen with a serum Na^+ concentration of 130 mEq/L if the change in concentration has been sudden. Thus, the patient's symptoms, if any, must be taken into account to determine the speed of correction of the serum sodium concentration.

3. The following is a **sample calculation** for a 10-kg child with no volume deficit but with serum Na^+ of 120 mEq who manifests irritability and diminished consciousness:

    a. 10 kg $\times$ 0.6 $\times$ (15 mEq deficit) = 90 mEq (total Na^+ deficit = 90 mEq)

    b. To raise Na^+ 5 mEq/L acutely requires 5 mEq $\times$ 0.6 $\times$ 10 kg = 30 mEq:

$$\text{Dose of 3\% NaCl} = \frac{30 \text{ mEq Na}^+}{0.513 \text{ mEq Na}^+/\text{ml}} = 60 \text{ ml}$$

$$\text{Dose of 5\% NaCl} = \frac{30 \text{ mEq Na}^+}{0.856 \text{ mEq Na}^+/\text{ml}} = 35 \text{ ml}$$

Following acute correction the patient's acidosis may worsen. Sodium bicarbonate (1 mEq/ml) may be mixed with the hypertonic saline to supply one-fourth of the Na^+ dose while also providing bicarbonate as the anion.

D. The therapy of **asymptomatic hyponatremia** requires gradual correction of the sodium deficit in increments of 10 mEq/L.

    1. The following is a **sample calculation** for a 10-kg child with 10% dehydration and serum Na^+ 125 mEq/L:

        a. Volume deficit = 10% $\times$ 10 kg = 1.0 L

        b. Volume maintenance = 100 ml $\times$ 10 kg = 1.0 L

        Total = 2.0 L

        c. Deficit Na^+ (see **III.B.3**)

        Na^+ = (10 kg $\times$ 0.6) (135 − 125) + (1.0) (125)

            = 6 (10) + 125

            = 185 mEq

        d. Maintenance Na^+ = 3 mEq/kg $\times$ 10

                        = 30 mEq Na

$$\text{Thus, } \frac{\text{total Na need} = 215 \text{ mEq/24 hr}}{\text{total volume 2.0 L/24 hr}} = \frac{108 \text{ mEq Na}}{1.0 \text{ L}}$$

$$= 3/4 \text{ normal saline}$$

    2. Administer one-half of the total fluid in the first 8 hr and the rest over the remaining 16 hr.

E. **Potassium** deficit and **acidosis** both require specific therapy for correction. Hemoconcentration and prerenal azotemia will resolve with restoration of fluids.

F. **Isotonic dehydration.** Children with enteric losses, taking an intermediate solute load (e.g., breast milk), arrive at a balanced dehydration. The deficit is lost both from ECF and ICF. For a given weight loss, symptoms will be less dramatic than for hypotonic dehydration—assume a weight loss of 5, 10, or 15% for clinical estimation of mild, moderate, and severe involvement respectively.

Treatment is similar to that for hypotonic dehydration (see **B.2**). However, a more leisurely tempo in completing deficit repair is acceptable. Aim to restore about two-thirds of the total estimated volume deficit during the first day. During day 2, the emphasis should be on restoring both potassium deficit and acid-base balance.

    1. After acute therapy, supply **maintenance** at 1,500 ml/M^2/24 hr (or 100 ml/kg for infants weighing < 10 kg) plus deficit from estimated weight loss.

    2. The solutions used are hypotonic, but since the normal kidney needs only 1/3 N solution for true maintenance, these 1/2 N solutions provide sufficient solute even for correction of isotonic losses.

G. **Hypertonic dehydration** results when inappropriately high solute loads are given as replacement fluid, or when a renal concentrating defect produces a large free-water loss. Usually, hypernatremia represents the principal excess solute, but agents such as glucose, urea, and mannitol can produce the same disturbance.

1. The **clinical presentation** in these infants can be deceptive. Shock is a late manifestation. When it supervenes, one can be certain that fluid loss exceeds 10% of body weight. Skin turgor does not exhibit the usual tenting of advanced dehydration, but is a thick, doughy consistency. Other findings include a shrill cry or mewling sound, muscle weakness, tachypnea, and intense thirst in toddlers. In assessing these infants, be sure to check *sugar* and *calcium*, since hyperglycemia is present in half the patients, and calcium deficiency has been noted in 10%.

2. **Treatment.** The total fluid deficit must be replaced slowly over 48 hr or more, dropping serum Na^+ by 10 mEq/L/day. Rapid correction floods the intracellular space with fluid, leading to cerebral (and sometimes pulmonary) edema. In general, the more dilute the solution being used to correct the deficit, the slower it should be infused.

   a. If shock is present, infuse 20 ml/kg of 5% albumin over 20–30 min.

   b. **First hour.** The goal is to reestablish satisfactory circulation and urine flow. Give 10–20 ml/kg of Ringer's lactate to reduce the chloride load in favor of lactate (alkali).

   c. **Over the next 4 hr,** the goal is to ensure urine output and reduce the serum Na^+. There is no best regimen. The rate of IV infusion is determined by the tonicity of the solution; i.e., isotonic solutions can be infused more rapidly. Infuse 10 ml/kg/hr of 5% D in Ringer's lactate, Ringer's lactate, or a mixture of 2½% dextrose and ½ N saline to which is added ¼ N bicarbonate (17 ml of 8% $NaHCO_3$/500 ml of solution), depending on the degree of acidosis or hyperglycemia. This should establish a steady urine flow, which then permits addition of potassium to the infusion.

   d. **The next 48 hr** are utilized to replenish the volume lost; infusion should proceed at a steady rate, based on calculated deficits. The deficit in a patient with severe hypernatremia will be approximately 10% of body weight, i.e., 1 L/10 kg.

   Calculation of water deficit:

   Water deficit (L) = usual body water − current body water

   Usual body water = current body water $\times \dfrac{\text{current Osm}}{\text{normal Osm}}$

   Current body water = current weight × 0.6

   Example: A dehydrated child who currently weighs 10 kg and whose serum Osm = 340 (Na^+ = 160):

   $$\text{Water deficit} = 10 \text{ kg} \times 0.6 \text{ L/kg} \times \frac{340}{290} - (10 \text{ kg} \times 0.6 \text{ L/kg})$$

   $$= 7 \text{ L} - 6 \text{ L}$$

   $$= 1 \text{ L}$$

   (1) Children with hypernatremic dehydration are usually not significantly deficient in Na^+. **Do not try to correct the water deficit rapidly** with sodium (½ N saline or greater) solutions, since it may lead to severe Na^+ overload and possibly to an increased serum Na^+ concentration.

   (2) **Do not allow the IV infusion to run rapidly,** because there is grave danger of CNS damage from acute osmotic shifts if fluid flow is unchecked. Also, it is unwise to attempt rapid control of hyperglycemia; the presence of extra glucose acts as an "osmotic buffer" under whose cover the necessary ion shifts can occur as reequilibration proceeds. Slow sugar metabolism then provides a continuous source of free water delivered at a gentle rate.

   (3) Treatment of acute salt poisoning requires dialysis or furosemide diuresis (1 mg/kg), replacing the urine output with a 10% D/W solu-

tion, monitoring sodium values q4h and repeating the administration of furosemide.

    e. If the serum Na^+ concentration is greater than 180 mEq/L, **dialysis** may be required to correct the abnormalities. In this case, peritoneal dialysis may be preferable to hemodialysis, since the correction is relatively slow. The peritoneal dialysate may be prepared with a relatively high Na^+ concentration initially (e.g., 165 mEq/L) and then reduced in a gradual stepwise fashion.

V. Monitoring fluid and electrolyte therapy

    A. Since the rationale for provision of maintenance and replacement of deficits and ongoing losses of fluids and electrolytes rests on several estimations and calculations, assess the results of therapy periodically and adjust accordingly.

    B. The usual variables to monitor include:

        1. Weight. The patient's weight should be increasing and decreasing as predicted by the calculations of treatment. It is frequently difficult to obtain accurate weights in sick patients. Weight is the single most accurate variable to follow in planning treatment.

        2. The **vital signs** indicate the stability of the vascular volume.

        3. Laboratory tests. Serum electrolytes, osmolality, blood sugar, BUN, creatinine, and urine electrolytes and osmolality

        4. Total inputs and outputs of both fluids and electrolytes

    C. A well-conceived **flow sheet** is an efficient means of assessing the adequacy of therapy and of making appropriate adjustments for patients with complications.

        1. Equally spaced time intervals are listed along the top of the flow sheet.

        2. The flow sheet should indicate both the interval and overall totals for both fluid and electrolytes.

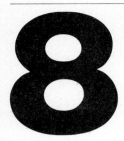

Renal Disorders

I. Acute renal failure

A. Prenatal failure. All patients with apparent acute renal failure must be assessed for a prenatal cause.

1. **Etiology.** Renal perfusion and intrarenal blood flow are reduced due to dehydration, hypovolemia, or hemodynamic factors.

2. **Evaluation**
   a. Review the history and physical findings for shock, dehydration, and heart failure.
   b. Measure the blood pressure and central venous pressure (CVP).
   c. Insert an indwelling bladder catheter to ascertain the urine output (< 0.5 ml/kg/hr indicates severe oliguria) and to obtain urine for urinalysis, Na^+, K^+, creatinine, and osmolality (see Chap. 7). Do not leave the catheter indwelling.

3. **The diagnosis** of prenatal failure is confirmed by
   a. Diuresis in response to an increase in intravascular volume and rehydration
   b. Improved renal function with improved cardiac function
   c. Urinary sodium less than 15 mEq/L
   d. Urinary potassium equal to or greater than 40 mEq/L
   e. A ratio of urine urea to plasma greater than 10:1, or of urine creatinine to plasma creatinine greater than 10:1

4. **Therapy.** The object of therapy is to restore urinary flow.
   a. Insert an IV line for infusion of fluids and solute and for the measurement of CVP.
   b. Reestablish an effective circulating blood volume (see Chap. 2).
   c. If, after restoration of extracellular fluid (ECF) volume, oliguria or anuria persists, mannitol, 0.5 gm/kg of a 20% solution, should be infused over 10–20 min. This should result in an increase in urine output of approximately 6–10 ml/kg over the next 1–3 hr. **If no increase in urine flow occurs, no further mannitol should be given.**
   d. A trial dose of furosemide, 1 mg/kg IV, should then be administered **after** the ECF volume is restored. Note that this agent will cause changes in urine electrolytes and osmolality, making a distinction between prenatal and renal oliguria more difficult.
   e. If marked oligoanuria persists, assess the patient immediately for intrinsic renal or postrenal failure (see **B**).

B. Intrinsic renal failure

1. **Etiology.** The causes are parenchymal injury due to acute tubular necrosis, severe or prolonged prenatal failure, vascular lesion, hemolytic uremic syndrome, or nephritis.

2. **Evaluation and diagnosis.** First, be sure the patient does not have prenatal or postrenal failure (see rest of this section). A history of decreased renal perfusion suggests acute renal failure due to acute tubular necrosis. Acute renal failure may be associated with acute glomerulonephritis, hemolytic uremic syndrome, accelerated hypertension, uric acid nephropathy, or vasculitis.

a. Stabilize the patient's condition prior to any invasive diagnostic procedures.

b. Obtain estimates of renal function (see Chap. 7).
(1) Urine plasma creatinine
(2) Creatinine clearance
(3) Urinary sodium concentration
(4) Fractional sodium excretion (FE_{Na})
(5) Obtain a radionuclide renal scan for estimate of renal perfusion and function when possible. Abdominal ultrasound will be helpful in ruling out obstruction and shows the characteristic patterns in chronic renal damage.

3. Therapy

a. The use of an indwelling catheter **should be discontinued** as soon as possible in a severely oligoanuric patient in whom intrinsic renal failure is established.

b. Weigh the patient bid (or use a metabolic bed with a scale).

c. Measure intake and output.

d. Fluid replacement
(1) Fluid and electrolyte replacement should be calculated as insensible losses (Table 7-5) plus urine output (if the patient is not edematous or does not have fluid overload).
(2) As many calories as possible are given, orally if practical. A peripheral IV line can tolerate 20% glucose; a central line can tolerate more.
(3) With fluid restrictions, weight should decrease by approximately 0.5% daily.
(4) When diuresis begins, increasing urine volume must be replaced with a solution containing approximately the same electrolytes as are being excreted. If the patient has been hyperkalemic, do not replace K^+ until the serum K^+ has returned to normal.

e. Nutrition. Optimal calories and protein nitrogen will help to decrease catabolism, lower BUN, ameliorate the uremic state, and improve healing and the immune response. With restricted fluids, little nitrogen and only 15–25% of calories can be given by a peripheral IV line.
(1) If the patient can take fluids PO, add Polycose, which gives 2 kcal/ml in solution (600 mOsm/L) with cream. Add an oral amino acid mixture such as Aminade.
(2) If the patient will be NPO for over a week and renal failure is profound, consider total parenteral nutrition (see Chap. 10).

f. Hyperkalemia
(1) If the serum K^+ is 5.5–7.0 mEq/L, Kayexalate in sorbitol at a dose of 1 gm/kg may be given PO or PR and repeated every hour until K^+ is lowered (see Chap. 7). **Warning.** 1 mEq of Na^+ enters the body for each milliequivalent of K^+ that is removed. Over time, hypernatremia may result.
(2) If the serum K^+ is above 7 mEq/L, or ECG changes, or arrhythmias, or both, are present, one or more of the following therapies is indicated immediately.
(a) Give sodium bicarbonate, 2.5 mEq/kg, as an IV push over 10–15 min.
(b) Give calcium gluconate, 10%, 0.5 ml/kg IV over 5–10 min, with ECG monitoring.
(c) Give 50% glucose, 1 ml/kg. Follow with a 30% glucose IV infusion.
(3) If hyperkalemia persists, insulin 0.5 U/kg IV, should be given while infusing 20% glucose. This dose may be repeated in 30–60 min if necessary. Prepare to dialyze the patient.
(4) Dialysis is usually necessary if K^+ is above 7.5 mEq/L, if the measures in **(2)** fail, or if **(3)** is needed.

g. Hypertension. If hypertension is acute and severe (3 S.D. above the age-appropriate norms), treat as outlined for hypertensive emergencies in sec. **III.A.** Note that in acute renal failure

(1) Antihypertensive agents with rapid onset of action should be selected.

(2) Phlebotomy, or dialysis, or both, should be used when hypertension is severe and unresponsive to medical management.

h. Congestive heart failure. See also Chap. 9.

(1) Congestive heart failure (CHF) can usually be prevented by proper **fluid restriction.**

(2) **There is no place for diuretics in the anuric patient.**

(3) Digitalis will not produce a dramatic effect.

(4) **Digitalization must be done slowly** and maintenance doses reduced as dictated by renal function. If CHF is severe, dialysis is indicated.

i. Acidosis can usually be alleviated by providing glucose for calories as well as 1–3 mEq/kg/day of exogenous bicarbonate, citrate, or lactate. **Warning.** A milliequivalent of bicarbonate contains 1 mEq of Na^+ or K^+. If acidosis is severe and treatment is difficult due to fluid overload, dialysis is indicated.

j. Seizures. See Chap. 20.

C. Postrenal failure

1. Etiology. Obstruction is usually due to congenital anomalies; urethral valves or stricture; hematuria with clots; tumor; or retroperitoneal fibrosis.

2. Evaluation and diagnosis. Obstruction is suggested by a history of genitourinary abnormalities, or lower abdominal trauma, or by the finding of flank masses or an enlarged bladder. Bilateral ureteral obstruction is suggested by absolute anuria.

a. If creatinine is less than 5 mg/100 ml, or the urine-plasma creatinine ratio is greater than 15, an intravenous pyelogram (IVP) may be attempted. (Do a nuclide scan, and an ultrasonogram if facilities are available.)

b. Urologic consultation should be obtained.

c. Cystoscopy with a unilateral retrograde pyelogram may be considered if anuria and obstruction are suggested.

3. Therapy consists in surgical correction or bypass, as required.

II. Chronic renal disease

A. Etiology. Almost half of chronic renal failure (CRF) cases are due to congenital causes: obstructive uropathy, renal dysplasia, juvenile nephronophthisis, or polycystic disease. About a third of cases of CRF in childhood are due to glomerulopathy. As a cause of CRF, chronic pyelonephritis is rare in the absence of an obstructive congenital lesion or marked reflux. Other causes include hemolytic uremic syndrome, malignant hypertension, interstitial nephritis, renal vein thrombosis, and nephrectomy for malignancy.

B. General therapeutic measures

1. Nutrition. Growth may be improved by appropriate dietary management. The limiting factor is the glomerular filtration rate (GFR).

a. Fluid. The aim is to replace insensible losses and urine output (see Chap. 7). **For the patient in chronic renal failure, fluid restriction may be more detrimental than overhydration.**

b. Calories. In fasting conditions, an obligatory loss of 25–35 cal/kg/day occurs. Since 50% is normally contributed by carbohydrates, the minimal administration of glucose necessary to avoid increased tissue breakdown is 400 gm/M^2 daily, or 3–4 gm/kg in the small child.

c. Protein

(1) The obligatory excretion of nitrogen through the kidney makes a progressive restriction of protein necessary. While the GFR remains above 25% of normal, any reasonable diet is usually tolerated.

(2) The progression of renal disease decreases osmotic tolerance, and some protein restriction is necessary. (Each gram of protein contains 6 mOsm urea.) As the GFR decreases from 25 to 10% of normal, a decrease of urinary concentration ability from 900 to 300 mOsm/L

occurs, forcing a restricted protein diet of 1.5–2.0 gm/kg/day. At these levels, proteins of high biologic value (egg, meat, milk) should be used in order to satisfy essential amino acid requirements.

(3) For infants, the use of human milk or a humanlike milk formula is lifesaving, and preferences for one could depend on the degree of renal failure (see Tables 5-2 to 5-5).

(4) As renal function falls below 10% of normal and approximates zero, further restrictions are necessary until dialysis is started.

  (a) If hemodialysis is instituted on a schedule of 3 times a week, liberalization of the protein intake is then possible to a daily intake of 2–3 gm of protein/kg (minimum), 2 gm of Na^+, and 2 gm of K^+.

  (b) A gradual increase in protein intake to 2 gm/kg or more daily can produce growth in a substantial number of children in renal failure.

d. Multivitamins. Daily administration of 1–2 standard multivitamin tablets or equivalent liquid preparations covers the basic requirements. Folic acid, 1–2 mg/kg/day, should be added as more severe renal failure supervenes.

e. Sodium

(1) To avoid arterial hypertension, sodium intake should be limited except when significant osmotic diuresis produces renal sodium wasting. A "no-salt-added" diet is usually the maximal restriction needed under these circumstances or with the nephrotic syndrome. It provides 40–90 mEq of Na^+/day (2–4 gm Na^+), depending on the amount used in cooking.

(2) If such a diet is insufficient, it may be combined with antihypertensive drugs, diuretics, or both.

(3) If salt wasting occurs, free salt intake may be necessary (see Chap. 7). Daily requirements are estimated by monitoring urinary sodium excretion and by the appearance of pitting edema and hypertension, indicating excessive salt administration. If sodium bicarbonate must be used, careful monitoring is necessary.

f. Potassium

(1) Hyperkalemia. Conditions usually leading to hyperkalemia include:

  (a) The onset of severe renal failure or sudden oliguria due to vomiting, diarrhea, or both, or to GI bleeding

  (b) The indiscriminate administration of aldosterone antagonists (spironolactone) or inhibitors of distal tubular sodium-potassium exchange (triamterene); use of captopril

  (c) Drugs containing K^+, such as potassium penicillin

  (d) Massive hemolysis or tissue destruction

  (e) Treatment. Serum K^+ levels below 5.8 mEq/L are usually well handled by further restrictions in potassium intake, using the following guidelines:

  Fruits high in K^+: Bananas, oranges (citrus), cantaloupe, watermelon, apricots, raisins, prunes, pineapples, and cherries

  Vegetables* high in K^+: Green leafy vegetables, potatoes, avocado, artichoke, lentils, and beets

  Meats and fish high in K^+: All have K^+ content (lowest are chicken liver, shrimp, and crab)

  Breads and flours highest in K^+: Pumpernickel, buckwheat, and soy

  Miscellaneous foods high in K^+: Chocolate, cocoa, brown (not white) sugar, molasses, nuts, and peanut butter

  The potassium content of commonly used beverages is given in Table 8-1. Serum levels above 5.8 mEq/L must be treated with an

*Cooking leaches out K^+; cook these foods.

Table 8-1. Potassium content of beverages

High K^+	mEq/L	Low K^+	mEq/L
Milk	36	Ginger ale	0.1
Cola	13	Pepsi-Cola	0.8
Orange juice	49		
Grape juice	31		
Tomato juice	59		

exchange resin to remove K^+ from the body, or by temporizing measures until dialysis can be started (see **I** and Chap. 7).

(2) Hypokalemia (see also Chap. 7). Hypokalemia is a common complication in the management of the patient with edema and secondary hyperaldosteronism (especially in the nephrotic patient during spontaneous or corticosteroid-induced diuresis and of the patient with polyuric renal disease complicated by an acute GI disorder). Unless renal failure supervenes, none of these patients will require any dietary potassium restrictions; rather, they will require potassium supplementation, as follows:

(a) Potassium chloride, a 300-mg tablet with 4 mEq/tablet, or a 1 mM/ml solution. **Enteric-coated tablets should not be used** because of their intestinal insolubility. Of the available preparations, K-Lor (a pineapple-orange-flavored powder, 25 mEq/packet) is the most palatable. If chloride is chosen because of alkalosis, K-Lor can be mixed in fruit juice and given in 3–4 doses over the day.

(b) Potassium bicarbonate, 300-mg capsules with 3 mEq/capsule, or Shohl's solution, 140 gm citric acid + 100 gm of sodium citrate or potassium citrate dissolved in water to 1 L

(c) The requirement may range from 1–2 to 2–5 mEq/kg/day and even higher in long-standing renal tubular disease.

(d) Triamterene (smallest available tablet = 50 mg) can aid in the prevention of urinary K^+ losses and works well for chronic conditions such as cystinosis or Bartter syndrome. (**Note.** In Bartter syndrome, inhibitors of prostaglandin synthetase [aspirin, indomethacin] have produced striking improvements in potassium balance.) Doses of 2–4 mg/kg daily or on alternate days can substantially reduce the need for K^+ supplements when urinary loss is a major factor.

(e) Prolonged hypokalemia will lead to secondary metabolic alkalosis and possible paradoxical aciduria if the patient also has a sodium deficit. If the hypokalemia is severe (<2 mEq/L serum), IV replacement should be given at 4–5 mEq/kg/day as potassium chloride (2 mEq/ml), at least in the first 24 hr, and continued according to the laboratory results and urinary output.

(f) In renal tubular acidosis, cystinosis, postobstructive diuresis, and acute tubular necrosis, serum K^+ levels of less than 1 mEq/L may be found, and the required replacement may exceed the maximal recommended IV fluid potassium concentration of 40–80 mEq/L and reach 150–200 mEq/L. (Such a concentration may be extremely caustic to the vessel wall, but lifesaving.)

2. Mineral metabolism in renal disease. Secondary hyperparathyroidism and metabolic bone disease occur in renal insufficiency (GFR < 25% of normal) unless vigorous measures are taken.

a. Hyperphosphatemia. If the serum phosphatase level is over 5 mEq/L, or if alkaline phosphate is elevated, dietary phosphate must be restricted

Table 8-2. Phosphate binders

Trade Name	Form	Description	Al (OH) (mg)	NA⁺ mg(mEq)
			Composition	
AlternaGEL	Suspension (5 ml)	Slightly lemon-flavored, white liquid; pleasant tasting, high potency	600	<2
Amphojel	Suspension (5ml)	Chalky, mint-flavored white liquid	320	6.9
	Tablets 0.3 gm	Aspirin-sized white tablets	300	1.4
	0.6 gm	Nickel-sized white tablets	600	2.8
Alu-Cap	Capsule	Easy to open and mix with food or fluid	475	
Basaljel	Capsule	Easy to open and mix with food or fluid	500	2.8
	Suspension	White liquid	400	1.8
Dialume	Tablet	Large, capsule-sized	500	
Nephrox	Suspension (5 ml)	Watermelon-flavored, pink liquid with chalky aftertaste; mineral oil 10% by volume.	320	

Source: Courtesy of Nancy Spinozzi, R.D., Renal Dietician, The Children's Hospital, Boston, Mass.

and oral phosphate binders administered. Once phosphate is normalized, vitamin D (as dihydrotachysterol or actual D_3 analogues) and oral calcium supplements are used.

Because of hypermagnesemia already present in patients with chronic renal failure, plain aluminum hydroxide (Amphojel, 300-mg and 600-mg tablets, 300 mg/5 ml liquid) is preferable as an **oral phosphate binder** (Table 8-2) to magnesium-containing preparations such as Gelusil. The dose is 300–1,800 mg, given immediately after meals. Phosphate binders must be given with or just after all meals and snacks to bind the phosphate in the diet; otherwise, they are ineffective. Other acceptable preparations are Basaljel, Alu-Caps, AlternaGEL, Nephrox, and cookies or bread made from these preparations (see Table 8-2). (AlternaGEL is especially tasty and is twice as potent as Amphojel.) If an antacid is needed, use Riopan, which is low in magnesium.

b. **Calcium balance.** In general, good control of serum phosphorus levels should precede the administration of calcium, but seizures or other complications make immediate treatment with calcium unavoidable.

(1) **Hypocalcemia.** See also Chap. 7.

(a) **Acute replacement** is needed only if the patient is symptomatic, i.e., has hypocalcemic seizures or tetany. Then 10–15 mg calcium/kg is given IV q4h as 10% calcium gluconate or 22% calcium glucceptate. The correcting effects last only a few hours, and a new infusion or further PO administration is required.

(b) **Oral preparations.** Calcium lactate is the oral preparation that is best tolerated. However, its low calcium content per weight (18%) requires ingestion of many tablets (each 300-mg tablet contains 54 mg of calcium) to provide the minimal allowance of 500–1000 mg/day. Cal-Sup contains 750 mg calcium carbonate (equivalent to 300 mg elemental calcium).

(2) Hypercalcemia. Although hypercalcemia is not common in renal disease, it is a possible complication of indiscriminate use of vitamin D, severe secondary hyperparathyroidism, and inappropriate dialysate concentration of calcium (see Chap. 7). If acute hypercalcemia occurs and immediate treatment is necessary, the following measures should be carried out:

(a) Reduce calcium intake. Special milk formulas are available with minimal calcium content ($<$ 100 mg/day). Discontinue the administration of vitamin D in any form (as in multivitamins).

(b) Administer IV saline. Use 1-2 L/M^2 in acute severe hypercalcemia if urine output is adequate.

(c) Decrease the absorption of calcium. Decrease gut absorption by administration of corticosteroids (prednisone, 1–2 mg/kg day). This takes days to act.

(d) Phosphate salts are best reserved for patients unresponsive to the preceding measures. Because IV infusion of sodium phosphate is itself dangerous, often producing metastatic soft tissue calcification and an abrupt fall in calcium, the preferred route of administration is P.R. Sodium phosphate (Phospho-Soda contains 3.3 gm/5 ml) may be given as an enema, or one can simply administer a Fleet enema.

(e) Hemodialysis may be used to control severe hypercalcemia.

c. Vitamin D

(1) The use of dihydrotachysterol is recommended to improve intestinal resorption and increase the parathyroid hormone-end-organ responsiveness, avoiding inappropriate hypertrophy of the parathyroid gland.

(a) Administration should start as soon as the GFR falls below 25–20% of normal and hyperphosphatemia is no longer present; the initial dosage should be conservative (0.125 mg/M^2/day), and follow-up should include periodic urinary calcium-creatinine ratios and serum calcium levels. These will be needed as long as dihydrotachysterol is administered and for 2–3 weeks thereafter.

(b) One milligram of dihydrotachysterol is approximately equivalent to 3 mg (120,000 units) of vitamin D$_2$.

(c) If vitamin D toxicity develops and is recognized early, the loss in renal function will probably be reversible.

(d) Patients should be cautioned to decrease their vitamin D intake when traveling or moving to areas that have higher sun exposure.

(2) 1,25-Dihydroxycholecalciferol (1,25-hydroxy vitamin D, calcitriol [Rocaltrol]) may be used. The initial dose is 0.25 μg/day for older children. Adult hemodialysis patients require 0.5–1.0 μg/day; the exact pediatric dose must be determined for each child. The advantage of calcitriol may be a short half-life, with pharmacologic activity lasting 3–5 days/dose.

3. Anticonvulsant therapy. See also Chap. 3, p. 59.

a. The usual causes for seizures in the renal patient with preserved renal function are hypertensive encephalopathy, severe metabolic alkalosis with relative hypocalcemia, or hypomagnesemia following hyponatremia underlying CNS complications.

b. In chronic renal failure the appearance of seizures is most probably due to acute acid-base and electrolyte changes, and a careful evaluation of acid-base and electrolyte status should always be done to provide adequate therapy.

c. Disequilibrium following dialysis may cause convulsions, which are best treated by a change in dialysis procedures.

d. Therapy depends on etiology.

4. Dialysis therapy. The indications for dialysis in renal failure are intractable congestive heart failure, increasing acidosis, intractable hyperkalemia, and continuing clinical deterioration. The decision to dialyze should not be made on the basis of one isolated laboratory value—each case should be individualized.

a. Peritoneal dialysis

(1) Disposable catheter sets are now available for pediatric peritoneal dialysis.

(2) After it is certain that the bladder is empty, the skin of the abdomen is prepared in a sterile fashion.

(3) To make insertion easier and decrease the risk of perforation of intraabdominal contents, the abdominal cavity is distended by an initial load of dialysis fluid (approximately 20 ml/kg) introduced through an 18- or 20-gauge needle inserted at the potential catheter site.

(4) The catheter is inserted, usually in the midline, one-third of the distance between the umbilicus and the symphysis pubis. It can then be advanced to the left lower or right lower quadrant and connected to the tubing.

(5) The usual amount of fluid exchanged is 20 ml/kg initially, with a gradual increase to 40–50 ml/kg per exchange. (The initial loading fluid is not removed. The presence of such a reservoir will ensure that all the holes in the catheter are under water and will prevent air block.) The fluid is usually warmed to body temperature, then permitted to run in as fast as is tolerated, allowed to equilibrate for 15–20 min, and then drained (usual time is 15–30 min). At every sixth cycle the abdomen is allowed to drain dry, a specimen is sent for culture, and the patient is weighed, unless a constant read-out bed scale is available.

(6) The usual dialysis is carried on for 36–72 hr, depending on the indications and the patient's clinical status. The danger of infection increases after 48 hr.

(7) Factors affecting peritoneal dialysis

(a) Clearance. Urea is cleared at the rate of 14–30 ml/min at 20°C. Creatinine is cleared at a slower rate of 10–15 ml/min.

(b) Temperature. Warming the solution to body temperature will decrease heat loss (especially important in small infants) and—more important—will increase urea clearance.

(c) Rate. Increasing the flow of the dialysis fluid will shorten the time for dialysis, but is expensive and will increase protein loss and aggravate hyperglycemia.

(8) Solutions

(a) Usually, 1.5% glucose and water with added electrolytes is used. Prepared solutions are available.

(b) Prepared solutions contain no potassium; K^+ should be added as required. In patients with hyperkalemia, except in those taking digitalis, no K^+ needs to be added to the initial three to five exchanges. Subsequently, 2.5–3.5 mEq/L may be added to the dialyzing fluid. The composition of a standard solution is given in Table 8-3.

(c) The 1.5% glucose solution as used in dialysis is hyperosmolar (372 mOsm/L) and thus can cause appreciable fluid loss (up to 200–300 ml/hr). For removal of excess fluid, glucose can be added to increase the osmolality of the solution as desired. However, the use of solutions of higher osmolality can rapidly dehydrate infants and children (4.25% glucose = 525 mOsm/L; 6.5% glucose = 678 mOsm/L).

(d) Heparin (500–1,000 units/L) should be added to the first liter of dialysate and continued if the fluid is not clear.

(e) When dialyzing for certain toxins, various additives such as albumin are useful in increasing removal.

Table 8-3. Composition of a standard peritoneal dialysis solution

Sodium	140 mEq/L
Chloride	101 mEq/L
Calcium	4.0 mEq/L
Magnesium	1.5 mg/L
Acetate	45 mg/L
Potassium	Added on individual basis

(9) Complications in peritoneal dialysis
   (a) Infection is usually due to *Staphylococcus aureus* and gram-negative organisms. Culture of fluid should be done every sixth cycle. Antibiotics are not advised for routine use, but treatment should be begun in a symptomatic patient even if culture results are not available (see Chap. 15, p. 362). If intraperitoneal antibiotics are used, they must be given with extreme care, since high blood levels can result from peritoneal absorption.
   (b) Hyperglycemia is a special problem in diabetic patients, but it can also occur in nondiabetic patients and result in nonketotic hyperosmolar coma. The blood sugar must be monitored routinely in patients dialyzed with a 4.25% solution.
   (c) Hypoproteinemia can occur; about 0.5 gm/L of protein is lost in dialysis.
   (d) Perforation. The risk of perforation of abdominal organs (e.g., bladder, bowel) can be reduced appreciably by distending the abdominal cavity with dialysate and emptying the bladder before catheter insertion [see **a.(3)**].
   b. Hemodialysis for childhood acute or chronic renal failure is practical and federally funded. Even small infants and neonates can be dialyzed without difficulty by experienced personnel. It is more efficient than peritoneal dialysis, permitting control of both clearance and ultrafiltration within narrow limits. A vascular access is necessary; a catheter placed in the femoral or subclavian vein is sufficient for a temporary access in older children. Permanent accesses consist of external connections between an artery and vein (shunt) or an internal connection (fistula). Children have been maintained on hemodialysis for years. Appropriate consultation and referral should be made.
      (1) Clearance on hemodialysis. Blood and dialysate flows are adjusted to give a urea clearance of 2–3 ml/min/kg of body weight.
      (2) Complications of hemodialysis. Common problems include dysequilibrium syndrome, bleeding, shock from too vigorous ultrafiltration, and infection of the vascular access site.
   c. Chronic ambulatory peritoneal dialysis (CAPD). This form of peritoneal dialysis, in which a patient with end-stage renal disease is dialyzed continually at a slow rate, is just beginning to be used in children. Episodes of peritonitis are a major complication. A variation of CAPD, continuous cycling peritoneal dialysis (CCPD), is also available. In CCPD, overnight cycling of dialysis fluid is performed automatically.
   5. Transplantation is preferable to chronic dialysis for most children with CRF. Any child with CRF should be considered a transplant candidate. Though transplantation cannot be considered curative, long-term survival is the rule, and transplantation offers the optimal chance for rehabilitation from CRF. Referral should be made to a transplantation center.
III. Hypertension. Hypertension in CRF prior to a need for dialysis should be treated with drugs (see below). In dialysis patients, hypertension is usually controlled with adequate ultrafiltration on hemodialysis.

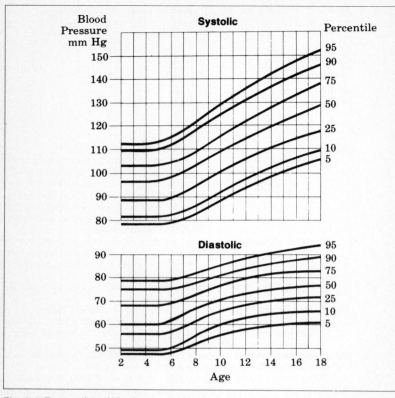

Fig. 8-1. Percentiles of blood pressure measurement in boys (right arm, seated). (From *Pediatrics* 59:803, 1977.)

Hypertension is suggested by blood pressure values (taken with a cuff of appropriate size covering two-thirds of the upper arm) that are 2 S.D. above the mean or above the 95th percentile for age. (Values for various age groups are depicted in Figs. 8-1–8-3.) *Any diastolic* blood pressure above 95 mm Hg in a small child or above 110 in a larger child requires immediate control. Such control is also necessary if blood pressure elevation has caused CNS or cardiac symptoms.

The curability of hypertension in children is greater than in adults. Primary (essential) hypertension in childhood has been identified in up to 30 percent in various series, but its natural history, both untreated and treated, remains to be delineated. Unless blood pressure is routinely recorded as part of the general physical examination, hypertension may be overlooked for considerable periods of time.

A. Hypertensive crisis. In acute, severe hypertension, the immediate short-term goal is control of blood pressure. Simultaneously, there should be a program of medical or surgical investigation, or both, and treatment aimed at long-term control. The usual effective doses of antihypertensive medications are given in **1–6**; many patients require less, some more. Diuretics (see **B.2** and Table 9-3) given concomitantly IV will often be helpful.

   1. Diazoxide (Hyperstat) is the most practical effective drug for acute hypertension now available. A benzothiazide with no diuretic effect, it acts directly

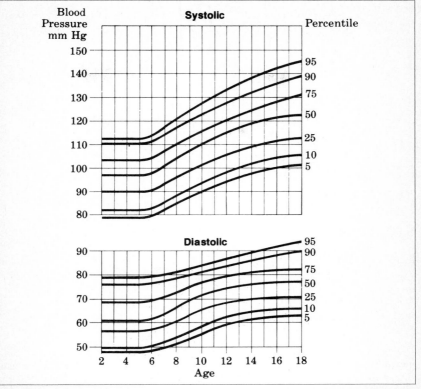

Fig. 8-2. Percentiles of blood pressure measurement in girls (right arm, seated). (From *Pediatrics* 59:803, 1977.)

on the vessels' smooth muscles, promptly and effectively reducing muscle tone. Diazoxide does not reduce renal blood flow.

  a. It is administered only IV (5 mg/kg/dose) **as fast as possible** to obtain minimal binding to serum protein and maximal action on the smooth muscle. The average fall in both systolic and diastolic pressures is 44 mm Hg, which occurs a few minutes after administration, and the effects last 3–15 hr. If the initial dose proves ineffective, a second can be tried after 15–20 min.

  b. Disadvantages. The effect of diazoxide cannot be titrated. It causes hyperglycemia and can cause sodium and fluid retention. Transient tachycardia often follows administration.

2. Sodium nitroprusside (Nipride) must be used as an IV drip with constant intensive care unit monitoring. It is universally effective, since it causes immediate vasodilation and lowers pressure. The effects disappear when the IV drip is stopped.

  a. The dose is 0.5–8.0 μg/kg/min. (**Note.** The prepared solution [look at method every time to avoid error] is inactivated by light. Do not use with other drugs in the same IV line.)

  b. Blood levels of thiocyanate must be checked daily, since nitroprusside is

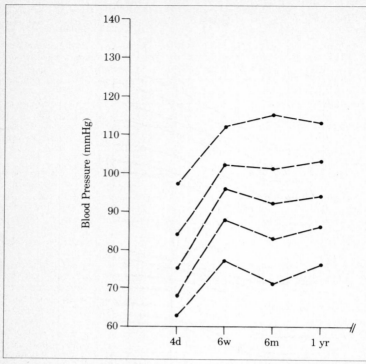

Fig. 8-3. Percentiles of blood pressure in infants awake (both sexes pooled) at age 4 days to 1 year (Brompton study). At age 6 weeks the percentile values were calculated from the 594 boys and 538 girls who were awake at the time of measurement. At ages 6 months and 1 year, all infants were awake. At age 4 days there were only 174 infants awake at the time of measurement, and the percentile values were therefore taken from these measurements plus the measurements made on the infants asleep after correction for wakefulness. (From M. de Swiet, P. Fayers, and E. A. Shinebourne, *Pediatrics* 65:1033, 1980.)

converted to thiocyanate by the hepatic enzyme rhodanase. **Caution** is necessary in the presence of hepatic insufficiency.

    c. Advantages. The onset of action is instantaneous. Nitroprusside is effective when all other drugs have failed. The rate of infusion can be titrated against desired blood pressure.

    d. Disadvantages. Nitroprusside requires constant supervision in the intensive care unit. Discontinuance of the IV drip means instantaneous loss of the pharmacologic effect.

3. Hydralazine (Apresoline). When hydralazine is given IM, the onset of action is within 15–30 min. Onset after IV administration is immediate.

    a. Dosage

        (1) Hydralazine is given parenterally at an initial dose of 0.15 mg/kg, which is progressively increased q6h to up to 10 times the initial dose, according to the response.

        (2) When given with diazoxide or reserpine, the dose needed may be smaller than when given alone.

        (3) For the oral dose, see **B.3.**

b. **Advantages.** Hydralazine does not reduce renal blood flow; it is effective fairly rapidly; and it seldom produces hypotension. It can be used with diazoxide, propranolol, methyldopa, or reserpine.

c. **Disadvantages.** The most important side effects are tachycardia, nausea, vomiting, headache, diarrhea, and positive lupus erythematosus (LE) and rheumatoid factor (RF) reactions (very rare in children). The drug should be avoided in patients with arrhythmias and heart failure. It is not consistently effective.

4. **Propranolol (Inderal)** is a beta-adrenergic blocker and is most safely given PO. It also has antirenin action. For discussion, see Chap. 9, p. 239).

5. **Methyldopa (Aldomet)** is an inhibitor of dopa decarboxylase and is metabolized to alpha-methyl norepinephrine, a weak pressor that displaces norepinephrine at nerve endings.

   a. **Dosage**

      (1) IV dosage is from 10–50 mg/kg daily, administered in 4 divided doses q6h, beginning with 10 mg/kg/24 hr and doubling each subsequent dose until the desired effect is obtained. It is recommended that it be diluted in 5% D/W and be given over 30–60 min. A paradoxical rise in blood pressure can be seen with too-rapid injection.

      (2) Oral dose. See **B.3.**

   b. **Advantages.** Gradual lowering of blood pressure. The renin level is also lowered.

   c. **Disadvantages.** Side effects are minimal but include drug fever and hemolytic anemia with a positive Coombs test, positive LE cell reaction, positive RF, granulocytopenia, and thrombocytopenia. Methyldopa is not recommended for patients with pheochromocytoma. Both methyldopa and its metabolites produce false-positive blood and urine tests for pheochromocytoma.

6. **Reserpine.** The *Rauwolfia* alkaloids deplete stores of catecholamines and 5-hydroxytryptamine in many organs. Depletion starts 1 hr after administration and becomes maximal by 24 hr. Tissue catecholamines are slowly restored, and repeated doses have a cumulative action even at intervals of a week or longer.

   a. **Dosage.** In acute hypertensive crisis, the recommended IM dosage is 0.07 mg/kg/dose q4-6h (in patients weighing over 25 kg, an initial dose of 1–2 mg should be given and subsequent doses based on the response), followed by an oral maintenance with 0.02 mg/kg/day. As the cumulative effect of the drug takes place, this dosage usually can be reduced to 0.1–0.5 mg/day, given in 1 dose.

   b. **Advantages.** Consistent and gradual lowering of blood pressure

   c. **Disadvantages.** Somnolence; mental depression is almost never seen in children; night terrors may occur. Nasal stuffiness is common and is generally well tolerated. However, reserpine should not be used in the neonate who is an obligate nose breather.

B. **Mild and/or chronic hypertension.** Symptomatic therapy should consist of

1. **Diet.** If blood pressure elevation is mild, a low-salt diet alone may be tried first. Weight reduction may help lower blood pressure.

2. **Diuretics** (see Table 9-3) may be used if mild hypertension fails to respond to diet.

3. **Antihypertensive agents** should be added if 1 and 2 do not control blood pressure *or* if hypertension is moderately to severely elevated (see **A**). The dosages are shown in Table 8-4.

IV. **Renal tubular acidosis (RTA).** This syndrome consists of hyperchloremic acidosis associated with normal or slightly decreased glomerular function and inappropriately alkaline urine.

A. **Proximal renal tubular acidosis**

1. **Etiology.** A tubular defect producing an abnormally low threshold for $NaHCO_3$ is present.

Table 8-4. Antihypertensive agents for oral use

Agent name	Tablet size or suspension[b]	Daily dosage (starting)	Dosage interval	Comments
Vasodilator				
Hydralazine (Apresoline)	10, 25, 50 mg	0.1–3.0 mg/kg	q4–q6	
Minoxidil[a] (Loniten)	2.5, 10 mg	0.2 mg/kg to start maximum 30–40 mg	Once daily to bid	For severe hypertension; hirsutism is problem
Central alpha stimulator				
Clonidine (Catapres)	0.1, 0.2 mg	0.05 mg–2.4 mg bid	q8–12h	Rebound hypertension may occur
Guanabenz[a] (Wytensin)	4, 8 mg	4 mg bid to start in adult, ? in child	bid	
Beta blockade[c]				
Propranolol (Inderal)	10, 40 mg	0.5 mg/kg/day to start	q6–12h	Long-acting capsule available but pediatric dosage not established
Metoprolol[a] (Lopressor)	50, 100 mg	2 mg/kg/day	q12h	Relatively cardiospecific
Nadolol[a] (Corgard)	40, 80, 120, 160 mg	40 mg/day in adult, ? in child	Once daily	Long acting
Atenolol[a] (Tenormin)	50, 100 mg	50 mg/day in adult, ? in child	Once daily	Long acting
Timolol[a] (Blocadren)	10 mg	0.3 mg/kg/day in adult, ? in child	q12h	
Pindolol[a] (Visken)	5–10 mg	0.3 mg/kg/day in adult, ? in child	q8–12h	Has some sympathomimetic activity

Peripheral alpha blockade				
Prazosin[a] (Minipress)	1, 2, 5 mg	1 mg tid in adult, ? in child	q8h	Also sometimes classified as vasodilator
Phenoxybenzamine[a] (Dibenzyline)	100 mg cap.	Individualized starting dose 2–5 mg; range 20–100 mg/day	q12h	For pheochromocytoma
False transmitter				
Methyldopa (Aldomet)	125, 250 mg tab or 25 mg/5 ml oral suspension	10 mg/kg/day	q6–12h	
Converting enzyme inhibitor				
Captopril[a] (Capoten)	25, 50, 100 mg	0.5–1 mg/kg/day	q6–12h	Beware of renal failure, hyperkalemia
Central inhibitor				
Reserpine (Sandril, Serpasil, Reserpoid)	0.1, 0.25 mg	0.02 mg/kg/day	Once daily	Maximum daily dosage 2.5 mg
Neuroeffector blockade				
Guanethidine (Ismelin)	10, 25 mg	0.2 mg/kg/day	Once daily	Postural hypotension, weakness, diarrhea may occur
Guanadrel[a] (Hylorel)	10, 25 mg	10 mg bid in adult, ? child	bid	Inhibits norepinephrine storage release *and* depletes from nerve endings

Note: Additional oral agents including calcium channel blockers and new converting enzyme inhibitors are in testing phases.
[a]Not specifically approved for use in childhood.
[b]Pharmacies can occasionally make specialized capsules on request.
[c]A large number of beta blockers are now available, but only propranolol is approved specifically for use in children.

2. Evaluation and diagnosis
   a. Growth failure is usually present.
   b. Arterial blood gases and serum electrolytes reveal a hyperchloremic acidosis with normal K^+ and Ca^{++} levels.
   c. Urine pH varies with the degree of acidemia. **All urine for pH should be collected under oil and measured while fresh.** A urine pH of less than 5.5 and a serum $NaHCO_3$ below the patient's renal threshold are seen in severe acidemia.
   d. A bicarbonate titration test may be done by infusing $NaHCO_3$ slowly (e.g., 1–2 mEq/kg over 1 hr) when the patient is acidotic and measuring serum HCO_3^- levels, urine pH, titratable acidity, and ammonium excretion. The renal threshold for HCO_3^- resorption in proximal RTA will be below the norms for children of comparable age.

3. Therapy
   a. Large doses of bicarbonate (10–15 mEq/kg/day) are required to maintain serum pH. In primary proximal RTA the dosage is decreased after 6 months to determine if the threshold is still abnormal, in which case acidosis will redevelop when therapy is stopped.
   b. A repeat bicarbonate titration test should be performed, since it appears that the disorder improves spontaneously after 2–3 years and some children will recover.

B. Distal renal tubular acidosis
   1. Etiology. A defect in the distal tubule is present, resulting in an inability to establish a hydrogen ion gradient between blood and tubular fluid.
   2. Evaluation
      a. The presenting symptoms are usually growth failure, polyuria, and polydipsia.
      b. Arterial blood gases and serum electrolytes reveal a hyperchloremic acidosis, with hypokalemia seen in a number of patients.
      c. The urine pH is rarely below 6.5, even in the face of severe existing acidemia.
      d. Concentrating ability is markedly impaired, with maximal urine osmolalities of less than 450 mOsm.
      e. Urinary calcium excretion is elevated (above 2 mg/kg/day).
      f. The GFR may be decreased.
      g. Ammonium chloride loading test. If the urine pH is spontaneously 5 or less even in an acidemic patient, this test is not necessary since the patient has proximal RTA. To distinguish proximal from distal tubule disease, an ammonium chloride loading test may be done (Table 8-5). The test is done by administering 75 mEq/M^2 of ammonium chloride PO followed by measurement of the urine pH, titratable acidity, and ammonium excretion; concomitant blood pH + CO_2 samples should be taken hourly for 5 hr. The serum HCO_3^- concentration should fall to 16 mEq/L

Table 8-5. Ammonium chloride loading test (normal values)

Age*	Urine pH	Titratable acid (μEq/min/1.73 M^2)	Ammonium excretion (μEq/min/1.73 M^2)
1–12 months	5.0	62 (43–111)	57 (42–79)
4–15 years	5.5	52 (33–71)	73 (46–100)

Source: Adapted from C. Edelmann et al., *Pediatr. Res.* 1:452, 1967; *J. Clin. Invest.* 46:1309, 1967.
*Although current data are sparse, normal values for ages 1–4 years appear to approximate those of older children.

or less. If it does not, a larger dose of ammonium chloride (150 mEq/M^2) should be given cautiously on a second testing day.

    h. X-rays will reveal nephrocalcinosis in some patients.

3. The **diagnosis** is confirmed by performing an ammonium chloride loading test. There is an inability to acidify the urine below 6.5, with depressed rates of excretion of titratable acid and ammonium. In proximal RTA, patients acidify urine when markedly acidemic.

4. Treatment

    a. Sodium and potassium bicarbonate and citrate in daily doses of 1–3 mEq/kg will correct the acidosis, improve growth, and normalize the GFR. However, they will not reverse nephrocalcinosis or improve concentrating ability.

    b. There is no indication at present that children will recover spontaneously from distal tubular acidosis, and therapy must be continued for life.

    c. The dosage of sodium and potassium bicarbonate and citrate should be adjusted according to the blood pH, and daily urine calcium excretion should be kept below 2 mg/kg. Plasma K^+ must be monitored, and some patients require all their bicarbonate as potassium bicarbonate.

V. Disorders with proteinuria

A. Etiology. Increased protein excretion occurs with or without renal pathology. Massive proteinuria ($> 2 \text{ gm/M}^2$/day) always indicates renal disease.

    1. Mild to moderate proteinuria (200–500 mg/day) may be seen with fever, dehydration, exercise, cold exposure, hypermetabolic states, heart failure, constrictive pericarditis, or lower urinary tract disease. **Orthostatic proteinuria** occurs without signs of renal disease.

    2. Casts or altered renal function may be seen with either minimal or massive proteinuria.

        a. Minimal proteinuria **with** hematuria suggests a focal nephritis, vascular disease, or an infectious process. **Without** hematuria, it suggests tubulointerstitial disease, "inactive" nephritis, congenital abnormalities of the kidneys, or drug toxicity.

        b. Massive proteinuria **with** hematuria suggests renal vein thrombosis, significant glomerulopathy (with or without systemic disease), or malignant hypertension. **Without** hematuria, it suggests minimal lesion nephrotic syndrome or membranous nephropathy and is consistent with the presence of amyloid, diabetic nephropathy, or myeloma.

B. Evaluation and diagnosis. In healthy adults, protein excretion is 30–100 mg/day; in children, 100 mg/day; in infants (1 month of age), 240 mg/M^2/day.

    1. Note how the sample was collected; look for fever, metabolic stress, etc., which might cause proteinuria. Recheck for protein on two more occasions to be certain that the patient is proteinuric.

    2. Look for orthostatic (postural) proteinuria: (a) Check A.M. and P.M. urines with a dipstick; A.M. should be negative. Obtain 12-hr daytime (active) urine and 12-hr nighttime (recumbent) urine collections. The recumbent urine collection should have **completely normal** protein excretion.

    3. Urinalysis and **culture** are necessary. Watch for false-positive reactions caused by Tolbutamide, penicillins, sulfonamides, radiologic contrast material, or zephiran. Recheck the patient after a suitable interval.

    4. Evaluation of the history, clinical features, and laboratory results suggests the diagnostic category.

    5. Persistent, constant (seen in all postures) proteinuria may require referral to a nephrologist for further evaluation and possible renal biopsy.

C. Treatment. No therapy is needed for orthostatic proteinuria. The therapy of proteinuria due to other causes depends on the diagnosis (Fig. 8-4).

VI. Nephrotic syndrome. The nephrotic syndrome is characterized by proteinuria, edema, hypoproteinemia, and hyperlipidemia. The incidence is 1.0 in 100,000 among whites and 2.8 in 100,000 among nonwhites under 16 years of age. The peak incidence is between 2–3 years (75% of cases occur in children under 5 years of age).

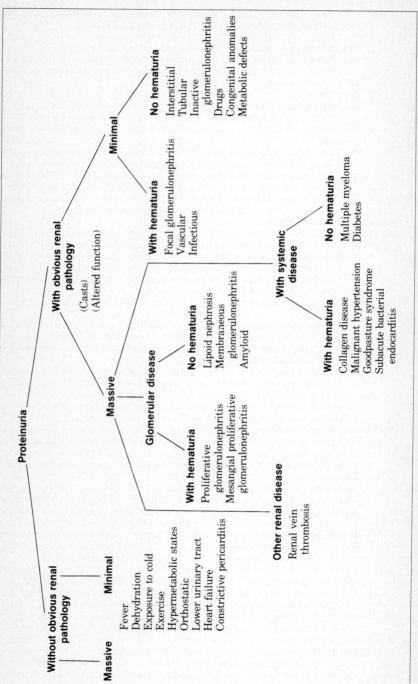

Fig. 8-4. Proteinuria with and without obvious renal pathology.

A. Etiology. The nephrotic syndrome can occur as part of the clinical course of any progressive glomerulonephritis, but the pathogenesis is unknown.

B. Evaluation

1. **History.** A history of infection or nephritis is sought.

2. **Physical examination.** A careful assessment should include weight, blood pressure, sites and extent of edema, and cardiac status.

3. **Laboratory evaluation** includes 24-hr urinary protein, serum protein and A/G ratio, urinary serum electrophoresis, serum lipid, BUN, electrolytes, creatinine clearance, C3, and selective protein index (ratio of IgG-transferrin clearances with selectivity [as opposed to nonselectivity] ≤ 0.2).

4. The presence of gross hematuria, a low C3, unselective proteinuria, an age of presentation below 1 year or over 10 years, a failure to respond to corticosteroids, elevated BUN, or elevated blood pressure should cast doubt on the diagnosis of lipoid nephrosis, and a renal biopsy should be performed.

C. Diagnosis. A combination of the defined clinical features with proteinuria in excess of 1 gm/M^2/24 hr confirms the diagnosis. **However, all features need not be present,** especially early in relapse.

D. Treatment

1. **Drugs** are generally for minimal lesion nephrotic syndrome only.

   a. **Corticosteroids** are the treatment of choice, usually 2 mg/kg/day of prednisone PO in divided doses (maximum dosage/day of 80 mg should not be exceeded). This regimen is continued until the urine is protein free for 3–10 days, or for up to 4–8 weeks if the urine fails to become protein free. (Lack of response by 8 weeks suggests corticosteroid resistance.) Following this, a further alternate-day regimen is generally given in a reduced dosage (1.0–1.5 mg/kg/day as 1 dose q48h) for a month, after which it is tapered over 2–3 weeks and discontinued.

   b. **Immunosuppression.** In patients who fail to respond to prednisone, a trial of immunosuppressive therapy may be indicated. Such therapy appears to be effective in patients who are frequent "relapsers" and require many or prolonged courses of prednisone; it appears less effective in those who show no response to corticosteroids. **Immunosuppressive therapy should only be undertaken after renal biopsy and consultation with a pediatric nephrologist.**

   c. **Diuretics and albumin.** See Table 9-3.

      (1) **The use of a diuretic alone can be hazardous in the presence of a low serum albumin,** since this can aggravate an already existing contraction of the circulating blood volume. However, diuretics may be used alone in the following circumstances:

         (a) Orally in patients who have problems with recurrent edema. Use furosemide, 1–2 mg/kg/day, adding triamterene, 0.7 mg/kg/24 hr, or thiazides, or both if need be.

         (b) Intravenously to mobilize edema fluid and alleviate symptoms from ascites, to help control infections while the patient is edematous, and to alleviate the aggravation of edema, which can occur when corticosteroids are first begun. **Caution.** If diuresis is ineffective, if pulse rate increases, or if blood pressure drops *or* goes up precipitously, discontinuation or use only with albumin is indicated.

      (2) When accumulation of edema fluid is severe, or when diuretics alone fail, salt-poor albumin may be given in a dose of 1 gm/kg IV slowly q12h, to be followed by IV furosemide, 1 mg/kg. **Caution.** Too-rapid administration of salt-poor albumin may cause pulmonary edema and congestive heart failure.

2. **General measures**

   a. **Diet.** There is no need for dietary restriction other than a low-salt diet (1–2 gm/M^2) during a period of edema. Fluid restriction will be self-imposed if salt is restricted. Prior to diuresis, fluid may be restricted to insensible losses plus urine output (or a bit less).

Table 8-6. Hemoglobinuria versus myoglobinuria

Observation	Myoglobin	Hemoglobin
Color of serum	Clear	Pink
Level of serum haptoglobin	Normal	Decreased
Mix urine with 80% $(NH_4) S_2O_4$ and filter	Pink	Clear
Muscle tenderness and elevated serum creatinine phosphokinase	Present	Absent
Clinical setting	Crush injuries, trauma, infection, rhabdomyolysis	Transfusion, disseminated intravascular coagulation

    b. Activity. No restriction of activity is required.

    c. Infection. Early and vigorous treatment of **bacterial** infection is important, since it can lead to relapses and was the leading cause of death prior to the advent of antibiotics.

    d. Instruction of family. Parents and child should be well informed about nephrosis and should be taught to test urine for albumin with dipsticks. A written diary of urine protein should be kept.

E. Prognosis

    1. In the usual type of minimal change nephrotic syndrome, 90–95% of children show an initial response to corticosteroids. Of these 85% will have further relapses.

    2. The rate of relapse in a group of children tends to decrease after the first 10 years. If a child remains free of a relapse for up to 3–4 years, there is a 95% chance he or she will remain free of relapses thereafter. However, after one relapse, the subsequent course cannot be predicted, and the number of relapses per se does not affect the ultimate outcome.

VII. Hematuria. Hematuria is defined as the presence of more than five red blood cells per high-power microscopic field on at least two properly performed urinalyses. Red urine and urine dipstick test results have a high false-positive rate. Thus, red urine, or a positive urine dipstick test, or both, mandate microscopic examination of the urine. The absence of red cells on microscopic examination suggests free hemoglobinuria or myoglobinuria (Table 8-6). Both pigments, hemoglobin and myoglobin, may be nephrotoxic, and full evaluation, with attempts at forced diuresis and urine alkalinization, should proceed.

A. Evaluation. Normal children excrete 200,000–500,000 red blood cells every 24 hr through the urinary system. High fever and vigorous exercise cause a transient, benign increase in red cell excretion rate. Based on average urinary volumes, it is abnormal to see more than a few red blood cells per high-power microscopic field on routine urinalysis.

The first step in evaluation is a complete history, physical examination, and baseline laboratory profile.

    1. History. Any possible precipitating event is noted.

        a. Particular attention is focused on symptoms of **cystitis** or renal colic.

        b. The **past medical history** focuses on any previous hemorrhagic tendencies and details of any drug or travel history.

        c. Any **family history** of tuberculosis, renal failure, or deafness is delineated.

        d. A **review of systems** includes recent rashes, arthralgias, arthritis, and abdominal pain and notes fevers, malaise, anorexia, weight loss, exercise pattern, and trauma.

2. A thorough **physical examination** is performed, with careful attention to height, weight, blood pressure, rashes, and edema. Anomalous features on abdominal or perineal examination are noted.

3. **Baseline laboratory profile.** Basic laboratory tests include a complete blood count, erythrocyte sedimentation rate, platelet count, prothrombin time, partial thromboplastin time, urinalysis with complete microscopic examination, urine culture, and a PPD skin test for tuberculosis.

B. **Differential diagnosis** (Fig. 8-5). The baseline investigations may provide the diagnosis **without further evaluation.** If not, all other causes of hematuria may be separated into the following distinct categories: symptomatic hematuria; hematuria associated with serious underlying systemic disease; asymptomatic hematuria; and complicated hematuria with significant proteinuria. Table 8-7 shows ways of distinguishing renal from nonrenal hematuria.

1. **Etiology suggested by baseline evaluation**
   a. Multiple telangiectasias and characteristic mucous membrane lesions indicate **hereditary hemorrhagic telangiectasia** (Rendu-Osler-Weber disease).
   b. An abdominal mass with hematuria requires exclusion of **Wilms' tumor** or **hydronephrosis.**
   c. Perineal excoriation or meatal inflammation implicates **local factors.**
   d. Hematuria occurs in association with sickle cell trait and S-C hemoglobin.
   e. A family history of asymptomatic hematuria suggests **benign familial hematuria,** while a family history of hematuria, deafness, and renal insufficiency suggests **Alport's hereditary nephritis.**

2. **Symptomatic hematuria**
   a. A clinical picture of **cystitis** accompanied by hematuria, mild proteinuria (trace to 1 + unless hematuria is gross), and leukocyturia is diagnostic of bacterial, viral, or traumatic involvement of the bladder or lower urinary tract. A **Gram stain** of the unspun urine and culture are done. When bacterial infection is documented, an **IVP** and **voiding cystourethrogram** are performed 4–6 weeks following successful antimicrobial therapy (see Chap. 15, pp. 396ff.).
   b. Culture-negative cystitis may be secondary to **viral infection.** Adenoviruses 11 and 21, influenza virus, and a papovalike virus have been implicated. Viral cystitis with resolution of hematuria and normal findings on urinalysis at follow-up requires no further investigation.
   c. Culture-negative cystitis may also be caused by **tuberculosis** and **schistosomiasis** and should be suspected in appropriate clinical and endemic settings.
   d. In addition to **gonococcal** or **nongonococcal urethritis,** vigorous masturbation and mechanical trauma to the urethra may also cause symptomatic hematuria with urethritis.
   e. In younger children with apparent cystitis, particularly in girls ages 2–6, urethral or vaginal foreign bodies may be present.
   f. Hematuria accompanied by moderate to severe abdominal pain is characteristic of **nephrolithiasis.** True renal colic is rare in the pediatric age group.
   g. Microscopic hematuria following abdominal or flank trauma is common and often benign. However, following gross hematuria, when persistent, or with hematuria following seemingly minor trauma, an IVP should be obtained to determine the extent of renal damage as well as structural abnormalities that might cause bleeding with minor trauma.

3. **Hematuria in systemic disease** (see Fig. 8-4). Attention should be focused on the evaluation and therapy of the **primary disorder.** The hematuria requires no further evaluation per se.
   a. Hematuria occurs with casts and protein in the critically ill child with catastrophic vascular diseases such as acute tubular necrosis, renal infarction, renal cortical necrosis, and renal vein thrombosis.

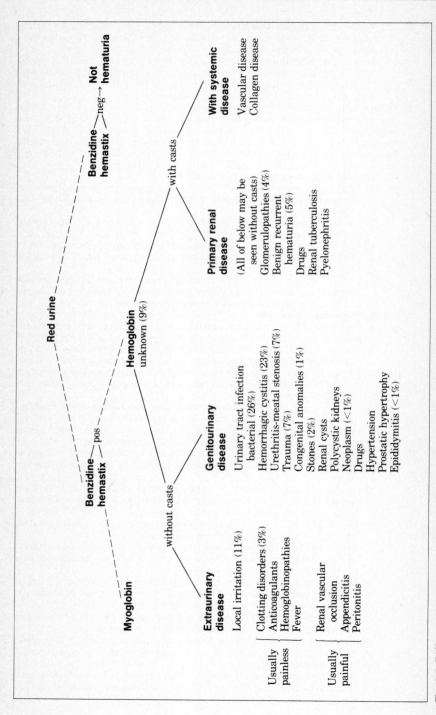

Fig. 8-5. Differential diagnosis of red urine. The percentages indicate the frequency of the category in an unselected population of pediatric patients.

Table 8-7. Distinguishing renal from nonrenal hematuria

Finding	Renal	Nonrenal
Urine color	Brown, smoky	Pink or red
Three-tube test	Same in each tube	Increased in 1 or 3
RBC casts	±	—
Clots	—	±
RBC morphology	Crenated	Fresh

    b. In subacute bacterial endocarditis and neurologic shunt infection, hematuria is immunologically mediated and represents focal areas of glomerulonephritis.

4. Asymptomatic hematuria

    a. Glomerulonephritis should be the first consideration in asymptomatic hematuria. Microscopic hematuria may be a manifestation of active subclinical disease or reflect a resolving, clinically apparent case. **Further evaluation** consists of

        (1) Antistreptolysin O (ASLO) titer and/or **anti-DNase B titer** in an attempt to document a group A β-hemolytic streptococcal infection.

        (2) Measurement of the **third component of complement,** which is depressed for 4–8 weeks in acute poststreptococcal glomerulonephritis and more persistently in most cases of membrano-proliferative glomerulonephritis.

    b. Family members should be screened with urinalyses to rule out benign **familial hematuria,** inherited as an autosomal dominant trait.

    c. Extraglomerular hematuria may be asymptomatic; anatomic lesions can be detected by an IVP. Hypercalciuria may be associated with microhematuria. Milk allergy may be associated with hematuria.

    d. Repeated episodes of gross hematuria with a normal IVP should be followed with a **voiding cystourethrogram** and cystoscopy.

    e. In a large group of patients, hematuria may persist without serologic or radiologic abnormalities. Such patients should be followed closely, with periodic examinations and urinalyses. During the follow-up period, the appearance of proteinuria, active urinary sediment with casts, deterioration in renal function, or development of hypertension suggests the need for renal biopsy.

    f. Asymptomatic microscopic hematuria that persists undiagnosed is regarded as **idiopathic.** Follow-up of such children has shown no deterioration in renal function. With careful longitudinal follow-up there is no indication for renal biopsy or invasive urologic investigations.

5. Complicated hematuria is asymptomatic hematuria in the presence of hypertension, active urinary sediment with casts, or proteinuria. All such patients should have the following laboratory studies: BUN and serum creatinine, ASLO titer, anti-DNase B titer, and serum complement level.

    a. Acute poststreptococcal glomerulonephritis (see sec. **VIII**) is easily recognized.

    b. Hypocomplementemia that persists suggests membranoproliferative glomerulonephritis or systemic lupus erythematosus (SLE) nephritis.

    c. Similarly, acute anaphylactoid purpura should be clearly apparent. Biopsy is reserved for atypical cases.

    d. When glomerulonephritis is present, an antinuclear antibody (ANA) test should be performed to delineate the subgroup with SLE nephritis. Renal biopsy is usually indicated to identify the histopathologic lesion and provide prognostic information.

(1) **IgG-IgA mesangial nephropathy (Berger's disease)** is characterized by recurrent episodes of macroscopic hematuria associated with respiratory illnesses on a background of persistent microscopic hematuria and proteinuria.

(2) **Focal sclerosing glomerulonephritis, membranoproliferative glomerulonephritis,** and **mesangial proliferative glomerulonephritis** are all chronic renal diseases. They are characterized by occasional clinical remissions, but generally progress to varying degrees of chronic renal failure.

VIII. Acute postinfectious glomerulonephritis

A. **Etiology.** A nephritogenic strain of group A β-hemolytic streptococci is the most common preceding infection. Other agents include influenza A, coxsackievirus B4, echovirus type 9, mumps, Epstein-Barr virus, and bacterial infections due to staphylococcal species (in infected shunts) and pneumococcus.

B. **Evaluation.** Edema, initially periorbital, hematuria, and hypertension are usually present, either singly or in combination. Some children present with abdominal pain, and hypoalbuminemia and hyperlipemia may occasionally be seen early in the course of the disease. Hypertension, hypertensive encephalopathy, and congestive heart failure are the common complications and should be sought in the initial evaluation.

C. The **diagnosis** is suggested by the finding of urine sediment containing red cell casts and protein, elevated BUN and creatinine, decreased C3, and evidence of preceding streptococcal infection. (The ASLO level may not rise if the initial infection is treated early with appropriate antibiotics.) A search for other agents should be undertaken if suggested by the clinical history.

D. **Treatment** is entirely symptomatic.

1. Appropriate antibiotics are given to eradicate the streptococcal infection (see Table 15-2).

2. A 1–2 gm salt diet is prescribed until the patient is asymptomatic, when a normal diet is resumed. There is no need for protein restriction in the usual case.

3. Bed rest is maintained until there is clinical improvement. Normal activity is resumed within a few weeks in most instances.

4. **Hypertension.** See sec. **III.**

E. **Prognosis.** The usual course ends in complete recovery. Up to 5% of patients who appear clinically to have acute poststreptococcal glomerulonephritis may have a continuously downhill course and progress to renal insufficiency. Renal biopsy in such patients usually reveals evidence of preexisting underlying chronic glomerular disease. The urine sediment may remain abnormal for a prolonged period; the proteinuria often clears up before the hematuria, which can persist for up to 2–3 years following the illness. However, even these patients make a complete recovery.

IX. Hemolytic uremic syndrome (HUS).
The triad of acute nephropathy, hemolytic anemia with fragmented red cells, and thrombocytopenia constitutes one of the most common syndromes of acute renal failure seen in childhood. It is endemic in Argentina, California, South Africa, and the Netherlands. It is often preceded by gastroenteritis or upper respiratory tract infection (URI).

A. **Etiology.** No discrete causes are known for the syndrome. Familial clustering has suggested that genetic predisposition is important.

B. **Evaluation.** Evaluate as for acute renal failure.

1. Do a CBC with a smear in any patient with acute renal failure.

2. Suspect HUS if preceding viral gastroenteritis or URI is found in a patient with renal failure or if marked pallor is present.

3. Separate into mild or severe categories, as follows:

a. **Mild.** No single 24-hr period of anuria. The patient may have oliguria, hypertension, or convulsions but not all.

b. **Severe.** Anuria or oliguria plus hypertension or convulsions is present.

C. **Diagnosis**

1. There is a history of prodromal illness.

2. Microangiopathic hemolytic anemia is found, including a low hematocrit, burr cells, helmet cells on smear, low platelets, and consumption coagulopathy.

D. Treatment is as for acute renal failure. In addition, note the following:

1. Early dialysis may be lifesaving.
2. Transfuse with only frozen glycerolated white cell-poor blood, since these patients may be renal transplant candidates in the future.
3. Control hypertension (see sec. **III.A**).
4. Do not use heparin or streptokinase, since studies to date indicate no benefit from either.
5. Antiplatelet agents are probably not indicated.

E. Prognosis. Mildly affected patients tend to do well, with little or no long-term proteinuria, hypertension, or azotemia. At least 20% of those with severe HUS will have long term sequelae, such as hypertension, proteinuria, and/or progressive renal insufficiency.

X. Wilms' tumor (nephroblastoma). Wilms' tumor accounts for a third of malignant intraabdominal tumors. The average age of presentation is 2 years. Most present as an abdominal mass. A fibroblastic cell or smooth muscle cell is the predominant tumor cell type. Some of the tumors are believed benign and are labeled *fetal renal hamartomas* or *congenital mesoblastic nephromas*.

A. The **etiology** is unknown, but its incidence is increased in congenital hemihypertrophy and in aniridia.

B. Evaluation. Proceed by evaluating abdominal mass (80–90% of patients present this way). (Other presentations include pain, fever, nausea, or anorexia. Hypertension may be present.) Radiologic studies should include the following:

1. Scout film and IVP. Abdominal ultrasound may be indicated to differentiate the lesion from cystic lesions (multicystic kidney) and hydronephrosis. An inferior venacavagram may aid in determining caval extension.
2. A liver scan (to search for hepatic metastases), a bone survey, and a chest x-ray. Radionuclide bone scans are superior to skeletal surveys for finding small lesions. Chest CT scan will find pulmonary metastases more sensitively than chest x-ray.

C. Treatment

1. Presurgical treatment with x-ray and chemotherapy may be indicated for a large or bilateral tumor.
2. Surgically remove and stage the tumor.
   a. **Stage I.** Limited to the kidney. Resect completely.
   b. **Stage II.** Local extension beyond the kidney or to local lymph nodes. Completely resect.
   c. **Stage III.** Residual gross or microscopic tumor in the abdomen after surgery or spill of tumor during surgery.
   d. **Stage IV.** Hematogenic metastases are present.
   e. **Stage V.** Bilateral renal involvement.
3. **Chemotherapy** (actinomycin D and vincristine)
   a. **Stage I.** Under 1 year
   b. **Stage II, III, IV, V**
4. Irradiation postoperatively for stages II–V
5. A bilateral complete nephrectomy is performed if there is continued disease in stage V.

D. Prognosis. The outlook has improved over the past decade. Nearly 90% of children under age 2 with stage I disease are free of signs of tumor 2 years later. Long-term survivors may have problems with hypertension, proteinuria, and/or interstitial nephritis.

XI. Neuroblastoma. This tumor is a common malignant neoplasm of infancy and childhood.

A. Etiology. Neuroblastoma arises from immature and undifferentiated neuroblasts from neural crest. It may be found wherever sympathetic nervous tissue is found, often in the adrenals. The kidneys may be displaced by tumor.

B. Diagnosis. The differential diagnosis of abdominal neuroblastoma includes

Wilms' tumor, cystic kidneys, and hydronephrosis. With bony symptoms, Ewing's tumor, lymphoma, sarcoma, or leukemic infiltrate of bone may be included in the differential diagnosis. CNS symptoms may be present.

C. Evaluation. Evaluate as for Wilms' tumor if an abdominal mass is present (see sec. **X.B**). Additionally,

1. A brain scan may be important in delineating the extent of the disease.
2. Cerebral and thoracic CT scans may be helpful.
3. Angiography may be indicated.
4. Measure urinary and plasma catecholamines and urinary cystathionine. All may be elevated.

D. Treatment. Surgery, chemotherapy, and irradiation are used in therapy.

1. Oncologic consultation is imperative.
2. Staging is helpful.
   a. **Stage I.** The tumor is confined to the organ or structure of the origin.
   b. **Stage II.** Local extension of ipsolateral nodes—no crossing midline
   c. **Stage III.** Extends past midline; lymph nodes may be involved bilaterally.
   d. **Stage IV.** Remote disease involvement: skeleton, parenchymatous organs, soft tissue, and/or distant nodes
   e. **Stage IV-S.** Patients whose tumors would be stage I or II but for remote disease confined to the liver, spleen, or bone marrow

E. The **prognosis** is best in stages I, II, and IV-S. Under 1 year of age the 2-year survival rate in these stages is 90% or better.

XII. Uric acid nephropathy

A. Etiology. Uric acid nephropathy may be seen in the following:

1. **Malignancies,** due to increased purine synthesis, as in leukemia and lymphomas. Especially seen with massive cytoreductive therapy.
2. **Regional enteritis,** due to increased intestinal absorption of uric acid.
3. **Gout.** This is unlikely to cause clinical problems and/or acute renal failure in childhood.

B. Evaluation

1. Determine **uric acid levels** in all children with malignancies, especially prior to and during cytoreductive therapy. Measure uric acid levels in patients with regional enteritis.
2. Measure **renal function** in all at-risk patients. If acute renal failure is developing, evaluate as in sec. **I.**

C. Therapy. The prevention of renal failure is the most important aspect of therapy.

1. Place children about to undergo massive cytoreductive therapy on **Allopurinol,** 4 mg/kg/day in 2 divided doses.
2. **Force fluids,** to 2–3 times maintenance.
3. **Alkalinize the urine,** so that its pH is above 6.5. Do this with sodium bicarbonate, starting at 1–2 mEq/kg/day, given IV, and increase as needed. (Uric acid is more soluble in alkaline urine.)
4. If oliguria or anuria develops, **hemodialysis** is indicated **early,** to remove uric acid and save the patient.

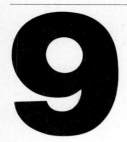

Cardiac Disorders

For a guide to management of cardiac disease in the newborn, see Chap. 6.

I. Cardiac arrhythmias

A. General considerations

1. Cardiac arrhythmias are caused by abnormalities of either automaticity or conduction. The specific characteristics of rhythm disturbances and their responses to therapeutic agents depend on the site of cardiac involvement and the underlying etiology.
2. Arrhythmias in the absence of underlying heart disease are usually benign. Care should be exercised lest the therapy that is undertaken become more of a hazard than the underlying arrhythmia.
3. Arrhythmias may be the manifestation of serious cardiac or metabolic disorders, as follows:
   a. Congenital or acquired heart disease
   b. Procedures such as cardiac catheterization, surgery, or general anesthesia
   c. Hypothermia
   d. Electrolyte disturbances, including sodium, potassium, calcium, and magnesium imbalances
   e. Systemic disorders of the musculoskeletal, endocrine, pulmonary, hematopoietic, or neurologic systems; in association with inherited disorders of metabolism, collagen diseases, or infectious diseases
   f. Drug toxicity or poisoning
   g. Neoplasia

B. Evaluation. The accurate diagnosis of an arrhythmia is usually possible from a careful analysis of the surface ECG. Occasionally, noninvasive studies such as carotid sinus massage, exercise electrocardiography, or ambulatory tape (Holter) monitoring are useful. Electrophysiologic studies with intracardiac catheters may be necessary in difficult cases.

C. Antiarrhythmic agents. See Table 9-1.

1. **Digitalis**
   a. **General considerations**
      (1) Digitalis is the most important single drug for the treatment of congestive heart failure (CHF) and may also be particularly useful in the treatment of arrhythmias.
      (2) Doses required for the treatment of arrhythmias may be higher than those used for CHF.
      (3) Although many digitalis glycosides are available, digoxin is the drug of choice for infants and children.
      (4) Variability in absorption, metabolism, excretion, and intracellular electrolyte concentrations necessitates *titration of each patient's correct dose.*
      (5) **A relatively narrow gap exists between optimal therapeutic doses and toxicity. Care must be taken to make certain that the correct dose has been ordered and given. Avoidable deaths have occurred because of a misplaced decimal point.**

Table 9-1. Antiarrhythmic agents for infants and children

Drug	Usual dose and interval	Route	Adverse effects	Therapeutic plasma level
Lidocaine	Bolus: 1 mg/kg every 20–60 min Infusion: 10–50 µg/kg/min	IV IV	Hypotension, CNS disturbances	1.5–6.0 µg/ml
Propranolol	10–20 µg/kg over 10 min q6–8h 1–8 mg/kg/day given q6h	IV PO	Hypotension, CHF, heart block, bronchospasm	Not established
Quinidine sulfate	15–60 mg/kg/day given q6h in 4 doses	PO	GI symptoms, cinchonism, thrombocytopenic rashes, hypotension, heart block, tachyarrhythmias	2–7 µg/ml
Procainamide	15–60 mg/kg/day given q4–6h in 4–6 doses	PO	Lupuslike syndrome, CNS disturbances, GI symptoms, rash, hypotension, arrhythmias, blood dyscrasias	4–10 µg/ml
Phenytoin	3–5 mg/kg over 5 min 3–8 mg/kg/day in 2–3 divided doses	IV PO	Ataxia, nystagmus, drowsiness, coma, blood dyscrasias, cardiac toxicity with rapid IV injection	5–20 µg/ml
Verapamil	*0–1 year:* 0.1 mg/kg over 2 min. May repeat dose 0.1–0.2 mg/kg in 30 min *1–15 years:* 0.1–0.3 mg/kg (maximum 5 mg) IV over 2 min. May repeat dose (maximum 10 mg) in 30 min	IV	Hypotension, severe tachycardia, atrial flutter or fibrillation, bradycardia, heart block, asystole, CHF, CNS effects	Not established

b. Indications include:
   (1) Control of ventricular rate in atrial fibrillation or atrial flutter
   (2) Supraventricular tachycardia
   (3) Ventricular premature contractions (occasionally effective)
c. Mechanisms of action
   (1) Inotropic effects. Digitalis appears to interfere with adenosine tri-phosphatase (ATPase) in the myocardial cell. The accumulation of sodium at the inner surface of the cell membrane allows for increased influx of calcium into the myofilament, thus potentiating myocardial contractility.
   (2) Antiarrhythmic effects. The cholinergic effects of digitalis *slow* the sinus rate, *prolong* the atrioventricular (AV) node refractory period, and *slow* AV conduction. Additionally, digitalis results in *hyper-polarization* of atrial conducting cells and decreases the slope of phase 4 depolarization, thus slowing or suppressing atrial ectopic impulse formation.
   (3) ECG changes. Digitalis prolongs the P–R interval, shortens the Q–T interval, and depresses the S–T segment.
d. Route of administration, absorption, and metabolism
   (1) Digoxin can be given PO, IM, or IV.
   (2) Orally, approximately 70–90% of the drug is absorbed, with peak levels within 1–3 hr.
   (3) The half-life is about 36 hr. Thus about one-third of the drug is excreted daily, and a steady state will be achieved when this amount is replaced.
   (4) Approximately 25% of the drug is bound to protein.
   (5) Digoxin is excreted primarily by the kidney.
e. Dosage
   (1) Before administration, a baseline ECG, electrolyte determinations (especially serum potassium), and some estimation of renal function are required.
   (2) The therapeutic plasma concentration is 1.0–2.4 ng/ml. However, individual variations in response can occur. Children with inflammatory disease of the myocardium may have enhanced sensitivity.
   (3) To avoid errors dosages should be calculated carefully and written in, for example, milligrams and milliliters.
   (4) Digoxin is usually administered in two stages: initial digitalization establishes the body stores; thereafter, one-fourth to one-third the total digitalizing dose (TDD) is given daily (usually in 2 divided doses 12 hr apart) to replace losses.
      (a) Variation of TDD with age
         (i) Prematures. 0.035 mg/kg PO over 24 hr. Usually, one-half the TDD is given, followed by one-fourth q12h twice.
         (ii) Newborn. 0.05 mg/kg
         (iii) Under 2 years. 0.05–0.07 mg/kg PO
         (iv) Over 2 years. 0.03–0.05 mg/kg PO. Parenteral doses should be about 75% of the oral dose.
      (b) Maintenance digoxin should be 25–33% of the TDD. In children with renal disease, maintenance should be calculated by using the following equation to determine the percentage of digoxin excreted per day.

$$\frac{14 \ + \ (\text{creatinine clearance})}{5} = \% \text{ digoxin excreted/day}$$

f. Toxicity
   (1) Cardiovascular. Virtually any arrhythmia may be a manifestation of digitalis toxicity. However, in children, supraventricular arrhythmias

predominate, while in adolescents and adults, ventricular arrhythmias are more common. The vagal actions may result in sinus node depression and AV conduction disturbances.

(2) **GI.** Complaints such as anorexia, nausea, vomiting, diarrhea, and abdominal pain are common.

(3) **Neurologic.** Fatigue, muscle weakness, and psychic disturbances are occasionally seen.

(4) **Visual.** Hazy vision, perceptual color (red and green), photophobia, and diplopia are occasionally seen in adults but are rare in children.

(5) **Treatment**

(a) Stop the drug.

(b) Check electrolytes. The administration of potassium may correct digitalis-induced arrhythmias, **but is contraindicated in the presence of AV block.**

(c) Lidocaine, phenytoin, and propranolol have been used for digitalis-induced arrhythmias.

(d) A temporary pacemaker may be necessary for high-grade AV block.

(e) If available, purified digoxin-specific "Fab" antibody fragments should be used for the treatment of advanced, life-threatening digitalis toxicity unresponsive to conventional therapy.

(f) Cardioversion should be used only as a last resort, since it may exacerbate rather than help and occasionally induces ventricular fibrillation.

g. **Drug interactions.** Concomitant administration of quinidine and digoxin can result in increased serum digoxin levels. When these drugs are used concurrently, digoxin dosage should be reduced, the patient observed for digitalis toxicity, and serum digoxin level monitored.

2. **Lidocaine**

a. **Indications.** Lidocaine is the drug of choice for emergency treatment of ventricular premature contractions (VPCs) or ventricular tachycardia. It is less effective against atrial or junctional arrhythmias. **It should not be used in the presence of complete heart block.**

b. **Mechanism of action.** Lidocaine depresses the automaticity of the heart and slows conduction. It shortens the Q–T interval on the surface ECG.

c. **Route of administration, absorption, and metabolism**

(1) Lidocaine should **not** be given PO, since the liver eliminates most of the drug before it reaches the systemic circulation.

(2) When it is given as an IV bolus, effective blood levels can be achieved in 5 min and last up to 2 hr, with a peak concentration at 30 min.

(3) Since lidocaine is almost entirely metabolized in the liver, patients with reduced hepatic function or diminished blood flow, as in heart failure or after cardiac surgery, should receive half the usual loading dose and should also be maintained at lower levels of IV lidocaine.

d. **Dosage**

(1) As a bolus, give 1.0 mg/kg IV; this may be repeated in 20–60 min.

(2) As a constant infusion, the dosage is 10–50 µg/kg/min.

(3) The therapeutic plasma concentration is 1.5–6.0 µg/ml.

e. **Toxicity**

(1) Lidocaine is the least cardiotoxic of the commonly used antiarrhythmic agents. However, at very high levels, hypotension and cardiovascular collapse can occur.

(2) At serum levels over 5 µg/ml, CNS disturbances such as drowsiness, lethargy, paresthesias, slurred speech, and diplopia can occur. At over 9 µg/ml, convulsions and coma have been reported.

(3) Discontinuation of the drug is the usual treatment for toxicity.

f. Drug interactions. A *prolonged* half-life occurs with propranolol, chloramphenicol, isoniazid, and norepinephrine. A *shortened* half-life occurs with isoproterenol and phenobarbital.

3. Propranolol is effective against a wide variety of atrial and ventricular arrhythmias.

a. Indications

(1) It may convert supraventricular tachycardia to sinus rhythm.

(2) It is used for prevention of supraventricular tachycardia.

(3) It reduces the ventricular response to atrial fibrillation and atrial flutter.

(4) It may be helpful in controlling ventricular arrhythmias, especially when used concurrently with other antiarrhythmic agents.

b. Mechanism of action. Propranolol is a beta-adrenergic blocking agent and works by reducing adrenergic tone and by depressing impulse formation and membrane responsiveness in the myocardial cell.

c. Route of administration, absorption, and metabolism

(1) Propranolol may be given PO or IV.

(2) Oral administration is accompanied by variable GI absorption, with a maximal blood level within 1–2 hr and a half-life of 2.5 hr.

(3) Plasma levels of 50–100 ng/ml are usually associated with blockade of beta-adrenergic receptors, but the therapeutic range for treatment of ventricular arrhythmias has not been determined.

(4) With IV administration the onset of action is within 2–5 min.

(5) Most of the drug is protein bound and is metabolized in the liver.

(6) The half-life of propranolol is prolonged in the presence of liver disease.

d. Dosage.

(1) The *oral* dosage is 1–8 mg/kg/day in 4 divided doses.

(2) The *IV* dose is 10–20 μg/kg over 10 min.

e. Toxicity

(1) Propranolol may cause hypotension and exacerbate CHF in patients with compromised cardiac status who depend on high circulating levels of catecholamines to maintain cardiac contractility. Sinus bradycardia with resting rates below 50 are not uncommon, and heart block may occasionally be seen.

(2) Other signs of toxicity include GI symptoms (nausea, diarrhea, cramps), bronchospasm, and hypoglycemia.

(3) Propranolol is contraindicated in patients with asthma.

(4) Treatment includes stopping the drug. Bradycardia can be treated with atropine, and hypotension with large doses of isoproterenol, a beta agonist.

f. Drug interactions. Negative inotropic or chronotopic effects may be accentuated by other antiarrhythmic or anesthetic agents.

4. Quinidine is effective against a variety of atrial and ventricular arrhythmias.

a. Indications include

(1) Treatment of repetitive atrial arrhythmias and VPCs

(2) Conversion of atrial fibrillation or flutter to sinus rhythm

(3) Preventing the recurrence of atrial fibrillation or flutter

b. Mechanism of action. Quinidine depresses automaticity and the refractory period in the cardiac cell and slows conduction. On the surface ECG these effects are manifested by lengthening of the P–R, QRS, and Q–T intervals.

c. Route of administration, absorption, and metabolism

(1) Oral absorption of quinidine sulfate is almost complete, with a peak plasma level in less than 2 hr and a half-life of approximately 6 hr.

(2) Approximately 80% of quinidine is bound to plasma protein.

(3) It is metabolized in the liver and excreted by the kidneys. Thus, blood levels are dependent on the integrity of both these systems. Patients who are in cardiac failure may require lower doses.

d. Dosage

 (1) The **dosage** of quinidine sulfate is 15–60 mg/kg PO in 4 divided doses.

 (2) The therapeutic plasma concentration is 2–7 μg/ml.

e. Toxicity is additive with procainamide or disopyramide.

 (1) Cardiovascular

  (a) Quinidine is a myocardial depressant, and its negative inotropic effect and weak alpha-blocking properties may produce *severe hypotension* or *exacerbate CHF*.

  (b) By altering phase 4 depolarization, serious *arrhythmias,* such as ventricular tachycardia and ventricular fibrillation, may be induced.

  (c) ECG changes associated with quinidine toxicity include an increase in the QRS duration of more than 50% and an increase in the Q–T interval of more than 0.10 sec.

  (d) Rarely, *syncope* and *sudden death* have been associated with quinidine use.

  (e) Quinidine may increase the ventricular response to atrial flutter or fibrillation; thus, concurrent digoxin or propranolol administration is usually recommended for treatment of these arrhythmias.

  (f) Arrhythmias and/or conduction disturbances caused by quinidine toxicity may be treated with sodium bicarbonate or molar sodium lactate.

 (2) GI toxicity is common, with diarrhea the usual manifestation. When symptoms are mild, the drug may be continued and symptomatic therapy used.

 (3) Cinchonism (blurred vision, tinnitus, altered color perception) may occur.

 (4) Other toxic manifestations include thrombocytopenia, hepatitis, hemolytic anemia, proteinuria, allergic reactions including anaphylaxis, and CNS symptoms, such as headaches, confusion, delirium, and psychosis.

 (5) Treatment is symptomatic after stopping the drug.

f. Drug interactions

 (1) The half-life is *reduced* by phenobarbital and phenytoin.

 (2) Quinidine *potentiates* the effects of coumarin and of the neuromuscular blocking action of anesthetic agents or antibiotics.

 (3) Digitalis levels are *increased* by concurrent administration of quinidine.

5. Procainamide is effective against the same arrhythmias and has the same mechanism of action as quinidine, but its metabolism and toxicity differ.

a. Indications. Although it is effective against the same arrhythmias as quinidine, procainamide is primarily used for *ventricular ectopy.*

b. Route of administration, absorption, and metabolism

 (1) The most common route is PO, although IV administration has been used in adults.

 (2) When it is given PO, 75–95% is absorbed, with peak levels appearing about 60 min later. The half-life is 3–4 hr.

 (3) Metabolism is primarily in the liver, with approximately half being excreted unchanged by the kidney.

 (4) Patients with diminished renal function should be treated with reduced dosages of procainamide and followed closely to detect QRS prolongation.

c. Dosage

 (1) The **dosage** is 15–60 mg/kg/day on a q4h schedule.

 (2) The therapeutic serum level is 4–10 μg/ml.

d. Toxicity is additive with quinidine or disopyramide.
- **(1)** The **cardiovascular effects** are the same as those for quinidine, but are less pronounced.
- **(2)** A **lupuslike syndrome** has been described in adults. Antinuclear antibodies (ANA) develop in more than 75% of adults after 3–6 months of procainamide therapy, but usually disappear when therapy is discontinued.
- **(3)** Thrombocytopenia, Coombs-positive hemolytic anemia, and GI symptoms occur occasionally.

6. Phenytoin (See also Chap. 20.)

a. Indications. Phenytoin is used primarily for the treatment of digitalis-induced arrhythmias, both ventricular and supraventricular. It is not very effective when used as a primary agent, although it may occasionally be useful in combination with other antiarrhythmic agents in controlling VPCs. Phenytoin may be especially effective for the treatment of VPCs in patients who have undergone correction of tetralogy of Fallot.

b. Mechanism of action. Some antiarrhythmic effects of phenytoin may be mediated, at least in part, by the CNS. It decreases automaticity in the specialized conducting system and also decreases the effective refractory period. ECG changes include shortening of the P–R and Q–T intervals.

c. Route of administration, absorption, and metabolism
- **(1)** When given PO, absorption is slow, with a maximal plasma level in 8–12 hr and a half-life of 15–24 hr. Without a loading dose, it takes 6–7 days to achieve a therapeutic plasma level.
- **(2)** The drug is metabolized in the liver and excreted into the GI tract. Resorption occurs, with only 5% excreted in the urine unchanged.
- **(3)** Its IV use should be reserved for emergencies and should be accompanied by constant ECG monitoring.
- **(4)** The therapeutic plasma level is 5–20 μg/ml.

d. The **dosage** is 3–8 mg/kg/day in 2–3 doses PO, or 3–5 mg/kg IV over 10 min (diluted in normal saline). Patients receiving phenytoin IV should have **ECG monitoring, frequent blood pressure measurements,** and observation for signs of **nystagmus.**

e. Toxicity
- **(1) Cardiovascular.** Mild hypotension, bradycardia, transient AV block, and ventricular fibrillation have been reported after IV use.
- **(2) CNS toxicity** includes ataxia, vertigo, drowsiness, confusion, respiratory depression, and even respiratory arrest.
- **(3) Other signs of toxicity** include hypersensitivity reactions such as leukopenia, thrombocytopenia, morbilliform rashes, and serum sickness.
- **(4) Gingival hyperplasia, megaloblastic anemia,** and **GI upset** occur occasionally.

f. Drug interactions
- **(1) Increased metabolism** is caused by concurrent administration of drugs that induce hepatic enzymes.
- **(2) Decreased metabolism** may result from concurrent administration of glucocorticoids, Coumadin, chloramphenicol, isoniazid, insulin, amphetamines, and phenylbutazone.
- **(3)** It increases the metabolism of **Coumadin.**
- **(4)** It increases the hepatic toxicity of **halothane.**

7. Verapamil

a. Indications include:
- **(1)** Conversion of paroxysmal supraventricular tachycardias to sinus rhythm, including those associated with accessory bypass tracts (e.g., Wolff-Parkinson-White syndrome)
- **(2)** Control of rapid ventricular rate in atrial flutter or atrial fibrillation

b. Its mechanism of action involves inhibition of the calcium ion influx through slow channels into conductile and contractile myocardial cells and vascular smooth muscle cells. By inhibiting calcium influx, verapamil slows AV conduction and prolongs the effective refractory period within the AV node.

c. Route of administration, absorption, and metabolism

(1) Verapamil is currently approved only for IV use.

(2) Following IV administration, verapamil is eliminated biexponentially, with a rapid early distribution phase (half-life 4 min) and a slower terminal elimination phase (half-life 2–5 hr).

(3) Approximately 70% of an administered dose is excreted in the urine, and 16% or more in the feces within 5 days. Approximately 3–4% is excreted as unchanged drug.

d. Dosage. The initial use of IV verapamil should be in a setting with monitoring and resuscitation facilities.

(1) 0–1 year. The initial dose is 0.1 mg/kg IV over 2 min under continuous ECG monitoring. The repeat dose is 0.1–0.2 mg/kg 30 min after the first dose if the initial response is not adequate.

(2) 1–15 years. The initial dose is 0.1 mg/kg (maximum dose 5 mg) IV over 2 min. Repeat the dose (0.1–0.3 mg/kg; maximum dose 10 mg) 30 min after the first dose if the initial response is inadequate.

e. Toxicity

(1) Hypotension is usually transient, but occasionally requires supportive therapy (IV fluids, Trendelenberg position) or IV drug therapy (see Chap. 3).

(2) Rapid ventricular response in atrial flutter or fibrillation occurs in approximately 1% of patients and may require cardioversion.

(3) Extreme bradycardia, heart block, or **asystole** may result from slowed conduction across the AV node. This is usually of brief duration, except in patients with sick sinus syndrome. Effective treatments include IV isoproterenol, IV levarterenol, IV atropine, and cardiac pacing (see Chap. 3).

(4) Worsening of heart failure may be seen in patients with moderately severe to severe cardiac dysfunction.

(5) Contraindications to the use of verapamil include severe hypotension; second- or third-degree heart block; sick sinus syndrome (except in patients with a ventricular pacemaker); severe CHF (unless secondary to SVT); wide-complex supraventricular tachycardia and concurrent IV administration of beta-adrenergic blocking drugs. Verapamil should be used with caution in neonates.

f. Drug interactions

(1) Concurrent use of IV beta-adrenergic agents or disopyramide with verapamil may exacerbate depressed myocardial contractility or AV conduction.

(2) Since verapamil is highly bound to plasma proteins, it should be administered with caution to patients receiving other highly protein-bound drugs.

D. Cardioversion is the use of a synchronized direct-current shock applied to the heart to convert certain arrhythmias to normal sinus rhythm.

1. Indications

a. Atrial fibrillation. Immediate cardioversion is indicated if atrial fibrillation is of short duration, if a rapid ventricular rate cannot be controlled, or if hemodynamic compromise exists. When cardioversion is elective, patients should receive anticoagulant therapy with a coumarin derivative for a period of 3 weeks *prior to* cardioversion. Cardioversion may be unsuccessful in restoring normal sinus rhythm in patients with an enlarged left atrium (e.g., mitral stenosis).

b. Atrial flutter converts easily to atrial fibrillation or sinus rhythm, often at low energy levels (0.5 watt-sec/kg). For this condition, cardioversion should be performed as an emergency procedure only in hemodynamically compromised patients; otherwise, cardioversion can be performed electively.

c. **Supraventricular tachycardia (SVT)** is often relatively resistant to cardioversion; thus, vagotonic manuevers and medical therapy should be used initially unless hypotension or CHF is present. If digitalis intoxication is suspected, cardioversion should begin at low energy levels, increasing until either cardioversion or signs of digitalis toxicity occur. Prophylactic lidocaine is often given (see **C.2**).

d. **Ventricular tachycardia.** Cardioversion is the treatment of choice for sustained ventricular tachycardia. During preparation for cardioversion, a bolus of IV lidocaine (1–2 mg/kg) may be given. Cardioversion is usually accomplished at low energy levels (50–100 watt-sec in an adult). However, in hypotensive patients, higher initial energy levels (e.g., in an adult, first 200 watt-sec, then 400 watt-sec) should be delivered.

e. **Ventricular fibrillation.** Immediate cardioversion with an unsynchronized discharge at an energy level of 2 watt-sec/kg is required for ventricular fibrillation in children (see Chap. 3, p. 41).

2. **Contraindications** include sinus tachycardia, digitalis-induced arrhythmias, multifocal atrial tachycardia, complete AV block, and the supraventricular arrhythmias associated with hyperthyroidism. Patients with sick sinus syndrome should have a temporary pacing wire placed prior to cardioversion.

3. **Techniques.** One must be prepared for complications, and the procedure should only be done in an intensive care unit. Cardioversion should be performed at the *lowest possible energy level* to minimize complications.

a. Analgesia should be obtained with IV administration of a short-acting barbiturate such as methohexital (Brevital, 0.5–1.0 mg/kg as a bolus in a 1% solution) or diazepam (0.25 mg/kg IV). **Use of these drugs for elective cardioversion should only be done in an intensive care unit with an anesthesiologist in attendance. The child should be preoxygenated prior to the procedure.** When the patient's lid reflex is lost, cardioversion can be attempted.

b. The cardioverter should be synchronized on the R wave to avoid the atrial and ventricular vulnerable periods. For treating ventricular fibrillation, the synchronizing switch must be turned off.

c. The electrode paddles should be liberally covered with conductive paste and placed in the 2nd right intercostal space and the 5th left interspace in the anterior axillary line in older children and adults or in the 3rd space in the parasternal area and below the left scapula in younger children.

d. Postconversion arrhythmias are not uncommon and include atrial and ventricular premature beats and delayed function of the sinoatrial node, manifested by slow junctional rhythm or sinus bradycardia. Occasionally, these must be treated. Lidocaine (IV), atropine (IV), and isoproterenol (IV) should be drawn up in advance and accessible for rapid delivery if necessary.

4. **Required energy levels.** Optimal energy levels for cardioversion of **infants** have not been well studied. Most pediatric cardiologists use a range of energy levels in children from 0.5–2.0 watt-sec/kg (maximum), depending on the arrhythmia.

E. **Specific arrhythmias.** See Table 9-2.

1. **Sinus mechanisms**

a. **Sinus tachycardia** is a normal response to exercise, fever, or fright, but may be associated with anemia, myocarditis, shock, CHF, or thyrotoxicosis.

(1) **Diagnosis.** A normal P wave is present, and AV conduction is normal. Although the heart rate normally varies with age, tachycardia is present when the heart rate exceeds 170 in a neonate, 140 in an infant, or 100 in a child.

(2) **Treatment** consists of management of the underlying condition, if any. Propranolol may be useful for the tachycardia of hyperthyroidism while the underlying disease is being treated (see Chap. 11, p. 304).

244

Table 9.2. Treatment of cardiac arrhythmias

Arrhythmia	Treatment of choice[a]	Alternative[a]	Remarks
Atrial flutter	Cardioversion	Digoxin to control ventricular rate	Propranolol may help slow ventricular rate. Quinidine may be used to maintain sinus rhythm. Digoxin may have adverse effect in patients with Wolff-Parkinson-White syndrome
Atrial fibrillation	Cardioversion	Digoxin to control ventricular rate	Same as atrial flutter
Supraventricular tachycardia	Vagotonic maneuvers	Verapamil Digoxin Propranolol	Optimal therapy depends on patient's hemodynamic status Cardioversion may occasionally be necessary
Ventricular premature contractions	Lidocaine[b]	Procainamide	A variety of agents may be used for long-term suppression: quinidine, propranolol, procainamide, digoxin, or phenytoin
Ventricular tachycardia	Cardioversion	Lidocaine	Same as VPC
Ventricular fibrillation	Cardioversion	See text	Cardiopulmonary resuscitation mandatory
Digitalis-induced tachyarrhythmias	Phenytoin or lidocaine	Procainamide[c] Propranolol[c]	Avoid cardioversion

[a]Optimal treatment may vary with the clinical situation.
[b]Reduce dosage in heart failure.
[c]May worsen heart block.

   b. Sinus bradycardia is associated with increased vagal tone. It may be a
      normal finding in athletic children, but can also be a manifestation of
      hypothyroidism, hypothermia, hypopituitarism, typhoid fever, or hyper-
      kalemia.
      (1) Diagnosis. A normal P wave and normal AV conduction are present,
         with a heart rate less than 100 in neonates (see Chap. 6, p. 149), and
         less than 60 in children and adolescents.
      (2) Treatment is unnecessary unless there is evidence of a low cardiac
         output. Atropine, 0.01–0.02 mg/kg IV, will increase the rate by reduc-
         ing vagal tone.
   c. Sinus arrhythmia is a normal finding and is a manifestation of peripheral
      and central circulatory reflexes.
      (1) Diagnosis. The P waves are normal, as is AV conduction, with vary-
         ing P–P intervals. The heart rate usually increases during inspira-
         tion and slows down during expiration.
      (2) Treatment is not necessary.
2. **Supraventricular mechanisms**
   a. Premature atrial contractions (PACs) may be an incidental finding in
      infants or children without other evidence of heart disease. When repeti-
      tive in groups of two or three, they may be a precursor to atrial flutter or
      fibrillation.
      (1) Diagnosis. PACs are characterized by a premature P wave, usually of
         a different configuration than the sinus P wave, followed by a QRS
         that is similar or identical to the normal QRS.
      (2) Treatment is unnecessary.
   b. Escape beats are usually a protective mechanisms when a higher
      pacemaker slows for any reason. They are commonly seen with a marked
      sinus arrhythmia but may be seen occasionally with the sick sinus syn-
      drome.
      (1) Diagnosis. The QRS is usually of normal configuration. The P waves
         may be normal, with a short P–R interval (nonconducted), or absent.
         In sinus arrhythmia with nodal escape, the escape rhythm is usually
         phasic with respiration.
      (2) Treatment is unnecessary.
   c. Atrial flutter may occasionally be seen in newborns or infants without
      other evidence of heart disease. In older children it is often associated
      with rheumatic heart disease or other diseases causing atrial dilatation.
      (1) Diagnosis. There is a rapid, regular atrial rate of 250–350 beats/min,
         with P (flutter) waves having a sawtooth pattern in leads II, III, aVғ,
         and V1 (but usually not in I). Conduction to the ventricles may be 1:1,
         2:1, 3:1, or 4:1.
      (2) Treatment
         (a) Digoxin (see **C.1**) is useful in controlling the rate by increasing
            block at the AV node.
         (b) DC cardioversion at very low energy is almost always successful
            in converting atrial flutter to normal sinus rhythm (see **D.1.b**).
   d. Atrial fibrillation is usually associated with significant heart disease and
      atrial dilatation. It may also be seen with hyperthyroidism or the Wolff-
      Parkinson-White syndrome.
      (1) Diagnosis. Irregular "f" waves are present at a rate of 400–600/min
         with an irregular ventricular response. The QRS usually appears
         normal, but some aberrant beats may be present.
      (2) Treatment
         (a) Digitalis is effective in slowing the rate (see sec. **I.C**)
         (b) While quinidine has been used in children in the past to convert
            sinus rhythm, electrical conversion is now often used instead (see
            D). Patients with atrial fibrillation for more than a few days
            should be given anticoagulants for 3 weeks prior to cardioversion
            to decrease the risk of embolism.

(c) Long-standing atrial fibrillation is likely to recur.

e. **Paroxysmal SVT** may be idiopathic or occur in association with cardiac catheterization or surgery, Wolff-Parkinson-White syndrome, emotional stress, or nyperthyroidism.

(1) **Diagnosis.** The rhythm is regular, at a rate of 160–260 beats/min, with a normal or slightly widened QRS. P waves, if present, are usually of a different configuration than sinus P waves.

(2) **Treatment**

(a) Reflex stimulation of the vagus by a Valsalva maneuver, gagging, placement of ice on the forehead, or unilateral carotid sinus massage may occasionally be effective in converting the heart to normal sinus rhythm.

(b) Verapamil, digoxin, or propranolol is the drug of choice. Verapamil should be used with caution in neonates.

(c) Increasing vagal tone by increasing systemic blood pressure using alpha-adrenergic drugs such as phenylephrine (0.005–0.01 mg/kg IV) or directly with edrophonium (0.1–0.2 mg/kg/IV) has been effective in children.

(d) In desperately ill patients or those resistant to drug therapy, electrical cardioversion may be effective (see sec. **D**).

3. **Ventricular mechanisms**

a. Premature ventricular contractions (PVCs) are commonly found in children without other evidence of heart disease. They may also occur secondary to myocardial inflammation or ischemia, hyperkalemia, sympathomimetic drugs, digitalis toxicity, cardiac tumors, or mitral valve prolapse.

(1) **Diagnosis**

(a) There is usually a wide QRS with opposite polarity of the T wave and a full compensatory pause before the next QRS complex. A preceding P wave is not seen.

(b) Characteristically, benign PVCs are unifocal, unassociated with other evidence of heart disease, disappear with exercise, and have a fixed coupling interval.

(c) Significant PVCs are usually associated with heart disease, are multifocal with a variable coupling interval, and are accentuated by exercise. A prolonged resting Q–T interval may be present.

(d) Ambulatory testing, either with exercise stress or 24-hr tape recordings, may be useful in assessing the significance of the PVCs and in judging the efficacy of treatment.

(2) **Treatment**

(a) Most PVCs in patients without heart disease are benign and require no treatment.

(b) The best treatment of significant PVCs is to remove the cause if possible.

(c) For the acute problem, lidocaine, 1 mg/kg IV in a bolus, is the drug of choice. Dose may be repeated every 5 minutes for 3 doses for loading or may be followed by continuous infusion of 10–50 μg/kg/min.

(d) Chronic suppression may be accomplished with quinidine, procainamide, disopyramide, propranolol, digoxin, or phenytoin. Each may be used alone or in combination with other antiarrhythmic agents.

b. **Ventricular tachycardia** is usually associated with severe congenital or acquired heart disease.

(1) **Diagnosis**

(a) **Intermittent.** Runs of three or more consecutive ventricular ectopic beats

(b) **Sustained.** A wide QRS and a rate of 140–200 beats/min are present. There may be evidence of separate atrial activity, such as

AV dissociation and intermittent ventricular capture, or fusion beats. The configuration of the QRS is often similar to that in isolated PVCs observed before the tachycardia.

(2) Treatment

(a) Acute

(i) For the intermittent form, a bolus of lidocaine, 1.0 mg/kg IV, is usually effective.

(ii) For the sustained variety, a sharp blow to the anterior chest may be tried. If this fails, DC cardioversion (0.5–2 watt-sec/kg) should be attempted, with a bolus of lidocaine, 1 mg/kg IV, delivered during the time taken to prepare for cardioversion.

(b) Chronic. Treatment is the same as for PVCs. Some children without heart disease may have repetitive episodes of ventricular tachycardia without symptoms and with reversion to normal sinus rhythm with exercise. The necessity for treatment in such children is controversial.

c. Ventricular fibrillation

(1) Diagnosis. Ventricular fibrillation is characterized by low-amplitude, rapid irregular depolarizations with no identifiable normal electrical activity.

(2) Treatment

(a) Consists of immediate cardioversion (unsynchronized mode) at the maximum energy level (2 watt-sec/kg)

(b) Acidosis and hypoxemia should be corrected.

(c) If cardioversion fails or fibrillation recurs, lidocaine, 1 mg/kg, may be given as an IV bolus and a continuous infusion of 10–50 μg/kg/min begun to enhance the effectiveness of cardioversion. When there is no response, IV epinephrine or isoproterenol may promote subsequent successful defibrillation.

4. Heart block

a. First-degree heart block is associated with increased vagal tone, inflammatory disease affecting the conduction system, and congenital heart disease, especially atrial septal defects, endocardial cushion defects, and Ebstein's anomaly.

(1) Diagnosis. *First-degree heart block* is defined as a P–R interval longer than rate- and age-corrected normal. A P–R interval greater than 0.14 sec in an infant, greater than 0.18 in a child, or greater than 0.20 in an adult represents first-degree heart block.

(2) Treatment. None is necessary.

b. Second-degree heart block

(1) Diagnosis

(a) Mobitz type I (Wenckebach) block consists of regular P waves with progressive prolongation of the P–R interval. The R–R interval becomes progressively shorter until a QRS is dropped.

(b) In **Mobitz type II block,** a normal P–R interval and QRS are followed by a P wave with no QRS. The next P wave is conducted normally. The dropped beats can occur every second, third, or fourth beat.

(2) Treatment is unnecessary, but progression to third-degree block may occur.

c. Third-degree (complete) heart block may be congenital or may be acquired in children with an otherwise normal heart. It also may be associated with congenital heart disease (corrected transposition of the great vessels) or acquired heart diseases, such as rheumatic fever, cardiac tumors, or endocardial fibroelastosis. Acquired heart block following cardiac surgery now occurs less often than previously.

(1) Diagnosis. Complete AV dissociation with the ventricular rate slower than the atrial rate is diagnostic. A wide QRS suggests block below the bundle of His.

(2) Treatment

(a) The need for therapy is dependent on the ventricular rate, the presence or absence of symptoms, and the stability of the inherent pacemaker.

(b) Congenital or acquired heart block in children without associated heart disease usually needs no therapy unless syncope or unremitting heart failure is present.

(c) Block acquired after cardiac surgery should always be treated with a **pacemaker.**

(d) Transvenous **pacemakers** in older children, or epicardial pacemakers in young children or those with right-to-left shunts, constitute the treatment of choice when raising the heart rate is necessary.

(e) Atropine, 0.01–0.02 mg/kg IV, or isoproterenol, 0.1 µg/kg/min may be effective in increasing ventricular rate while awaiting insertion of a temporary or permanent pacemaker.

II. Congestive heart failure. Congestive heart failure (CHF) is a clinical syndrome in which the heart is unable to supply an output sufficient to meet the metabolic requirements of the tissues.

A. Etiology includes:

1. Congenital diseases of the heart, usually with large left-to-right shunts or obstructive lesions of the left or right ventricle.

2. Acquired diseases of the heart, including myocarditis, acute or chronic rheumatic heart disease, and infectious endocarditis.

3. Arrhythmias, including paroxysmal atrial tachycardia, atrial fibrillation or flutter, or complete heart block.

4. Iatrogenic causes, including damage to the heart at surgery (ventriculotomy), fluid overload, or doxorubicin (Adriamycin) therapy.

5. Noncardiac causes, such as thyrotoxicosis, systemic arteriovenous fistula, acute or chronic lung disease, glycogen storage disease, or connective tissue or neuromuscular disorders.

B. Clinical manifestations. The signs and symptoms of CHF fall into the following three categories:

1. Signs of impaired myocardial performance. These include growth failure, sweating, cardiac enlargement, gallop rhythm, and alterations in peripheral pulses, including pulsus paradoxus and pulsus alternans.

2. Signs of pulmonary congestion include tachypnea, dyspnea with effort, cough, rales, wheezing, and cyanosis.

3. Signs of systemic venous congestion include hepatomegaly, neck vein distension, and peripheral edema.

C. Treatment. Whenever possible, the precipitating causes (e.g., arrhythmia) and underlying causes (e.g., structural abnormalities) of CHF should be removed. Control of CHF may be achieved by (1) *increasing cardiac contractile performance,* (2) *reducing cardiac workload,* and (3) *reducing the volume overload* responsible for congestive symptoms.

1. Increasing cardiac contractile performance

a. Digitalis therapy increases cardiac output by directly enhancing the myocardial contractile state. The inotropic effect of digoxin increases linearly with increasing dose until toxicity is reached. The optimal dose should be dictated by the patient's response and must be individualized. Guidelines for digoxin use are detailed in sec. **I.C.1.**

b. Other cardiotonic agents. When CHF is associated with hypotension or is refractory to other modes of therapy, additional inotropic support may be achieved with the following:

(1) Dopamine. The usual therapeutic dose is 5–10 µg/kg/min by continuous IV infusion. Therapy is begun at a low dose (2 µg/kg/min) and gradually increased until the desired effect is achieved. At low doses (< 2 µg/kg/min), dopamine causes renal vasodilation. At higher doses (> 10 µg/kg/min), dopamine may have the undesirable effects of increasing total peripheral resistance and heart rate. Relatively high doses of dopamine (e.g., 15 μg/kg/min) are usually necessary to achieve effectiveness in neonates.

    (2) Isoproterenol. The usual therapeutic dose is 0.1 μg/kg/min, but should be titrated by the patient's response.

2. Reducing cardiac workload

  a. General measures

    (1) Restriction of physical activity and periods of **bed rest** reduce metabolic requirements in older children and adolescents. Activity restriction is usually counterproductive in young children.

    (2) Cool, humidified oxygen by tent, mask, or nasal prongs may be useful in hypoxic patients.

  b. Afterload reduction. Vasodilator therapy, which decreases peripheral resistance and ventricular filling pressures, is used in patients with CHF refractory to digoxin and diuretics. Vasodilator agents are most effective in patients with extremely decreased cardiac index, high systemic vascular resistance, and pulmonary congestion. Agents that alter arteriolar resistance have the greatest effect on cardiac index, while agents that increase venous capacitance reduce congestive symptoms caused by elevated ventricular filling pressures.

    (1) Acute therapy. Sodium nitroprusside affects both arteriolar resistance and venous capacitance, thus treating both low output and congestive symptoms. Continuous IV infusion is usually begun at 0.5 μg/kg/min and increased until the desired effect is achieved or until arterial pressure falls by 10%. The average dose is 3 μg/kg/min. Sodium nitroprusside should be administered in an intensive care unit setting with monitoring by an arterial line and a thermodilution Swan-Ganz catheter, with supervision by a physician experienced in its use. *Thiocyanate levels should be measured when the drug is used for an extended period.*

    (2) Long-term maintenance

      (a) Hydralazine preferentially dilates the peripheral arteriolar bed, thus augmenting cardiac output. The initial dosage is 1 mg/kg/day PO given in 3–4 divided doses, with a gradual increase until the desired effect is achieved or adverse effects occur.

      (b) Isosorbide dinitrate, which dilates the venous bed and reduces congestive symptoms (e.g., from pulmonary edema), is used only rarely in children.

3. Reducing volume overload

  a. Sodium restriction. No-added-salt diets are used in children. Infants should receive a high-calorie, low-sodium formula.

  b. Fluid restriction is necessary only when dilutional hyponatremia complicates far-advanced CHF. Formula intake should **not** be restricted in infants.

  c. Diuretics. The effectiveness of a diuretic is dependent on renal perfusion and electrolytes and acid-base balance. Diuretic agents may cause profound changes in electrolyte composition, and therefore frequent electrolyte evaluations should be made. In the presence of shock or acute renal failure, diuretics will have little effect. **Potassium depletion, especially in the digitalized patient, is dangerous and may be lethal.**

  The characteristics of commonly used diuretics are given in Table 9-3.

    (1) Thiazides are sulfonamide derivatives that share moderate potency and low toxicity. Those most commonly used in pediatrics are chlorothiazide (Diuril) and hydrochlorothiazide (HydroDIURIL).

      (a) Mechanism. The thiazide diuretics inhibit resorption of sodium and chloride at the cortical diluting site of the ascending loop of Henle and the early distal convoluted tubule.

Table 9-3. Dosages and characteristics of various diuretics

Drug	Dosage	Action				Contraindications	Adverse reactions	Mechanism of action
		Onset	Peak	Duration				
Furosemide (Lasix)	IV: 1.0 mg/kg/dose (over 1–2 min) PO: 2–3 mg/kg/day	5 min	30 min	2 hr	Anuria	Hypovolemia	Blocks resorption of Cl^- in ascending loop of Henle
Ethacrynic acid (Edecrin)	IV: 1 mg/kg/dose PO: 2–3 mg/kg/day	1 hr 5 min	1–2 hr 45 min	4–6 hr 3 hr	Hypersensitivity Women with child-bearing potential	Hypokalemia Hyperuricemia Ototoxicity	
Chlorothiazide (Diuril)	PO: 20–30 mg/kg/day in 2 doses	30 min 2 hr	2 hr 4 hr	6–8 hr 6–12 hr	Anuria, progressive renal insufficiency	Hypokalemia	Blocks resorption of Na^+ in ascending loop of Henle
Hydrochlorothiazide (Hydro-DIURIL)	PO: 2–3 mg/kg/day in 2 doses	2 hr	4 hr	6–12 hr	Hypersensitivity to this or other sulfonamide-derived drugs	Hyperuricemia Hypersensitivity Dermatitis Photosensitivity	
Spironolactone (Aldactone)*	PO: 1–3 mg/kg/day in 2 doses		Several days		Renal insufficiency	Headaches Gynecomastia Nausea and vomiting Rashes	Blocks aldosterone exchange of K^+ for Na^+
Acetazolamide (Diamox)	PO: 5 mg/kg/day	1 hr	2 hr	24 hr	Hypokalemia Anuria Renal insufficiency Hyperchloremia Acidosis	Drowsiness Paresthesias Hypersensitivity	Carbonic anhydrase inhibitor

*Spironolactone is rarely given alone, but its potassium-sparing effect makes it useful in combination with other agents.

(b) Route of administration, absorption, and metabolism. The thiazides are rapidly absorbed from the GI tract and begin to have a diuretic effect within 1 hr. The duration of action of chlorothiazide is about 6–12 hr, while that of hydrochlorothiazide is 12 hr or more. Excretion is via the kidney, with some subsequent resorption.

(c) Dosage. Give chlorothiazide, 20–30 mg/kg/day PO in 2 divided doses, or give hydrochlorothiazide, 2–3 mg/kg/day PO in 2 divided doses.

(d) Toxicity

    (i) Potassium depletion may occur with long-term use. Alternate-day therapy, intake of foods high in potassium, administration of liquid potassium, or the addition of a potassium-sparing diuretic such as spironolactone or triamterene may protect against potassium depletion. However, periodic measurements of serum potassium are necessary, especially early in therapy.

    (ii) Allergic reactions, such as thrombocytopenia, leukopenia, or vasculitis, are rarely seen. **Hyperglycemia** and **aggravation of preexisting diabetes or hyperuricemia** may occur.

(2) Furosemide (Lasix) and ethacrynic acid (Edecrin). These potent diuretics are different structurally from each other but have similar diuretic effects. Because of the massive diuresis that may be produced, they should rarely be used in previously untreated children unless careful observation of electrolytes, especially serum potassium, and blood volume is possible.

    (a) Mechanism. Both furosemide and ethacrynic acid inhibit active chloride transport in the ascending limb of the loop of Henle, where 25% of sodium resorption occurs.

    (b) Route of administration, absorption, and metabolism

        (i) Both drugs are well absorbed PO or may be given IV.

        (ii) When they are given PO, effects can be expected within 30–60 min. The onset of action after parenteral administration is within 5 min for furosemide and within 15 min for ethacrynic acid.

        (iii) The duration of action for the parenteral dose is 2–3 hr and 6–8 hr for the PO dose.

        (iv) Both drugs are bound to plasma protein, with approximately two-thirds excreted by the kidney.

    (c) Dosage

        (i) Ethacrynic acid is given in a 1 mg/kg/dose IV over 1–2 min IV and 2–3 mg/kg/day PO. *Or*

        (ii) Furosemide can be given as 1 mg/kg/dose over 1–2 min IV or 2–3 mg/kg/day PO.

    (d) Toxicity. Both drugs are potent, and clinical toxicity is usually manifested by **hypovolemia** or **hypokalemia.** Both drugs competitively inhibit urate secretion in the proximal tubule and may cause **hyperuricemia** and, in susceptible persons, gout. Transient or even permanent deafness has been reported, especially with ethacrynic acid (possibly due to electrolyte changes in the endolymph). **GI disturbances, bone marrow suppression, skin rashes,** and **paresthesias** have been reported occasionally.

(3) Spironolactone (Aldactone) is a weak diuretic by itself but may be useful as an addition to diuretics previously discussed, both because of its different site of action and because of its potassium-sparing effects.

    (a) Mechanism. The diuretic properties of spironolactone result from its structural similarity to aldosterone. It is a competitive inhibitor of the mineralocorticoids that normally stimulate sodium resorption and potassium excretion in the distal tubules.

  (b) Route of administration, absorption, and metabolism. Spironolactone is absorbed orally, but the diuretic effects may not be
  manifested for 2–3 days. Its effects may persist for 2–3 days after
  cessation of therapy.
  (c) The **dosage** is 1–3 mg/kg/day PO.
  (d) Toxicity. The major complication is **hyperkalemia,** resulting from
  inhibition of potassium secretion with normal or increased potassium intake. Careful monitoring of serum potassium will avoid
  this problem. Spironolactone has been shown to be **oncogenic** in
  chronic toxicity studies in rats. Gynecomastia may be seen in
  adolescents.

III. Hypoxic or cyanotic spells. Paroxysmal dyspnea with marked cyanosis often occurs
in infants and young children with tetralogy of Fallot. Rarely, it may occur in other
types of cyanotic congenital heart disease. It is characterized by increasing rate and
depth of respirations with increased cyanosis, progressing to limpness, loss of consciousness, and, in the more severe cases, convulsions, cerebrovascular accidents,
and even death.

  A. Etiology
  1. Cyanotic spells are due to an acute reduction of pulmonary blood flow, in-
     creased right-to-left shunting, and systemic hypoxemia.
  2. "Spasm" of the infundibulum of the right ventricular outflow tract has been
     suggested. Other explanations include inadequate systemic venous return,
     decreased systemic vascular resistance, and a vicious cycle of arterial hypox-
     emia due to hyperpnea.
  3. Anemia, either absolute or relative to the child's oxygen saturation, may
     predispose to cyanotic spells.

  B. Diagnosis
  1. **Signs and symptoms** include:
     a. Reduction in intensity or disappearance of the pulmonary ejection mur-
        mur
     b. Hyperpnea
     c. Increased cyanosis
     d. Irritability, often leading to unconsciousness and occasionally to convul-
        sions due to cerebral anoxia
  2. **Laboratory findings** include:
     a. Hypoxemia and acidosis
     b. Diminished pulmonary blood flow on x-ray
     c. Increased voltage of the P wave on the ECG

  C. Treatment
  1. Place the child in a knee-chest position.
  2. Give **oxygen** by hood or mask at 5–8 L/min.
  3. Give **morphine sulfate,** 0.1–0.2 mg/kg IM or SQ.
  4. If the spell is severe, give **sodium bicarbonate,** 1 mg/kg IV.
  5. If the hemoglobin is less than 15 gm/100 ml, a **transfusion** (5 ml/kg) should
     be given.
  6. **Propranolol,** 0.1 mg/kg IV, may be effective in a protracted spell that does
     not respond to the preceding measures.
  7. **Surgery** (corrective or palliative) may be necessary to increase pulmonary
     blood flow, or to prevent recurrence of spells, or both.

IV. Recognition of the innocent murmur. The innocent murmur is one that occurs in
the absence of either anatomic or physiologic abnormalities of the heart and lacks
association with future cardiovascular disease. Innocent murmurs are audible in the
majority of children.

  A. Clinical characteristics of innocent murmurs
  1. **General**
     a. Systolic in time and of short duration
     b. Loudest along the left sternal border; transmission is usually not wide-
        spread; loudness may change with position but not respiration and is
        usually grade III or less and increases with exercise.

  c. Other heart sounds are normal (importantly, there is a normal split of the second sound). Thrills are absent.

  d. The ECG and chest x-ray are normal.

2. Specific

  a. Still's murmur is usually grade I–III. It is a vibratory, buzzing, or musical systolic ejection murmur, loudest in the 2nd to 5th left intercostal spaces and maximal in the supine position. It may intensify with exercise, excitement, and fever. It is not associated with a thrill.

  b. Pulmonic systolic murmur. A grade I–III, high-pitched, crescendo-decrescendo murmur, usually peaking in the first half of systole. It is maximal in the 2nd left intercostal spaces, radiating upward and to the left. It is not associated with a thrill. It is best heard in the supine position and more apt to be heard in aesthenic persons, especially those with narrow anteroposterior diameter. It originates in the pulmonary trunk.

  c. Cardiorespiratory murmurs are of extracardiac origin; usually located at the heart-lung margin. They are not well transmitted—seem to originate close to the ear. Their variable loudness and timing are associated with cardiac and respiratory cycles, and they often disappear in expiration. Their incidence is associated with intraabdominal masses or ascites, thoracic-cage deformities, and pleural or pericardial adhesions.

  d. Cervical venous hum. This is a grade I–VI continuous murmur with diastolic accentuation and is maximal in the supraclavicular fossa lateral to the sternocleidomastoid muscle. It may radiate below the clavicle, where it may be confused with the murmur of patent ductus arteriosus. It is elicited by turning the patient's head away from the side of the murmur and elevating the chin while in a sitting position. It is abolished by recumbency, turning the head to the ipsilateral side of the murmur, or by digital compression of the ipsilateral internal jugular vein.

  e. Supraclavicular arterial bruit. This is a crescendo-decrescendo early systolic ejection murmur. It is maximal over the supraclavicular fossa and prominent in the suprasternal notch. It may generate a carotid thrill. Radiation is better to the neck than to below the clavicles. The murmur is accentuated by exercise and abolished or diminished by hyperextension of the shoulders.

B. Specific diagnosis. The innocent murmur should be distinguished from the following lesions.

 1. Mitral valve prolapse

  a. Clinical evaluation. Most commonly, mitral valve prolapse is characterized by an isolated variable mid- to late systolic click or a midsystolic click followed by a late systolic murmur. However, it may also present as an early systolic click, isolated late systolic murmur, pansystolic murmur, or precordial honk or whoop. Since the click in mitral valve prolapse is not always evident, auscultation should be carried out in four positions: supine, left decubitus, sitting, and standing. The click and murmur occur earlier with maneuvers that decrease left ventricular volume and/or increase left ventricular contractility (e.g., inspiration, standing, a Valsalva maneuver, isoproterenol, amyl nitrate inhalation). Opposite maneuvers (e.g., squatting, propranolol, phenylephrine) delay the onset of the click and murmur. Regurgitant murmurs become louder with maneuvers that raise arterial pressure and diminish with those that decrease it.

  b. Laboratory data. In approximately one-third of patients with mitral valve prolapse seen by cardiologists, the **ECG** shows T wave inversion with or without minimal S–T segment depression, characteristically noted in leads II, III, and aVf with frequent additional involvement of the left precordial leads. A **chest x-ray** reveals a normal heart size in the absence of mitral insufficiency. The **M-mode echocardiogram** is abnormal in approximately 80% of subjects with the auscultatory findings of mitral valve prolapse.

  c. Complications. Although the prognosis in patients with mitral valve prolapse is generally excellent, rare complications include progression of mitral insufficiency, bacterial endocarditis, malignant arrhythmias, cerebral ischemic events, and sudden death. Antibiotic prophylaxis against infective endocarditis should be used in patients with late or pansystolic murmurs (see Table 15-9, p. 370). Their prophylactic use in patients with an isolated click is controversial.

2. **Idiopathic hypertrophic subaortic stenosis.** Auscultation is characterized by a harsh midsystolic ejection murmur that is maximal between the apex and left sternal border and results from left ventricular outflow tract obstruction. Frequently, there is a separate pansystolic regurgitant murmur maximal at the apex, caused by mitral regurgitation. The systolic ejection murmur is augmented by maneuvers that increase contractility, decrease preload, or decrease afterload, i.e., Valsalva maneuvers, standing, postextrasystole, exercise, digitalis, amyl nitrite, or isoproterenol. Conversely, the murmur diminishes with squatting, isometric hand grip, alpha-adrenergic stimulation, or beta-adrenergic blockade.

V. Cardiac infections
A. Myocarditis
1. **Etiology.** Infectious myocarditis is a common cause of acute congestive cardiomyopathy and may be caused by a variety of infectious agents, including viruses, rickettsiae, bacteria, mycobacteria, spirochetes, fungi, or parasites. Myocardial damage is effected by either invasion of the myocardium (e.g., echoviruses or coxsackieviruses), production of a myocardial toxin (e.g., diphtheria), or autoimmune mechanisms (e.g., rheumatic fever). In North America, the most common etiologic agents are viruses. Myocarditis may be either acute or chronic.
2. **Presentation and evaluation.** The clinical presentation of infectious myocarditis ranges from the asymptomatic state to fulminant CHF, depending on the severity of myocardial involvement.
   a. **Symptoms** on presentation include fatigue, dyspnea, palpitations, and chest pain (usually secondary to associated pericarditis). **Signs** include tachycardia, protodiastolic gallop, and clinical evidence of CHF in severe cases.
   b. The **ECG** often shows S–T and T wave changes, arrhythmias, conduction defects, and occasionally a pattern consistent with myocardial infarction.
   c. On **chest x-ray,** heart size ranges from normal to markedly enlarged.
3. The **diagnosis** depends in part on the features of the associated systemic illness. Viral etiology should be evaluated by obtaining viral cultures of throat washings, blood, feces, and pericardial fluid, as well as by acute and convalescent sera for virus neutralizing antibody, complement fixation, or hemagglutination inhibition titers.
4. **Treatment**
   a. Treatment of infectious myocarditis should be supportive, with maintenance of adequate oxygenation.
   b. Monitoring and treatment, preferably in an intensive care unit, should be provided for arrhythmias, conduction abnormalities, and CHF.
   c. Since patients with myocarditis may be sensitive to digitalis glycosides, digoxin should be administered cautiously at a reduced dose.
   d. Patients should remain at bed rest for 10–14 days, and exercise probably should be limited for 3 months.
   e. **Corticosteroids are contraindicated in the acute phase of viral myocarditis.**
   f. Specific therapy should be appropriate to the cause.

B. Pericarditis
1. **Causes**
   a. **Bacterial.** Bacterial pericarditis may occur by hematogenous or contiguous spread. The most common causative organisms are staphylococci, pneumococci, *Haemophilus influenzae,* meningococci, streptococci, and *Mycobacterium tuberculosis.*
   b. **Viral.** Viral pericarditis is often preceded by a history of upper respiratory tract infection and occurs as part of the spectrum of viral myopericarditis.

The most common causative agents are coxsackievirus, echovirus, adenovirus, influenza virus, mumps virus, varicella–zoster virus, vaccinia, or Epstein-Barr virus (i.e., infectious mononucleosis).

    c. Noninfectious causes include collagen diseases, uremic fibrinous pericarditis, radiation-induced pericarditis, and malignant pericardial effusion.

2. Diagnosis

    a. Presenting clinical signs and symptoms depend in part on the etiology, age of the patient, associated infection or systemic disease, and presence of tamponade.

    b. The **ECG** is characterized by diffuse S–T and T wave abnormalities. Echocardiography establishes the presence of fluid in the pericardial space.

    c. The chest x-ray often shows an increase in the size of the cardiac silhouette with normal pulmonary vascular markings; associated infection of the lung or pleural space may be evident.

    d. Pericardiocentesis for culture and examination of pericardial fluid should be performed in all patients who appear toxic, have evidence of tamponade, or in whom the cause of the pericarditis is uncertain.

    e. Additional studies should be done as appropriate to the cause (e.g., blood cultures; viral cultures of blood, urine, throat, and feces; tuberculin skin test; test for connective tissue disorders; BUN and creatinine; CBC and differential; cold agglutinins; heterophils; fungal serology; thyroid studies; rheumatic fever assessment).

3. Treatment

    a. General measures include bed rest, analgesia, and observation for and treatment of tamponade or cardiac decompensation.

    b. Specific therapy should be directed toward the etiology (e.g., antimicrobial agents, chemotherapy, dialysis). In acute purulent pericarditis, antibiotic therapy appropriate to the sensitivities of the causative organism should be combined with effective pericardial drainage (e.g., subxyphoid pericardial window, anterior pericardiectomy with tube drainage).

C. Subacute bacterial endocarditis. See Chap. 15, p. 406.

D. Rheumatic fever is covered in Chap. 15, p. 407.

Gastroenterology

I. General principles
A. Nutrition
  1. Assessment
    a. Height and weight (specifically the following indices):
      (1) Weight/age
      (2) Height/age
      (3) Weight/height (see Chap. 2, pp. 13ff.)
    b. Anthropometrics
      (1) Triceps skin fold
      (2) Arm circumference
      (3) Head circumference
    c. Blood tests
      (1) CBC with lymphocyte count
      (2) PPD and *Candida*
      (3) Total protein, albumin, transferrin, and globulins
      (4) Liver function tests and alkaline phosphatase
      (5) Iron and total iron binding capacity
      (6) Minerals
    d. Urine tests
      (1) Creatinine × creatinine/height index (*Pediatrics* 46:696, 1970)
      (2) Nitrogen
      (3) Minerals
  2. Diets prescribed for the management of a specific nutritional deficiency may be obtained by writing to the Nutrition Department at Children's Hospital, Boston, MA 02115. For patients in whom the oral route is not appropriate, nasogastric or nasojejunal feedings are indicated, utilizing elemental formulas (see Table 10-1).
  3. Values for daily dietary allowances for different ages can be found in Chapter 2, p. 20, and Table 2-2.
  4. Therapy
    a. General approach. Remember that patience is the most important principle in the management of malnourished patients. The following measures are suggested:
      (1) Correction of fluid and electrolyte disorders (hyponatremia, hyposmolality, acidosis, hypomagnesemia, hypokalemia)
      (2) Therapy for infections
      (3) Protein load. Start with 1 gm/kg/day, and increase as tolerated.
      (4) Caloric load. Start with 80–100 cal/kg/day, and increase as tolerated.
      (5) Use formulas without lactose to prevent diarrhea secondary to dissacharidase insufficiency.
      (6) If the infant is anorectic, nasogastric feeding should be considered.
      (7) Vitamin and mineral supplementation
    b. Total parenteral nutrition (TPN). *Intravenous alimentation* is delivery of a mixture of hypertonic dextrose and crystalline amino acid solutions utilizing a central high-flow vein. This method should be used if the

Table 10-1. Enteral hyperalimentation chart

	General			Milk-Base		
	Formula 2	Compleat-B	Vitaneed	Meritene	Carnation Instant Breakfast	Nutri 1000
Calories/cc	1	1	1	1	1	1
Carbohydrate source	Lactose, sucrose	Maltodextrin, lactose, sucrose	Corn syrup solids, maltodextrins	Lactose, corn syrup, sucrose	Sucrose, corn syrup, lactose	Sucrose, lactose, corn syrup solids
Protein source	Wheat, beef, egg, milk	Beef, skim milk, vegetable	Beef caseinate	Skim milk	Milk, sodium caseinate, soy protein isolate	Skim milk
Fat source	Egg yolk, corn oil, beef fat	Corn oil, beef fat	Soy oil, soy lecithin	Corn oil	Whole milk	Corn oil
Protein (gm/L)	38	40	35	60	58	40
Fat gm/L	40	40	40	33	31	55
Carbohydrate gm/L	123	120	130	115	135	101
mOsm/kg	435/510	390	400	550	500	500
Na/K mEq/L	26/45	68/33	24/32	40/42	41/70	23/39
Residue	High	High	High	Medium	Medium	Medium
Vitamin content	Yes	Yes	Yes	Yes	Yes	Yes
Producer	Cutter	Doyle	Organon	Doyle	Carnation	Cutter
Flavors	Orange	Natural flavor	Natural flavor	Varied	Varied	Chocolate, vanilla
Form	Ready to use	Ready to use	Ready to use	Ready to use	Powder	Ready to use
Uses/features	Blenderized tube feeding, requires digestion & absorption	Blenderized tube feeding, requires digestion & absorption	Blenderized tube feeding, requires digestion & absorption, low Na, lactose free	High protein, supplemental, tube feeding, requires digestion & absorption	Supplemental, easily available, requires digestion & absorption	Supplemental, tube feeding, requires digestion & absorption

Table 10-1 (continued)

	Lactose-Free								
	Sustacal	Citrotein	Nutri 1000 LF	Isocal	Osmolite	Renu	Ensure	Ensure Plus	Magnacal
Calories/cc	1	66	1	1	1	1	1	15	2
Carbohydrate source	Sucrose, corn syrup	Sucrose, maltodextrin	Sucrose, corn syrup	Glucose, oligosaccharides	Corn syrup	Corn syrup solids, maltodextrins	Corn syrup, sucrose	Corn syrup, sucrose	Corn syrup solids, maltodextrin, sucrose
Protein source	Skim milk, calcium & sodium caseinate soy protein isolates	Egg albumin	Calcium & sodium caseinates, soy protein isolates	Calcium & sodium caseinates, soy protein isolates	Calcium & sodium caseinate, soy protein isolates	Caseinate, soy protein isolates	Sodium & calcium caseinate, soy protein isolates	Sodium & calcium caseinate, soy protein isolates	Caseinate
Fat source	Partially hydrogenated soy oil	Partially hydrogenated soybean oil	Corn oil	Soy oil, MCT oil	MCT oil, corn oil, soy oil	Soy oil, soy lecithin	Corn oil	Corn oil	Soy oil, soy lecithin
Protein (gm/L)	60	43	40	34	35	33	37	55	70
Fat gm/L	23	2	55	44	34	40	37	53	80
Carbohydrate gm/L	138	129	101	130	138	130	145	197	250
mOsm/kg	625	496	380	300	300	330	450	600	520
Na/K mEq/L	39/53	31/19	23/39	22/33	22/23	22/32	32/32	46/48	43/32
Residue	Low	Low	Low	Low	Low	Low	Low	Low	Low
Vitamin content	Yes	Yes	Yes	Yes	Yes	Yes	Yes	Yes	Yes
Producer	Mead Johnson	Doyle	Cutter	Mead Johnson	Ross	Organon	Ross	Ross	Organon
Flavors	Varied	Orange, grape	Chocolate, vanilla	Unflavored	Unflavored	Vanilla	Varied	Varied	Vanilla
Form	Ready to use	Powder	Ready to use	Ready to use	Ready to use	Ready to use	Ready to use	Ready to use	Ready to use
Uses/features	High protein, supplemental, tube feeding, requires digestion & absorption	Supplemental, lactose, gluten, cholesterol free, clear liquid supplement	Supplemental, tube feeding, lactose free, low Na, requires digestion & absorption	Tube feeding, requires digestion & absorption, low Na, lactose free	Supplemental, tube feeding, lactose free, low Na, requires digestion & absorption	Supplemental, tube feeding, requires digestion & absorption, low Na, lactose free	Supplemental, tube feeding, lactose free, requires digestion & absorption	Supplemental, tube feeding, lactose free, requires digestion & absorption	Supplemental, tube feeding, lactose free, requires digestion & absorption, high calcium, high protein

260

Table 10-1 (continued)

	Chemically Defined Formulas					Elemental		
	Precision Isotonic	Precision LR	Precision HN	Flexical	Vital	Vivonex	Vivonex HN	Vipep
Calories/cc	1	1	1	1	1	1	1	1
Carbohydrate source	Glucose, oligosaccharides, sucrose	Maltodextrin, sucrose	Maltodextrin, sucrose	Corn syrup, modified tapioca starch	Glucose oligopolysaccharides	Glucose oligosaccharides	Glucose oligosaccharides	Corn syrup, sucrose, corn starch
Protein source	Egg albumin	Egg albumin	Egg albumin	Casein hydrolysate, crystalline amino acids	Whey, soy & meat protein, hydrolysate, free essential amino acids	L-amino acids	L-amino acids	Peptides of 2–4 amino acid units, 4–14 amino acid units, free amino acids
Fat source	Soybean oil	Soy oil	Soy oil	Soy oil, MCT oil	Sunflower oil	Safflower oil	Safflower oil	MCT oil, corn oil
Protein (gm/L)	30	26	44	23	42	21	42	25
Fat gm/L	31	0.8	0.5	34	10	1	1	25
Carbohydrate gm/L	150	249	218	152	185	226	210	176
mOsm/kg	300	525	557	550	450	550	844	520
Na/K mEq/L	35/26	30/22	43/23	15/32	17/30	37/30	34/18	33/22
Residue	Low	Low	Low	Low	Low	Low	Low	Low
Vitamin content	Yes	Yes	Yes	Yes	Yes	Yes	Yes	Yes
Producer	Doyle	Doyle	Doyle	Mead Johnson	Ross	Eaton	Eaton	Cutter
Flavors	Vanilla, orange	Varied	Citrus	Varied	Varied	Varied	Varied	Varied
Form	Powder	Powder	Powder	Powder	Powder	Powder	Powder	Powder
Uses/features	Supplemental, tube feeding, lactose free, isotonic, absorbed in upper gut	Supplemental, tube feeding, lactose free, absorbed in upper gut	Supplemental, tube feeding, lactose free, absorbed in upper gut, high protein	Supplemental, tube feeding, lactose free, absorbed in upper gut	Supplemental, tube feeding, absorbed in upper gut, low Na	Supplemental, tube feeding, lactose free, no pancreatic stimulus, absorbed in upper gut	Supplemental, tube feeding, lactose free, absorbed in upper gut, high protein	Supplemental, tube feeding, uses free amino acid peptide carrier system, lactose free, absorbed in upper gut

Table 10-1 (continued)

	Special Formulations				Caloric Additives			
	Amin-aid	Hepatic-aid	Microlipid	Controlyte	Polycose (powder)	Polycose (liquid)	Sumacal	Sumacal Plus
Calories/cc	19	16	45	5 cal/gm 2 cal/cc	4 cal/gm	2 cal/cc	2	25
Carbohydrate source	Maltodextrose, sucrose	Maltodextrins, sucrose		Corn starch	Hydrolysis of corn starch	Hydrolysis of corn starch	Glucose syrup solids, maltodextrins	Maltodextrins, glucose syrup solids
Protein source	Crystalline essential amino acids	Branch chain and aromatic amino acids						
Fat source	Partially hydrogenated soybean oil	Soy oil, lecithin, mono & diglycerides	Safflower oil, soy lecithin	Vegetable oil				
Protein (gm/L)	19	43		trace				
Fat gm/L	66	36	500	96				
Carbohydrate gm/L	330	287		286		500	500	625
mOsm/kg	900	900	32	590		570	680	890
Na/K mEq/L	<8/ <8			2.6/0.4		27	9/6	9/8
Residue	Low	Low	Low	Low	Low	Low	Low	Low
Vitamin content	No	No	No	No	No	No	No	No
Producer	McGaw	McGaw	Organon	Doyle	Ross	Ross	Organon	Organon
Flavors	Varied	Varied	Unflavored	Unflavored	Unflavored	Unflavored	Cherry, lemon & lime	Unflavored
Form	Powder	Powder	Ready to use	Powder	Powder	Liquid	Ready to use	Ready to use
Uses/features	Supplemental, tube feeding, low electrolytes, essential amino acids, lactose free, indicated for renal disease	Supplemental, tube feeding, high branched-chain amino acid formula, low electrolytes, lactose free, indicated for liver disease	Supplemental, pure fat emulsion, low osmolarity, low electrolytes, lactose free	Supplemental, low electrolytes, low protein, lactose free	Supplemental, lactose free	Supplemental, lactose free	Supplemental, lactose free	Supplemental, lactose free

enteral route is not possible. Intravenous alimentation should be used in all patients who will be allowed nothing by mouth for 2 weeks or more. Periods of poor intake from 2–3 days to 2 weeks should be managed with peripheral IV alimentation.

(1) Nitrogen sources are generally provided as either protein hydrolysate or a mixture of pure crystalline amino acids. The usual daily requirement of each is 2–4 gm/kg in infants and children. The bulk of the caloric content of hyperalimentation fluid is derived from glucose. The amount required in most infants is 25–30 gm/kg/day. The rest of the metabolic needs (i.e., water, electrolytes, minerals, and vitamins) are provided in the customary amounts.

(2) Intralipid (soybean oil), a fat emulsion that provides 1.1 cal/ml, is necessary to prevent essential fatty acid deficiency and should be given as 5–10% of the total calories. The following are the recommended rates:

    (a) 5–10 ml/kg for first 10 kg

    (b) 2.5–5.0 ml/kg for second 10 kg

    (c) 1.25–2.5 ml/kg for all weights above 20 kgs

The maximum amount is 40 ml/kg/day. It is inadvisable to begin Intralipid at the same time as other parenteral nutrition solutions.

(3) Caloric densities utilized:

    (a) Amino acids, 3.33 cal/gm

    (b) 10% Dextrose, 0.34 cal/ml

    (c) 20% Dextrose, 0.68 cal/ml

    (d) PN 10, 0.39 cal/ml

    (e) PN 20, 0.73 cal/ml

(4) Indications for TPN. Any patient unable to maintain nutrition adequate for metabolic needs is a candidate for TPN. Specific disease states in which TPN is employed include:

    (a) Chronic diarrheal states

    (b) Inflammatory bowel disease with growth failure or fistulas

    (c) Postoperative status

    (d) Chronic pancreatitis and pseudocyst

    (e) Short-bowel syndrome

    (f) Esophageal injury

(5) Management of hyperalimentation program

    (a) A central venous catheter is placed and its position checked radiographically.

    (b) A 10% glucose solution is given IV at a rate 1½ times maintenance fluid as tolerated (see Chap. 7, p. 197). Adequate electrolytes should be provided. Continue the infusion for 12–24 hr.

    (c) A 20% glucose-amino acid solution is then given at ¾ maintenance fluid requirement for 12 hr.

    (d) The infusion rate is increased approximately 10% q12h until fluid intake is 135 ml/kg/day, irrespective of age. An infusate with 20% glucose and 3 gm/100 ml of protein provides the equivalent of 110 cal/kg/day. Generally, no more than 200 ml/kg/day is used in infants. It may be necessary to decrease the protein content of the infusate at such rates.

    (e) Intralipid infusion

        (i) Intralipid is administered via a peripheral vein and does not require "breaking" the central venous circuit for administration.

        (ii) The initial rate of Intralipid infusion via a peripheral vein should provide 15 ml/kg/day given over 6–12 hr. If the patient's serum is not lipemic, the infusion is increased by 5 ml/kg/day until 30–40 ml/kg/day is attained.

(6) Monitoring the patient receiving TPN
  (a) Daily weights should be measured.
  (b) Intake and output is charted and qualitative sugar and acetone measured on all urine specimens.
  (c) Na, K, Cl, BUN, and glucose are determined daily while increasing fluid and then weekly when fluid requirements have been reached.
  (d) CBC, Mg, Ca, P, and total protein are measured initially and then weekly.
  (e) SGOT, SGPT, LDH, alkaline phosphatase, bilirubin, and creatinine are measured initially and then weekly.
  (f) Copper, zinc, and iron levels are measured at the beginning of therapy and then monthly.
  (g) Lipemia checks daily
  (h) 24-hr urine for creatinine, Ca^{2+}, PO_4^{2+}, and Mg^{2+} every 2 weeks
(7) Complications of TPN
  (a) Infection is the most serious complication of TPN.
    (i) The incidence of this complication increases dramatically if less than scrupulous care is applied to maintaining the integrity of the central venous line.
    (ii) Unexplained glycosuria may be the first clue. Fungi (usually *Candida albicans*) and bacteria are the infecting agents. Several blood cultures should be obtained from the patient and from the line. When sepsis is documented, the central venous line should be withdrawn if possible. Although appropriate antibiotics should be used for documented sepsis, chemotherapy may not be necessary for *Candida* infection.
  (b) Hepatic complications. Abnormalities in liver function test results are common during the course of TPN. Hepatomegaly with elevations of serum transaminases (often to high levels, with prolongation of prothrombin time (PT) and partial thromboplastin time (PTT) may be seen, and liver biopsy reveals a fatty liver. Cholestatic liver disease frequently develops in premature infants.
  (c) Metabolic complications
    (i) Hyperglycemia is common in septic patients, premature infants, and patients with renal disease.
    (ii) Hypoglycemia is a common and severe complication *if TPN is stopped abruptly.*
    (iii) Acidosis occurs in patients with renal compromise or prematurity when large (4 gm/kg/day) protein loads are administered.
    (iv) Hypomagnesemia may occur in patients with low endogenous magnesium stores (e.g., those with chronic diarrhea).
    (v) Hyperlipemia occurs with excess Intralipid administration.
    (vi) Hyperammonemia
    (vii) Hypocalcemia
  (d) Trace metal deficiency
    (i) Copper deficiency is not uncommon and is manifested by anemia, neutropenia, and rash.
    (ii) Zinc deficiency is common and is manifested by an erythematous, maculopapular rash (acrodermatitis enteropathica) (see Chap. 22) involving the face, trunk, metacarpophalangeal joints, and perineum. *Low* serum alkaline phosphatase is common.
  (e) Mechanical complications
    (i) Arrhythmias may occur with an improperly placed catheter.
    (ii) Venous thrombosis is rare.

(iii) **Air embolus** occurs only after accidental coupling of the IV line.

(f) **Local complications. Skin sloughs** may occur from infiltration of peripheral venous infusions.

(g) **Complications of Intralipid administration**

   (i) **Pulmonary.** It may decrease oxygen diffusion at the alveolar-capillary junction.

   (ii) **Bilirubin.** Intralipid displaces bilirubin from albumin and is contraindicated in jaundiced infants.

   (iii) **Eosinophilia** may be present.

(h) **Contraindications to the use of Intralipid** include hyperlipemic states and severe liver disease.

B. Evaluation of gastrointestinal disease

1. Examination of the stool

a. Examine the stool for consistency, odor, blood, and mucus. The presence of gross blood and mucus indicates colitis. Use saline and Lugol's solution to look for parasites.

b. **Clinitest to detect the presence of reducing substances**

   (1) Mix 1 part **fresh** stool in 2 parts water (to detect sucrose intolerance); hydrolyze with 1 N HCl, boiling for 30 sec.

   (2) Centrifuge and add 15 drops of supernatant to 1 Clinitest tablet.

   (3) The test is positive if 0.5% or more of reducing substance is present. The presence of reducing substance is always abnormal and indicates sucrose or disaccharide intolerance, or both.

c. **pH**

   (1) Normal stool pH is 7–8.

   (2) A decreased pH suggests the presence of organic acids, as seen in disaccharide intolerance.

   (3) An increased pH suggests secretory diarrhea.

d. **Hemoccult** or **guaiac test** for blood

e. **Sudan stain for fat.** Place a representative sample on two slides. On the first slide, put 2 drops of 95% ethyl alcohol and several drops of Sudan black III. Place a cover slip and examine for neutral fats. On the second slide, put 2–4 drops of 35% acetic acid and several drops of Sudan black III. Place a cover slip, heat the slide to boil, and examine for split fats (*N. Engl. J. Med.* 264:85–87, 1961). A positive test will result in the presence of fat (red) globules in the slide. The amount of fat globules correlates with the 72-hr fecal fat assay.

f. **Fecal leukocytes**

   (1) Stain with Loeffler's methylene blue, or Wright's or Gram stains.

   (2) Diseases associated with leukocytes include the following:

      (a) **Shigellosis.** Polymorphonuclear, 84%

      (b) **Salmonellosis.** Polymorphonuclear, 75%

      (c) **Typhoid fever.** Mononuclear, 95%

      (d) **Invasive *Escherichia coli*.** Polymorphonuclear, 85%

      (e) **Ulcerative colitis and Crohn's disease.** Polymorphonuclear, 88%

g. **Ova, parasites, and cultures**

2. Fecal fat excretion. Although often distasteful to patient and clinician, this is the best method for detecting steatorrhea.

a. All stools are collected for 72 hr.

b. Since fecal fat excretion is expressed as a percentage of intake, the patient must keep a diary of food intake during this period, so that the amount of fat in the diet can be estimated.

Coefficient of absorption:

$$\frac{\text{dietary fat} - \text{fecal fat}}{\text{dietary fat}} \times 100 =$$

c. **Normal values.** (Values for breast-fed infants are lower but are not precisely known.)

Normal C.A.:
  Prematures: 60–75%
  Newborns: 80–85%
  10 mo–3 yr: 85–95%
  Older than 3 yr: 95%

3. **D-Xylose excretion.** This test reflects enteric mucosal absorption.
   a. Give 14.5 gm/M^2 after an overnight fast.
   b. Measure serum xylose at 1 hr; above 25 mg/100 ml is normal.
   c. Delayed gastric emptying is a variable that may cause falsely low levels. The reliability of this test for detecting mucosal disease is controversial. However, it remains a useful screening test.

4. **Breath tests** include three stages: delivery of a substrate; enzymatic metabolism of the substrate by bacteria, or body cells, or both; and the measurement of the products. A number of different breath tests are in current use or trial. The **breath hydrogen test** for lactose and sucrose malabsorption is well studied.
   a. After an overnight fast, the patient is given a loading dose of the disaccharide to be studied.
   b. A nasal prong is inserted, and 3–5 ml of expired air is collected in a syringe at 30-min intervals for 3 hr.
   c. H_2 excretion is measured; excretion of 11 ppm H_2 indicates disaccharide malabsorption.
   d. False-positives and false-negatives may be seen due to natural or antibiotic-induced changes in bacterial flora. No antibiotics should be administered within 1 week prior to the test.

5. **Jejunal biopsy** is a safe, well accepted, and invaluable tool for the diagnosis of intestinal mucosal disease. Specimens are obtained with a multipurpose Rubin or Crosby capsule.
   a. All patients must have a platelet count, PT, and PTT prior to the procedure.
   b. After an overnight fast, patients over 6 months of age and under 6–7 years are premedicated with chlorpromazine (Thorazine), 1 mg/kg IM, and pentobarbital, 4 mg/kg. Older patients require no premedication; instead, an anesthetic spray (e.g., tetracaine [Pontocaine or Cetacaine]) is used to anesthetize the pharynx.
   c. The biopsy specimen is sent for histologic examination and assay of small-intestine disaccharidases. The values at Children's Hospital (normal values vary from laboratory to laboratory) are:

   Lactase 30.5 ± 16.6 Units/gm protein
   Sucrase 62.8 ± 26.7 Units/gm protein
   Maltase 203.6 ± 75.2 Units/gm protein

   The biopsy is invariably of diagnostic value in gluten-sensitive enteropathy, Whipple's disease, abetalipoproteinemia, and agammaglobulinemia.

6. **Duodenal fluid** should be obtained by a nasogastric tube or at the time of biopsy. The fluid is examined for parasites, especially *Giardia lamblia,* and sent for bacterial culture (aerobic and anaerobic).

7. **Sweat test.** Pilocarpine iontophoresis for sweat electrolytes diagnoses cystic fibrosis in 99% of cases. Sweat weight should be greater than 100 mg. A chloride level above 60 mEq/L or a sodium level above 60 mEq/L is abnormal.

8. **The Schilling test** is a technique devised to measure the ability to absorb ingested vitamin B_{12}. It is used in gastroenterology to evaluate patients with

pernicious anemia, ileal dysfunction syndromes, malabsorption, pancreatic insufficiency, bacterial overgrowth, and Crohn's disease.

   a. The patient is given PO 0.5 microcuries of cyanocobalamin tagged with ^{57}Co and 2 hr later is given 1 mg of nonradioactive cyanocobalamin.

   b. The urine is collected 24 hr prior to the test and 24 hr after the cyanocobalamin is given.

   c. Stages of the test

     (1) Without intrinsic factor

     (2) With intrinsic factor

     (3) With orally administered antibiotics (tetracycline)

     (4) Pancreatic enzymes

     Stage 1 and stage 2 can be continued. Less than 12% absorption indicates an abnormal test.

  9. Esophageal manometry is a procedure designed to evaluate the motility characteristics of the esophagus and the upper and lower esophageal sphincter pressures. It provides information in diseases such as scleroderma, achalasia, diffuse esophageal spasm, and abnormal gastroesophageal reflux.

  10. Rectal manometry is a procedure designed to evaluate the relaxation and pressure of the rectal sphincters. It is very useful in the diagnosis of Hirschsprung's disease.

  11. Radiologic evaluation

    a. An **upper GI series** and small bowel follow-through

    b. Barium enema

    c. Oral cholecystogram

    d. Percutaneous transhepatic cholangiogram

  12. Nuclear medicine and ultrasound

    a. A liver and spleen scan to evaluate liver and spleen size as well as filling defects

    b. Technetium-99 scans for evaluation of pathologic gastroesophageal reflux, aspiration pneumonia, or gastric emptying

    c. Bida/Hida and rose bengal scans for evaluation of bilirubin excretion

    d. Abdominal ultrasound to evaluate the liver parenchyma, biliary tree, and pancreas

  13. Endoscopy

    a. Esophagogastroduodenoscopy

    b. Proctosigmoidoscopy

    c. Colonoscopy

    d. Endoscopic retrograde cholangiopancreatography

  14. A CT scan

II. Specific entities

  A. Malabsorption. The three phases of digestion and absorption are shown in Table 10-2. Because fat absorption depends on all the phases of digestion, the presence of steatorrhea (fat malabsorption) is the best indicator of a malabsorptive defect. Further tests will permit the localization of specific sites of abnormality.

  B. Diarrheal disease. Diarrhea is among the most common symptoms in pediatrics, and in underdeveloped countries it is the most common cause of morbidity and mortality in childhood.

  Evaluation of chronic diarrhea includes a history, with particular attention to blood or mucus in the stools, weight loss, failure to thrive, associated symptoms (fever, recurrent infection), drugs taken, particularly antibiotics, GI surgical procedures, family history, travel, age, and race.

  A **physical examination** should be done, with attention to nutritional status, hydration, edema, protuberant abdomen, abdominal masses, muscular habitus, rectal prolapse, and affect, particularly irritability. The cardiopulmonary system and neurologic status should be carefully evaluated.

  Laboratory studies include a CBC, erythrocyte sedimentation rate (ESR), urinalysis, serum protein analysis (SPA), stool examination, and sweat test. If the results of malabsorption screening are positive, the steps listed in this subsection should be followed.

Table 10-2. Mechanisms of digestion and absorption

Diet	Intraluminal phase — Pancreatic	Intraluminal phase — Biliary	Mucosal phase	Removal phase
Fat				
Triglycerides →	Monoglycerides (MG) Fatty acids (FA)	FA, MG Bile acids } Micelle →	Chylomicrons	Lymphatics
Medium-chain triglycerides →		→		
Protein →	Small peptides Amino acids	→	Amino acids	Portal vein
Carbohydrate →	Oligosaccharides Disaccharides	→	Monosaccharides	

Table 10-3. Common causes of acute diarrhea in childhood

Viral enteritis (rotavirus)

Bacterial enteritis
  Enterotoxin associated (*E. coli,* cholera, *Clostridium perfringens,*
    Staphylococcus)
  Nonenterotoxin associated* (*Salmonella, Shigella, E. coli, Yersinia*)

Parasitic enteritis (amebiasis,* giardiasis)

Extraintestinal infection (e.g., otitis media, urinary tract infection, sepsis)

Antibiotic induced* (*Clostridium difficile*)

Hemolytic-uremic syndrome*

Inflammatory bowel disease* (ulcerative colitis, Crohn's disease)

*May be associated with blood in the stool.

1. **Acute nonspecific gastroenteritis**
   a. **Etiology.** This common condition has many causes. These are listed in Table 10-3.
   b. **Evaluation.** This condition is often manifested by a sudden onset of vomiting, followed by diarrhea. It is most often self-limited. Fever may or may not be present, but with a reduction of fluid intake and abnormal losses, dehydration may occur, especially in children under 3 years of age.
      (1) **History.** In evaluating the patient with gastroenteritis, record the following: weight loss, duration, presence of blood or mucus, type and frequency of stools, type and amount of feedings, frequency of urination, presence or absence of tears, associated symptoms (e.g., fever, vomiting, localized abdominal pain), and current family illnesses.
      (2) **Physical examination** should include a description of the skin turgor, mucous membranes, fontanelles, eyes, presence or absence of tears, activity state, irritability, and associated rashes.
      (3) **Laboratory tests** can be minimized in the milder clinical states, but stool cultures and Wright's stain for neutrophils may be helpful, and urinary specific gravity is a useful sign of early dehydration. (For further workup in cases of diarrhea, see **D.**)
   c. **Therapy**
      (1) Children with acute diarrheal disease and minimal dehydration are treated most effectively with clear fluids, including water, Coca-Cola, or ginger ale *with the bubbles shaken out,* apple juice, diluted tea, and Jell-O. In the initial vomiting stage in infants or small children, large-volume feedings should be avoided. Small amounts (1–2 oz qh) as tolerated are sufficient initially.
      (2) Water may be sweetened with sugar, or a 5% glucose solution can be used.
      (3) Oral electrolyte solutions (Table 10-4) may be administered for up to 24 hr.
      (4) **Boiled skim milk has a very high solute load and can cause hypernatremia.**
      (5) Frequent large feedings stimulate the gastrocolic reflex and may aggravate the problem.
      (6) Clear fluids alone should not be continued more than 48 hr, or reactive loose stools may be passed. Bland solids can then be added, such as rice cereal, banana flakes, applesauce, saltines, Ritz crackers, dry cereal, or toast with jelly for older children.
      (7) The value of drugs such as kaolin and belladonna-containing compounds remains unproved, and their use should be discouraged. In the rare case when an **antispasmodic** is considered, diphenoxylate

Table 10-4. Approximate electrolyte content for fluid replacement or oral administration of electrolytes

Solution	Calories per ounce	Carbohydrate source	Carbohydrate (gm/100 ml)	Na$^+$	K$^+$	Cl$^-$	Osmolarity	Osmolality	Estimated renal solute load (mOsm/L)
Lytren (Mead Johnson)	9	Glucose	7.6	30.0	25.0	25.0	440	536	106
Pedialyte (Ross)	6	Glucose	5.0	30.0	20.0	30.0	405	(Estimated)	116
5% Glucose	6	Glucose	5.0				278	293	
10% Glucose	12	Glucose	10.0				562	625	
Pedialyte RS		Glucose	2.5	60.0	20.0	50.0	290		
Infalyte		Glucose	2.5	50.0	20.0	40.0	280		
WHO solution		Glucose	2.0	90.0	20.0	80.0	331		

Table 10-5. Causes of chronic diarrhea

Chronic nonspecific diarrhea (irritable bowel syndrome)

Chronic infections: *Salmonella, E. coli, Giardia, C. difficile*

Cystic fibrosis (*Yersinia, Campylobacter*)

Gluten-sensitive enteropathy (celiac disease)

Disaccharide deficiency (particularly lactose intolerance)

Inflammatory bowel disease

Immunodeficiency states

Anatomic causes
    Short-bowel syndrome
    Malrotation
    Hirschsprung's disease

Endocrine
    Hyperthyroidism
    Addison's disease
    Congenital adrenal hyperplasia

Others
    Urinary tract infections
    Acrodermatitis enteropathica
    Neuroblastoma and ganglioneuroma

(Lomotil)* or camphorated opium tincture (paregoric, 0.2 ml/kg/ dose) may be used sparingly. Even when spasm is reduced, fluid losses continue to occur into the lumen of the gut, but are not measurable and give a false sense of security. In toxogenic diarrhea the elimination of the toxin is also delayed by these agents.

(8) Antiemetics such as promethazine (Phenergan) or dimenhydrinate (Dramamine) (6–12 years, 12.5–25.0 mg tid) suppositories or capsules in 1 or 2 doses are useful adjuncts when simple gastroenteritis is established as the cause of vomiting. The side effects of these drugs preclude their long-term use. If vomiting persists, more vigorous evaluation and management are indicated.

(9) Close follow-up, including daily weights, is imperative, particularly in smaller infants, who may rapidly become dehydrated.

(10) **Specific therapy for acute diarrhea**

   (a) **Enterotoxigenic *Escherichia coli.*** Bismuth subsalicylate (Pepto-Bismol)

   (b) ***Shigella* species.** Trimethoprim-sulfamethoxazole (Bactrium)

   (c) ***Campylobacter fetus.*** Erythromycin

   (d) ***Clostridium difficile.*** Vancomycin, cholestyramine

   (e) ***Giardia.*** Quinacrine, metronidazole (Flagyl), bacitracin

   (f) ***Entamoeba histolytica.*** Metronidazole (Flagyl)

2. **Chronic gastroenteritis.** Diarrheal symptoms lasting more than 2 weeks are chronic. The causes of chronic diarrhea are listed in Table 10-5.

   a. **Nonspecific diarrhea** is the most common cause of chronic diarrhea in childhood.

      (1) The **etiology** is unknown. Psychosocial and family stress is often implicated.

      (2) **Evaluation and diagnosis.** The classic history is of profuse, watery diarrhea with multiple formula and dietary changes in the age group

---

*Diphenoxylate should not be used in children **under** 2 years of age. The dosage is as follows: 2–5 years, 6 mg/day; 5–8 years, 8 mg/day; 8–12 years, 10 mg/day.

1–5 years. On close questioning, parental discord or another social stress is often revealed. The physical findings and growth are normal. The findings of routine urinalysis and stool cultures are negative. The diagnosis is based on exclusion of other causes of diarrhea.

(3) Therapy. The goal of therapy is to stop diarrhea.

  (a) The family should be reassured that the illness is not too serious.

  (b) Often, past dietary manipulations may have contributed to the production of symptoms, and correction of the diet may result in relief of the diarrhea. A decrease in the intake of fructose and sucrose-containing drinks, or changing the diet, may function as a placebo.

  (c) Should reassurance and dietary adjustment fail, hospitalization may be necessary. The disappearance of diarrhea during hospitalization will help convince the family of the absence of significant disease and permit the examination of psychosocial factors.

  (d) Antidiarrheal medication is not indicated.

  (e) X-ray contrast studies should be done when it is necessary to rule out anatomic abnormalities.

C. Cystic fibrosis and Shwachman-Diamond syndrome

  1. Cystic fibrosis is an automosal recessive disorder with a gene frequency of 1:20 in which there is a dysfunction of the exocrine mucous glands. The incidence is 1 in 1,600 in whites and 1 in 2,000 in blacks. It is characterized by a diffuse chronic obstructive pulmonary disease, a pancreatic failure in approximately 80% of cases, and a threefold to fivefold increase in the Na^+ and Cl^- in sweat.

  a. The **etiology** is unknown.

  b. Clinical manifestations

    (1) Gastrointestinal

      (a) Pancreatic insufficiency occurs in 85% of patients with cystic fibrosis. These patients usually present with a history of chronic diarrhea with foul-smelling stools and failure to thrive. There are many GI manifestations of cystic fibrosis, and the disease should always be excluded in patients presenting with these features.

      (b) Meconium ileus presents with intestinal obstruction, often associated with ileal atresia, in the immediate neonatal period (see Chap. 6, pp. 184ff.) in 15% of patients. The sweat test is often not diagnostic in the first week of life, and thus the diagnosis may not be definitive until later.

      (c) Rectal prolapse is a common presenting feature.

      (d) Meconium ileus equivalent (intestinal obstruction in the older child or adult) presents with abdominal pain and may be associated with intussusception.

      (e) Cirrhosis of the liver develops in 15–20% of patients. An elevated alkaline phosphatase is often the first sign of liver involvement. Subsequent development of portal hypertension is common.

      (f) Diabetes mellitus. Overt diabetes occurs in 1% of patients with cystic fibrosis. Ketoacidosis is rare.

      (g) Gallstones occur in nearly one-third of all cystic fibrosis patients, although acute cholecystitis develops in only a few.

    (2) Pulmonary

      (a) Infancy. Cough, slight increase in the AP diameter, tachypnea, and retraction; often presents with the picture of bronchiolitis

      (b) Childhood and adolescence. A widespread process of bronchial plugging and large areas of segmental lobar atelectasis. Bronchiectasis is present as well.

      (c) Pulmonary function tests. The findings range from normal to the pattern of obstructive lung disease:

        (i) An increase in residual valine

     (ii) An increase in total lung capacity
     (iii) A decrease in vital capacity
     (iv) Decreased flow rates
     The earliest pulmonary functional change is reduction in the PO_2.
- **(d) Chronic pulmonary infection,** thick viscous sputum, frequently rich in *Pseudomonas aeruginosa* and *Staphylococcus aureus*
- **(e)** Pneumothorax (see Chap. 3, p. 54)
- **(f)** Cor pulmonale
- **(g) Hemoptysis.** Bleeding is due to rupture of small aneurysms from bronchopulmonary arterial shunts. This problem is treated with gel from embolization. Follow-up evaluation is needed.
- **(h)** Reactive airway disease and allergic aspergillosis

c. Diagnosis. Pilocarpine iontophoresis for sweat electrolytes. The results are abnormal when Cl^- is more than 60 mg/L with appropriate volume of collected sweat.

d. Therapy

(1) Treatment of GI disorder
- **(a) Pancreatic preparations.** All patients with cystic fibrosis who have steatorrhea (85%) require pancreatic enzymes. Although fat absorption improves with these agents, it does not return to normal even with massive doses.

     Various pancreatic preparations are available. The dosage can be established only by trial. Excessive dosage may result in the "meconium ileus equivalent," i.e., recurrent abdominal pain, palpable fecal masses, and obstruction. Rough dosage schedules for various pancreatic preparations are as follows:

     (i) Viokase (powder and tablets):

          Newborn, $\frac{1}{4}$–$\frac{1}{2}$ tsp/bottle
          1–2 years, $\frac{1}{2}$–1 tsp/meal, $\frac{1}{4}$ tsp/snack
          After age 3, 2–4 tablets/meal
          Adolescents, 8–12 tablets/meal

     (ii) The **Cotazym** dose is roughly $\frac{1}{2}$ that for Viokase. Cotazym can be taken before meals. The dose is titrated on stool frequency, degree of steatorrhea, and growth.
     (iii) The **Pancrease** dose is roughly one-fourth that of Viokase.
- **(b) Diet.** A low-fat diet (about 30–40 gm fat/day in older children) is indicated. Medium-chain triglycerides (MTCs), which are more readily absorbed than long-chain fats, are an important source of calories. MCT supplementation is indicated in patients with poor weight gain. Infant formulas such as Pregestimil and Portagen, supplemented with MCT, are utilized for infants with cystic fibrosis.
- **(c) Vitamins.** Multivitamins are given daily. Vitamin E and vitamin K are given as follows:
     (i) Vitamin E, until age 2–3 years, 50 IU/day; over age 3,100 IU/day
     (ii) Vitamin K, until age 1, 2.5 mg biweekly. Over age 1, vitamin K is indicated only if liver disease is present or when the PT is prolonged.
- **(d) Salt supplementation.** In hot weather, supplementary sodium chloride, 3–5 gm/day, should be given.

(2) Treatment of pulmonary disorder
- **(a)** Adequate hydration is of primary importance, and mobilization and loosening of secretions are essential.
- **(b)** Mist tents are no longer used in many institutions. Studies demonstrating lack of particle deposition in the small airways and

worsening pulmonary function tests in some patients when tents were used support the discontinuation of this practice.
- **(c) Aerosol drugs.** Any generator properly suited to deliver medications can be used. Most of the preparations include normal saline as the base solution.
- **(d)** Acetylcysteine
- **(e)** Bronchodilators
- **(f)** Expectorants
- **(g)** Chest physiotherapy can be carried out by the patient, a therapist, or an electric vibrator.
- **(h) Antimicrobial agents.** Hospitalized patients receive IV therapy (carbenicillin, gentamicin). Ambulatory patients receive a wide variety of agents, such as dicloxacillin, erythomycin, clindamycin, and cloramphenicol.
  - **(i)** Electrolyte abnormalities (e.g., hypochloremic alkalosis) are seen more frequently in patients receiving large doses of carbenicillin, and hypocalcemia and hypomagnesemia are occasionally seen in association with gentamicin.
  - **(ii) Prognosis.** The average life expectancy is now in excess of 18 years, and an optimistic outlook must be maintained.

2. Shwachman-Diamond syndrome (congenital hypoplasia of the pancreas) is a rare disease characterized by exocrine pancreatic insufficiency, growth retardation, metaphyseal dyschondroplasia, bone marrow hypoplasia, neutropenia, anemia, or thrombocytopenia. After cystic fibrosis it is the most common cause of pancreatic insufficiency in childhood.
- **a. Etiology.** This condition is probably hereditary.
- **b. Evaluation.** The **history** includes failure to thrive, chronic diarrhea, and recurrent infection. Physical examination reveals a small, malnourished child. Laboratory investigation includes a sweat test, stool examination, CBC, platelets, 72-hr stool-fat test, pancreatic function test, bone x-rays, bone marrow examination, and liver function tests.
- **c. Diagnosis**
  - **(1)** The findings of a sweat test are normal.
  - **(2)** A blood count reveals cyclic or constant neutropenia. Some patients have anemia and thrombocytopenia as well.
  - **(3)** A stool examination reveals positive Sudan stain.
  - **(4)** A 72-hr stool-fat test reveals steatorrhea.
  - **(5)** The bone marrow shows maturation arrest of the neutrophils.
  - **(6)** A bone x-ray reveals metaphyseal dysostosis in 10–15% of patients.
- **d. Treatment**
  - **(1)** Replace pancreatic enzymes [see **1.d.(1)(a)**].
  - **(2)** Give antibiotic therapy for recurrent infections.

D. Gluten-sensitive enteropathy (GSE, celiac disease) is manifested clinically by malabsorption and morphologically by a flat intestinal lesion. Both improve on a gluten-free diet and are reexacerbated by the reintroduction of gluten into the diet. It is a lifelong disease that presents most frequently between 9 and 18 months of age (earlier in formula-fed infants), but can be seen at any age.
- **1. Etiology.** The mechanism of gluten sensitivity is unknown. Genetic factors play an important role. It is more common in Ireland (1:200) than in the rest of the world (United States estimate is 1:3000). Theories as to its cause include immune mediation of gluten toxicity and an enzymatic defect.
- **2. Evaluation**
  - **a.** Relevant features in the **history** may include a family history of GSE, failure to thrive, irritability, anorexia, and chronic diarrhea.
  - **b.** The **physical examination** classically reveals an irritable, malnourished child with a pot belly and proximal muscle wasting, characteristically including the buttocks. However, some patients present atypically with features only of a selective malabsorption, i.e., only growth failure, anemia, and rickets.

   c. **Laboratory investigations** should include a blood count, serum albumin, immunoglobulin, folate, iron, iron-binding capacity, stool examination, and sweat test. **Jejunal biopsy is mandatory for the diagnosis of GSE.**
3. **Diagnosis**
   a. The finding of a **stool examination,** including culture, ova, and parasites, is negative. Clinitest findings are variable. Sudan stain and a 72-hr stool-fat test reveal steatorrhea.
   b. The results of D-xylose absorption test and lactose H_2 breath tests are abnormal.
   c. Jejunal biopsy reveals a flat, villous lesion. This is not a pathognomonic finding.
   d. **Clinical and morphologic improvement on a gluten-free diet** and exacerbation on a gluten challenge confirm the diagnosis.
4. **Treatment**
   a. A gluten-free diet is begun immediately. Rye, oats, and barley should also be excluded.
   b. Lactose should be omitted for the first 6 weeks to ameliorate the secondary disaccharide intolerance that is usually associated with GSE. Pregestimil or a soy-based formula will accomplish this purpose in infants.
   c. Irritability is the first symptom to respond to therapy; diarrheal symptoms may linger for up to 6 weeks. If diarrhea persists, it may be necessary to alter the sugar base of the formula prescribed.
   d. Vitamins and minerals should be replaced according to specific losses. A multivitamin preparation and iron are usually administered for 2–3 months, after which resolution of malabsorption permits normal dietary replacement. Common specific deficiencies are vitamin D, folic acid, vitamin K, and iron.
   e. **A gluten-free diet is maintained for life.** For this reason, confirmation of the diagnosis must be as clear as possible. It is presently accomplished by **gluten challenge.** This is done after the patient has returned to a normal growth pattern and is symptom free, usually a minimum of 1 year after the initial diagnosis.
      (1) A jejunal biopsy is performed to demonstrate a return to normal morphology.
      (2) Gluten-containing foods are reintroduced using at least two slices of white bread each day.
         Parents are often reluctant to reintroduce gluten, remembering their child's previous symptoms. On the other hand, once the child (*particularly* older children) tastes previously restricted foods, he or she may resist a return to gluten restriction. To obviate this problem, gluten powder, where available, may be sprinkled into food in a dose of 10 gm/day. In the absence of this material, gluten-rich flour may be substituted. In any case, the clinician must be resourceful, since a positive gluten challenge is the only available confirmatory test for GSE.
   f. The challenge is done for up to 6 weeks, at which time (or earlier if symptoms recur) a third jejunal biopsy is done. It is *unusual* for overt diarrheal symptoms to occur during the challenge period. If the biopsy demonstrates evidence of active enteritis, the diagnosis is confirmed. If the biopsy findings are negative, celiac disease is almost certainly not present. A subsequent biopsy may yet be needed after 1 year on the normal diet if symptoms recur.
5. **Prognosis**
   a. On adequate gluten restriction, patients achieve normal life expectancy and fertility.
   b. Spontaneous remission does not occur.
   c. Recent reports indicate an increased incidence in the subsequent development of GI malignancy in patients with GSE.

E. Disaccharidase deficiency may be primary (genetic) or secondary to intestinal mucosal damage. The most clinically relevant disaccharidases are lactase and sucrase.

1. **Lactose intolerance (primary).** Primary lactase deficiency is extremely common and an important cause of recurrent abdominal pain in childhood.
   a. **Etiology.** The condition is genetic.
   b. **Evaluation**
      (1) Lactase deficiency usually presents in blacks over 3 years of age and whites over 5 years of age. Detection of lactose intolerance prior to these ages indicates a secondary lactose intolerance.
      (2) The **history** includes recurrent abdominal pain and flatulence or diarrhea, or both.
      (3) The **physical examination** usually reveals no abnormality.
      (4) **Laboratory tests** include a stool examination, lactose tolerance test, and lactose breath test. Jejunal biopsy is usually not indicated.
   c. **Diagnosis**
      (1) The stool may be positive for reducing substances.
      (2) The results of the lactose tolerance test are usually, but not always, positive.
      (3) Jejunal biopsy shows a normal morphologic picture and normal disaccharidase levels except for lactase.
      (4) The **lactose breath test** is an easy, reliable, noninvasive test for the diagnosis of lactase deficiency.
      (5) There is usually a dramatic response to milk withdrawal in both primary and secondary lactase deficiency. It does not distinguish one from the other.
   d. **Therapy**
      (1) A lactose-free diet is begun immediately.
      (2) A calcium supplement may be needed for long-term therapy (see Food and Drug Administration requirements). This can be supplied in patients over 5–6 years of age by commercially available calcium-containing antacid tablets (e.g., Tums, Rolaids).
      (3) Lactase deficiency persists for life. However, patients may reintroduce lactose in small amounts until symptoms supervene. Lact-Aid, a commercially available lactase, appears to be of value in some patients who wish to try a limited amount of lactose.

2. **Sucrase-isomaltase deficiency**
   a. **Etiology.** This is a rare autosomal recessive disorder.
   b. **Evaluation**
      (1) **History.** These patients present with chronic diarrhea that starts with the introduction of sucrose-containing foods.
      (2) The physical findings are usually normal. Failure to thrive is not a feature of this disease.
      (3) **Laboratory tests** include stool examination, sucrose tolerance and breath tests, and jejunal biopsy.
   c. **Diagnosis**
      (1) The stools may be positive for reducing substances.
      (2) Sucrose tolerance test findings are usually positive.
      (3) The sucrose breath test is a reliable indicator of the presence of sucrase-isomaltase deficiency.
      (4) Jejunal biopsy shows a normal histologic picture and, except for low to absent sucrase-isomaltase, normal disaccharide levels.
   d. **Treatment**
      (1) A sucrose-free diet is instituted immediately, usually with a dramatic response.
      (2) Sucrose-isomaltose restriction is lifelong.
      (3) Dietary supplements are not indicated.

F. Food sensitivity. The most common food sensitivities associated with GI disease are cow's milk and soy protein.

1. **Cow's milk protein sensitivity.** The incidence of cow's milk protein sensitivity is estimated at 0.5–1.0% of infants under 6 months of age.
   a. **Etiology.** Systemic sensitivity (e.g., anaphylaxis, wheezing) to cow's milk appears to be mediated by immediate hypersensitivity (IgE), whereas GI disease **appears not to be mediated in this manner.** GI involvement is usually limited to the upper GI tract or to the colon.
   b. **Evaluation.** Sensitivity to cow's milk usually presents in infants.
      (1) The **history** may include pallor, edema, irritability, vomiting, diarrhea, colic, and failure to thrive.
      (2) The **physical examination** may reveal a pale, edematous child. Some infants may present with a colitislike picture with profuse, bloody diarrhea.
      (3) **Laboratory tests** include a CBC, serum albumin and immunoglobulins, serum iron, iron-binding capacity, IgE, radioallergosorbent test (RAST) to milk sensitivity, gastric and intestinal biopsy, sigmoidoscopy, and rectal biopsy (if the patient has grossly bloody diarrhea). **Occult blood is always present in the stool.**
   c. **Diagnosis**
      (1) The CBC shows iron deficiency anemia and eosinophilia.
      (2) Serum protein analysis (SPA) reveals low serum albumin and immunoglobulins.
      (3) IgE levels are normal and the RAST is negative in GI disease alone, but usually not in systemic allergic disease.
      (4) Gastric biopsy may reveal a gastritis with eosinophilic infiltration.
      (5) Small-intestine biopsy reveals a patchy, flat, villous lesion.
      (6) In patients with colonic involvement, sigmoidoscopy reveals colitis.
      (7) Withdrawl of milk protein (not lactose) produces a dramatic clinical and morphologic response. Reintroduction of milk protein after remission produces exacerbation of clinical and morphologic abnormalities. Unlike GSE, this disease is transient, and milk protein can be tolerated after the age of 2. A **milk challenge should not be attempted in patients with a history of milk anaphylaxis.** In patients with GI disease who have negative skin tests and normal serum IgE, mild challenge is a safe technique.
   d. **Therapy**
      (1) A milk-free diet is instituted immediately.
      (2) In view of associated secondary disaccharidase deficiency, a disaccharide-free formula or diet is introduced.
      (3) An iron supplement should be provided.
2. **Soy protein sensitivity.** The incidence of isolated soy sensitivity is unknown. It is estimated that 10% of patients with milk sensitivity have associated soy sensitivity.
   a. **Etiology.** The cause is unknown.
   b. **Evaluation.** The history, physical examination, and laboratory investigations are similar to those carried out in patients with cow's milk sensitivity. The syndrome is usually seen in infants for whom soy formulas have been prescribed.
   c. **Diagnosis**
      (1) The CBC shows iron deficiency anemia and eosinophilia.
      (2) SPA reveals low levels of serum albumin and immunoglobulins.
      (3) IgE levels are normal. The RAST reaction is negative in GI disease alone but positive in systemic allergic disease.
      (4) Gastric biopsy may reveal a gastritis with eosinophilic infiltration.
      (5) Small-intestine biopsy reveals a patchy, flat, villous lesion.
      (6) Sigmoidoscopy reveals colitis.
      (7) Withdrawal of soy protein produces a dramatic clinical response.
      (8) Rechallenge after remission will reproduce abnormalities in a manner similar to that occurring with milk challenge.
      (9) It is unknown whether this lesion is transient or permanent.

d. Therapy
   (1) A soy protein-free diet is instituted.
   (2) An iron supplement is indicated.
3. Eosinophilic gastroenteritis
   a. Etiology. The cause is unknown.
   b. Evaluation
      (1) The history reveals the onset of systemic allergy (usually asthma) and abdominal pain.
      (2) Growth failure is a prominent part of the syndrome. The physical findings may also include pallor and edema.
      (3) Laboratory investigations include a stool guaiac test, CBC, SPA, IgE, serum iron, and skin and RAST test reactions to various foods (see Chap. 19, p. 479).
   c. Diagnosis
      (1) The CBC reveals peripheral eosinophilia and iron deficiency anemia.
      (2) SPA reveals hypoalbuminemia and hypogammaglobulinemia.
      (3) Serum IgE is elevated.
      (4) RAST and skin test reactions to many foods are positive.
      (5) Gastric biopsy reveals gastritis with eosinophilic infiltration.
      (6) Jejunal biopsy reveals a patchy, flat, villous lesion.
      (7) An upper GI series reveals an abnormal antrum and abnormal gastric mucosa.
   d. Treatment
      (1) Dietary manipulations may alleviate acute symptoms (anaphylaxis) but have no effect on the chronic course of disease.
      (2) Initially, prednisone in a dose of 1–2 mg/kg/day is used. Then alternate-day corticosteroids may be used.
      (3) Vitamins and iron supplements are indicated.
      (4) Unlike cow's milk sensitivity, eosinophilic gastritis (like GSE) appears to be a lifelong condition.
G. Inflammatory bowel disease
   1. Ulcerative colitis
      a. Etiology. Ulcerative colitis is a chronic inflammatory mucosal disease of unknown origin. Genetic, environmental, psychological, infectious, and immunologic mechanisms have been implicated.
      b. Evaluation
         (1) The **history** usually includes bloody diarrhea and recurrent abdominal pain.
         (2) Systemic manifestations, including arthritis, erythema nodosum, uveitis, episcleritis, and liver disease, may precede or accompany the GI symptoms.
         (3) The findings on **examination of the abdomen** are usually benign, unless local complications of toxic megacolon or perforation have occurred. Growth failure may be present. Laboratory tests include CBC, stool examination, cultures, ova and parasites, SPA, sigmoidoscopy, rectal biopsy, barium enema, and upper GI series.
      c. Diagnosis
         (1) Stool examination reveals blood and fecal leukocytes.
         (2) Sigmoidoscopy reveals colitis, confirmed by rectal biopsy.
         (3) Stool cultures are negative, and ova and parasites are not present.
         (4) The CBC reveals anemia, leukocytosis with left shift, thrombocytosis, and elevated ESR.
         (5) Serum albumin levels may be low or normal.
         (6) A barium enema reveals colitis (the findings may be normal in the early stages of the disease). An upper GI series reveals nothing abnormal.
      d. Treatment depends on the severity of the symptoms and signs.
         (1) Sulfasalazine (Azulfidine) is usually the drug of choice in mild to moderate cases. Therapy is begun at 500 mg/day and increased over

4–5 days to 2–3 gm/day in 3 divided doses. Under the age of 5 years 50 mg tid should be sufficient. Side effects include leukopenia agranulocytosis, hemolytic anemia, arthralgia, headache, rash, and rarely, lower GI bleeding.

(2) Corticosteroids are the mainstay of therapy in inflammatory bowel disease. In the moderate case in which sulfasalazine alone is inadequate, prednisone, 1–2 mg/kg/day in a daily dose, is given. In patients requiring IV therapy, methylprednisolone sodium succinate (Solu-Medrol), 1–2 mg/kg/day in 2–4 divided doses is indicated. In limited rectal disease methylpredisolone (Medrol) enemas are prefered to systemic therapy.

(3) Parenteral alimentation should be used in all patients requiring IV therapy.

(4) Psychiatric consultation may be required to assist the patient, or the parents, or both to cope with chronic ulcers.

(5) Surgery. Colectomy is curative. The indications are:
  (a) Perforation
  (b) Toxic megacolon
  (c) Massive bleeding
  (d) Severe corticosteroid side effects that preclude further use
  (e) Malignancy. There is a definite risk of the development of colon cancer in patients with long-standing ulcerative colitis. Appropriate screening, such as colonoscopy and rectal biopsy, should be performed annually for more than 10 years on patients with the disease. Any sign of dysplasia on biopsy is an absolute indication for colectomy.

2. Crohn's disease
  a. Etiology. This is a chronic transmural and predominantly submucosal inflammatory disease of unknown etiology that can affect any part of the GI tract from mouth to anus, most often affecting the distal ileum and colon while sparing the rectum.
  b. Evaluation
    (1) The **history** commonly includes growth failure, recurrent fever, abdominal pain, and diarrhea. Systemic symptoms include arthritis and erythema nodosum.
    (2) Physical examination may reveal evidence of malnutrition, localized abdominal signs or perianal disease on rectal examination, and blood and mucus. Laboratory tests include a CBC, ESR, SPA, electrolytes, iron, iron-binding capacity, folate, sigmoidoscopy, barium enema, and upper GI series.
  c. Diagnosis
    (1) Stools. Cultures are negative for bacteria, ova, and parasites. Leukocytes are present. The guaiac test findings are positive if colitis is present.
    (2) A CBC reveals anemia, leukocytosis with left shift, and thombocytosis. The ESR is elevated.
    (3) Serum iron and folate are low, and iron-binding capacity is increased.
    (4) SPA reveals a serum albumin that may be low.
    (5) Sigmoidoscopy may show colitis (if the colon is involved).
    (6) A barium enema, or upper GI series, or both, may show involvement.
    (7) Growth failure. Severe growth failure occurs in 30% of patients with Crohn's disease. Less than 5% of patients have malabsorption. The cause of growth failure is believed to be lack of caloric intake.
    (8) Periodic flare-ups are very common in the clinical course.
    (9) The Schilling test might be abnormal.
  d. Treatment
    (1) Colonic Crohn's. Sulfasalazine (Azulfidine) and corticosteroids as in ulcerative colitis

able 10-6. Clinical, pathologic, and radiographic
eatures of ulcerative colitis and Crohn's disease

'eatures	Ulcerative colitis	Crohn's disease
)iarrhea	Severe	Moderate or absent
tectal bleeding	Common	Rare
bdominal pain	Frequent	Common
Veight loss	Moderate	Severe
irowth retardation	Mild	Severe
:xtraintestinal man- ifestations	Common	Common
'ercentage with bowel involvement		
Anus	15	85
Rectum	95	50
Colon	100	50
Ileum	0 (except for backwash ileitis)	80
)istribution of lesions	Continuous	Skip areas
'athologic features	Diffuse mucosal disease	Granulomas; focal disease
tadiographic features	Loss of haustra Superficial ulcers No skip areas	Thumbprinting Skip areas String sight
:ancer risk	High	Less than with ulcerative colitis but still increased

(2) **Ileal Crohn's.** Corticosteroids are the drug of choice. Sulfasalazine is not useful for this specific disease. Azathioprine (Imuran) and 6-mercaptopurine have been used with satisfactory results in patients with dependence or undesirable side reactions to corticosteroids.

(3) **Perianal fistula.** Metronidazole (Flagyl), 250 mg PO tid, has been used with benefit.

(4) Antispasmodics have no place in the management of acute disease. However, in chronic disease, with diarrhea and tenesmus, their use is recommended (deodorized tincture of opium, diphenoxylate and loperamide hydrochloride).

(5) The use of elemental formula supplementation has proved of benefit for patients with Crohn's disease and growth failure.

(6) Total parenteral nutrition has been used with good success in prepubertal patients to promote growth and initiate puberty in those who fail to respond to corticosteroids. It does not, however, modify the course of acute disease.

(7) **Psychiatric consultation** is useful for the patients and their families in managing this chronic, often debilitating, disease.

(8) The **indications for surgery** are less clear-cut than for ulcerative colitis because of the chronic nature of this disease. They include:

(a) Perforation

(b) Obstruction

(c) Extensive perianal or rectal disease unresponsive to other therapeutic modalities

(d) Severe growth failure, in which a localized segment may be removed. (See Table 10-6 for a comparison of the features of ulcerative colitis and Crohn's disease.)

H. Hirschsprung's disease (congenital, aganglionic megacolon). Congenital absence of the intrinsic ganglionic plexus of Auerbach and Meissner, which involves varying lengths of the rectum and colon. The incidence is estimated at 1 in 5,000. A family incidence exists in 10% of cases.

1. **Etiology.** The cause is unknown.
2. **Evaluation.** The **neonatal history** includes failure to pass meconium in the first 24 hr of life or bile-stained vomiting in the first week of life. In late infancy and childhood the history is of increasing constipation. **Rectal examination** classically reveals an empty rectum followed by an explosive gush of stool and gas. In the neonatal period abdominal distention is a prominent feature, whereas in the older child, fecal masses are palpable. **Laboratory investigations** include a kidney-ureter-bladder (KUB) study, barium enema, rectal manometry, and rectal biopsy.
3. **Diagnosis**
   a. X-rays of the abdomen reveal dilated loops of bowel on an anteroposterior film. Rectal air is absent.
   b. The **barium enema** is usually diagnostic, revealing a narrow aganglionic segment with a dilated colon above. In the immediate neonatal period this typical pattern may be absent. An important clue will be a 24-hr film showing that the barium is still present. Rarely, in "low segment" Hirschsprung's disease, the barium enema findings may be normal or nondiagnostic.
   c. Rectal manometry may reveal absence of the normal relaxation reflex of the internal sphincter.
   d. **Rectal biopsy** is the definitive method of diagnosis. If a suction biopsy does not reveal ganglion cells, a full-thickness surgical biopsy is necessary. Rarely, if symptoms persist when laboratory findings are normal, a second or even a third biopsy may be needed.
4. **Treatment**
   a. The neonate is often extremely ill, with enterocolitis, shock, and sepsis.
      (1) A nasogastric tube is passed for decompression.
      (2) Urgent rehydration is begun.
      (3) Antibiotics are indicated.
      (4) An emergency colostomy is performed in an area of the colon where ganglion cells are seen.
      (5) Resection of the aganglionic segment is delayed for 6 months to 2 years.
   b. In infants and children who are relatively well, the definitive surgery may be performed with a diverting colostomy.
   c. **Surgical management.** Three types of operations have been in vogue.
      (1) **Swenson.** Aganglionic colon is resected, and the ganglion-containing bowel is anastomosed to the rectal stump.
      (2) **Duhamel.** A longer piece of rectum, usually 5–7 cm, is left and closed proximally. Ganglionic bowel is pulled down retrorectally to 1 cm from the mucocutaneous junction, leaving part of the internal sphincter intact. Colorectal anastomosis is achieved by clamping the posterior wall of the rectum to the anterior wall of the colon.
      (3) **Soave.** This operation leaves 10–20 cm of rectal stump. The mucosa is stripped and the ganglionic bowel pulled through.
   d. **Surgical complications**
      (1) **Following colostomy**
         (a) Circulatory collapse resulting in severe enterocolitis may occur following colostomy for decompression. Treatment is supportive, i.e., fluid and electrolyte replacement and antibiotics.
         (b) Persistent diarrhea, which is often due to disaccharide deficiency, may occur. A Clinitest is positive, and a change in the type of sugar in the formula will alleviate symptoms.

Table 10-7. Causes of hepatic failure in childhood

Infections
　Viral hepatitis, particularly hepatitis B, non-A, non-B hepatitis (rare
　　in Type A)
　Leptospirosis
　Adenovirus
　Coxsackievirus
　Infectious mononucleosis
　Q fever
　Disseminated herpes simplex virus
　Clostridium perfringens

Metabolic abnormalities
　Reye syndrome
　Wilson's disease

Drugs, chemicals, poisons
　Acetaminophen
　Salicylates
　Tetracycline
　Carbon tetrachloride
　Ethanol
　Phosphorus
　Anesthetic agents
　　Halothane (fluothane)
　　Methoxyflurane (penthrane)
　Mushrooms (*Amanita phalloides*)

Ischemia and hypoxia
　Acute circulatory failure
　Acute Budd-Chiari syndrome
　Acute pulmonary failure
　Ligation of hepatic artery
　Heat stroke

---

　　(2) After definitive surgery. Segmental obstruction with overflow incon-
　　　tinence is often a problem, especially in the first few months after
　　　surgery.
I. Hepatic failure
　1. Etiology. Acute hepatic failure is a clinical syndrome resulting from severe
　　hepatic dysfunction or massive hepatic necrosis. The causes are listed in
　　Table 10-7.
　2. Evaluation
　　a. The **history** may reveal evidence of a previous viral infection; exposure to
　　　blood products, drugs, or chemicals; circulatory collapse; preexisting liver
　　　disease, or a family history of liver disease.
　　b. The **physical examination** reveals progressive jaundice (except in Reye
　　　syndrome), asterixis ("liver flap"), fetor hepaticus, mental confusion, or
　　　coma.
　　c. **Laboratory investigations** include urinalysis, CBC, platelet count, re-
　　　ticulocyte count, monospot test, PT, PTT, BUN, electrolytes, glucose,
　　　creatinine, ammonia, SGOT, SGPT, alkaline phosphatase, bilirubin,
　　　blood gases, serum albumin, serologic tests for hepatitis B, slit-lamp ex-
　　　amination for Kayser-Fleischer rings, serum copper, ceruloplasmin, 24-
　　　hr urine copper, alpha$_1$-antitrypsin level, and toxic screen.

3. Diagnosis
   a. The blood count may reveal leukocytosis, or hemolytic anemia, or both. (Always rule out Wilson's disease when liver disease and hemolytic anemia occur.)
   b. PT and PTT are prolonged. Serum albumin may be low. These measurements reflect impaired liver synthetic function.
   c. SGOT and SGPT are increased and reflect liver structural damage, with leakage of enzymes from hepatocytes.
   d. Alkaline phosphatase may be normal or increased.
   e. Serum bilirubin is usually increased except in Reye syndrome. The increase is usually both in direct and indirect bilirubin fractions.
   f. Blood glucose may be low.
   g. BUN and electrolytes may reflect electrolyte imbalance, especially hypokalemia and hyponatremia.
   h. Blood gases may reveal a metabolic alkalosis or, less commonly, acidosis.
   i. Serologic tests for hepatitis B (HbsAg, HbsAb, HbcAg, HbcAb) may be positive.
   j. Serum copper may be low. Ceruloplasmin is low, with increased 24-hr urinary copper excretion. These findings may suggest Wilson's disease and further diagnostic tests (e.g., slit-lamp examination for Kayser Fleischer rings and liver copper) are needed.
   k. The findings of a toxic screen may be positive if ingestion has occurred.
4. Treatment. The purpose of therapy is to alleviate the systemic effects of liver failure and promote liver cell regeneration.
   a. Prepare a flow sheet to record laboratory data and daily intake and output.
   b. Give a 10–15% glucose solution IV at a rate dependent on renal function. Monitor blood glucose.
   c. Give vitamin K, 5–10 mg/day IV, for 3 days or while PT remains prolonged. If therapy is needed for more than 3 days, reduce this vitamin K dose to 1–2 mg daily. Fresh frozen plasma may be required to control bleeding.
   d. To decrease ammonia production, do the following:
      (1) Initially, give 10 gm of protein/day if the patient is able to take food orally.
      (2) Give lactulose, 1 ml/kg q6h, or neomycin, 50 mg/kg/day q6h, or both, to reduce the activity of endogenous flora.
      (3) Prevent constipation with magnesium citrate (4–8 gm).
   e. Pass a nasogastric tube to identify GI bleeding and as a route for medication.
   f. A central venous pressure line is needed to maintain fluid balance.
   g. Avoid all sedatives, especially those metabolized by the liver (e.g., barbiturates).
   h. Always culture urine, blood, and ascitic fluid.
   i. Treat GI bleeding vigorously. If gastritis or peptic ulcer disease is present, start cimetidine, 300 mg IV q6h (children under 12 years, 5–10 mg/kg q6h). Monitor gastric pH > 5. If bleeding is due to varices, use a Sengstaken-Blakemore tube, or a vasopressin infusion may be necessary. In certain circumstances, emergency surgery may be undertaken.
   j. Monitor serum and urinary electrolytes daily. Characteristically, low urinary sodium and high urinary potassium with urine osmolarity greater than plasma osmolarity are found. Table 10-8 gives the differential diagnosis of renal impairment in severe liver failure.
   k. If intravascular volume and serum albumin are low, give albumin, 1.75 gm/kg. This dose will increase serum albumin 1 gm/100 ml.
J. Pathologic gastroesophageal reflux is defined as the abnormal clearance of acid from the distal esophagus. It differs from the *chalasia of infancy,* which is defined as the regurgitation of gastric contents into the esophagus without pathologic complications.

Table 10-8. Differentiation of renal disorders associated with hepatic failure

Feature	Renal circulatory failure	Acute tubular necrosis	Preexisting renal disease
Liver function	Severely impaired	Variable	Variable
Ascites	Usually	Sometimes	Sometimes
Encephalopathy	Usually	Sometimes	Sometimes
Precipitating factors	Diuretics Paracentesis GI bleeding	Hypotension	Variable
Course	Slow	Rapid	Slow
Hypotension	Late	Early	None
Oliguria	Gradual	Acute	Variable
Urine sediment	Normal	Abnormal	Abnormal
Urine osmolarity	Greater than plasma	Low, fixed	Low
Urine sodium	Very low	Moderate	Moderate
Kidney size	Normal	Normal or large	Small
Renal pathologic findings	None	Often	Yes

Source: Adapted from W. P. Baldus, *Prog. Liver Dis.* 4:251, 1972.

1. The **etiology** is unknown.
2. **Clinical manifestations** include (also see *Gastroenterology* 81:376, 1981):
   a. Recurrent emesis
   b. Recurrent pneumonia
   c. Asthma
   d. Sudden infant death syndrome, apnea
   e. Failure to thrive
   f. Sandifer syndrome
   g. Heartburn (pyrosis)
   h. Dysphagia
   i. Nocturnal cough and wheeze
   j. Hematemesis
   k. Rumination
   l. Iron deficiency anemia
3. **Diagnosis**
   a. The **continuous intraesophageal pH probe study** is the best test to evaluate acid clearance. It is positive when a sustained pH less than 4 lasts for more than 4 min. It should be over an 18- to 24-hr period.
   b. **Esophageal manometry** to assess esophageal motility and lower esophageal sphincter pressure
   c. **Upper GI series** to assess anatomy, the presence of strictures, and the gastric outlet
   d. **A technetium 99-m scan** (milk scan) to assess pathologic reflux, regurgitation of gastric contents into the lungs, and gastric emptying
   e. **Endoscopy** and **biopsy** to evaluate the presence of esophagitis (basal zone hyperplasia, infiltration of neutrophils, and the presence of intraepithelial eosinophils)
   f. **Treatment for children with chalasia of infancy.** Upright posturing and frequent small, thickened feedings are sufficient. For children with abnormal acid clearance, the following therapy is recommended:
      (1) **Antacid therapy** (alternating AlternaGEL and Mylanta). The dose is 0.5–1.0 ml/kg 1 and 3 hr after meals and at bedtime.

Table 10-9. Clinical and laboratory manifestations in Wilson's disease, by stage

Stage	Description	Kayser-Fleischer rings	Serum copper	Ceruloplasmin	Urine coppe
I	Hepatic copper accumulation	0	D	D	N,I
IIA	Hemolytic anemia	0, +	N,I	D	I
IIB	Hepatic failure	0, +	N,I	D,N,I	N,I
III	Cerebral copper accumulation	0, +	D	D	I
IV	Neurologic disease	+	D	D	I
V	Copper balance on therapy	0	D	D	I

0 = absent; + = present; D = decreased; I = increased; N = normal.
Source: R. J. Grand et al., *J. Pediatr.* 87:1161, 1975.

    (2) Therapy to increase sphincter pressure. Bethanechol chloride (Urecholine), 2.9 mg/M^2/dose PO q8h. The maximum single dose is 50 mg.

    (3) Therapy to lower sphincter pressure and enhance gastric emptying. Metoclopramide (Reglan), 0.25–0.5 mg/kg/day PO.

    (4) Therapy to block acid secretion. Cimetidine (H$_2$ blocker) is used. The recommended dosage is 5–10 mg/kg/dose q6–8h. A bedtime dose is indicated when the medication is tapered down. If intensive medical therapy fails, surgical intervention is indicated (Nissen fundoplication).

K. Wilson's disease (Table 10-9) is a autosomal recessive metabolic disorder, associated with consanguinity, characterized by cirrhosis of the liver, bilateral softening of the basal ganglia of the brain, and greenish brown pigmented rings in the periphery of the cornea (Kayser-Fleischer rings).

    1. The **etiology** is unknown.

    2. Clinical manifestations include:

      a. Onset

        (1) The majority of patients become symptomatic between 6–20 years of age.

        (2) The presenting features are variable and include the liver, kidney, and CNS.

        (3) Clinical disease rarely presents before age 4–5 years.

      b. Modes of presentation include:

        (1) Acute hepatitis

        (2) Chronic active liver disease

        (3) Cirrhosis

        (4) Fulminant hepatic failure

        (5) Hemolytic anemia

        (6) Neurologic disease

          (a) "Clumsiness," poor handwriting, tremors

          (b) Slurring of speech, dysarthria, behavioral disturbances

          (c) Dystonia, fixed facial expression, rigidity, athetoid movements

        (7) Renal disease

          (a) Renal tubular acidosis

          (b) Reduced GFR

          (c) Increased urate clearance, decreased serum uric acid levels

          (d) Aminoaciduria (threonine, crystine), glycosuria, proteinuria

          (e) Hyperphosphaturia

      (8) Bones and joints

          (a) Osteoporosis

          (b) Osteoarthritis

3. Diagnosis

    a. Clinical history and **family history,** especially regarding psychiatric or neurologic disease and childhood deaths

    b. Neurologic and general physical examination

    c. Examination with slit lamp for Kaiser-Fleischer ring. Gross inspection is inadequate.

    d. Laboratory

      (1) Blood. Hemoglobin, reticulocytes, smear, iron, haptoglobin, ceruloplasmin, other proteins, and PT

      (2) Liver. Liver function tests and ^{99m}Tc scan

      (3) Copper. Serum levels, 24-hr urine value, and hepatic content

      (4) Urine. Aminoaciduria, protein, sugar, uric acid, and 24-hr copper level

4. Treatment

    a. Penicillamine (β_1 β-dimethylcysteine) is the treatment of choice. The dosage is 1.2 gm of D-penicillamine hydrochloride PO qid before meals. If there is no improvement, the dosage can be increased to 2 gm daily.

      (1) The side effects of penicillamine include skin rashes, leukopenia, aplastic anemia, nephrotic syndrome, a lupuslike syndrome, and hemolytic anemia.

      (2) An alternative agent, trilene (triethylene tetramine), can be used, but it has more side effects.

    b. Diet

      (1) Avoid organ meats, shellfish, dried beans and peas, whole wheat, and chocolate.

      (2) Allow scotch or whiskey in adults.

      (3) Try to limit copper intake to 1 mg/day.

      (4) Measure tap water for copper.

L. Acute pancreatitis is a systemic disease characterized by acute inflammation of the pancreas. On a pathologic basis it is divided into two distinct entities: edematous (or interstitial) and hemorrhagic (or necrotic) pancreatitis.

  1. Etiology

    a. Trauma: blunt, penetrating, or surgical

    b. Infectious. Mumps, coxsackievirus B, rubella, measles, *Mycoplasma,* and septic shock

    c. Systemic disease. Diabetes mellitus, systemic lupus erythematosus, periarteritis nodosa, uremia, hypercalcemia, Henoch-Schönlein purpura, Reye syndrome, and cystic fibrosis

    d. Drugs and toxins. Azathioprine, thiazides, sulfonamides, furosemide, tetracycline, corticosteroids, L-asparginase, ethanol

    e. Obstruction to flow

      (1) Congenital. Absence of pancreatic duct, absence of common bile duct, stenosis of ampulla of Vater, and choledochal cyst duplications

      (2) Acquired. Trauma, gallstones, tumors, pseudocyst, infection in the ducts, *Ascaris*

    f. Hereditary. Hyperlipoproteinemia (types I and V), hyperparathyroidism

    g. Miscellaneous. Postoperative, graft versus host disease, idiopathic, penetrating peptic ulcer

  2. Clinical manifestations include abdominal pain, nausea and vomiting, fever, ileus, and shock. It can also present as chronic upper abdominal pain and epigastric tenderness, ascites of unknown etiology, or following abdominal trauma.

Table 10-10. Hepatomegaly

Mechanism	Entity
Inflammation	TORCH infections
	Hepatitis B, A, non-A non-B
	Hepatic abscess (pyogenic, amebic)
	VLM, schistosomiasis, liver flukes
	Toxin and drug injury
	Intra- and extra-hepatic
	Biliary tract obstruction
Congestion	Hepatic cirrhosis/Wilson's disease
	Stenosis or thrombosis of portal of splenic vein
	Myeloid metaplasia
	Vinyl chloride
	Biliary atresia
Storage	Glycogen storage disease
	Mucopolysaccharidoses
	Gaucher's disease
	Niemann-Pick disease
	Gangliosidosis M_1
	Alpha$_1$-antitrypsin deficiency
	Amyloidosis
	Porphyrias
	Wilson's disease
Infiltrative lesions	Erythroblastosis fetalis
	Metastatic tumor
	Histiocytosis
	Leukemia
	Lymphoma
	Hepatomas
	Hemochromatosis
	Amyloid
	Extramedullary hematopoiesis
Intrinsic	Cirrhosis, PBC
	Congenital hepatic fibrosis
	Multicystic liver and kidney disease
	Hereditary hemorrhagic telangiectasia
Kupffer cell hyperplasia	Sepsis
	Granulomatous hepatitis
	Hypervitaminosis A

Source: Modified from W. A. Walker, et al. *Pediatr. Clin. North Am.* 22:929, 1975.

3. **Diagnosis**
   a. Elevated serum or urine **amylase** or **lipase** only supports rather than proves the diagnosis of pancreatitis. Remember that amylase can be detected in other organs (parotid gland, fallopian tube, small intestine).

   b. $Cam/Cr = \dfrac{\text{amylase (urine)}}{\text{amylase (serum)}} \times \dfrac{\text{creatinine (serum)}}{\text{creatinine (urine)}}$

   $\times$ 100 should be less than 4%. Values above 6.5% are suggestive of pancreatitis.
   c. Liver function tests (SGOT, SGPT, alkaline phosphatase)
   d. CBC, BUN, creatinine, and electrolytes
   e. Glucose and Ca should be monitored.

Table 10-11. Splenomegaly

Inflammation or immunologic	Subacute bacterial endocarditis
	Brucellosis
	Tuberculosis
	Mononucleosis
	TORCH infections
	Malaria
	Schistosomiasis
	RA, SLE, Felty syndrome
	Sarcoidosis
	Typhoid fever
	Sepsis
Congestion	Congestive heart failure
	Budd-Chiari syndrome
	Congestive pericarditis
	Cavernous transformation
Sequestration	Sickle cell disease
	Thalassemia
	RBC enzyme deficiencies
	Rh and ABO incompatibility
	Autoimmune hemolytic anemia
	Galactosemia
	Wolman's disease
	Reye syndrome
	Tetracycline toxicity
Infiltrative lesions	Leukemia
	Lymphoma
	Histiocytosis
	Metastatic neuroblastoma
	Polycythemia
	Myelofibrosis
Other	Splenic trauma
	Splenic hemangiomas or cysts

Source: Modified from M. K. Younoszai, et al. *Clin. Pediatr.* 14:378, 1975.

      f. Abdominal ultrasound
      g. A CT scan (abdomen)
      h. A chest x-ray to detect pleural effusion and pulmonary edema
   4. Treatment
      a. Treat fluid and electrolyte imbalance, specifically hypovolemia, hypocalcemia, and hyperglycemia.
      b. Stop enteral feeding until there is no amylase and no evidence of abdominal pain.
      c. Relieve pain using meperidine q3–4h by the IV route.
      d. Aspiration by nasogastric tube (to reduce pancreatic stimulation and prevent paralytic ileus)
      e. Use of total parenteral nutrition (peripheral or central)
      f. Anticholinergics, antacids, and H_2 blockers are very controversial, but can be used.
      g. Monitor for respiratory insufficiency and renal failure.
      h. Other medications, such as calcitonin, glucagon, somatostatin, and proteinase inhibitors have been used without any good evidence for their benefit.
      i. Remember to be aware of further complications such as pancreatic pseudocyst and pancreatic fistula.

M. Hepatomegaly and splenomegaly. Differential diagnoses for childhood hepatomegaly and splenomegaly are listed in Tables 10-10 and 10-11.

N. Protein-energy malnutrition. Sustained deficits in the daily intake of protein or energy in relationship to specific requirements for nitrogen-amino acids and calories will result in the clinical syndrome of protein energy malnutrition. This broad spectrum of protein-energy deficiency is conditioned by several factors: the severity of the deficiency, the duration, the age of the host, the cause of the deficiency, and the relative severity of protein versus energy deficiency (*Am. J Clin Nutr.* 23:67, 1970). It is essential to understand that adequate nutrition is the most important aspect of therapy in acute and chronic illness.

  1. Classification

  a. A child with **marasmus** has a caloric deficiency and an expected weight for age of less than 60% of normal. The clinical characteristics include the following:

  (1) The age of maximal incidence is 6–18 months.

  (2) No clinical evidence of edema with normal serum albumin ("skin and bones")

  (3) Poor nitrogen retention

  (4) No fatty infiltration of the liver

  (5) A slow response to dietary therapy during the first 4 weeks

  b. Kwashiorkor is predominantly a protein deficiency, usually with the child having a minimum weight not less than 60% of expected weight for age. It has the following characteristics:

  (1) The age of maximal incidence is 12–48 months.

  (2) Clinical evidence of edema with low albumin

  (3) Fatty infiltration of the liver

  (4) Initial weight loss with delivery of edema

  c. Intermediate protein-energy malnutrition occurs in children weighing less than 60% of the expected weight but without the salient features of either marasmus or kwashiorkor (see *Br. Med. J.* 3:566, 1972).

  2. Diagnosis. See **A.l** for assessment of malnutrition.

  3. Therapy. See **4.a.**

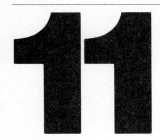

Disorders of the Endocrine System

I. General approach to endocrine disorders. Deviations from the normal rate or sequence of growth and development are frequent reasons that endocrine disorders are suspected in pediatric patients. Morphologic aberrations and behavioral changes are common in endocrine abnormalities.

A. The endocrine history

　　1. A more directed history is frequently necessary, expanding the review of systems to include such items as a detailed summary of intake, sleep patterns, bowel and bladder habits, activity level, and school performance.

　　2. The **family history** can be used to help assess the patient's growth and development. Actual somatic measurements of family members improve the accuracy of examination.

B. The physical examination assesses somatic growth, sexual development, and the rate and sequence of bodily changes documented by serial measurements. Measurements are compared to normative data (see Chap. 2, Figs. 2-5 and 2-6; and Tables 11-1 and 11-2) and considered in light of the family growth history.

C. Screening laboratory tests. Few screening tests can be recommended as a routine. Rather, specific laboratory studies are suggested on the basis of the history and physical examination.

　　1. Bone age of the left hand and wrist reflects a composite of biologic growth. Comparison of bone age to height age, as well as to chronological age, may differentiate normal from pathologic conditions.

　　2. Twenty-four-hour urine collections should be obtained from 8 A.M. to 8 A.M. the following day. Since most hormones are subject to cyclic secretion, a 24-hr interpretation of their metabolites minimizes temporal variation. Adequacy of collection may be estimated by measuring the milligrams of creatinine per total volume. (Normal ranges of urinary creatinine excretion are between 10 mg/kg/day in infants and 20–22 mg/kg/day in adults.)

D. Therapy

　　1. Since most endocrine disorders are chronic diseases, **parent and patient education (and reeducation)** are essential if life-styles are to be as normal as possible. The social effects of an often highly visible condition must be approached with concern and support. The importance of relating the child to his or her chronological age, despite size or sexual development, should be emphasized.

　　2. Hormonal therapy is at best an artificial replacement, is not as sensitive as endogenous secretion, and is always dependent on compliance.

　　3. Personality and behavior may be affected directly by hormonal excess or deficiency. It may be difficult to determine the relative contributions of organic factors and psychological problems incurred because of a chronic disease.

　　4. Medic Alert bracelets or **necklaces** should be worn by patients with diabetes mellitus, diabetes insipidus, congenital adrenogenital hyperplasia, and adrenal insufficiency.

II. Disorders of growth

A. Short stature

　　1. Etiology. See Table 11-3.

　　2. Evaluation of patients with short stature should determine whether or not the patient has a disorder for which therapy is available.

Table 11-1. Tanner stages of sexual development

Stage	Characteristics	Age at onset
Genital stages: male		
1	Prepubertal	
2	Scrotum and testes enlarge	11.4 ± 1.1 yrs
	Skin of scrotum reddens and rugations appear	
3	Penis lengthens	12.9 ± 1.0 yrs
	Testes enlarge further	
4	Penis growth continues in length and width	13.8 ± 1.0 yrs
	Glans develops adult form	
5	Development completed; adult form	14.9 ± 1.1 yrs
Breast development: female		
1	Prepubertal	
2	Breast buds appear	11.2 ± 1.1 yrs
	Areolae enlarge	
3	Elevation of breast contour	12.2 + 1.1 yrs
	Areolae enlarge	
4	Areolae and papilla for a secondary mound on breast	13.1 ± 1.2 yrs
5	Adult form	15.3 ± 1.7 yrs
Menarche		13.5 ± 1.0 yrs
Pubic hair: both sexes		
1	Prepubertal	
	No coarse hair	
2	Longer, silky hair appears at base of penis or along labia	F—11.7 ± 1.2 yrs
		M—12.0 ± 1.0 yrs
3	Hair coarse, kinky, spreads over pubic bone	F—12.4 ± 1.1 yrs
		M—13.9 ± 1.0 yrs
4	Hair of adult quality but not spread to junction of medial thigh with perineum	F—13.0 ± 1.1 yrs
		M—14.4 ± 1.1 yrs
5	Spread to medial thigh	F—14.4 ± 1.1 yrs
		M—15.2 ± 1.1 yrs
6	"Male escutcheon"	Variable if occurs
Maximum growth rate		
Males at 14.1 ± 0.9 years		
Females at 12.1 ± 0.9 years		

  a. **Weight.** Hormonal abnormalities usually result in patients who are overweight for their height.
  b. **Rate and pattern of growth.** In patients with "organic" causes of growth failure, the rate of growth is decreased. A decelerating growth rate may indicate a change in factors controlling growth.
  c. **Family history.** For most patients the genetic potential for growth is ascertained by an evaluation of **mid–parental height.** Generally, the final height of the patient should be within 2 inches of the mid–parental height.
    (1) For males, mid–parental height = paternal height + (maternal height + 13 cm) divided by 2.
    (2) For females, mid–parental height = (paternal height − 13 cm) + maternal height, divided by 2.
    (3) Exact measurement of parental height improves the accuracy of such predictions.

Table 11-2. Penis length and testicular volume index

Age	Penis length Length (cm)	Testicular index (cm^2) (length (cm) $\times$ width (cm))
0–2	2.7 ± 0.5	Approx. 1.0
2–4	3.3 ± 0.4	Approx. 1.0
4–6	3.9 ± 0.9	0.9–1.8
6–8	4.2 ± 0.8	0.8–2.2
8–10	4.9 ± 1.0	0.8–3.6
10–12	5.2 ± 1.3	1.2–8.4
12–14	6.2 ± 2.0	1.6–16.0
14–16	8.6 ± 2.4	7.4–12.6
16–18	9.9 ± 1.7	7.6–11.8
18–20	11.0 ± 1.1	
Adult	12.4 ± 1.6	

   3. Diagnosis
      a. Laboratory tests (Table 11-4). The somatomedin C level in plasma has become used extensively in evaluation of growth hormone (GH) status. If the somatomedin C determination is normal, a GH deficiency is unlikely.
      b. Constitutional short stature is a diagnosis of exclusion and is supported by a normal history, normal physical findings and growth velocity, bone age equal to or greater than height age, and, often, a family history of short stature.
      c. Hormonal deficiencies that result in short stature include hypothyroidism, GH deficiency, and hypercortisolism. Inadequate quantities of GH result in slow growth rates, delayed bone age, and a weight greater than expected for height. The diagnosis is usually confirmed with provocative GH testing. Commonly used tests are arginine and insulin tolerance tests.
      d. Normal variant short stature is present when no direct cause of short stature can be found and predicted adult stature is 2 S.D. below the population norms.
      A subpopulation of patients with normal variant short stature who have an abnormal GH can be detected.
      (1) The serum is normal; somatomedin C low.
      (2) These patients respond to GH administration as if they had a GH deficiency.
   4. Treatment. Normal growth velocity may be restored if the underlying cause is treated effectively. No treatment is currently available that increases the mature height of children with constitutional short stature.
B. Tall stature
   1. Etiology
      a. Organic causes include growth hormone–producing tumors (see secs. III–VII); cerebral gigantism; Beckwith, XXYY, Klinefelter, and Marfan syndromes; homocystinuria; lipodystrophy; neurofibromatosis; and hyperthyroidism. Patients with sexual precocity may have accelerated growth velocity.
      b. Constitutional tall stature is the most frequent diagnosis.
   2. Evaluation and diagnosis
      a. The probable diagnosis should be established following a history and physical examination.
      b. Past growth data and bone age are necessary to evaluate velocity and predict mature height. Skull x-rays, fasting growth hormone, insulin, blood glucose determinations, and karyotyping may be indicated.

Table 11-3. Causes of short stature

Familial factors
Constitutional[a]

Congenital factors
Prader-Willi syndrome
Male Turner or Noonan syndrome[a]
Progeria
Laurence-Moon-Biedl syndrome[a]

Chromosomal disorders
Down syndrome[a]
Trisomies 13, 18
Turner syndrome

Intrauterine growth retardation
Infection
Placental insufficiency
Congenital anomalies (Russell-Silver, Seckel, Bloom syndromes)
Congenital without associated anomalies

Skeletal disorders
Achondroplasia[a]
Osteogenesis imperfecta[a]
Rickets
Osteochondrodystrophy[a]
Metaphyseal dysostosis

Nutritional factors
Low caloric or protein intake
Persistent vomiting
Malabsorption, celiac disease, cystic fibrosis[a]

Endocrine factors
Hypothyroidism[a]
Psychosocial deprivation
Growth hormone deficiency[a]
Abnormal growth hormone[b]
Corticosteroid excess
Androgen or estrogen excess
Diabetes insipidus[a]
Somatomedin deficiency[a]

Metabolic disorders
Acidosis
Unavailability of glucose
Altered mineralization
Fanconi syndrome
Galactosemia[a]
Aminoacidurias
Glycogen storage diseases
Mucopolysaccharidoses
Mucolipidoses[a]
Sphingolipidoses[a]

Pseudohypoparathyroidism[a]
Pseudopseudohypoparathyroidism

CNS disorders
Microcephaly
Mental retardation
Diencephalic syndrome

Hematologic disorders
Chronic anemia
Fanconi anemia
Blackfan-Diamond anemia

Cardiovascular abnormalities
Cyanotic congenital heart disease

Pulmonary conditions
Asthma,[a] bronchiectasis, tuberculosis, cystic fibrosis

GI disease
Regional enteritis or ulcerative colitis

Renal disease
Chronic renal failure
Renal acidosis

Chronic infection

Immune deficiencies[a]

[a]May have a genetic origin.
[b]Normal variant short stature with abnormal growth hormone.

Table 11-4. Screening tests in children with growth failure

Renal function tests: urine pH and specific gravity; BUN; serum creatinine; CO_2; electrolytes

Test for rickets: calcium, phosphorus, alkaline phosphatase

Serum thyroxine

Somatomedin C

Karyotype (girls)

Hand and wrist x-rays for bone age

X-ray views of the sella turcica

Source: L. Underwood, et al., *Pediatr. Clin. North Am.* 27:771, 1980.

3. **Treatment**
   a. Treatment of a pituitary tumor follows the guidelines outlined in sec. **IV.B.4.**
   b. Occasionally, patients with constitutional tall stature will demand therapy. This should be approached carefully because of its questionable efficacy and potential risks.
   c. Psychological support is important. This may enable the patients to forego therapy.

C. **Obesity**
   1. **Etiology**
      a. **Idiopathic (exogenous) obesity** is characterized by excessive food intake for the patient's caloric demands. Psychosocial stress is often present. A family history of obesity is frequently obtained. Recent studies have demonstrated that caloric requirements in some obese patients are lower than predicted. This seems to be related to decreased Na^+-K^+–adenosine triphosphatase activity. This has been found to show familial trends, suggesting a possible genetic component of obesity.
      b. **Organic conditions** associated with obesity include hypothyroidism; pseudohypoparathyroidism; the Cushing, Turner, Prader-Willi, and Laurence-Moon-Biedl syndromes; and hypothalamic lesions.
   2. **Evaluation**
      a. A person who is at least 10% overweight for his or her height is considered obese.
      b. Most children with idiopathic obesity are of normal or tall stature. Patients with organically caused obesity are usually short or have a deceleration in height velocity.
      c. The **history** should elicit the age of onset of obesity, a complete dietary history (preferably of a 3-day diet with a calorie count), unusual eating or drinking patterns, food preferences, exercise habits, history of past CNS injury or disease, intellectual ability, and symptoms suggestive of hypothyroidism, tetany, or the Cushing syndrome.
      d. The **severity of obesity** should be assessed.

      $$Kg \; overweight = current \; weight - ideal \; weight$$

      $$\% \; Overweight = \frac{no. \; kg \; overweight}{current \; weight} \times 100$$

      e. Particular attention should be directed to the distribution of body fat, muscle and bone, facial abnormalities, fundoscopic changes, presence of a goiter, abnormal sexual development, tetany, skin texture, short 4th metacarpal, and polydactyly. Striae and a buffalo hump may be present in patients with either idiopathic or organic obesity.
   3. **Diagnosis** of organic conditions should be made primarily by clinical evaluation, with confirmation pursued as indicated.

    a. Growth data should be obtained in all cases.

    b. Documentation of bone age, T_4, RT_4, and fasting and 8 P.M. cortisol may be a helpful screen.

    c. Elevated insulin levels, a "diabetic" response to glucose challenge, impaired growth hormone release, and elevated urinary 17-ketosteroids may be observed in the obese state, but may revert to normal when normal weight is attained.

  4. Treatment of hypothyroidism or Cushing syndrome often results in weight loss. The only therapy for other forms of obesity is caloric restriction and increased activity.

    a. In older children and adolescents, dietary intake should be restricted to a level that will make the patient forego approximately 300 cal/day. This will allow a loss of about 0.5 kg every 10 days (utilization of 3,000 cal of stored energy is necessary to lose 0.5 kg).

    b. Medications are often ineffective and potentially dangerous.

    c. Surgical therapy with intestinal bypass and oral occlusion have been attempted successfully in some patients. Serious long-term side effects have occasionally developed.

III. Disorders of sexual development

  A. Ambiguous genitalia

    1. Etiology. See Table 11-5.

    2. Evaluation and diagnosis

      a. The **history** includes documentation of maternal hormone ingestion or production, family history of ambiguous genitalia, infant deaths, sexual precocity, amenorrhea, or infertility.

      b. The **physical examination** should concentrate on ascertaining the presence of testes or a uterus. The phallus should be carefully examined and measured, and the urethral position should be noted. The degree of labioscrotal fusion and the amount of rugation are also noted. The uterus is searched for by a gentle rectal examination. Finally, stigmata suggesting chromosomal abnormalities are documented. Care must be taken not to overinterpret the significance of the external anatomy of the phallus and labioscrotal folds. If present, the testes and uterus provide useful clues to the genetic sex of the infant.

      c. Serum cortisol, 17-hydroxyprogesterone, electrolytes, buccal smear or karyotype, and a 24-hr urine for 17-ketosteroids should be obtained. Retrograde x-ray studies, laparoscopy, gonadal biopsy, or surgical exploration may be appropriate.

    3. Treatment

      a. An **accurate determination of the cause** of ambiguous genitalia is critical to sex assignment in the newborn period in order to maximize the potential for sexual and reproductive function. In general, designing a vagina is less complicated than reconstructing an adequate phallus and penile urethra. However, each case should be considered individually.

      b. Operations on the female genitalia are usually performed early in the first year; second-stage vaginoplasty is completed at adolescence.

      c. Reconstruction of the penis and correction of hypospadias may require four to six operations from infancy to age 9–10. To preserve valuable tissue for reconstruction, **circumcision is contraindicated.**

      d. Intraabdominal or inguinal testes should be sought and removed to avoid future malignant degeneration or virilization of a phenotypic female at adolescence.

      e. Growth and sexual development should be monitored closely and **hormonal therapy** instituted as indicated (see **B.4.b**).

      f. The diagnosis and prognosis for sexual and reproductive function should be discussed frankly with the parents and later with the patient. Psychological support, guidance, and repeated explanations, especially when the patient has reached adolescence, are of critical importance.

Table 11-5. Etiologic classification of causes of ambiguous genital development

Primary abnormality	Phenotype	Buccal smear
I. Gonadal		
A. *Structural*		
1. Gonadal dysgenesis or destruction	Male, female, or ambiguous	±
2. True hermaphroditism	Ambiguous	±
3. Tubular fibrosis (Klinefelter syndrome) or atrophy (Reifenstein syndrome) and germinal aplasia	Male or ambiguous	±
4. Secondary to neuroendocrine dysfunction (hypopituitarism, Kallman syndrome)	Male (micropenis, small testes)	−
B. *Functional**		
1. Male pseudohermaphroditism (including feminizing testicular syndrome and congenital adrenal hyperplasia due to 3β-oldehydrogenase deficiency)	Ambiguous female	−
2. Female pseudohermaphroditism? (cystic ovaries of newborn—Stein-Leventhal syndrome?)	Ambiguous	+
II. Extragonadal (female pseudohermaphroditism)		
A. *Congenital adrenocortical hyperplasia*	Ambiguous	+
B. *Maternal ingestion of virilizing hormones*	Ambiguous	+
C. *Maternal virilizing lesions* (e.g., arrhenoblastoma)	Ambiguous	+
III. End organ: defects of the external genitals without an apparent gonadal abnormality (e.g., extrophy of the bladder, cleft scrotum). Often associated with urinary tract abnormalities	Ambiguous	±

*Includes patients who may have a defect in gonadal steroid synthesis or an end-organ insensitivity owing to an abnormality of extragonadal steroid hormone metabolism or some other factor. This fact must be kept in mind when assigning the sex of the patient.

B. Delayed puberty
  1. Etiology
    a. Constitutional delay of pubertal development occurs more frequently in males than in females. A characteristic growth pattern is seen, with the pubertal growth acceleration shifted by several years. In many patients, there is a family history of delayed pubertal development.
    b. CNS abnormalities such as pituitary and hypothalamic tumors, congenital vascular anomalies, severe trauma, birth asphyxia, psychosocial deprivation, and Kallmann and Laurence-Moon-Biedl syndromes result in pubertal delay.
    c. Systemic conditions, such as anorexia nervosa; severe cardiac, pulmonary, renal, or GI disease; malabsorption syndromes; weight loss or weight gain; sickle cell anemia; thalassemia; chronic infection; hypothyroidism; or Addison's disease, are associated with an increased incidence of delayed or incomplete sexual development.
    d. Primary gonadal insufficiency may be caused by the following: Turner, Noonan, Klinefelter, Reifenstein, and Sertoli-cell-only syndromes; tes-

ticular feminization; pure or mixed gonadal dysgenesis; cryptorchidism and anorchism; trauma, infection, pelvic radiation, and surgical castration.

2. **Evaluation.** Although there are normal variations in the time of onset of puberty, differential diagnosis of delayed puberty should be considered when a girl over 14 or a boy over 15 lacks any secondary sexual characteristics, or when an adolescent has not completed maturation over a period of 5 years.

   a. The **history** should concentrate on the details and chronology of any sexual development, previous growth pattern, CNS symptoms, including anosmia, and nutrition. Any **family history** of abnormal puberty, amenorrhea, infertility, or ambiguous genitalia should be elicited.

   b. The **physical examination** should include all growth measurements (height, weight, span, upper-lower ratio), sexual staging, careful observation of the genitalia for ambiguity, palpation for inguinal masses, a pelvic examination (or at least a rectal), and a search for stigmata suggesting a syndrome. Signs of virilization in the female or incomplete masculinization in the male strongly imply an underlying pathologic cause that must be pursued.

   c. **Review of past growth data** is mandatory; a subtle growth spurt may be the first indication of impending sexual development. Conversely, abnormal deceleration may be a sign of active disease.

   d. The initial **laboratory evaluation** usually includes a CBC, urinalysis, luteinizing hormone (LH), follicle-stimulating hormone (FSH), estrogen, testosterone, dehydroxyandrosterone (DHEAS), bone age, and skull films. A karyotype is sometimes indicated.

3. **Diagnosis.** A specific diagnosis of the cause of delayed puberty is essential to ensure maximal realization of sexual and reproductive function, to provide genetic counseling, and to protect the patient against potential malignancy.

   a. The diagnosis of constitutional or hereditary delay in an otherwise normal patient is always tentative, since it can be confirmed only after normal sexual development has evolved.

   b. Patients with hypothalamic or pituitary deficiencies have low (usually prepubertal) levels of LH, or FSH, or both. An LH-releasing hormone test may differentiate hypothalamic from pituitary lesions.

   c. In systemic conditions, an absence of cyclic levels of FSH-LH is sometimes observed.

   d. In primary gonadal failure, gonadotropins are usually elevated by age 12–13 years. A precise diagnosis of the gonadal abnormality requires clinical acumen and appropriate investigation.

4. **Treatment.** Before therapy is begun the patient's height, growth potential, emotional needs, and the risks of treatment must be considered.

   a. **Constitutional and genetic delay.** The patient and family should be reassured that no abnormalities are apparent, that normal development is anticipated, but that continued surveillance is important. Progression of development should be monitored and emotional support offered. For certain patients, temporary hormone replacement therapy may be justified.

   b. **CNS abnormalities**

      (1) In patients with hypogonadotropic hypogonadism (decreased production of LH and FSH), hormonal therapy is often necessary. With the availability of LH-releasing hormone analogues, a new concept in therapy for these patients is being investigated. If the pituitary is intact, treatment with LH-releasing hormone analogues enables a more normal progression through puberty. In some patients, fertility has resulted.

      (2) Therapy is first directed to the indicated surgical or radiation treatment of the lesion.

      (3) **In females** the replacement regimen includes an oral conjugated estrogen, e.g., Premarin, 0.3 mg/day, with the dosage gradually in-

creased to 1.25 mg/day over 9–12 months; Provera, 10 mg/day on days 1–5 of each month, is then added to induce cyclic bleeding.

(4) In males, ideal therapy consists of human chorionic gonadotropin (HCG), 1,000–2,500 IU IM q5 days. Serum testosterone may be helpful in monitoring dosage needs.

  c. **Systemic conditions.** Improvement of the underlying medical condition may be followed by normal puberty. Replacement therapy as outlined in **b** may be necessary, but its efficacy varies in different conditions.

  d. **Primary gonadal insufficiency**

(1) In females, treatment consists of estrogens and progesterone (see **b.(3)**)

(2) In males, a therapeutic trial of HCG should be attempted if there is a possibility of testicular function. If no response is demonstrated, testosterone enanthate, 100–200 mg IM every 2–4 weeks, may be prescribed. Testicular prostheses should be offered if necessary. The prognosis for fertility should be evaluated and discussed frankly.

C. Sexual precocity
  1. **Etiology.** See Table 11-6.
  2. **Evaluation** should focus on the points emphasized in **B.2.** In addition, a careful search should be made for an abdominal or testicular mass (if necessary, under anesthesia), galactorrhea, and hyperpigmentation. A kidney-ureter-bladder film (KUB), adrenal photoscan, serum HCG, DHEA, and androstenedione determinations or a dexamethasone-suppression test may be indicated. Hormonal levels should be interpreted in relation to the stage of sexual development and age.
  3. **Diagnosis.** See Table 11-7.

Table 11-6. Causes of sexual precocity

Idiopathic (constitutional)
Familial
Central nervous system
  Tumor (teratoma, astrocytoma, ependymoma, pinealoma, craniopharyn-
    gioma, optic glioma, hamartoma, other)
  Infection (tuberculosis, meningitis), postencephalitic scarring
  Hydrocephalus
  Neurofibromatosis
  Tuberous sclerosis
Androgen- and/or estrogen-producing tumors
  Ovarian (granulosa or theca cell tumor, theca-lutein or follicular cyst)
  Testicular (Leydig cell, adrenal rest tumors)
  Adrenal (adenoma, carcinoma, hyperplasia)
Gonadotropin-producing tumors
  Ovarian (chorioepithelioma, teratoma, dysgerminoma)
  Testicular
  Teratoma (CNS, presacral)
Endocrine dysfunction
  Hypothyroidism
  Congenital adrenal hyperplasia
Exogenous hormones
  Birth control pills
  Estrogens (cosmetics, poultry, cattle)
  Androgens
  HCG
Syndromes
  Russell-Silver
  Polyostotic fibrous dysplasia (McCune-Albright syndrome)

Table 11-7. Laboratory evaluation of precocity

Isosexual
  Hormonal
    Circulating LH, FSH, estradiol, testosterone, dehydroepiandro-
    sterone-sulfate (DHEA-S), βHCG; response to LH-releasing
    hormone stimulation (6-hr monitoring of LH, FSH)
  Radiographic
    Bone age
    Head CT scan, only if CNS tumor is suspected
    Abdominal ultrasound or CT scan if indicated
Premature thelarche
  (Tests usually not indicated if examination is negative.)
  Hormonal
    Circulating estradiol
  Urinary
    Cytologic study for vaginal index
  Radiologic
    Bone age
    Abdominal ultrasound to assess uterine size and ovarian contour
Precocious adrenarche
  Hormonal
    Circulating DHEA-S, Δ^4-androstenedione, testosterone, 17-hydroxy-
    progesterone
  Radiologic
    Further studies only as indicated

- a. **Isosexual precocity** refers to an abnormally early onset (girls < 8 years of age, boys < 9 years of age) of sexual characteristics appropriate to the child's sex, with eventual attainment of full sexual maturation. In girls, isosexual precocity is usually idiopathic; organic and often malignant conditions are responsible in males. Inappropriate precocity, i.e., masculinization in the female or feminization in the male, is always pathologic and requires investigation.
- b. **Precocious adrenarche (pubarche)** consists of the early appearance of pubic hair, axillary hair, and/or apocrine odor, which are effects of adrenal androgens.
- c. **Precocious thelarche** refers to the premature development of one or both breasts in females, without vaginal estrogenization or any other signs of sexual development.
- d. The **differential diagnosis** should be narrowed down by determining the source(s) of hormone (e.g., CNS, adrenal or gonadal) and intensifying investigation of that limited area.
- 4. **Treatment.** Unless eradication of the specific cause of the precocity is possible, no satisfactory treatment to prevent progression of sexual changes is currently available. Patients should be followed closely to monitor growth and development, to examine for treatable lesions, and to offer psychological guidance. Long-acting LH releasing hormone analog therapy has been used experimentally to stop isosexual precocity. This therapy may soon be widely available.
- D. **Gynecomastia**
  - 1. **Etiology**
    - a. **Idiopathic gynecomastia** occurs in 65% of all normal males carefully examined during puberty. This usually resolves within 2 years and is not associated with galactorrhea.
    - b. **Iatrogenic sources** may be estrogens, androgens, HCG, desoxycorticosterone acetate, isoniazid, digitalis, reserpine, spironolactone, phenothiazines, meprobamate, and amphetamines.

      c. Organic conditions include true or male pseudohermaphroditism (e.g., Klinefelter or Reifenstein syndromes), estrogen-producing tumor, hypothyroidism, hyperthyroidism, acromegaly, diabetes mellitus, hepatic disease, nephritis, paraplegia, primary testicular failure, and testicular tumors.

  2. Evaluation

      a. The **history** should concentrate on measures of sexual development and function, symptoms of pain, tenderness, galactorrhea, hair loss, iatrogenic sources, and systemic illness.

      b. The size and configuration of ductular tissue, color of the areolae, presence of galactorrhea (best elicited with the patient in the sitting position), dimensions and consistency of the testes, and stage of sexual development should be noted.

  3. Diagnosis. If abnormalities are present, measurement of FSH, LH, estrogen, testosterone, buccal smear and/or karyotype, and cortisol and/or 24-hr urinary 17-ketosteroids and 17-hydroxycorticosteroids may be indicated.

  4. Treatment. Spontaneous regression occurs in most normal boys after 1–3 years. Removal of the hormonal or pharmacologic agent usually results in disappearance of ductular tissue. If the gynecomastia is unusually severe or contributing to significant psychological problems, mammoplasty may be warranted.

IV. Disorders of the pituitary

  A. Hypopituitarism. Pituitary function depends on the integrity of the entire hypothalamic-pituitary axis.

    1. Etiology

      a. Tumors of the pituitary and suprasellar tumors (especially, craniopharyngioma) may disrupt pituitary function.

      b. Tissue damage due to a trauma, hemorrhage, neurofibromatosis, previous irradiation, and infarction may cause isolated or multiple hormonal defects.

      c. Psychosocial deprivation alters pituitary function. Up to 6 months of supportive care may be necessary before normal hormonal status is regained.

      d. Isolated GH deficiency occurs as an X-linked recessive disorder.

      e. Isolated gonadotropin deficiency occurs in association with Kallmann syndrome (anosmia and color blindness) and Laurence-Moon-Biedl syndrome (mental retardation, polydactyly, obesity, retinitis pigmentosa, nerve deafness, short stature, and diabetes insipidus [DI]).

      f. Isolated deficiencies of thyroid-stimulating hormone (TSH) and adrenocorticotropic hormone (ACTH) have been reported.

    2. Evaluation. Systemic investigation of all anterior and posterior pituitary hormones is necessary to determine the status of current function and establish a baseline for future alterations.

      a. The **history** should cover past growth, CNS symptoms (anosmia, visual changes, symptoms of increased intracranial pressure), and previous head or neck illnesses or therapy.

      b. The **physical examination** should include precise growth measurements, staging of sexual development, a neurologic survey, including visual fields and fundoscopy, and a search for the signs of hypothyroidism and hypoadrenalism.

      c. Further evaluation should include a carefully plotted height and weight curve and bone age. If pituitary insufficiency is suggested, an evaluation of both anterior and posterior pituitary hormonal status includes circulating levels of somatomedin C, LH, FSH, thyroxine, and ACTH. Serum and urine values of sodium and potassium and osmolality should be obtained.

      d. A CT scan of the pituitary fossa and suprasellar regions is useful in evaluating structural lesions. It is best to secure the advice of a competent radiologist to guide this and further evaluation.

3. **Diagnosis**
   a. Patients with isolated growth hormone deficiency have a normal birth weight and length; growth velocity begins to decrease at 6-12 months of age.
      (1) Patients with GH deficiency have a growth rate of less than 4 cm/year.
      (2) The weight age is usually greater than the height age, and the facies and body proportions are immature and associated with a high-pitched voice.
      (3) No rise in GH occurs with the following stimuli known to increase circulating levels of immunoreactive GH in healthy individuals: fasting, exercise, stress, third-stage rapid-eye-movement sleep, hypoglycemia, arginine, propranolol, and glucagon.
   b. **Deficiencies of LH and FSH** may not become apparent until puberty. However, micropenis, apparent at birth in males, may be present in hypogonadotropic states.
   c. Deficiency of TSH may be responsible for mild to severe clinical hypothyroidism without a goiter. Thyroid function tests, including tests for TSH, reveal low levels.
   d. Patients with ACTH deficiency often have a relatively mild form of adrenal insufficiency that may go undetected until they are under stress. These patients are differentiated from patients with Addison's disease by the lack of hyperpigmentation or salt craving. Serum cortisols may be low or even within normal range, but a significant response to metyrapone or diurnal variation of adrenocortical activity is absent.

4. **Treatment**
   a. Surgical or radiation treatment of the underlying condition should be carried out as indicated.
   b. **GH** is available commercially and through the National Pituitary Agency. Because GH is in limited supply, each source has criteria that must be met before a patient can obtain the hormone. GH, 0.12 unit/kg/dose, administered weekly by deep IM injection, is the standard replacement therapy.
   c. **TSH deficiency** is treated with L-thyroxine (as discussed in sec. **V**).
   d. **ACTH deficiency** usually requires no treatment except with the stress of surgery, trauma, or infectious illness with temperatures greater than $38.5°C$ ($101°F$). In these cases, treatment with cortisone acetate, 50 mg/M^2/day IM, is recommended. An additional 100 mg/M^2 of hydrocortisone sodium solution is usually administered IV during surgery.

B. **Hyperpituitarism**
   1. **Etiology.** Excessive levels of GH, TSH, ACTH, or prolactin result from autonomous hormone production by a primary pituitary tumor or by altered regulation at a hypothalamic level.
   2. **Evaluation**
      a. Clinical states reflecting hypersecretion may be a result of elevated serum levels of the hormone or of uninterrupted secretion within a "normal" range.
      b. **Evaluation** consists in documenting the onset of observed changes (serial photographs are very helpful), determining current CNS and pituitary function, and measuring the ability of pharmacologic stimuli to suppress pituitary secretion.
   3. **Diagnosis**
      a. **GH excess** results in an accelerated growth rate in the growing child—or in acromegaly when the epiphyses have fused.
         (1) **Physical findings and symptoms** include weakness, thickened skin, hypertrichosis, headaches, excessive perspiration, and joint pains.
         (2) **Laboratory diagnosis** is established by elevated circulating levels of somatomedin C, and the inability of a glucose load to suppress the level of immunoreactive GH. Diabetic glucose tolerance test findings

may be seen, along with elevations in circulating levels of immunore-active insulin.

  b. Excess TSH results in a clinical picture of hyperthyroidism, with elevated thyroid hormone levels and elevated TSH.

  c. Cushing's disease in which the basic defect is hypercortisolism secondary to excessive or inappropriate secretion of ACTH presents with the clinical picture of the Cushing syndrome as a result of a CNS tumor (see sec. **VI**).

  d. Patients with **hyperprolactin states** usually present with galactorrhea, oligomenorrhea, or amenorrhea.

4. Treatment

  a. Complete eradication of the tumor is often difficult and may require two approaches. These are surgery (transphenoidal or frontal approach) and cryosurgery plus radiation (x-ray, proton beam, isotope implantation).

  b. Cushing's disease may not be successfully treated by pituitary surgery alone. Partial or complete adrenalectomy may be necessary, either surgically or with ortho-para dichlorodiphenyldichlorethane (O′-P′DDD).

  c. Bromocriptine is useful in treating **hyperprolactinemia.** Dosages of 2.5 mg/day are used at the inception of therapy; this is increased in 2.5-mg increments (maximum is usually 7.5 mg/day) by increasing the frequency of dosage (schedule: qd, bid, tid). Bromocriptine may cause an underlying adrenal insufficiency to be unmasked. For this reason it is usually prudent to perform a metyrapone test before beginning therapy. If adrenal insufficiency is unmasked, glucocorticoid replacement at 13 mg/M^2/day PO with hydrocortisone acetate should be begun. When large tumors are present, surgery and radiation therapy may be necessary.

C. Diabetes insipidus

  1. Etiology. The causes of DI include hypothalamic or posterior pituitary antidiuretic hormone (ADH) deficiency, or both; it may be idiopathic or a result of CNS tumor (especially Hand-Schüller-Christian disease or postoperative craniopharyngioma), infection, infarction, trauma, or familial (autosomal dominant, ADH deficiency, or X-linked dominant) nephrogenic diabetes insipidus.

  2. Evaluation

   a. Although the onset of symptoms may be abrupt, a cycle of polyuriapolydipsia may allow the older child to remain well compensated. Infants, however, may present with severe failure to thrive and dehydration. Evidence of CNS or pituitary abnormalities may not be present.

   b. Polyuria is investigated by a record of 24-hr urine input and output, urinalysis with specific gravity, serum Na, K, BUN, creatinine Ca, P, and AP, concomitant serum and urine osmolality (random or following a defined fast), and 24-hr urine tests for Na, K, and Ca creatinine.

  3. Diagnostic evaluation. It is necessary to document excess water intake and output. Output is usually greater than 3.0 L/M^2/day. Serum osmolality is increased relative to urine osmolality. Hypercalcemia may mimic ADH deficiency.

   a. Water deprivation. The patient is placed on an npo regimen at bedtime. Baseline urine and serum osmolalities are obtained. Urinary specific gravities are monitored. In patients with DI the urinary osmolality or specific gravity does not rise (above 300 mOsm/L or 1.010) despite a decrease in weight of 5%. Serum sodium increases during the deprivation.

   b. Vasopressin clearance. In some institutions it is possible to assess vasopressin clearance by obtaining 2-hr urine specimens and a plasma sample to determine vasopressin levels. This is the most accurate means of diagnosis and allows quantitation of partial ADH deficiency.

   c. Vasopressin test. A single dose of 1-deamino-8-D-arginine vasopressin (0.05 ml by nasal applicator) will yield a rise in urinary osmolality and specific gravity in ADH deficiency. In nephrogenic DI, such a rise is not found.

4. Treatment

a. Acute. DI may occur in postsurgical or posttraumatic injuries of the hypothalamic-pituitary region. The initial treatment consists of fluid management. The goal of this management is to compensate for water losses without providing an excessive urinary osmotic fluid load. Fluids should contain only the amount of glucose and electrolytes that would be given in maintenance fluids. The remainder of the fluid should be free water. The fluid volume should be related to urine output, but should not exceed 3.0 L/M^2.

b. Chronic therapy. Replacement therapy with DDAVP is recommended. Therapy is begun at night, when the chances of the patient becoming water intoxicated are least. Dosages of 0.025 ml, delivered intranasally, are begun. This is increased by 0.025 ml until an adequate response occurs. The final dose is usually 0.05 ml/day in patients 1–6 years old and 0.1 ml/day in patients 6–10 years of age. In patients over 10 years of age, 2 daily doses are frequently necessary.

c. Nephrogenic DI is treated with a low-salt diet. Chlorpropamide and thiazide diuretics may also be beneficial.

D. Inappropriate ADH (ADH excess) (IADH)

1. Etiology. Usually, this disorder is encountered following trauma to the head or intracranial surgery. Intracranial tumors, infections, and intrathoracic surgery may result in excessive ADH secretion.

2. Presentation. There is a decrease in urine output, weight gain, and altered states of consciousness if excess free water is retained. Occasionally, a patient with a lesion in the hypothalamic area will present with a chronic picture of IADH. Although rare in children, the ectopic production of ADH, especially by lung neoplasms, is seen in them.

3. The **laboratory findings** in inappropriate ADH include a decreased serum sodium and osmolality with increased urinary sodium and osmolality. The presence of normal renal and adrenal function must be documented. There must be no evidence of hypovolemia.

4. Treatment

a. The most effective treatment is **prevention.** This is done by limiting fluids to urine output while not allowing fluid intake to be less than 800 ml/M^2/24 hr (the amount of fluid needed to excrete 24 hours' worth of solute load). Inappropriate ADH secretion may alternate with DI.

b. In patients with both ADH excess and DI, fluid intake should be

(1) Matched to urine output

(2) A minimum of 800 ml of water/M^2/24 hr

(3) A maximum of 3,000 ml of water/M^2/24 hr

(4) Contain only maintenance glucose, sodium (2–3 mEq/kg/24 hr), and potassium (1–2 mEq/kg/24 hr).

c. Therapy should be monitored carefully with frequent weights and serum electrolyte determinations.

V. Disorders of the thyroid

A. Neonatal hypothyroidism

1. Etiology

a. Endemic

b. Embryonic errors in development (thyroid dysgenesis)

c. Idiopathic, with the majority of cases remaining unexplained

d. Maternal hyperthyroidism. Administration of iodides, radioactive iodine, or propylthiouracil during pregnancy may be the cause of inadequate fetal thyroid hormone production.

e. Inherited inborn errors of thyroid hormone production are usually transmitted as an autosomal recessive trait. Abnormal thyroid function may begin in the neonatal period or in early childhood.

2. **Evaluation.** In view of the significant neurologic sequelae, the possibility of hypothyroidism should be considered in an infant with any suggestive signs or symptoms.
   a. With neonatal thyroid screening, many children are considered normal until the test is returned. Parents are very disturbed when informed of these abnormalities.
   b. The **history** may include postmaturity, unusually placid behavior (e.g., "a good baby who never cries"), somnolence, hypotonia, feeding difficulties, constipation, and prolonged jaundice.
   c. **Physical features** may include hypothermia, abnormal movement (as if in slow motion), hypotonia, enlarged anterior and posterior fontanelle, macroglossia, coarse facial features, umbilical hernia, and cool, dry, mottled skin. The thyroid may be enlarged or absent.
3. **Diagnosis.** Laboratory evaluation has usually been done in screening programs prior to the initial visit. When T_4 is low, or TSH is elevated, or both, patients are referred for evaluation. The recommended work-up follows.
   a. Repeat thyroid studies determining T_4, TT_3, T_3 resin (or thyroid-binding globulin index).
   b. Obtain a thyroid scan and radioactive iodine uptake.
   c. If the TSH is low, a thyroid-releasing hormone stimulation test is recommended (7 μg/kg of thyroid-releasing hormone is given IV with TSH measured at time 0 and at 90 min after injection).
   d. Bone age films are useful in diagnosis and in determining the results of therapy.
4. **Treatment** should be begun immediately if there is clinical or laboratory evidence present for diagnosis.
   a. L-Thyroxine (7 μg/kg/day) is recommended. This should be adjusted as necessary based on thyroid function tests obtained at 2 weeks, 1 month, 6 weeks, 3 months, and 6 months after the onset of therapy. Treatment should maintain the T_4 between 10–14 μg/100 ml and TSH at less than 20 μU/ml.
   b. A trial without therapy is attempted at age 4–5 years.
B. **Neonatal hyperthyroidism**
   1. **Etiology**
      a. Women with **Graves' disease** may have offspring with hyperthyroidism, presumably secondary to transplacental passage of long-acting thyroid stimulation.
      b. Patients with "idiopathic" disease may have a family history of thyroid disease.
   2. **Evaluation.** A goiter is usually present.
   3. **Treatment.** When the mother has Graves' disease, the possibility of **respiratory obstruction secondary to fetal goiter** should be anticipated prior to delivery. Resection of the thyroid isthmus or tracheostomy may be necessary.
C. **Acquired hypothyroidism**
   1. **Etiology**
      a. **Idiopathic**
      b. **Thyroiditis** is the most common cause. Many patients in the idiopathic group may be patients with thyroiditis which is no longer clinically apparent.
      c. **TSH deficiency**
      d. **Exogenous causes** include thyroidectomy, radioactive iodine, iodine excess or deficiency, fluorine, lithium, cobalt, perchlorate, thiocyanate, para-aminosalicylic acid, propylthiouracil, phenylbutazone, resorcinol (in skin creams), and certain foods in large amounts (e.g., cabbage, turnips, cauliflower, rutabaga, soybeans).
      e. Rarely, **thyroid carcinoma** may produce hypothyroidism.
   2. **Evaluation and diagnosis**
      a. Iodine goiters are very hard. Goiters associated with thyroiditis may be moderately firm, granular, and suggested by a Delphian node. A discrete,

hard mass (or masses) may be a malignant tumor or adenoma. Absence of a goiter suggests TSH deficiency or, rarely, ectopic thyroid tissue.

   b. Laboratory findings include decreased T_4, and elevated TSH. Thyroid antibodies are frequently positive in thyroiditis. A thyroid scan is helpful in evaluating a nodule if one is palpated. It may also be helpful if an ectopic gland is suspected.

3. Treatment

   a. Treatment with L-thyroxine is begun with 0.025 mg/day, with the dosage gradually increased by 0.025 mg every 1–2 weeks until the appropriate dosage is attained. Most children require 0.1 mg/day from age 1–9 and 0.15 mg/day from age 10 to adolescence. Adults usually require 0.15–0.2 mg/day.

   b. Thyroid function tests may be done to monitor the appropriateness of the dosage, or compliance, or both. TSH may be the most sensitive guide to the adequacy of therapy.

   c. Striking alterations in personality and behavior may be observed initially, but such problems eventually resolve as the patient and family adapt to the euthyroid state.

D. Acquired hyperthyroidism

1. Etiology

   a. Elevated thyroxine (T_4) may be seen in Graves' disease (hyperthyroidism with exophthalmos), diffuse toxic goiter, thyroid adenoma, thyroiditis, or, very rarely, hyperfunctioning thyroid carcinoma or a TSH-producing tumor.

   b. In T_3 toxicosis, only triiodothyronine is excessive, while T_4 is normal.

2. Presentation. Patients present with increased activity, increased appetite, a noticeable goiter, exophthalmos (in Graves' disease), heat intolerance, diminished sleep, and poor coordination. Physical examination reveals a rapid heart rate and elevated blood pressure with a widened pulse pressure. The thyroid gland is usually firm and may be tender. Neurologic examination reveals hyperreflexia, chorea, and restlessness. *Thyroid storm* is severe hyperthyroidism with cardiac decompensation and a decreased state of consciousness. T_4 is usually over 20 μ/100 ml.

3. Laboratory evaluation should include T_4, T_3, and T_3 uptake and TSH. In patients with pheochromocytoma and T_3 toxicosis, there is an elevated T_3 with a normal T_4.

4. Treatment

   a. Thyroid storm is a rare medical emergency. When it is diagnosed, treatment should include the following:

   (1) Control of thyroid hormone production by giving a large dose of propylthiouracil (PTU) (200–400 mg).

   (2) Iodide PO or sodium iodide IV is given in a dose of 1–2 gm.

   (3) Hydrocortisone, 200 mg/M^2/day, is given.

   (4) Propranolol, 2–4 mg IV, may reverse severe decompensation. This dose may be repeated q2h until consciousness is regained. At this point the patient is placed on 0.50–2.5 mg/kg/dose given PO q6h.

   (5) A cooling blanket may be necessary to control body heat.

   b. Thyrotoxicosis

   (1) PTU is given as 150 mg/M^2/day in 3 divided doses. This dose may need to be increased if the desired effect is not achieved. Usually, 100 mg tid is given initially. This is then decreased to 50 mg tid as a maintenance dose.

   (2) Methimazole (Tapazole) can be used instead of PTU. The initial dose is 10 mg tid, with a daily maintenance dosage of 10–15 mg after 6–8 weeks (neutropenia may occur with either medication).

   (3) In patients with poor compliance, surgery is an option. Hypothyroidism is a frequent complication of surgery.

   (4) Radioactive iodine therapy is used in some centers; the safety of this therapy is still in question.

VI. Disorders of the adrenals
   A. Adrenocortical hypofunction
   1. Etiology. The causes include the following:
      a. Congenital adrenal hyperplasia
      b. Adrenal hemorrhage
      c. Hypoplasia or aplasia of the adrenals
      d. Congenital unresponsiveness to ACTH
      e. Fulminating infections, especially meningococcemia
      f. Addison's disease
      g. Familial (associated with diabetes mellitus, hypoparathyroidism, candidiasis, thyroiditis)
      h. Iatrogenic chronic adrenal suppression
   2. Evaluation
      a. Personality changes, increased pigmentation, salt craving, hypotension, anorexia, nausea, vomiting, diarrhea and weight loss, menstrual abnormalities, and hypoglycemia may be present for months before the diagnosis is made. GI symptoms may mimic those of influenza or simulate an acute abdominal condition.
      b. In adrenal crisis, often precipitated by mild stress, vomiting, dehydration, hypoglycemia, and hypotension may lead to coma and shock.
   3. Diagnosis
      a. Decreased Na, increased K, hypochloremic acidosis, hypoglycemia, increased urinary Na, and decreased urinary K
      b. Eosinophilia and relative neutropenia may be documented, depending on the severity of the illness.
      c. Serum cortisol and aldosterone may be low or within normal range, but ACTH levels are significantly elevated in primary adrenal insufficiency, especially if they are obtained at the time of maximal stress.
      d. Urinary 17-hydroxycorticosteroids are usually less than 3.0 ± 1.0 mg/M^2/day.
      e. The findings of metyrapone and water-loading tests are abnormal, but do not distinguish primary from secondary glucocorticoid deficiency.
      f. The diagnosis is confirmed when serum cortisol and aldosterone and 24-hr urinary 17-hydroxycorticosteroids and 17-ketosteroids do not respond adequately to exogenously administered ACTH.
   4. Therapy
      a. Shock must be treated by rapid volume expansion (20 ml/kg of normal saline IV stat). If hypoglycemia is suspected (or documented with a Dextrostix), 1–2 gm/kg of dextrose solution is given IV. Hydrocortisone sodium succinate (Solu-Cortef), 25–50 mg, should be given IV stat; the equivalent of 150 mg/M^2/day should be given IV in divided doses q4–6h and continued over the next 24 hr. Pressor agents usually are not necessary if adequate fluids are administered.
      b. For patients with **mild symptoms,** 1.5–2 times the amount of maintenance fluids (see **c**) may be sufficient to equilibrate the electrolytes and allow diagnostic tests to be carried out.
      c. Maintenance therapy consists of the equivalent of 13 mg/M^2/day of hydrocortisone in divided doses tid, or fludrocortisone (Florinef), 0.05–0.1 mg/day, and table salt ad lib, especially in the summer.
      d. During periods of stress the hydrocortisone dosage should be doubled or trebled and the frequency of administration increased to q6h. Patients, or parents, or both, should know how to use cortisone acetate, 25–50 mg IM, in emergencies. Patients should wear a Medic Alert identification tag.
      e. For **surgery** or **severe stress,** see **IV.A.4.d**).
   B. Congenital adrenal hyperplasia (androgenital syndrome)
   1. Etiology
      a. Congenital adrenal hyperplasia is an autosomal recessive enzyme defect of cortisol synthesis. The five most common enzyme deficiencies and clinical presentations are shown in Table 11-8.

Table 11-8. Evaluation and diagnosis of congenital adrenogenital hyperplasia

| Enzyme deficiency | External genitalia | | Symptoms | Diagnostic abnormalities | |
	Female	Male		Urine	Serum
21-Hydroxylase	Virilized	Virilized	½–⅓ have salt losing	Increased 17-ketosteroids Increased pregnanetriol	Increased 17-hydroxyprogesterone
11-β-Hydroxylase	Virilized	Virilized	Hypertension	Increased 17-ketosteroids Increased pregnanetriol	Compound S (11-desoxycortisol compounds)
3-β-Hydroxysteroid dehydrogenase	Mildly virilized	Incompletely masculinized	Salt losing	± Increased 17-ketosteroids	Increased dehydroepiandosterone
20, 20-Desmolase	Normal	Incompletely masculinized	Salt losing	Normal or decreased 17-ketosteroids	
17-Hydroxylase	Normal	Incompletely masculinized	Hypertension	Increased pregnanetriol	

   b. Two enzyme deficiencies, 18-hydroxylase and 18-dehydrogenase, result only in deficiencies of aldosterone synthesis.

2. **Presentation and evaluation.** See also Table 11-8.
   a. Hypertension is present in patients with 11-hydroxylase and 17-hydroxylase deficiencies.
   b. There is often a family history of spontaneous abortion or early infant death.

3. **Laboratory evaluation and diagnosis**
   a. The abnormality most readily detected is an elevated level of 17-hydroxyprogesterone. This will be present in patients with 21-hydroxylase deficiency and in most patients with 3-β-hydroxysteroid dehydrogenase deficiency. Circulating ACTH is elevated. In virilizing defects, urinary 17-ketosteroids (derived from degradation of adrenal androgens) will be elevated ($>$2 mg/24 hr in the newborn). Serum cortisol and aldosterone may be normal or low.
   b. Often, a buccal smear or karyotype is of help in identifying sex in patients who are partially virilized.

4. **Treatment**
   a. **Salt-losing crisis** is treated with infusion of normal saline. Hypotension is treated with a fluid bolus of 20 ml/kg followed by 1.5 times maintenance fluids until the patient's condition is stable. Frequently, diurnal weight changes are dramatic. Fludrocortisone, 0.05 mg/day, is used for mineralocorticoid replacement. This is begun when the patient's condition has stabilized and he or she is ready for oral intake. Dosages of 0.05 mg bid may be necessary in some infants. Salt supplementation of 2–4 gm/day may be necessary for stabilization. This can be added to the formula or solids until the child is capable of ad lib salt supplementation.
   b. **Initial glucocorticoid therapy** may require 3–4 times the maintenance dosage to suppress ACTH levels, especially during stress. Newborns may be treated with 5 mg of hydrocortisone q8h for 3 days. The dosage is then tapered to 2.5 mg q8h and continued for the first 6–12 months. Patients with congenital adrenal hyperplasia seem to require 15–20 mg/M^2/day of hydrocortisone or its equivalent, given tid to provide adequate glucocorticoid replacement, to suppress ACTH and to allow for normal growth and development. Desoxycorticosterone acetate may also be needed. Optimal dosage timing may vary among patients.
   c. Females with virilization may require an operation on the clitoris, or vagina, or both. If necessary, this procedure should be performed as early in infancy as is feasible.
   d. Patients should be followed at intervals of 3–4 months to monitor growth, urinary 17-ketosteroids, and bone age. The medication should be adjusted as necessary.

C. **Cushing syndrome**
   1. **Etiology.** Glucocorticoid excess may be caused by adrenal tumors, adrenal hyperplasia, an ACTH-producing tumor of the pituitary (Cushing's disease), or prolonged treatment with corticosteroids.
   2. **Evaluation**
      a. **Manifestations** of glucocorticoid excess include an initial increase then a decrease in appetite, weight gain, slowing or arrest of height velocity, weakness, fatigue, and personality changes.
      b. Fat deposition occurs in the facial, nuchal, shoulder, and abdominal areas, producing the characteristic "moon" facies and "buffalo hump." The extremities often appear thin, the result of muscle wasting.
      c. Hypertension, plethora, purplish red striae, ecchymoses, and weakness may be present.
      d. Signs of excess adrenal androgens (acne, pubic hair, enlarged clitoris or phallus) may indicate a mixed tumor or hyperplasia secondary to excess ACTH.

3. Diagnosis

a. Serum F (cortisol), urinary 17-hydroxycorticosteroids, and free cortisol are usually increased. Serum androgens and urinary 17-ketosteroids may be increased in the virilized patient, but the most specific diagnostic feature is the **absence of the normal diurnal variation in cortisol level.** Serum ACTH should be low in primary adrenal tumors and inappropriately elevated in CNS or ectopic ACTH-producing tumors.

b. Glucocorticoid excess may be accompanied by a hypokalemic hypernatremic alkalosis, polycythemia, eosinopenia, and abnormal glucose tolerance with hyperglycemia, or glucosuria, or both. Bone age may be less than height age and chronological age. Osteoporosis may be present.

c. Dexamethasone suppression and metyrapone tests, CNS evaluation, an intravenous pyelogram, and an adrenal arteriogram may be necessary to determine the cause of the syndrome.

4. Treatment

a. Resection of an adrenal tumor may be complicated by the patient's clinical state (hypertension, obesity, poor wound healing). When a demonstrable pituitary tumor, especially with visual field changes, is demonstrated surgery, radiation, or both, must be considered.

b. Recently, metyrapone (which blocks the synthesis of cortisol), or mitotane (Lysodren) (an adrenolytic drug), or both, have been used to eliminate the effects of glucocorticoid excess, either to prepare for surgery or to perform a "medical" adrenalectomy, with preservation of mineralocorticoid activity.

D. Pheochromocytoma

1. Etiology. The adrenal medulla is derived from the ectoderm of the neural crest and secretes the catecholamines epinephrine and norepinephrine. Overproduction of the catecholamines may be due to tumors of the adrenal medulla or of accessory chromatin tissue. In children, as many as 20–30% of pheochromocytomas are extramedullary in location, and, in 25% of patients more than one tumor may be found.

2. Evaluation. The **clinical manifestations** most commonly noted are hypertension, headache, tachycardia, weight loss, visual changes, palpitations, nervousness, abdominal or chest pain, hyperhydrosis, anxiety, fatigue, facial pallor, polydipsia, polyuria, and tremors. A **family history** of autoimmune disease, neuroectodermal dysplasias, medullary carcinoma of the thyroid, and parathyroid tumors should be explored.

3. Diagnosis. Typically, symptoms and signs are intermittent. The diagnosis is usually made by the detection of an increased concentration of epinephrine, norepinephrine, or metanephrine in the urine or blood, or of increased urinary vanillylmandelic acid. Localization of the tumor(s) may be difficult, and surgical exploration may be necessary.

4. Treatment. The hypertension should be brought under control with dibenzamine prior to invasive diagnostic procedures or surgery. Blood pressure must be monitored carefully during surgical resection.

VII. Disorders of calcium homeostasis

A. Hypoparathyroidism

1. Etiology

a. Idiopathic

(1) Early onset of hypoparathyroidism (first year)

(a) X-linked recessive (mild)

(b) Congenital absence of parathyroids (3rd and 4th pharyngeal pouches [embryonic] syndrome = DiGeorge syndrome)

(2) Later onset. Males and females are equally affected.

(a) Associated with Addison's disease and candidiasis

(b) Isolated hypoparathyroidism

b. Iatrogenic (following surgery)

c. Neonatal hypoparathyroidism

2. **Presentation.** Patients with hypoparathyroidism have a decreased ability to excrete phosphate, decreased calcium absorption, and decreased bone resorption, resulting in hypocalcemia and hyperphosphatemia, tetany, blepharospasm, conjunctivitis, papilledema, and increased intracranial pressure. Prolonged hypocalcemia results in trophic changes of the nails and skin.
3. **Laboratory evaluation** should include:
   a. Serum Ca, P, Mg, and alkaline phosphatase
   b. Circulating parathyroid hormone (PTH) and circulating vitamin D metabolites
   c. $3'$-$5'$-Cyclic adenosine monophosphate (AMP) clearance
4. **Diagnosis**
   a. The serum calcium is usually 7–8 mg/100 ml, with a serum phosphorus of above 5.5 mg/100 ml.
   b. Circulating PTH is decreased (nondetectable or low normal) despite the low calcium (normally a stimulus for PTH secretion).
   c. **PTH infusion.** Using 200 IU of bovine PTH IV will lead to a rise in serum Ca and urinary phosphate. A rise in urinary cyclic AMP will also be found. This distinguishes hypoparathyroidism from pseudohypoparathyroidism.
5. **Treatment**
   a. **Tetany** is treated with an IV solution of calcium gluconate; $CaCl_2$, 2 ml/kg, is given slowly IV. ECG monitoring is essential during infusion. If the heart rate decreases, the infusion should be slowed or stopped.
   b. When tetany has cleared, the patient can be maintained on oral calcium gluconate at 200 mg/kg/day divided into 4–6 doses.
   c. In **chronic hypoparathyroidism,** therapy with vitamin D is recommended. Vitamin D therapy should be withheld in postsurgical hypoparathyroidism until a chronic deficiency is documented (the parathyroid function may be suppressed up to 120 hr and still return to normal).
      (1) **Dihydrotachysterol,** 0.25–0.75 mg/day. The compound remains in the bloodstream for 10–14 days after the medication is withdrawn.
      (2) 1,25-Dihydroxy vitamin D (calcitriol) in dosages of 0.25–1.0 μg/day. Each capsule contains 0.25 μg. If more than one capsule is used, 0.25 μg/day bid, tid, or qid should be administered.
   d. Vitamin D therapy should be monitored with a 24-hr urine for calcium and creatinine excretion and with frequent serum calciums. If the calcium-creatinine ratio exceeds 0.3, or if the serum calcium exceeds 10.5 mg/100 ml, the vitamin D preparation parameters return to normal. The medication should be restarted at a lower dose.
B. **Pseudohypoparathyroidism** is a genetic disorder resulting from an abnormality in the adenyl cyclase enzyme complex that mediates the response to levels of PTH.
   1. **Presentation.** The disorder is familial, with the usual transmission, appearing to be X-linked dominant. Albright's hereditary osteodystrophy (obese with a round face, mental retardation, metastatic calcification, especially of the basal ganglia, shortened 4th and 5th metacarpals and metatarsals) is present in many patients with this disorder. The manifestations of hypocalcemia are similar to those previously described.
   2. **Laboratory findings and diagnosis** are similar to those in hypoparathyroidism except that circulating levels of immunoreactive PTH are elevated. **PTH infusion** is the definitive test. In pseudohypoparathyroidism, no rise in phosphate excretion or increase in serum calcium is seen.
   3. **Treatment** is the same as for hypoparathyroidism.
C. **Hypercalcemia** is defined as a calcium greater than 11 mg/100 ml.
   1. **Etiology**
      a. **Idiopathic hypercalcemia of infancy** (Williams syndrome), when associated with supravalvular aortic stenosis, mental retardation, and "elfin" facies), presents in early infancy. Hypercalcemia **usually** resolves by 1 year of age.

b. **Hyperparathyroidism** may be primary. In this case, association with other endocrinopathies should be sought in the patient or family members (multiple endocrine adenomatoses type I [acromegaly, insulinoma, peptic ulcers] or type II [medullary thyroid carcinoma, pheochromocytoma, and mucosal neuromas]).

c. **Secondary hyperparathyroidism** is usually due to renal failure, but it may be encountered in long-term malabsorptive conditions.

d. **Vitamin D toxicity**

e. **Vitamin A toxicity**

f. **Immobilization** hypercalcemia occurs predominantly in adolescents following trauma.

2. **Presentation.** Hypercalcemia results in nausea, constipation, weight loss, headaches, personality changes, renal stones, bone pain, hypotonia, polyuria, and polydypsia. Infants with hypercalcemia secondary to neonatal hyperparathyroidism (rare) are usually critically ill.

3. **Evaluation** should include the following:

a. Serum Ca, P, Mg, CO_2

b. Circulating PTH and vitamin D metabolites

c. A 24-hr urine for Ca, P, Mg, Cr, cyclic AMP

d. Bone films, including skull and pelvis

e. Vitamin A

4. **Diagnosis**

a. **Hyperparathyroidism** is diagnosed by the presence of an elevated circulating PTH level, decreased serum phosphate, and bone films showing evidence of irregular surfaces and bone cysts (osteitis fibrosa cystica). Differential cannulation of vessels supplying the parathyroid may be necessary to localize a parathyroid adenoma.

b. **Williams syndrome** is diagnosed on the basis of clinical presentation. An echocardiogram may be helpful in establishing the diagnosis.

c. **Vitamin A toxicity** is rare but may occasionally be diagnosed on the basis of a careful dietary history (intake of liver) or by measurement of serum levels of retinoic acid.

5. **Treatment**

a. **Acute** hypercalcemia should be treated with the infusion of 0.9% NaCl solution and with the administration of furosemide, 1 mg/kg. Glucocorticoids are also useful in lowering serum calcium.

b. In **primary hyperparathyroidism**, surgical correction of the condition is frequently necessary. This is true if an adenoma is found and in neonatal hyperparathyroidism. In this latter disease, surgery in the first weeks of life may be lifesaving.

c. In **secondary hyperparathyroidism** due to renal failure, improvement is usually seen when the patient's calcium balance is restored. This is accomplished by a combination of 1,25-dihydroxy vitamin D therapy and phosphate control (binding or dialysis).

d. Immobilization hypercalcemia resolves when weight bearing can be tolerated. In severe cases, fluid therapy with furosemide and/or calcitonin may be needed.

D. **Rickets**

1. **Etiology**

a. **Vitamin D deficiency** may result from inadequate intake (vegetarians, breast-fed infants, infants on TPN), malabsorptive states, anticonvulsive therapy, renal disease, and inadequate renal production of 1,25(OH)2D (vitamin D dependency).

b. **Excessive renal phosphate loss** also causes rickets. This is seen in X-linked hypophosphatemia (vitamin D–resistant rickets), Fanconi syndrome, Lowe syndrome.

c. **Renal tubular acidosis** has also been associated with rachitic changes.

2. **Laboratory evaluation** should include the following:
   a. Circulating vitamin D metabolites, especially 25-hydroxy vitamin D and 1,25-dihydroxy vitamin D
   b. Circulating levels of PTH
   c. Serum Ca, P, Mg, alkaline phosphatase, and total CO_2
   d. Knee and wrist films
   e. Urinary Ca, P, Mg, pH, creatinine, and amino acids
3. **Evaluation**
   a. Patients with vitamin D–deficient rickets present with a history of bone pain, anorexia, slowed growth, and alterations in the long bones, with widening of wrists and knees, bowed legs, and muscle weakness. A rachitic rosary (enlarged costochondral junctions) and craniotabes may be noted.
   b. Patients with hypophosphatemic syndromes usually have a family history of rickets.
4. **Diagnosis**
   a. **Radiologic findings** of rickets include irregular cortices and bony margins, widened metaphyses, widened growth plates, and osteopenia.
   b. In **vitamin D–deficient rickets,** serum Ca is normal or low, phosphorus is low, but over 3.0 mg/100 ml, alkaline phosphatase is elevated, and urinary phosphate excretion is not excessive. An elevated level of PTH and a decreased 25-hydroxy vitamin D level confirm the diagnosis.
   c. In **hypophosphatemic rickets,** renal phosphate wastage is increased (renal tubular resorption of phosphate is less than 80%). Serum phosphate is usually less than 3.0 mg/100 ml. Serum calcium and circulating levels of PTH and vitamin D metabolites are normal, and alkaline phosphatase is elevated.
5. **Treatment**
   a. In **vitamin D–deficient or –dependent rickets,** the treatment is vitamin D replacement. Dietary rickets in infants heals when they are given 1,000 IU/day of cholecalciferol PO. In malabsorptive syndromes and renal disease, calcitriol 1,25-dihydroxy vitamin D is recommended. Therapy should begin with 0.25 µg/day. If there is an inadequate response, this may have to be increased by 0.25 µg/day by adding doses.
   b. In **hypophosphatemic disorders** the administration of potassium acid phosphate in dosages ranging from 1.0–5.0 gm/day may be necessary to improve the rickets. Treatment with 0.25 µg/day of calcitriol is recommended to maintain adequate calcium absorption during phosphate therapy.
   c. To avoid the side effects of hypercalcuria and hypercalcemia, frequent monitoring (every 2–3 months) of blood and urinary calcium levels should be done.
VIII. **Hypoglycemia.** Hypoglycemia is the most common metabolic abnormality in childhood. This may be due in part to the child's limited ability to store significant quantities of glucose. *Hypoglycemia* (outside of neonatal hypoglycemia) is generally defined as a glucose of less than 40 mg/100 ml.
A. **Etiology.** See Table 11-9.
B. **Presentation.** The signs of hypoglycemia are predominantly those of epinephrine release: tremor, sweating, increased heart rate, abdominal pain, lethargy, nausea, light-headedness, headache, blurred vision, and seizures (rare). In small children, drowsiness may be seen.
   1. **Hyperinsulin** states usually present before age 2 years. A family history of hypoglycemia may be present. Physical examination may be completely normal.
   2. **Ketotic hypoglycemia** occurs after a prolonged fast (the so-called "Sunday morning" syndrome) in children between 18 months and 4 years of age. Presentation beyond this age is rare. Children with ketotic hypoglycemia tend to be small for their age.

Table 11-9. Classification of hypoglycemia

Neonatal hypoglycemia
Hypoglycemia associated with the small-for-gestational-age infant
Transient hyperinsulinemia of the newborn infant
  Infant of the diabetic mother
  Infant with erythroblastosis
Hypoglycemia of infancy and childhood
Hyperinsulinemia
  Beta-cell hyperplasia
  Beta-cell tumors
  Nesidioblastosis
  Functional beta-cell secretory defects
Substrate limited
  Ketotic hypoglycemia
  Hypoglycemia associated with endocrine disorders
    Panhypopituitarism
    Isolated GH deficiencies
    ACTH deficiency
    Addison's disease
    Hypothyroidism
Hepatic enzyme deficiencies
  Glycogen storage diseases
    Glucose 6-phosphatase
    Amylo 1,6-glucosidase
    Defects of the phosphorylase enzyme system
  Disorders of gluconeogenesis
    Fructose 1,6-diphosphatase
    Pyruvate carboxylase
  Other enzyme defects
    Glycogen synthetase
    Galactose 1-phosphate uridyl transferase
    Fructose 1-phosphate aldolase

Table 11-10. Evaluation of hypoglycemia

Test ordered[a]	Results expected in		
	Ketotic hypoglycemia	Excess insulin	Endocrine abnormalities
Blood sugar	↓	↓	↓
Insulin	↓	↑↑	Normal
Proinsulin	Normal	↑ % or normal	Normal
GH	Normal or ↑	↑	↑ [b]
Cortisol, ACTH	Normal or ↑	↑	↓ [b]
T₄, TSH	Normal	Normal	↓ [b]
Free fatty acids	↑↑	↓ or normal	↓ [b]
Ketones	↑↑	Negative	↑ or negative
Alanine	↓↓	↓	Normal or ↓

[a] Obtained at time of hypoglycemia episode or after an 8- to 12-hr fast.
[b] GH deficiency, ACTH deficiency, and TSH deficiency may occur as multiple or as isolated deficiencies.

   3. **Endocrine disorders** present with signs and symptoms of the primary deficiency. One note should be made: Severe hypoglycemia associated with a microphallus suggests a hypopituitary state.
C. **Laboratory evaluation and diagnosis.** See Table 11-10.
   1. **Glycogen storage disease** usually presents with organomegaly. If suspected, the glucose response to glucagon, 0.03 mg/kg given SQ, will show little or no rise in glucose 6-phosphatase deficiency and a number of other storage diseases.
   2. The various entities responsible for hyperinsulin states cannot be differentiated on the basis of serum tests. Radiographic techniques or selective cannulation of pancreatic vessels may aid in diagnosis. However, surgical exploration is frequently necessary.
D. **Treatment** is dependent on the etiology.
   1. Hyperinsulin states due to **neoplastic** or **hypoplastic disorders** require surgical intervention with removal of the lesion or subtotal pancreatectomy. In hyperplasia, this frequently will still provide inadequate control. Glucocorticoid administration at low doses, 15 mg/M^2/day may provide substantial stabilization.
   2. **Ketotic hypoglycemia** is usually a mild, self-limited disorder. Frequent feedings and avoiding prolonged overnight fasts are usually adequate to prevent further episodes.
   3. Hormonal replacement improves the hypoglycemia found in patients with **endocrine disorders,** especially in GH and cortisol deficiencies.
   4. **Glycogen storage diseases** are best treated by providing a relatively constant carbohydrate intake. This can be accomplished in most patients with frequent (q3h) feedings during the day and with an overnight glucose infusion. Both should deliver an average of 0.5 gm of glucose/kg/hr.

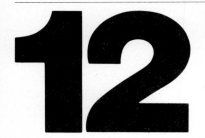

Prepubertal and Adolescent Gynecology

Pregnancy and venereal disease are common among adolescents. Pediatric and adolescent gynecologic complaints should be investigated and initially treated in the familiar setting of the pediatrician's office. This setting may eliminate much of the emotional and physical discomfort otherwise associated with these procedures.

I. **Gynecologic evaluation**

A. The **pelvic examination** should be carefully explained before it is begun, with no surprises in store for the patient. The use of plastic models of pelvic organs is helpful in demonstrating the procedure. As the examination proceeds, each step should be reexplained. Alert the patient to expect mild discomfort, e.g., on insertion of the speculum. Show the instruments to be used and allow the patient to touch them. This will be especially helpful with the younger child and may allay many of the parent's fears as well. Whether or not a parent remains in the room depends on the parent-child relationship. Little girls usually prefer to have the mother readily accessible. The adolescent, however, should be examined alone if the examiner is female, or with a chaperon present if the examiner is male.

1. **Examining the young child**

   a. **Inspecting the external genitalia.** The child is told that the procedure will not hurt. She is placed on her back, with the knees wide apart and the soles of the feet touching each other. As the external genitalia are inspected, the patient is asked to help by holding the labia apart. This allows her to participate and have a sense of control.

   Note the presence or absence of pubic hair, clitoral size, character of the introitus, and perineal hygiene. The premenarcheal clitoris should not exceed 3 mm in length and 2 mm in transverse diameter.

   b. **Visualizing the vagina.** Placing girls over 2 years old in the knee-chest position allows the examiner to view the vagina and cervix without instrumentation. The patient is told to "lie on her tummy with her bottom in the air." She is reassured that the examiner is only going to look with the help of the otoscope light. She is allowed to see and touch the light. As the child takes a few deep breaths and allows her spine and stomach to "sag like an old horse," the vaginal orifice falls open. The otoscope provides the necessary light and magnification needed to visualize the cervix.

   c. **Rectal-abdominal examination.** While the child is lying on her back, a gentle rectal-abdominal examination is carried out. The index or fifth finger of one hand is inserted into the rectum. The other hand is placed on the abdomen for bimanual palpation. The example of a rectal thermometer can be used to explain how the examining finger will feel.

   The examiner will feel only a "button" of a cervix. The ovaries are not palpable in the prepubertal child; hence, if an adnexal mass is felt, a cyst or tumor should be suspected.

2. **Examining the adolescent.** The psychological implications of a pelvic examination in a teenager warrant taking the time to establish a trusting relationship before proceeding.

   a. **Preparations.** The patient is given an examining gown and told to remove all her clothes and put the gown on while the physician is out of the room. Respect for the patient's privacy is essential, and the procedure

Table 12-1. Specula for use in the adolescent age group

Type of speculum	Usage
Huffman ($\frac{1}{2} \times 4\frac{1}{2}$ inches)	Small hymeneal opening
Pederson ($1 \times 4\frac{1}{2}$ inches)	Sexually active adolescent
Graves ($\frac{5}{8} \times 3$ inches)	Sexually active adolescent

should be explained. She is then placed on the table in stirrups and draped. Older adolescents often prefer no draping and appreciate watching the examination with the help of mirrors.

b. Inspecting the external genitalia. The Tanner staging of pubic hair is noted, along with size of the clitoris (the normal glans is 2–4 mm in width; 10 mm indicates significant virilization) and the appearance of the introitus.

c. Speculum examination. Two types of specula are available for use in the adolescent age group (Table 12-1).

   (1) The appropriate speculum, once selected, is shown to the patient. If possible, the speculum is warmed and touched to the patient's thigh before insertion.

   (2) Before the speculum is inserted in the virginal teenager, a slow, one-finger examination is done to demonstrate the size of the introitus and location of the cervix.

   (3) With a finger, the introitus is gently depressed and spread, and the speculum is slowly slipped into the vagina. After a moment's pause the speculum is carefully opened, the cervix located, and the speculum secured in place.

   (4) Note the appearance of the cervix and vaginal mucosa. Cultures and smears may be taken at this time. The speculum is then removed.

d. Bimanual examination. After the speculum is removed, lubricant is applied to the index and middle finger before insertion into the vagina.

   (1) The fingers are placed just under the cervix, and with the other hand on the abdomen, the uterine size and location are determined. The adnexae are then checked.

   (2) In tense or obese patients it may be difficult to identify ovarian tissue by touch. A confirmatory rectovaginal examination is done by placing the index finger in the vagina, the middle finger in the rectum, and the other hand on the abdomen. The patient is warned that she will feel as though she is having a bowel movement.

   (3) When the examination is completed and the patient has dressed, the examiner's findings are discussed with her.

B. Breast examination. Breast cancer will develop in 1 in 13 women. Adolescents should be taught how to do a breast self-examination and should become familiar with their breasts, so that when an unusual lump is noted, they will seek prompt medical attention. Cancer of the breast is extremely rare in children and adolescents. In girls with a strong family history of breast cancer, particularly in the maternal line, the importance of self-examination should be stressed.

   1. Methods of self-examination

      a. Supine. Lying on her back, she places the left hand under the head. The fingertips of the right hand are placed on the left breast at 12 o'clock. The breast is gently palpated clockwise. The examination is repeated for the right breast, using the left hand for palpation, with the right hand under the head.

      b. Upright. The procedures described above are repeated in a standing position (usually in the shower, since the wet skin is easier to manipulate). The breasts should be examined each month, just at the *end* of the menstrual flow. If periods are irregular, an arbitrary day each month is selected, e.g., the first Monday of the month.

2. Findings

a. Some evidence of **benign cystic change** is found in 85% of women.

b. Mild **asymmetry** of the breasts is normal. However, when the unequal size results in an obvious cosmetic deformity, plastic surgery may be indicated.

c. **Lack of development** may be secondary to a congenital absence (amastia) or to a systemic disorder, e.g., malnutrition, congenital adrenal hyperplasia, gonadal dysgenesis, or hypogonadotropic hypogonadism. In Western society, where breast size is often used as a measure of femininity, girls with normal, small breasts may need reassurance. (You might remind them that there would not be so many size 32A bras to choose from if they were the only ones who need that size!)

d. **Accessory nipples or breasts** occur in 1–2% of healthy patients. No therapy is indicated.

e. **Nipple discharge** is rare. Galactorrhea is seen in patients on phenothiazines, reserpine, methyldopa, and oral contraceptives. Amenorrhea with galactorrhea requires evaluation to rule out a CNS tumor. A periareolar follicle may drain brownish fluid for several weeks; no treatment is needed.

f. **Periareolar hair** is not uncommon in healthy adolescents. No treatment is indicated.

C. Diagnostic studies

1. A **Papanicolaou smear** should be done on all young women who have a speculum examination.

a. With the speculum in place, an Ayer wooden spatula is scraped around the cervix, and the collected material is spread on a slide. In addition, a cotton-tipped applicator moistened with saline is swirled in the endocervical canal (¼ inch through the cervical os) and streaked on the frosted side of a glass slide.

b. The slide is then placed in a bottle of Papanicolaou fixative or sprayed with fixative and sent to the cytology laboratory.

c. The results are classified as follows:
  I. Negative
  II. Benign aplasia (also negative)
  IIR. Atypical cells
  III. Dysplasia
  IV. Suspicious cells, probably carcinoma in situ
  V. Definite tumor cells

d. Treatment
  (1) Class I or II. Annual Papanicolaou smears should be done.
  (2) Class IIR. The atypical cells seen may be secondary to infection (*Trichomonas, Candida albicans*) or endometrial cells (present when the smear was taken at the end of the menstrual period). Treat the vaginitis and repeat the smear in 2–3 months at midcycle.
  (3) Class III, IV, V. Refer the patient to a gynecologist.

2. In the absence of infection, a **vaginal smear for estrogen** is useful for evaluating the patient's hormonal status. When the speculum is in place, the side wall of the vagina is scraped with a tongue depressor or a Q-tip moistened with saline. When the speculum is not used, a Q-tip is inserted directly through the introitus. The material obtained is streaked on a glass slide and placed in Papanicolaou fixative.

3. The **cervical mucus** can be used to evaluate the patient's estrogen status. First, swab the cervix with a large, cotton-tipped applicator. Then obtain a small sample of cervical mucus with a long forceps or saline-moistened Q-tip. On day 8–9 of the menstrual cycle the mucus is scant and watery. On day 14–16 it is profuse, clear, and elastic. On day 20 it is thick and sticky. Spread the collected cervical mucus on a glass slide, allow it to air-dry for 10–

20 min, and examine it under the microscope. The late proliferative phase of the menstrual cycle is characterized by *ferning* of the cervical mucus. The presence of ferning in sexually active patients with secondary amenorrhea indicates a persistent proliferative phase suggesting an anovulatory cycle not pregnancy. Ferning will not occur when progesterone is present.

4. **Wet preparations** are used in determining the cause of a vaginal discharge
   a. **In the prepubertal child,** the sample is collected with a saline-moistened Q-tip or eyedropper while the patient is supine.
   b. **In the adolescent,** the specimen is collected from the vaginal pool while the speculum is in place. The Q-tip is taken from the vaginal pool to a slide, where it is mixed with 1 drop of saline, and then is placed on another slide, where it is mixed with 1 drop of 10% potassium hydroxide (KOH).
   c. A cover slip is promptly applied, and the slides are examined under the microscope (low and high dry power).
      (1) **Trichomonas** infection is indicated by the presence of lively, flagellated organisms.
      (2) In **Gardnerella vaginalis** infection, refractile bacteria, large epithelial cells ("clue cells"), and leukocytes are seen.
      (3) In **Candida albicans** infection, budding hyphae and yeast forms are present.
5. **Gram stain.** In symptomatic gonorrhea the smear may reveal gram-negative intracellular diplococci. However, because saprophytic *Neisseria* organisms are normally present in the vagina, only a positive culture establishes the diagnosis.
6. **Cultures.** Sexually active adolescents should have a routine cervical culture for gonorrhea every 6 months. The sites of culture in the symptomatic patient or a contact are the urethra, cervix, rectum, and pharynx.
   a. Swab the area to be cultured with a Q-tip and streak directly on a slide, using a Transgrow, modified Thayer-Martin-Gembec, or Thayer-Martin medium.
   b. To confirm yeast vaginitis, swab the vagina and streak on Nickerson's medium.
   c. Leave the cap of the bottle with the medium partially unscrewed and incubate the tube in your office at room temperature. The appearance of brown colonies in 3–7 days confirms the diagnosis.
7. **Progesterone test.** Progesterone is used as a diagnostic test in the evaluation of primary and secondary amenorrhea; it is not a test for pregnancy. Medroxyprogesterone (Provera), 10 mg PO, is given for 5 days, or progesterone-in-oil, 50–100 mg, is given IM. If the endometrium is estrogen primed and the patient is not pregnant, withdrawal bleeding will result in 3–7 days.
8. **Pregnancy tests**
   a. Several 2-min urine pregnancy tests (Gravindex, Pregnosticon Accuspheres, Pregnosis, and the UCG slide test) are available. These tests detect human chorionic gonadotropin (HCG) 10–14 days after the first missed period. Tube tests done in commercial laboratories and hospitals require 2 hr and become positive 1 week earlier than the 2-min tests.
   b. **Blood test.** The Beta subunit test measures HCG in serum and is positive within 5–10 days of conception.
   c. **False-negative and false-positive tests**
      (1) **Urine.** False-negative tests occur when the patient is less than 6 weeks pregnant and in ectopic pregnancies. False-positive tests are seen with detergent residue on the glassware, significant proteinuria, and some drugs (e.g., methadone, phenothiazines, and progestational agents).
      (2) **Blood.** False-negative tests are obtained very early in pregnancy when HCG is less than 0.2 IU/ml of serum. The presence of choriocarcinoma or hydatidiform mole may result in false-positive tests in young women.

9. **Buccal smear.** The patient rinses her mouth with water, and a tongue depressor is then scraped along the buccal mucosa.
   a. The material is streaked on a glass slide and placed in Papanicolaou fixative or a 3:1 methanol–acetic acid solution.
   b. The chromatin-positive material (Barr body) represents the second X chromosome. Normal Barr-body counts vary from 10–49%. The absence of Barr bodies indicates XO or XY; a low count suggests a mosaic; XXX or XXXY causes two Barr bodies per cell.
10. The **basal body temperature chart** is used primarily for infertility patients, although it is also helpful in determining when ovulation occurs in a patient with oligomenorrhea or a mosaic Turner syndrome. Instruct the patient to keep a thermometer by the bedside, place the thermometer in her mouth as soon as she awakens, and record the temperature on a chart. There is a drop in the basal body temperature at the time of ovulation.

II. **Common gynecologic complaints of children and adolescents**
   A. **Vulvovaginitis in the prepubertal child**
      1. **Etiology.** Poor perineal hygiene is likely after the age of 3, when mothers are not directly involved with toileting.
         a. Pinworm infestation with the subsequent anal scratching can contaminate the vaginal area; an adult pinworm may migrate to the vagina and produce vaginal irritation and discharge.
         b. Bubble bath and harsh soaps cause vulvitis and secondary vaginitis.
         c. Tight-fitting nylon underpants worn in hot weather cause maceration and secondary infections, usually yeast.
         d. *Trichomonas, Neisseria gonorrhoeae,* group A beta-hemolytic streptococci, and pneumococci are specific agents causing vulvovaginitis.
      2. **Evaluation**
         a. A careful history should be traced, questioning the child about the etiologic factors listed in **1.** Ask about the quantity, duration, and type of discharge. Determine the direction in which the child wipes the anal area. Ask about the use of bubble baths, the type of soap used, symptoms of anal pruritus, and whether or not there is exposure to an infected adult through sexual contact or indirectly by sharing a bed, towels, and so on.
         b. Examine the child in the knee-chest position to rule out the presence of a foreign body.
         c. When a vaginal discharge is persistent or purulent, Gram stains, wet preparations, and cultures should be done. If the amount of discharge is scant, use brain-heart broth and Thayer-Martin-Gembec as media. If the discharge is copious, use Thayer-Martin-Gembec and either brain-heart infusion or send the swab to the laboratory for culture on blood, McConkey, and chocolate agar.
         d. Do a wet preparation for yeast and *Trichomonas.* Yeast infection is rare, but when found, check the urine for glucose to rule out diabetes. Do the Scotch Tape or pinworm paddle test to confirm the presence of pinworm infestation.
      3. **Diagnosis.** A **history of exposure** to offending agents, the presence of **symptoms** (itching, discomfort, vaginal discharge), the **character of the discharge,** and the **physical findings** aid in establishing the diagnosis of vulvovaginitis.
      4. **Therapy**
         a. **Nonspecific vaginitis** (culture shows *E. coli,* other gram-negative enteric organisms, or normal flora) is treated with the following measures:
            (1) Instruct the child to
               (a) Improve perineal hygiene.
               (b) Wear white cotton underpants.
               (c) Avoid bubble baths and harsh soaps.
               (d) Take sitz baths tid in plain warm water. Wash the vulvar area with mild soap (Basis, Oilatum, Castile) and pat dry. Allow for

further drying by lying on the back with the legs spread apart for 10 min.
   (2) If there is no improvement in 3 weeks, treat the child with oral antibiotics (such as amoxicillin, ampicillin, or cephalexin) for 10–14 days
   (3) If improvement still does not occur, treat the child with an estrogen containing cream for 2–3 weeks (reversible breast tenderness and vulvar pigmentation may occur).
   b. Acute severe edematous vulvitis
   (1) Sitz baths should be taken q4h, without soap and with air drying.
   (2) Witch hazel pads (Tucks) should be used instead of toilet paper.
   (3) After 2 days, sitz baths should be alternated with painting of the vulva with a bland solution, e.g., calamine lotion.
   (4) For *pruritis,* hydrocortisone cream 1%, Neo-Cortef Cream 1%, or Vioform-Hydrocortisone cream should be applied to the vulva.
   c. Specific vaginitis
   (1) Gonococcus. See Chap. 15, p. 398.
   (2) For **group A beta-hemolytic streptococci or pneumococci:**
   (a) Penicillin, 125–250 mg PO qid for 10 days, or
   (b) Erythromycin, 30–50 mg/kg/day PO tid.
   (3) For **Trichomonas,** Metronidazole (Flagyl), 125 mg tid PO for 5 days, or 1–2 gm PO in 1 dose, is recommended.
   (4) Pinworms. See Chap. 16, p. 427.
   (5) *Candida albicans.* Nystatin cream (for moist lesions) or ointment (for dry scaly lesions) should be applied to the vulva tid for 2 weeks. For persistent yeast infections, nystatin, 100,000 units PO qid for 2 weeks, or 1 ml in the vagina tid for 2 weeks, is recommended.
   (6) Condyloma acuminatum is often seen in association with *Trichomonas* vaginitis. Examine the lesions by biopsy to establish a definitive diagnosis, and treat with podophyllin (see **B.3.f**).
   (7) Labia adhesions can occur in girls 2–6 years of age. The cause is unknown. In mild cases, no treatment is required. When vaginal or urinary drainage is impaired, Premarin cream is applied bid for 2 weeks and lubrication with K-Y Jelly should be continued for several months to prevent the adhesions from re-forming. **The labia should not be forced apart.** This is traumatic to the child and leads to further adhesion formation.
B. Vulvovaginitis in the adolescent
   1. Etiology. Unlike prepubertal vaginitis, which is nonspecific most of the time, vaginitis in the adolescent usually has a specific cause and is often related to sexual contact, e.g., *N. gonorrhoeae, Trichomonas, Candida, Haemophilus vaginalis,* or herpesvirus. However, the most common cause of discharge in the adolescent is physiologic leukorrhea (normal desquamation of epithelial cells).
   2. Evaluation and diagnosis. A pelvic examination is required, with wet preparations and cultures.
   a. *Trichomonas.* A wet preparation (saline) reveals flagellated organisms dancing under the microscope. Small punctate hemorrhagic spots may be seen on the cervical and vaginal cells.
   b. *Candida.* A wet preparation (potassium hydroxide) reveals budding hyphae. Nickerson's medium is used for culturing.
   c. Nonspecific vaginitis. A wet preparation reveals large epithelial cells coated with small refractile bacteria (clue cells). To identify *G. vaginalis,* the discharge is streaked on chocolate agar and incubated under increased CO_2 tension.
   d. Gonorrhea. The discharge should be cultured.
   e. Leukorrhea. A wet preparation reveals epithelial cells only.
   f. Condyloma acuminatum. Wartlike growths are inspected.
   g. Herpes vulvitis (see Chap. 15, pp. 414ff.). The vesicles are inspected and the base of the lesion is scraped and stained with Wright's stain. A smear

reveals multinucleated giant cells and inclusions. Viral cultures are available in hospital and commercial laboratories.

h. Pediculosis pubis (crabs). Firmly attached flakes will be seen on the pubic hair. (The flakes are adult lice or nits.)

i. Pinworms. See Chap. 16, p. 427.

j. Foreign body. Inspect the patient for the presence of a foreign body. In the adolescent, this is often a forgotten tampon.

3. Treatment

a. For *Trichomonas* vaginitis, give metronidazole, 2 gm PO, all in 1 dose or 250 mg tid for 7 days. Treat sexual partners at the same time. Instruct the patient not to drink alcohol while on metronidazole, since vomiting often results.

b. For **candidal (monilial) vaginitis,** miconazole (Monistat) vaginal cream, 1 applicatorful intravaginally for 7 nights, or Mycostatin, a vaginal suppository, 1 bid for 14 days, is recommended.

c. For nonspecific vaginitis, therapy is still controversial. Recent studies suggest metronidazole, 500 mg bid PO for 7 days for patient and partner. Alternate but less effective treatment is ampicillin 500 mg qid for 10 days.

d. Gonorrhea. See Chap. 15, p. 398.

e. Leukorrhea. Reassure the patient and recommend good perineal hygiene and the wearing of *white* cotton underpants.

f. Condyloma acuminatum. Treating the associated vaginitis often results in spontaneous regression of the lesions. If the associated vaginitis is not treated, the warts will recur.

    (1) Apply podophyllum resin (25%) in tincture of benzoin to the lesions. Do not touch the normal skin. Tell the patient to wash the lesions 2 hr later.

    (2) If burning occurs, use petrolatum (Vaseline) or lidocaine (Xylocaine) 2% jelly topically.

    (3) Treat the lesions once a week. If they are larger than 1 cm in diameter, refer the patient for excision, fulguration, or cryocautery.

g. Herpes vulvitis. Soothing relief may be obtained with Betadine povidone-iodine (1%) solution and/or lidocaine (Xylocaine) 2% jelly plus sitz baths. Urinating in the shower or tub may be necessary for patients with severe pain.

h. Pediculosis pubis. Kwell lotion should be used on all hairy areas. **Do not exceed recommended dosage as lindane can be absorbed through the skin with potential CNS toxicity.** Clothing and bedding should be washed.

i. Pinworms. See Chap. 16, p. 427.

C. Delayed sexual development. See Chap. 11, p. 295.

D. Secondary amenorrhea

1. Etiology

a. The most common causes are pregnancy and stress caused by fever, emotional turmoil, weight change, change in environment (camp, boarding school, college).

b. Also consider anorexia nervosa, obesity, Stein-Leventhal syndrome, thyroid disease, ovarian tumor, and diabetes.

2. Evaluation

a. Pregnancy. When a sexually active patient's period is 2 weeks late, the patient should have a pelvic examination and a pregnancy test.

b. Stress. The history will elicit areas of stress in a patient's life.

c. Anorexia nervosa. No specific laboratory test is available. Psychiatric evaluation is essential.

d. Obesity. Determine whether or not weight gain (often rapid) is correlated with cessation of periods.

e. Stein-Leventhal syndrome. A pelvic examination will determine the size and characteristics of the ovaries. If the syndrome is present, serum testosterone and LH are usually elevated. The FSH is normal. Urinary

17-ketosteroids are normal to moderately elevated. The diagnosis i confirmed by laparoscopy.

   f. Thyroid disease. See Chap. 11, p. 302.
   g. Ovarian tumor. A pelvic examination should be done.
   h. Diabetes mellitus. See Chap. 13.
3. Diagnosis
   a. Pregnancy is indicated by an enlarged uterus and a soft, blue cervix, and is confirmed by a positive pregnancy test.
   b. Stress. A stressful situation in the patient's life is identified and cor related with the onset of amenorrhea.
   c. Anorexia nervosa. The classic history of prolonged weight loss secondary to poor intake, coupled with excessive activity, amenorrhea, and emo tional problems, confirms the diagnosis of anorexia nervosa.
   d. Obesity. Documentation of excessive weight gain with resultant amen orrhea is required.
   e. Stein-Leventhal syndrome. The diagnosis is considered in a patient with a history of oligomenorrhea, the physical findings of hirsutism, obesity and enlarged cystic ovaries on pelvic examination, and abnormal hor monal levels. It is confirmed through pelvic ultrasound or at laparoscopy when the ovaries demonstrate the typical findings of a thickened capsule and multiple cysts.
   f. Thyroid disease. See Chap. 11, p. 302.
   g. Ovarian tumor. The presence of an adnexal mass on pelvic examination is confirmed by direct visualization and histologic study of sections in estrogen-deficient patients.
   h. Diabetes mellitus. See Chap. 13.
4. Therapy of secondary amenorrhea. Identify the cause and eliminate it when possible.
   a. Stress. Provera 10 mg PO for 5 days. Withdrawal bleeding will result in 3 to 7 days after completing the medication.
   b. Anorexia nervosa. Regaining sufficient weight is critical for the individual's hypothalamic suppression to cease. Interestingly, the final weight at which menstruation spontaneously recurs is usually higher than what the patient weighed at menarche. If the youngster insists on having a period she can be cycled with Premarin 1.25 mg qd from day 1 through day 21 and Provera 10 mg qd from day 17 to day 21.
   c. Obesity. Loss of excessive weight initiates spontaneous periods. Provera in the usual dose is effective in producing withdrawal bleeding.
   d. Stein-Leventhal syndrome. Provera, 10 mg qd for 5 days monthly, is given to prevent endometrial hyperplasia. In patients with enlarged ovaries and elevated testosterone, birth control pills are the treatment of choice. Clomiphene citrate and/or wedge resection are reserved for patients desirous of becoming pregnant.
   e. Thyroid disease. See Chap. 11, p. 302.
   f. Ovarian tumor. Surgical removal of the tumor mass when feasible. If a bilateral oophorectomy is done, cycle the patient on Premarin and Provera as described above (see **b**).
   g. Diabetes mellitus. See Chap. 13.
E. Dysfunctional uterine bleeding
   1. Etiology. One of the most common gynecologic complaints in the adolescent is irregular, prolonged menstruation.
      a. In the **young adolescent** the cause is anovulatory cycles (unopposed estrogen) with incomplete shedding of the proliferative endometrium.
      b. In the **older adolescent** it is secondary to anovulatory cycles from stress or illness.
   2. Evaluation
      a. Pelvic examination
      b. Complete blood count with platelet estimate
      c. Cultures for gonorrhea

       d. Tine test

       e. Pregnancy test

       f. Drug ingestion (warfarin), birth control pills

   3. Diagnosis. A past history of painless irregular periods occurring every 2–3 weeks suggests anovulatory bleeding. Any positive findings in the evaluation procedures suggest specific diagnoses.

   4. Treatment

       a. For irregular periods of short duration with normal hemoglobin and if patient is not bleeding at the time of the visit, Provera 10 mg bid for 7 days. Repeat in 1 month.

       b. For **persistent vaginal bleeding** without significant anemia or no response to **a**, do the following:

          (1) Give Ortho-Novum 1/50   21, 1 pill q4h until the bleeding stops, then one bid until the package is finished.

          (2) The bleeding should stop in 24 hr, followed by withdrawal flow in 2–4 days after the last pill.

          (3) Then cycle the patient with Provera, 10 mg daily PO for the first 5 days of the month for 3 months.

       c. For **heavy vaginal bleeding** with anemia, do the following:

          (1) Give Ortho-Novum 1/50, 2 mg q4h, until bleeding stops, or

          (2) Enovid-E, 2.5 mg q4h, until bleeding stops.

          (3) Once bleeding stops, 1 tablet is taken bid until the package is gone. Withdrawal flow follows the last tablet in 2–4 days.

          (4) Then cycle the patient with Ortho-Novum 1/50 21, or 1/80 21 if breakthrough bleeding occurs, for 2–3 months.

          (5) If bleeding does not stop in 36–48 hr, consult a gynecologist.

F. Dysmenorrhea

   1. The etiology is unclear. It is theorized that prostaglandins released during the menstrual flow stimulate the contractility of the endometrium.

   2. Evaluation. Review the menstrual history, premenstrual symptoms, timing of cramps, and how the patient deals with cramps. In a virginal girl of 13–14 years, inspect the genitalia to rule out a hymenal abnormality. Patients with severe dysmenorrhea require a pelvic examination.

   3. Diagnosis. Cramping lower abdominal pain usually starts 1–4 hr before a period and lasts up to 24 hr. Some girls experience dysmenorrhea 2 days before the onset of menstrual flow, and the pain can last 4–6 days. Nausea and vomiting may accompany the cramps. Dysmenorrhea is functional in 95 percent of patients. Organic lesions associated with dysmenorrhea include chronic pelvic inflammatory disease, vaginal agenesis, rudimentary uterine horn, paramesonephric cysts, and endometriosis.

   4. Treatment is directed at symptomatic relief.

       a. Pain

          (1) Aspirin, 300–600 mg q4h

          (2) Naprosyn, 250 mg q8h

          (3) Empirin with Codeine, 15–30 mg q4h

          (4) Motrin, 400 mg q4h

       b. Nausea and vomiting

          (1) Prochlorperazine (Compazine), 5–10 mg q4h

          (2) Chlorpromazine (Thorazine), 25 mg PR q6h

       c. Bed rest, use of a heating pad, and clear fluids can be helpful.

       d. See the patient every 3 months to evaluate the effectiveness of therapy and foster the physician-patient relationship.

       e. If analgesics fail, give a 6-month course of birth control pills, which eliminate or substantially reduce cramps.

       f. If the cramps persist despite oral contraceptives, refer the patient for a laparoscopy to rule out endometriosis.

G. Mittelschmerz is the pain experienced at the time of ovulation.

   1. Etiology. It is thought to be secondary to spillage of fluid from the rupturing follicular cyst, which irritates the peritoneum.

    2. Evaluation. The patient usually complains of midcycle, unilateral dull and aching lower quadrant abdominal pain lasting from a few minutes to 6–8 hr. Rarely, the pain can be severe, mimicking appendicitis, torsion or rupture of an ovarian cyst, or an ectopic pregnancy. Refer the patient for laparoscopy to rule out these diagnoses.

    3. Diagnosis. The midcycle nature of the pain and absence of significant disease establish the diagnosis.

    4. Treatment. Explain the benign nature of the pain to the patient. A heating pad and mild analgesics are helpful.

H. Diethylstilbestrol exposure in utero

    1. Etiology. Diethylstilbestrol (DES) was given as an antiabortant to women during the 1950s and 1960s. The development of clear cell adenocarcinoma in girls exposed to DES in utero was reported in 1970. Adenosis (glandular epithelium of müllerian origin) of the vaginal wall has been described in 36–90 percent of girls exposed to DES. Although adenosis is a benign condition because of its cytologic similarity to adenocarcinoma, regular follow-up is required. Abnormal uterine shape and incompetent cervix are associated with an increased miscarriage rate among DES-exposed offspring.

    2. Evaluation

        a. Obtain a history of all drugs taken by the girl's mother during pregnancy.

        b. Refer known DES-exposed patients at age 15 to a gynecologist.

        c. Stress the importance of gynecologic follow-up.

    3. The **diagnosis** must be made by a gynecologist.

    4. Treatment. Patients with adenosis should be followed up every 6–12 months.

III. Adolescent sexuality. The care of adolescents includes dealing not only with their physical and emotional well-being, but also with their emerging sexuality. The spectrum of adolescent sexual concerns ranges from homosexual fears to an unwanted pregnancy. To be able to allay these concerns, the pediatrician must establish a confidential, trusting relationship with the teenager, which requires time and patience. Most adolescents are reluctant to initiate sexual discussions. However, sexuality introduced in the context of the system review eliminates the mutual embarrassment often felt by both physician and patient.

A 15-year-old male experiencing spontaneous erections while roughhousing with a male friend fears he is a homosexual. A 14-year-old girl missing her period after a session of heavy petting is convinced she is pregnant. A 16-year-old boy has been taught that masturbation is a sin, yet he continues, convinced he is beyond redemption. A 16-year-old girl is having unprotected intercourse in the belief that she is too young to use any type of birth control.

These are but a few of the issues adolescents will raise as they progress in their normal psychosexual development. By not patronizing them because of their lack of sexual expertise and sophistication, but providing respectful reassurance, the pediatrician can correct most sexual misconceptions.

The decision whether or not sex becomes a part of a teenage relationship rests ultimately with the persons involved. Young people are influenced in such a decision by the family standards, religion, society's expectations, peer pressure, internal needs, drug and alcohol usage, and partner availability. The pediatrician's role is not to judge the patient's behavior, but to provide sufficient information to permit the teenager to make a responsible decision.

The issue of whose obligation it is to educate adolescents about sexuality has not been resolved. The young person has three readily available sources of information: parents, peers, and school. Some parents are uncomfortable discussing sexuality with their children. An equal number of children cannot tolerate discussing sex with their parents. Parents who hand their child a book on sex and say "Read it" have not fulfilled their role in educating their child. As important as the mechanisms of sex are, the feelings involved are of equal value. To understand sexuality, the "why" of sex must be explored, and this is not available in a book. It is during frank discussions between parent and child that the psychology of sex is taught.

Peers as an information source are often a cause of confusion. Why then do children turn to their friends? They are available, approachable, willing to listen, and rarely make moral judgments. Their lack of expertise is rarely seen as a drawback.

Schools in general cannot provide the subtle sensitivity needed to explore adolescent sexuality. Most sex education classes are limited to the mechanics of intercourse. Many states still prohibit the schools from teaching the available methods of birth control. The feelings involved in a sexual experience, the expectations, fantasies, fulfillment, and disappointments are virtually ignored.

The dilemma of adolescent sexuality has not been resolved, which is one reason why teenage pregnancy has reached epidemic proportions in this country. Pediatricians have the opportunity and responsibility to educate and counsel their patients on sexual issues.

IV. Birth control. Statistics clearly show that more than half of all first sexual encounters among teenagers are unprotected. Despite the availability of contraceptives, adolescents often refrain from using them because they detract from the spontaneity of the act. Question your patients on their sexual activity (teenagers rarely volunteer this type of information). If asked in a direct, nonjudgmental manner, most adolescents are willing to share this information and to request a method of birth control that is most appropriate for them.

A. Oral contraceptives. The "pill" is viewed by some as the salvation of women, liberating them from the fear of pregnancy. Others see it as consisting of dangerous chemicals that poison those who use it. There is some truth to both points of view. The pill, taken as prescribed, will prevent pregnancy with over 99 percent efficiency. This is not achieved without complications, however.

1. The **complications and side effects** of oral contraceptive use include the following:
   a. Nausea, bloating, and weight gain
   b. Breakthrough bleeding
   c. Headaches
   d. Hypertension
   e. Thrombophlebitis
   f. Fluid retention, which may increase frequency of epileptic seizures
   g. Scanty or absent periods
   h. Depression
   i. Dry eyes secondary to lack of tearing or corneal edema
   j. Birth control pills containing 50 μg or more of estrogen produce abnormal results on glucose tolerance tests in some patients. Diabetic patients on the pill may have increased insulin requirements.
   k. The pill has produced false-positive LE prep and arthralgias in normal patients. Both of these findings disappear when the pill is stopped.

2. **Contraindications.** The pill is contraindicated in patients with lupus erythematosus, chemical diabetes, and cholestatic jaundice of pregnancy.

3. **Indications for estrogen-dominant pill**
   a. Hirsutism
   b. Acne
   c. Scanty periods (on or off the pill)
   d. Increased appetite and weight gain on the pill
   e. Early-cycle spotting on the pill

4. **Indications for progesterone-dominant pill**
   a. Mucorrhea
   b. Cervical erosion
   c. Nausea or bloating on pills
   d. Fibroids
   e. Fibrocystic breast disease
   f. Cyclic weight gain
   g. Dysmenorrhea
   h. Hypermenorrhea
   i. Late-cycle spotting on the pill

Table 12-2. The hormonal content of commonly used oral contraceptive pills

Product	Estrogen	Progestin
Combination pills		
Enovid-E	Mestranol 0.1 mg	Norethynodrel 2.5 mg
Enovid 5 mg	Mestranol 0.075 mg	Norethynodrel 5 mg
Ortho-Novum 1/35	Ethinyl estradiol 0.05 mg	Norethindrone 1 mg
Norinyl 1 + 35	Ethinyl estradiol 0.035 mg	Norethindrone 1 mg
Ortho-Novum 1/50, Norinyl 1 + 50	Mestranol 0.05 mg	Norethindrone 1 mg
Ortho-Novum 1/80, Norinyl 1 + 80	Mestranol 0.08 mg	Norethindrone 1 mg
Ortho-Novum 2 mg, Norinyl 2 mg	Mestranol 0.1 mg	Norethindrone 2 mg
Norlestrin 1/50, Zorane 1/50	Ethinyl estradiol 0.05 mg	Norethindrone acetate 1 mg
Norlestrin 2.5/50	Ethinyl estradiol 0.05 mg	Norethindrone acetate 2.5 mg
Ovulen	Mestranol 0.1 mg	Ethynodiol diacetate 1 mg
Demulen	Ethinyl estradiol 0.05 mg	Ethynodiol diacetate 1 mg
Ovral	Ethinyl estradiol 0.05 mg	Norgestrel 0.5 mg
Ovcon-50	Ethinyl estradiol 0.05 mg	Norethindrone 1 mg
Ovcon-35	Ethinyl estradiol 0.035 mg	Norethindrone 0.4 mg
Brevicon	Ethinyl estradiol 0.035 mg	Norethindrone 0.5 mg
Lo/Ovral	Ethinyl estradiol 0.03 mg	Norgestrel 0.3 mg
Loestrin	Ethinyl estradiol 0.02 mg	Norethindrone acetate 1 mg
Mini-pills		
Nor-Q.D., Micronor		Norethindrone 0.35 mg
Ovrette		Norgestrel 0.075 mg

Source: Modified from S. J. H. Emans and D. P. Goldstein, *Pediatric and Adolescent Gynecology* (2nd ed.). Boston: Little, Brown, 1982.

5. **Changes in common laboratory values**
   a. T_4 is increased, and resin T_3 is decreased. Free T_4 is unchanged.
   b. There is a slight increase in coagulation factors II, VIII–X, and XII and a moderate increase in factor VII.
   c. Triglyceride, cholesterol, and phospholipid levels are increased in some patients.
   d. Serum folate is decreased in some patients and is rarely associated with megaloblastic anemia.
   e. The ESR is increased slightly.
6. **Prescribing the pill**
   a. **Patient evaluation** requires the following:
      (1) A complete history and physical examination, including a pelvic examination.
      (2) **Laboratory studies.** Hemoglobin and Papanicolaou smear. In patients with a family history of arteriosclerotic heart disease or stroke, cholesterol and triglyceride levels should be determined. In sexually active patients, test for syphilis once a year and culture for gonorrhea every 6 months.
   b. **Choice of pill.** See Table 12-2.
      (1) A medium-dose pill (e.g., Norinyl 1/35 or 1/50, Ortho-Novum 1/35 or 1/50) can be prescribed for girls with regular periods and no special indication for an estrogen-dominant or progesterone-dominant pill.
      (2) A low-dose pill (e.g., Brevicon, Lo/Ovral, Loestrin) can also be given. Although girls on low- to middle-dose pills often experience midcycle breakthrough bleeding, the elimination of weight gain secondary to fluid retention is considered worth the aggravation. However, if the

bleeding persists for more than three cycles the next higher dose pill is prescribed. Because of the higher incidence of breakthrough bleeding in the low-dose pill, many girls prefer the medium-dose pill.

(3) Pills for 21-day and 28-day cycles are available. Since, with the latter, the teenager is taking a pill *every* day, the chances that she will forget to take it are reduced.

c. **Follow-up.** The patient should be seen in 3 months for a blood pressure and weight check. At this visit, any problems she may be having can also be explored. Thereafter, she is seen every 6 months.

d. **The mini-pill** is a progestogen-only pill. The pregnancy rate on this pill is higher than on combination pills (1.5–3.0 pregnancies/100 woman-years), and irregular menstrual bleeding occurs.

B. **Intrauterine devices (IUDs)** that are available include the Cu_7 (copper), Lippes Loop, Saf-T-Coil, and Progestasert. Because of the risk of infection the IUD should be considered only in nulliparous patients who cannot or will not use other means of contraception.

1. **Complications**
   a. **Irregular bleeding and cramps**
   b. **Expulsion** (most common in the first month after insertion)
   c. **Infection** (increased risk of pelvic inflammatory disease)
   d. **Pregnancy.** The rate is 1.1–2.5 pregnancies/100 women-years.
   e. **Perforation** occurs in less than 1/2000 insertions.
   f. **Mortality** is 2 in 100,000 insertions.

2. **Patient evaluation**
   a. Check the strings attached to the IUD once a week for 1 month, then after each period.
   b. Have the patient return in 6 weeks, then every 6 months–1 year. Replace the Cu_7 in 36 months.

C. **Diaphragms.** The use of a diaphragm should be limited to adolescents who are highly motivated, feel comfortable with their bodies, and are not offended by inserting a mechanical device into the vagina in anticipation of intercourse.

1. **Fitting.** Fitting rings of various sizes are inserted into the vagina to determine the appropriate size. A correctly fitting diaphragm covers the cervix snugly without discomfort to the patient.

2. **Instructions.** The following written instructions are given to the patient on the use and care of the diaphragm:
   a. Put 1 tbsp of contraceptive cream in the cup of the diaphragm.
   b. Insert the diaphragm no more than 2 hr prior to intercourse, checking that the cervix is covered.
   c. If more than 2 hr have passed since insertion, place an applicatorful of contraceptive cream in front of the diaphragm.
   d. Leave the diaphragm in place at least 6 hr after intercourse.
   e. After removing the diaphragm, wash it with a mild soap (cornstarch may be used after washing).
   f. Check the diaphragm once a week for holes by holding it up to the light.
   g. A weight change of 10 lb requires a refitting.

D. **Foam** is a readily available form of birth control that requires no prescription. The adolescent is given the following instructions:

1. Insert the contraceptive foam into the vagina 1 hr or less *before* intercourse. It is not effective after intercourse.
2. Do not douche for 6 hr after intercourse.
3. When possible, have the partner use a condom with foam to lessen the risk of pregnancy.

E. **Condoms** are the only birth control devices that lessen the risk of venereal disease dissemination. Condom usage allows the male to participate actively in birth control.

F. **Administration of the "morning-after" pill.** High-dose estrogens (DES) after unprotected intercourse is an effective means of lowering the risk of pregnancy. However, it should be used only in cases of rape and after first intercourse because of possible risk of uterine carcinoma. Because of the risk of giving it to a patient who is already pregnant by previous exposure, estrogen therapy should be prescribed only to those patients who would have an abortion if already pregnant at the time of unprotected intercourse.

1. **Administration.** DES is taken within 24–72 hr after intercourse.
2. **Dosage.** DES, 25 mg bid for 5 days
   Premarin, 25 mg bid for 5 days
   Estinyl (ethinyl estradiol), 2 mg bid for 5 days
3. **Complications**
   a. **Nausea.** All high-dose estrogens are associated with nausea and vomiting. Prochlorperazine, 5–10 mg PO, given 2 hr prior to estrogen, reduces the nausea.
   b. **Fluid retention**
   c. **Headache, dizziness**
   d. **Menstrual irregularities**
   e. **Breast soreness**

V. **Pregnancy.** Each year, more than 1 million girls 15–19 years of age become pregnant. Unfortunately, the "it can never happen to me" philosophy still prevails. The majority of pregnant teenagers are neither emotionally disturbed nor promiscuous, but psychological issues often precipitate the pregnancy. The baby is seen as a love object and is used to replace a recent loss by death, separation, or divorce. The baby is expected to love the teenager and provide the stability needed to maintain the relationship with her boyfriend. Threatened with punishment if she becomes pregnant, an adolescent may become pregnant to test her parents' love. Thus, pregnancy is a plea for someone to care. Unless these complex emotional issues are resolved, another pregnancy is likely to follow the first.

A. **Diagnosis.**
1. Many girls cannot bring themselves to express concern over a missed period, and many will deny that the possibility of pregnancy even exists. Every girl should be questioned about her menstrual cycles and sexual activity.
2. A pregnancy test is given to confirm the suspected diagnosis (see sec. **I.C**).
3. Pelvic examination and sizing of the uterus
   a. An 8-week pregnant uterus is the size of an orange.
   b. At 12 weeks the uterus is the size of a grapefruit at the symphysis pubis.
   c. At 16 weeks the uterus is felt midway between the umbilicus and symphysis pubis.
   d. At 20 weeks the uterus is palpable at the umbilicus.

B. **Mortality and morbidity complications**
1. The **death rate** from the complications of pregnancy, delivery, and the postpartum period is 60 percent higher for girls who become pregnant before the age of 15 years than for those who became pregnant at a later age.
2. The **causes of death** include the following:
   a. **Toxemia,** resulting from:
      (1) An immature endocrine system
      (2) Emotional stress
      (3) Poor nutrition
      (4) Inadequate prenatal care
   b. **Hemorrhage**
   c. **Infection**
3. Pregnancy is a common cause of school dropout; 9 of 10 girls whose first delivery occurs at age 15 or younger never complete high school.
4. Couples who marry because of pregnancy have a higher divorce rate than that of the general population.

C. **Abortion**
1. **Methods**
   a. **Suction curettage** is done before 12 weeks (in many hospitals to 15 weeks) under local or general anesthesia. **Complications** include perforation and hemorrhage (secondary to incomplete removal of the products of conception), and infection.

b. **Saline or prostaglandin infusion** is done at 16–24 weeks of pregnancy. **Contraindications** to saline infusion are chronic renal disease, cardiac disease, and severe anemia. **Complications** include infection, retained products of conception, coagulopathy, and mortality.

2. **Counseling.** Explore thoroughly with the pregnant teenager the options of abortion, adoption, or keeping the child. She must participate in the decision-making process. Once she has reached a decision, it should be supported by the health professionals caring for her.

VI. Rape. By definition, rape is the introduction of the penis within the genitals of the victim by force, fear, or fraud. Statutory rape is intercourse with a female below the age of consent (usually 16 years). Sexual molestation is noncoital sexual contact without consent.

A. Patient evaluation

1. Carefully collect and record the medical data.
2. The history should include the time, place, circumstances, and witnesses, if any, as well as efforts to resist the attack.
3. Inquire if the patient has bathed, douched, or urinated since the attack.
4. Record the patient's menstrual history and the type of contraceptive used, if any.
5. Consent forms for all procedures should be signed and witnessed.
6. **Physical examination**
   a. The patient's appearance (e.g., torn, bloody clothing) and emotional state should be noted and recorded.
   b. The physical examination should include inspection for evidence of trauma.
   c. In the pelvic examination, the vulvar area, urethra, and anus should be carefully inspected. A water-moistened speculum should be used (do not use a lubricant).
7. **Laboratory tests**
   a. Swab the vaginal pool and vulvar area (place the swab in a test tube and give to the police if an officer is investigating).
   b. Swab the vaginal pool and streak on slides labeled with the patient's name and the date and numbered 1 and 2.
      (1) **No. 1 slide.** No. 1 is placed in Papanicolaou's fixative for hematoxylin and eosin staining (permanent record).
      (2) **No. 2 slide.** Mix 1 drop of saline with the swab on the slide and cover with a cover slip. Using high dry power on the microscope, check for red blood cells or motile sperm. Motile sperm indicate sexual contact within 24 hrs; nonmotile sperm persist in the vagina up to 48 hrs. (If the smear is positive, place it in Papanicolaou's fixative.) **The absence of sperm does not eliminate the possibility of rape;** ejaculates contain no sperm in men with primary azoospermia or who have had a vasectomy.
   c. Endocervical, urethral, rectal, and pharyngeal cultures for gonorrhea and a serologic test for syphilis should be done.
   d. A pregnancy test should be done to detect a preexisting pregnancy.
   e. A CBC should be done.

B. Treatment

1. If the patient agrees to be treated prophylactically for syphilis, gonorrhea, and pregnancy, treat with
   a. Procaine penicillin G, 4.8 million U IM. Give probenecid, 1 gm PO, immediately before the injection.
   b. Give diethylstilbestrol or conjugated estrogen (Premarin) (see sec. **IV.F.2).**
   c. A follow-up visit should be made 1 week later to assess healing. In the second visit, at 6 weeks, repeat the serologic test for syphilis, the pregnancy test, and the cervical culture (if obtained automatically at the time of pelvic examination).
2. The patient should be counseled by health professionals skilled in rape management.

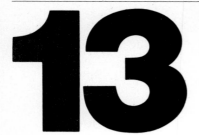

Diabetes Mellitus

I. General features and classification of diabetes mellitus. Diabetes has recently been categorized into two subtypes: type I, insulin-dependent diabetes mellitus (IDDM), and type II, non-insulin-dependent diabetes mellitus (NIDDM); 1.9 in 1,000 children and adolescents ages 5–18 are diabetic, and the overwhelming majority have type I disease, which is characterized by the metabolic derangements secondary to partial or complete insulin deficiency. Type II is the most common type diagnosed in adults and features sluggish insulin secretion and/or insulin-receptor defects.

In mild cases of insulin deficiency, the metabolic consequence is a decreased capacity to assimilate ingested foodstuffs, resulting in glucose intolerance. In severe insulin deficiency, hyperglycemia, ketogenesis and protein wasting occur.

Although a positive family history is found in both types, only type I has been associated with an increased incidence among certain HLA haplotypes. Over 90% of patients carry HLA DR3 and/or DR4.

The development of type I diabetes is the consequence of viral or toxic insults to the pancreatic islets of the genetically predisposed child. Finding islet cell antibodies in the blood of newly diagnosed patients suggests that the immune system is involved in the beta cell destruction, and by the time of clinical presentation over 90% of insulin-producing cells are nonfunctioning. Although diabetic symptoms may develop suddenly, the initial insult may have preceded hyperglycemia by months to years.

II. Clinical course

  A. The **initial phase** from the onset of clinical symptoms to the time of diagnosis lasts anywhere from 1 day to several weeks. It is often precipitated by infection, emotional upset, or physical trauma.

  B. The **recovery phase** usually occurs a few days following therapy, when the stress is controlled and tissue sensitivity to insulin increases.

  C. The **remission phase** is typical of type I. It usually occurs 1–3 months following the introduction of insulin therapy. The duration is variable, lasting anywhere from weeks to months.

  D. The **intensification phase** follows the remission phase and occurs about 6–18 months after the initial diagnosis. Endogenous insulin is depleted. About one-third of the total type I population bypasses the remission phase.

III. Diagnosis

  A. Clinical presentation. The possibility of diabetes is usually brought to medical attention by one or more of the following situations:

   1. Family history. First-degree relatives of a type I diabetic patient have a 1.5–18% risk of the development of the disease. HLA typing may reveal the relative risk.

   2. Symptoms. Polydipsia, polyuria, weight loss with polyphagia, enuresis, recurrent infections, and candidiasis.

   3. Glycosuria on routine examination. Screening is best performed during the stress of infection.

   4. Ketoacidosis and coma.

  B. Diagnostic tests. It would be easy to make the diagnosis in the situations in **A.3** and **A.4**, but in the asymptomatic patient the diagnosis of diabetes mellitus, particularly of the subclinical, or chemical type, is dependent on the demonstra-

Table 13-1. Normal oral GTT percentiles for children (whole blood) (mg/100 ml)

Time sampled (hr)	Percentile		
	3rd	50th	97th
0 (fasting)	56	83	111
½	80	131	183
1	66	110	172
2	64	100	140
3	48	82	126

tion of carbohydrate intolerance. A series of carbohydrate function tests, namely, the oral glucose tolerance test (OGTT), and the intravenous glucose tolerance test (IVGTT), may be necessary to make the definite diagnosis. For the standardization of testing conditions the patient should be on a diet high in carbohydrates for 3 days prior to the test and should then be tested in a fasting and basal state.

1. The **OGTT** is still generally accepted as a standard test for the initial workup in asymptomatic diabetes mellitus (**not** indicated in fasting hyperglycemia).
   a. A loading dose of 1.75 gm of glucose/kg of body weight is given (maximum dose, 100 gm).
   b. Blood samples are obtained at 0, ½, 1, 1½, 2, and 3 hr for glucose determination by the Somogyi-Nelson or ferrocyanide method and for insulin by immunoassay. When possible, urine is obtained simultaneously for glucose determination. **"Whole blood" sugars are 10–15% lower than serum values.** Normal OGTT percentiles for children (whole blood) are given in Table 13-1.
2. **IVGTT** (**not** indicated in fasting hyperglycemia)
   a. A loading dose of 0.5 gm of glucose/kg of body weight at 0 time is given by IV push within 2 minutes.
   b. Blood samples are obtained at -30, 0, 1, 3, 5, 15, 30, 45, 60, 90, 120, 150, and 180 min for the determination of sugar and immunoreactive insulin (IRI). The result of blood sugar is expressed by the glucose disappearance rate (K-rate). A K-rate below 1.2%/min is usually suggestive of carbohydrate intolerance. A blunted and decreased insulin response is suggestive of the early diabetic state.
3. **Individual variations in tolerance and response to carbohydrate function tests.** The carbohydrate tolerance in the same person may vary from time to time. Also, different responses may be elicited from different tests. Some patients are thus required to go through multiple and repeated tests in order to elicit carbohydrate intolerance.
4. The **glycosylated hemoglobin test (hemoglobin A₁)** provides an index of blood glucose concentrations during the weeks prior to sampling. Values are found to be elevated in virtually all children with newly diagnosed diabetes. The test is unreliable in hemolytic states and hemoglobin variants, including fetal hemoglobin.

IV. **Therapy**
   A. **General objectives in management**
      1. Maintenance or establishment of optimal physical and emotional growth and development
      2. Education of the patient, family, and school personnel to a full understanding of diabetes and their role in its management
      3. **Short-term goals**
         a. Control of insulin-deficient metabolic alterations (hyperglycemia, glycosuria, infections, weight loss, ketoacidosis)
         b. Control of the effects of insulin therapy: hypoglycemia and lipodystrophy

4. The **long-term goal** is to prevent or delay the onset of complications.
   a. Control of blood sugar to **as normal a level as can be obtained** within the limits of available therapy. Hyperglycemia may be responsible for microangiopathic complications resulting from glycosylation and thickening of capillary basement membranes and neuropathy, via accumulation of end products of the altered pathways of glucose metabolism.
   b. Avoidance of other cardiovascular risk factors: hyperlipidemia, hypertension, obesity, and cigarette smoking.

B. **Management of diabetic acidosis and coma**
   1. The basic principles of management of these conditions are:
      a. Maintaining an adequate insulin administration program
      b. Proper handling of precipitating factors (e.g., infection)
      c. Prompt correction of dehydration and the prevention and control of complications such as shock, oliguria, cardiac arrhythmias, and potassium deficiency
   2. There is no rigid guide for insulin or fluid and electrolyte therapy. The clinical response and the improvement of biochemical status dictate subsequent management in the individual patient.
   3. **Guidelines for the treatment of severely acidotic and dehydrated comatose children** include the following:
      a. Thoroughgoing **history,** particularly of the event leading to the onset. Recent weight and the last insulin administration in the known diabetic patient should be noted. A **physical examination** (for signs of infection and physical trauma) should be done.
      b. **Accurate body weight**
      c. **Baseline studies.** Venous blood glucose; serum acetone (serial dilutions on Acetest tablets, which detect acetoacetic and *not* betahydroxybutyric acid); pH; total CO_2; BUN; electrolytes; Ca, phosphate; CBC; urinalysis; ECG (T waves); and appropriate cultures.
      d. **Urine bagging** for constant collection to avoid catheterization except in the comatose patient. Urine samples should be collected q1–2h for sugar and acetone determination.
      e. Determination of **blood sugar** q1–2h and **venous pH, TCO_2, electrolytes,** and **acetone** q2–3h until the patient is out of danger
      f. A **flow sheet** containing hourly intake and output, insulin administered, urinary sugar and acetone, blood chemistries, body weight (q12h), and mental status
      g. An **IV infusion** (cutdown or central venous catheter if the patient is in shock) (see Chap. 3, p. 89)
      h. **Serial ECG monitoring** (lead II), to detect T wave changes of hyperkalemia and hypokalemia
      i. **Administration of regular (crystalline) insulin.** Various methods are effective (Table 13-2). Low dose (IV and IM) methods now constitute the treatment of choice and require hourly monitoring and immediate reporting of blood glucose. The half-life of insulin injected IV is only 8 min in new diabetics. Reliability of the IV line is essential.
      j. **Treatment of infection if present**
      k. **Alertness to the signs and symptoms of acute cerebral edema,** a rare (1% incidence) but ever-present risk, especially in hyponatremic patients. It often occurs *after* a semicomatose patient becomes alert. The prognosis is grim.
   4. **Fluid and electrolyte program for the first 24 hr** (see also Ch. 7, pp. 201ff.). The fluid deficit in severe diabetic acidosis is about 10–15 percent of ideal body weight (100–150 ml/kg). The deficit consists of equal amounts of extracellular (ECF) and intracellular (ICF) fluid.
      a. The amount of fluid replacement for the first 24 hr consists of 75% of the total deficit (100% of ECF lost; 50% of ICF lost) plus maintenance and continuing losses (NG tube drainage, etc.).

Table 13-2. Methods of regular insulin administration

Method and dose	Advantages	Disadvantages
Low-dose IV 0.1–0.5 U/kg IV push, then 0.1 U/kg/hr. IV drip or pump (mix with albumin or preflush 25% infusate to prevent adherence of insulin to glassware and tubing). Give SQ insulin ½ hour before discontinuing infusion when acidosis improving and blood glucose ≅ 300 mg/100 ml	Steady reduction in blood glucose and serum hypertonicity Less risk of sudden hypokalemia Total ability to adjust rate of insulin	Accurate infusion pump necessary Infiltrated IV yields negligible dose to patient Low dose may be insufficient in severe infection Hourly monitoring of blood glucose essential
Low-dose IM 0.1–0.5 U/kg IV push, then 0.1 U/kg/hr IM. (When blood glucose ≅ 300 mg/100 ml, give SQ insulin.)	As effective as IV in reducing blood glucose and reversing acidosis *if* IV priming dose given No infusion pump	Repeated injections necessary Less ability to discontinue insulin in case of "overshoot" Reduced absorption in hypotensive patient
SQ 0.5–1.0 U/kg (½ IV push and ½ SQ), then 0.25–0.5 U/kg SQ q2–4h	Most physicians and hospitals familiar with method	Delayed absorption in markedly dehydrated or poorly perfused patient Late hypoglycemia and sudden hypokalemia common

   b. **First hour.** The main goal is treatment and prevention of hypovolemic shock. Give 20 ml/kg/hr of normal saline and continue at this rate until the patient is out of shock.
   c. **Hours 2–8.** Replace the remainder of ECF loss (50% of total deficit) as N saline. Switch to 5% dextrose in ½ N saline when blood sugar falls to 250 mg/100 ml.
   d. **Hours 9–24.** Give the remainder of the calculated requirement (50% of ICF lost, plus maintenance and continuing losses which are increased by hyperpnea and osmotic polyuria). 5% Dextrose in ⅓–½ N saline. 2.5–10% Dextrose may be necessary to **maintain** blood sugar at 200–250 mg/100 ml, the therapeutic range for the first 24 hr.
5. **Potassium.** When urinary output is established, give K^+, 40–80 mEq/L, as equal amounts of potassium chloride and potassium phosphate (Table 13–3). (Phosphate replaces erythrocyte 2,3-DPG concentrations.) Overzealous phosphate replacement can produce hypocalcemia, and thus serum calcium levels and the ECG (Q–T interval) must be monitored.
6. **Sodium.** Assume a loss of 7–8 mEq/kg in the typically isotonic dehydration of ketoacidosis (70–80 mEq/L of fluid loss).
7. **Bicarbonate** should be administered **only** when the pH is ≦ 7.10, since infused bicarbonate increases plasma osmolality and may **increase** tissue hypoxia (via a shift of the O_2-hemoglobin dissociation curve), hypokalemia, and cerebrospinal fluid acidosis. For replacement, 0.7 mEq $NaHCO_3^-$/kg

Table 13-3. Potassium replacement

Serum K$^+$ (mEq/L)*	Infusion rate (mEq/hr)
<3	40
3–4	30
4–5	20
5–6	10
>6	K$^+$ withheld

*Monitor ECG continuously for T wave changes if serum K$^+$ is < 3.5 mEq/L or > 5.0 mEq/L.

raises the CO_2 content (TCO$_2$) 1 mEq/L. Give 1.0 mEq/kg sodium bicarbonate IV stat, then give 40 mEq in each 500 ml of IV solution until the pH reaches **7.10. Then stop.**

C. **Insulin**
   1. **Insulin preparations** are divided into three categories according to promptness, duration, and intensity of action following SQ administration. They are classified as fast, intermediate, and long-acting types (Table 13–4).
   2. **Insulin selection.** In general, NPH is preferred as the intermediate-acting insulin. All new diabetic patients should use the U-100 strength (100 units/ml) of a purified pork or "human" insulin. Smaller syringes (0.5-ml capacity) are also available for patients taking small doses.
      a. Some new diabetic patients can be controlled on a single daily dose of intermediate-acting insulin, but most require combinations of intermediate and regular (⅔–¾ intermediate, ¼–⅓ regular).
      b. Better control is achieved in most patients, particularly adolescents, with twice-daily injections; with ⅔–¾ of the total daily dose given before breakfast, the remainder before supper. Each dose may contain a combination of intermediate and regular, as outlined in **a**.
      c. Regular insulin is required during acidosis and other acute situations in which the patient's food intake is variable.
   3. **Insulin therapy.** The administration of insulin therapy is based on the various phases of the clinical course of diabetes mellitus.
      a. **Initial phase (newly diagnosed patient with moderate to severe ketoacidosis or coma).** The administration of adequate quantities of rapidly acting insulin (regular) is essential for recovery from diabetic ketoacidosis.
         (1) **Initial dosage.** See Table 13–2.
         (2) **After ketoacidosis is reversed**
            (a) Give regular insulin SQ q4–6h, the amount depending on the clinical and chemical response. Each dose should be specifically ordered, rather than preprogrammed by a sliding scale. Finger-stick bedside glucose monitoring is preferable to urine glucose determinations.
            (b) As a rule of thumb, the maximum dose administered (for blood glucose ≥ 400 mg/100 ml and high urine acetone) is ¼–½ unit/kg/dose.
         (3) The insulin dosage is adjusted until the total daily requirement can be estimated moderately well, which is usually after 48 hr of initial therapy. Then ⅔ of the total daily requirement is given as a single dose of an intermediate preparation (or in a split dose as outlined in **2.a**).
         (4) Further adjustments in dosage will be necessary, based on the results of blood sugars obtained preprandially and before bedtime.

Table 13-4. Insulin preparations

Type	Appearance	Action	Peak activity* (hr)	Duration* (hr)	Composition	Compatible in use with regular insulin
Regular (crystalline)	Clear	Rapid	2–4	5–7		
NPH (neutral protamine Hagedorn)	Turbid	Intermediate	6–12	24–28	Protamine, zinc, insulin	Yes
PZI (protamine zinc)	Turbid	Prolonged	14–24	36+	Same as NPH	No
Semilente	Turbid	Rapid	2–4	12–16	Zinc, acetate buffer, insulin (no protein modifier)	Yes
Lente (30% Semilente, 70% Ultralente)	Turbid	Intermediate	6–12	24–28	Same as Semilente	Yes
Ultralente	Turbid	Prolonged	18–24	36+	Same as Semilente	No

*Insulin kinetics are highly variable, since insulin-binding antibodies develop in most patients within months of therapy.

(5) In mild to moderate ketoacidosis, insulin therapy should be less vigorous (initial dose, 0.25–0.5 unit/kg) because of the danger of inducing hypoglycemia in these glycogen-depleted patients.

(6) For patients presenting with mild or moderate diabetes without significant ketosis, treatment may be started with an arbitrary amount (0.25–0.5 unit/kg/day) of an intermediate preparation; further adjustments are made as dictated by the response.

b. The **remission phase** usually occurs after the patient's discharge from the hospital. At this stage the insulin requirement decreases, and the patient should be on a gradually decreasing dosage to avoid hypoglycemia. If there is no glycosuria, consider maintenance on a minimum dose of intermediate-acting insulin (2–4 U/day), and prescribe a dietary regimen to avoid the emotional trauma of discontinuing and then reintroducing insulin.

c. Stabilized (intensification) phase

(1) In general, the range of the average requirement for exogenous insulin as the patient approaches the stage of "total" diabetes usually rises slowly and unevenly, eventually stablizing between 0.6–1.0 U/kg/day.

(2) Sexual maturation and the adolescent growth spurt increase the requirement for insulin in many children, up to 0.8–1.2 U/kg/day. There is a variable decline in the requirement for exogenous insulin after attainment of full growth and sexual maturation.

4. Insulin regulation

a. Preprandial second-voided urines and 24-hr fractionated urine glucose measurements assist in the adjustment and dosage of insulin during follow-up care.

b. Generally, preprandial urine sugar tests are maintained at negative to 0.5%. If the 24-hr urine sugar falls between 5–10% of the daily carbohydrate intake, regulation is accepted as good, provided the patient is free of frequent or severe reactions.

c. Home blood glucose monitoring using an Autolet or other blood-letting device should be taught to all patients. Ideal blood glucose concentrations should range between 80–120 mg/100 ml fasting, 80–150 mg/100 ml before lunch, supper, and bedtime, and no lower than 80 mg/100 ml during sleep. To avoid severe hypoglycemia in preschool children, blood glucose levels 20–40 mg/100 ml higher are acceptable.

d. Glycosylated hemoglobin (HgbA$_1$) tests evaluate overall blood glucose regulation over a period of weeks and should be performed every 3 months, with a goal towards values < 11%.

5. Problems in insulin therapy

a. Hypoglycemia is a major and common complication of insulin therapy and may be manifested acutely by behavioral changes (inattention, confusion, or hyperactivity), headaches, perioral pallor, or "glassy stare," diaphoresis, anxiety, or tremor and may progress to convulsions and coma if untreated. Hypoglycemia may result from

(1) Excessive dosage of insulin due to visual failure, mismatched insulin and syringe, inappropriate site of injection, or deliberate overdose.

(2) A reduced need for insulin, resulting from increased exercise (insulin is absorbed more quickly from an injection site that is exercised); diminished caloric intake; development of concomitant endocrinologic or systemic disease; recovery from "stress states" (infection, ketoacidosis, surgery); and the use of drugs with a hypoglycemic effect.

(3) **Treatment**

(a) Simple sugars such as 4–7 Life Savers, orange juice and soft drinks should be given if the patient can swallow, or concentrated dextrose gels may be squirted into the cheek pouch and can be absorbed directly into the circulation. Glucagon (0.03 mg/kg body weight SQ—maximum, 1 mg) is useful for raising the blood sugar temporarily at home. Nausea often follows its administration, however.

(b) Carbohydrate input should be continued until sugar appears in the urine. In severe cases, it is necessary to administer 50% glucose IV (0.5 gm/kg, or 1 ml/kg in 50% D/W).

b. Lipodystrophy. Fat atrophy at the site of injections develops in some childhood diabetics. Injection of "single peak" pure pork or human insulins into the edges of atrophic areas has been beneficial.

c. Allergic reaction. Transient, localized urticarial lesions may occur during the first few weeks of insulin therapy and later disappear. Generally, no change in regimen is needed. Pure pork and human insulin may be useful alternatives.

d. The **Somogyi phenomenon** is the establishment of a pattern of inapparent hypoglycemia, followed by reactive hyperglycemia and ketonuria. It results from administration of excessive insulin.

(1) The mechanism of the hyperglycemia and ketonuria is increased concentration of hormones (catecholamine, glucocorticoid, growth hormone) with actions antagonistic to insulin, so that insulin hyposensitivity develops.

(2) The Somogyi phenomenon should be suspected when continual increases in the dosage of insulin do not produce beneficial results. This factor is also considered if the total insulin dose exceeds 1.2 units/kg/day.

(3) In spite of apparently poor control, these patients usually gain weight, are rarely ketoacidotic, and handle infections reasonably well. Hepatomegaly (from glycogen deposition) may develop. To stabilize the situation, a reduction in insulin dosage is necessary.

e. Persistent **insulin resistance** is a rare event in the treatment of diabetes mellitus. In the adult, it is defined as an insulin requirement in excess of 200 units/day in the absence of acidosis. A change from beef to pork or human insulin may be effective in reducing the requirement.

6. Recent developments in insulin therapy

a. Purified single peak pork and human insulins are less antigenic than beef or beef-pork combinations. Although more expensive, they usually require lower doses. A therapeutic benefit has yet to be established except in insulin allergy, lipoatrophy, and true insulin resistance.

b. Human insulin is produced by recombinant DNA technology. The perfect amino acid composition further reduces antigenicity and may render a more predictable absorption and half-life. Human insulin will also improve worldwide availability for the growing diabetic population

c. Insulin infusion pumps are "open-loop," battery-operated pumps that inject a constant flow of subcutaneous insulin plus premeal bolus doses. Since the patient must act as glucose "sensor," frequent blood glucose monitoring, strict attention to the total regimen, and close follow-up by a team familiar with the equipment are essential. Carefully selected patients have experienced improved blood glucose regulation, improved growth, and lower blood cholesterols. Multiple daily injections, however, have produced similar results. These pumps should never be expected to bring a patient through ketoacidosis or surgery. Severe hypoglycemia is a major concern with current devices.

Individual patients who fail to respond to conventional or intensified therapy and are unwilling to undertake the major self-monitoring requirements are courting significant risk with open-loop pump technology. Optimal insulin-glucose regulation requires a glucose sensor capable of signaling insulin delivery from a reservoir. Such an implantable device has yet to be developed.

D. Oral hypoglycemic agents (sulfonylureas) have **no** place in the treatment of children with type I diabetes. For children with type II disease, dietary regulation, with emphasis on the maintenance of normal weight, will suffice. Oral agents may improve blood glucose control in obese type II patients who fail to comply with a dietary regimen.

E. Guidelines for the diabetic diet

1. **The aim of the diabetic diet** is to permit the patient to lead a comfortable, asymptomatic life and to attain normal growth and development. The nutritional needs of diabetic children are essentially no different from those of nondiabetic children. The diabetic diet is thus a normal, well-balanced diet with concentrated carbohydrates eliminated. Dietary manipulation is sometimes used as an adjunct to the insulin adjustment in the regulation of urinary sugar.

   The emphasis in the diabetic diet is on the regularity of meals and snacks and the consistency of quantity of foods eaten, rather than on a strictly controlled regimen. It is not recommended that foods be weighed, but rather that the food exchange and diabetic food lists be followed. The simplicity of this approach seems to aid acceptance of the disease by patient and family.

2. **Planning the diabetic diet.** A normal, well-balanced diet should contain representative proportions of each of the following four basic food groups:

   a. **Skim milk,** three or more glasses/day for children (small glasses for those under age 6) and four or more glasses for teenagers

   b. **Meat or fish,** two or more servings

   c. **Vegetables and fruit,** four or more servings

   d. **Bread and cereals,** four or more servings

   e. These foods should be taken in sufficient amounts to provide the following:

      (1) **Calories.** It is desirable to keep the diabetic patient's weight in an ideal range for height and body build. The rule of thumb in caloric estimation is by age: 1000 calories daily at 1 year, plus 100 for each additional year up to 18 years for males, 15 years for females.

      (2) **Protein.** Because of fat restriction in the diabetic patient, protein intake is usually increased to approximately 20% of the calories.

      (3) **Carbohydrates** are maintained at about 45–50% of the calories, largely by avoiding sweets and foods containing concentrated sugars.

      (4) **Fat.** The fat allowance is moderately restricted, to about 30–35% of the dietary calories, to make up the balance of daily caloric needs.

   f. **Snacks.** The daily diet is usually planned to include three meals and two or three snacks.

      (1) The main purpose of snacks in a diabetic diet is to provide additional carbohydrate coverage at the peak of the insulin reaction and to aid in the prevention of possible nighttime hypoglycemia.

      (2) Snacks are usually scheduled midmorning, midafternoon and at bedtime.

      (3) Athletes may require a carbohydrate snack before exercising.

V. Education. Patients and parents are taught the fundamentals of the pathophysiology and management of diabetes. Insulin preparation, injection technique, and a program for the management of acute illness are introduced. They are also made aware of the symptoms of hypoglycemia, its oral treatment, and the use of glucagon. Qualitative urine tests for sugar and acetone and quantitative fingerstick blood monitoring are taught. Patients are encouraged to participate in activities normal for their age. The importance of understanding the dietary instructions, exchange lists, and food preparation guidelines should be pointed out. All patients are advised to carry a diabetic card and Medic Alert bracelet or necklace.

VI. Special problems of diabetes mellitus

A. Physical growth and maturation. In general, diabetic children follow the normal growth pattern. However, there may be a diminished growth rate in those whose diabetes is poorly controlled.

B. Problems in emotional adjustment. Diabetic patients often become overly dependent and demonstrate anxiety and hostility. Understanding, patience, education of both patient and family, and, occasionally, psychiatric counseling are necessary in these cases. Heavy responsibilities (e.g., the administration of insulin) should not be levied on a diabetic child who is not mature enough to accept them. Summer camps for diabetic children have been invaluable in this regard.

C. Infection

1. The incidence of urinary tract infections, subcutaneous abscesses, candidal vulvitis, and cystitis is higher in teenage girls with diabetes than in non diabetic female adolescents.
2. Pyelonephritis is more common in diabetic patients than in the nondiabetic.
3. If infection occurs, adequate doses of appropriate antibiotics and antifungal agents should be administered promptly, and the establishment of good diabetic control should be emphasized.
4. Diabetic children should receive pneumococcal and influenza vaccines.

D. Surgery presents special challenges via increased stress hormones (cortisol, catecholamines) that antagonize insulin action. Frequent blood glucose monitoring is critical, and a physician familiar with type I diabetics should supervise the medical management.

1. Elective surgery should be performed in the early morning in patients whose blood glucose regulation has been good for several days preoperatively. A blood glucose is drawn, a glucose-containing IV drip is started by 8 A.M., and one-half the usual dose of NPH or Lente is given. Short-acting insulin is given q4–6h only if necessary to maintain a blood glucose of 150–250 mg/100 ml. Glucose-containing IV lines should be left in postoperatively until the patient has demonstrated an ability to ingest calories.
2. Oral surgery and procedures requiring even brief general anesthesia are best performed in a hospital.
3. Emergency surgery should be delayed until metabolic acidosis is corrected. When this is not possible, a constant IV insulin infusion (0.1 units/kg/hr) should be maintained perioperatively (see Table 13-2).

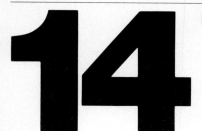

Metabolic Diseases

I. **Newborn screening.** Newborn screening allows certain metabolic diseases to be diagnosed and treated in the newborn period **before** the onset of clinical symptoms. In several metabolic disorders, early therapy prevents the development of significant clinical morbidity.

    A. Screening varies from state to state (Table 14-1). Infants are screened for phenylketonuria (PKU) and congenital hypothyroidism in most areas. **Do not assume that there is screening for any other disorder.**

    B. Procedure

        1. **A filter paper blood sample should be obtained from every newborn infant prior to discharge from the nursery regardless of the age at discharge.**

            a. Blood samples should be obtained from any full-term or premature infant **no later than the first week of life.**

            b. Infants who are not cared for in a newborn nursery should have blood samples taken at the first possible opportunity.

            c. If the initial blood sample is taken at less than 24 hr of age or before at least three protein feedings, a follow-up blood sample should be obtained at 2–4 weeks of age.

            d. Samples obtained prior to 48 hr of age or before protein feeding probably identify infants with PKU or congenital hypothyroidism, though infants with mild hyperphenylalaninemia (MHP) or other metabolic disorders may be missed.

        2. Follow-up testing is not necessary if an appropriate initial test is performed.

        3. Screening of urine obtained at 3–4 weeks of age is performed in a few areas and allows diagnosis of a larger variety of metabolic diseases.

        4. If a positive newborn screening test is reported, **additional testing must be done to confirm the diagnosis.** Newborn screening is designed to eliminate false-negative results that cause an infant with a metabolic disease to be missed. This produces many false-positive results.

        5. **Some cases are missed by newborn screening.** As many as 10–20% of newborns may not receive appropriate screening even in areas where newborn screening is routine. **Metabolic testing should be repeated if clinical symptoms suggest a metabolic disorder.**

II. **Clinical presentations of metabolic disease.** (See Table 14-2.)

    A. **Acute presentations of metabolic disease constitute a medical emergency. The diagnosis and timely treatment of metabolic disease requires a high index of suspicion in the presence of unusual clinical events.**

    B. **In the newborn,** metabolic disease usually presents within the first few days of life or several days after feeding has begun. Metabolic disease should be considered in any child with unexplained **lethargy, vomiting, hypoglycemia, neurologic depression, respiratory distress, metabolic acidosis,** or **hepatic dysfunction.** Special attention is required if there is a **family history** of metabolic disease, neonatal death, childhood death due to "sepsis," or parental consanguinity and in populations in which certain metabolic diseases are particularly common.

Table 14-1. Routine screening practices in the United States*

State	PKU	THY	GAL	MSUD	HOMO	TYR	SS	HIS
Alabama	Yes	Yes						
Alaska	Yes	Yes	Yes	Yes	Yes	Yes		
Arizona	Yes	Yes	Yes	Yes	Yes			
Arkansas	Yes	Yes						
California	Yes	Yes						
Colorado	Yes	Yes	Yes	Yes	Yes	Yes	Yes	
Connecticut	Yes	Yes	Yes					
Delaware	Yes	Yes						
District of Columbia								
Florida	Yes	Yes						
Georgia	Yes	Yes	Yes	Yes	Yes	Yes		
Hawaii	Yes	(Yes)						
Idaho	Yes	Yes	Yes	Yes	Yes	Yes		
Illinois	Yes	Yes						
Indiana	Yes	Yes						
Iowa	Yes	Yes						
Kansas	Yes	Yes						
Kentucky	Yes	Yes	Yes				Yes	
Louisiana	Yes	Yes						
Maine	Yes	Yes	Yes	Yes	Yes			
Maryland	Yes	Yes	Yes	Yes	Yes			
Massachusetts	Yes	Yes	Yes	Yes	Yes			
Michigan	Yes	Yes						
Minnesota	Yes	Yes	Yes					
Mississippi								
Missouri	Yes	Yes						
Montana	Yes	Yes	Yes	Yes	Yes	Yes		
Nebraska	Yes							
Nevada	Yes	Yes	Yes	Yes	Yes	Yes		
New Hampshire	Yes	Yes						
New Jersey	Yes	Yes						
New Mexico	Yes	Yes	Yes	Yes	Yes			
New York	Yes	Yes	Yes	Yes	Yes	Yes	Yes	Yes
North Carolina	Yes	Yes					Yes	
North Dakota	Yes	Yes						
Ohio	Yes	Yes	Yes		Yes			
Oklahoma	Yes	Yes						
Oregon	Yes	Yes	Yes	Yes	Yes	Yes		
Pennsylvania	Yes	Yes						
Rhode Island	Yes	Yes	Yes	Yes	Yes			
South Carolina	Yes	Yes						
South Dakota	Yes							
Tennessee	Yes	Yes						
Texas	Yes	Yes	Yes		Yes			
Utah	Yes	Yes	Yes					

Table 14-1 (continued)

State	PKU	THY	GAL	MSUD	HOMO	TYR	SS	HIS
Vermont	Yes	Yes						
Virginia	Yes	Yes						
Washington	Yes	Yes						
West Virginia	Yes	Yes						
Wisconsin	Yes	Yes	Yes	Yes				
Wyoming	Yes	Yes						

*As of February 1981.
PKU = phenylketonuria; THY = congenital hypothyroidism; GAL = galactosemia; MSUD = maple syrup urine disease; HOMO = homocystinuria; TYR = tyrosinemia; SS = sickle cell disease; HIS = histininemia.

    C. In older children, metabolic disease is suggested by **failure to thrive, feeding intolerance, developmental delay, loss of developmental milestones,** or recurrent episodes of acidosis, hypoglycemia, or hyperammonemia.

    D. Many metabolic diseases that are subclinical or chronic in nature may be punctuated by acute metabolic crises caused by dietary change, infection, or stress. Such metabolic crises can be life-threatening and can inflict permanent damage. In these situations the signs of metabolic disease are often superimposed on the clinical features of the precipitating event.

III. Laboratory tests. (See Table 14-3.)

    A. Spots tests on urine provide a rapid diagnosis.

        1. Reducing substance (Clinitest, Benedict's reagent) for galactosemia and fructosemia. It is also positive in glucosuria of renal Fanconi syndrome.

        2. Glucose (Clinistix and glucose oxidase)

        3. Urine ketones (Ketostix) for maple syrup urine disease (MSUD) and organic acid disorders

        4. Ferric chloride test for PKU, tyrosinemia, and MSUD

        5. Nitroprusside test for homocystinuria and cystinuria. It is weakly positive in the generalized aminoaciduria of renal Fanconi syndrome.

        6. Berry spot test for mucopolysaccharidoses

    B. Urine tests

        1. Qualitative screening by paper chromatography is the first test for metabolic disorders involving amino acids, organic acids, or the urea cycle. Different stains are required for the diagnosis of different disorders, so communication of a provisional diagnosis to the laboratory is essential.

        2. Quantitative analysis for amino acids should be performed on collected urine to confirm the results of qualitative analysis.

        3. Quantitative organic acid analysis by gas chromatography should be performed for disorders involving organic acids and certain amino acids.

    C. Serum tests

        1. Quantitative amino acid analysis should be performed for the diagnosis of disorders involving amino acids, organic acids, or the urea cycle.

        2. Fatty acid analysis should be performed for the diagnosis of disorders of organic acids.

    D. In many diseases, a definitive diagnosis requires assay of **enzyme activity** from an affected tissue, erythrocytes, leukocytes, or a skin fibroblast culture.

    E. Carrier (heterozygote) detection is available for many metabolic diseases and is an important adjunct to genetic counseling. Carrier testing should be considered in families of persons with metabolic disease and in populations in which the incidence of specific metabolic diseases is high. **Screening for carriers of Tay-Sachs disease should be performed prior to childbearing age for all Jews of eastern European (Ashkenazi) ancestry.**

Table 14-2. Clinical features of metabolic disease

Disease	Neonatal presentation	Failure to thrive	Mental retardation	Vomiting	Seizures	Hepatomegaly	Eye findings	Renal involvement	Sepsis	Rickets	Dysmorphology
Phenylketonuria	—	—	X	—	X	—	—	—	—	—	—
Galactosemia	X	X	X	X	—	X	X	X[a]	X	—	—
Maple syrup urine disease	X	X	X	X	X	—	—	—	—	—	—
Tyrosinemia	—	—	—	—	—	X	—	X[a]	X	X	—
Homocystinuria	—	—	X	—	—	—	X	—	—	—	X
Cystinosis	—	X	—	—	—	—	X	X	—	X	—
Cystinuria	—	—	—	—	—	—	—	X	—	—	—
Fructosemia	X	X	X	X	—	X	—	X[a]	X	X	—
Urea cycle	X	X	X	X	X	X	—	—	—	—	—
Organic acid	X	X	X	X	X	X	—	—	X	—	—
Glycogen storage	—	X	—	—	—	X	—	—	—	—	—
Lipid storage	—	X	X	—	X	X	—	—	—	—	X
Wilson's disease	—	—	—	—	—	X	X	X[a]	—	—	—
Mucopolysaccharide	—	X	X	—	X	X	—	—	—	—	X

[a]Renal Fanconi syndrome: glucosuria, generalized amino aciduria. X = incidence.

F. Prenatal diagnosis of many metabolic diseases can be performed using amniocentesis to study metabolites in amniotic fluid and the activity of enzymes in cultured amniotic fluid cells.

G. If a child dies before the diagnosis of metabolic disease is confirmed, a postmortem diagnosis may be made from samples of serum and urine, fresh frozen (unfixed) tissue, or skin fibroblast cultures.

IV. Treatment for acute metabolic disease. Early therapy is important and should be started if metabolic disease is suspected, even before a specific diagnosis is made.

A. Discontinue feedings of protein and milk (lactose, galactose).

B. Provide **caloric support** with parenteral glucose infusions to prevent catabolism and provide an energy source. This requires 60–100 cal/kg/day. Parenteral fat emulsions (Intralipid) can provide supplemental calories, particularly if large fluid volumes cannot be tolerated. If glucose infusions cause hyperglycemia, insulin should be given to ensure utilization of glucose as an energy source.

C. Treat fluid and electrolyte abnormalities. The primary treatment for acidosis due to the accumulation of abnormal metabolites is correction of fluid and electrolyte imbalances and administration of an energy source. Bicarbonate may compromise the ability to generate a compensatory respiratory alkalosis and should be used only for critical acidosis (pH < 7.2).

D. Treat for **sepsis.** Many metabolic diseases are associated with impaired immune function and predispose to gram-negative sepsis (see Chap. 15, p. 351 ff).

E. Hyperammonemia associated with neurologic symptoms should be treated aggressively. Elimination of protein from the diet is of primary importance. Lactu-

Table 14-3. Laboratory findings in metabolic disease

Disease	Acidosis	Hypoglycemia	Hyperammonemia	Urine tests Glucose	Reducing substances	Ferric chloride	Nitroprusside	Berry spot test	Ketones[b]	Organic acids	Amino acids	Serum tests Amino acids	Fatty acids
PKU	—	—	—	—	—	X	—	—	—	X	X	X	—
GAL	—	X	—	X[a]	X	—	X[a]	—	—	—	X[a]	—	—
MSUD	X	X	X	—	—	X	—	—	X	—	X	X	—
TYR	—	X	—	X[a]	X[a]	X	X[a]	—	—	X	X	X	—
HOMO	—	—	—	—	—	—	X	—	—	—	X	X	—
CYSOSIS	—	—	—	X[a]	X[a]	—	X[a]	—	—	—	X[a]	—	—
CYSURIA	—	—	—	—	—	—	X	—	—	—	X	—	—
FRUCT	—	X	—	X[a]	X[a]	—	X[a]	—	—	—	X[a]	—	—
UREA	—	—	X	—	—	—	—	—	—	—	X	X	—
ORGANIC	X	X	X	—	—	—	—	—	X	X	X	X	X
GLYCOGEN	X	X	—	—	—	—	—	—	—	—	—	—	—
MPS	—	—	—	—	—	—	—	X	—	—	—	—	—

PKU = phenylketonuria; GAL = galactosemia; MSUD = maple syrup urine disease; TYR = tyrosinemia; HOMO = homocystinuria; CYSOSIS = cystinosis; CYSURIA = cystinuria; FRUCT = fructosemia; UREA = urea cycle disorders; ORGANIC = organic acid disorders; GLYCOGEN = glycogen storage diseases; MPS = mucopolysaccharidoses.
[a]Renal Fanconi syndrome may complicate the clinical picture, giving glycosuria (reducing substance positive) and generalized amino aciduria (with weakly positive nitroprusside due to cystine).
[b]Ketoacidosis and ketonuria secondary to clinical morbidity frequently accompany acute metabolic disease.

lose or oral aminoglycosides should be given except in the newborn, whose GI tract is not yet colonized with bacteria. Infusion of **arginine hydrochloride** (4 mmol/kg) is effective in lowering ammonia levels when hyperammonemia is associated with low arginine levels. Sodium benzoate (250–500 mg/kg/day) is also effective in lowering ammonia levels.

 F. **Dialysis** or **exchange transfusion** is indicated for the treatment of extreme hyperammonemia and either is effective in eliminating other toxic circulating metabolites. **Hemodialysis** is the treatment of choice for severe hyperammonemia, but peritoneal dialysis is also effective. **Exchange transfusion** is sometimes effective in treating hyperammonemia if the ammonia accretion rate is low.

 G. Pharmacologic doses of **vitamins** should be administered for vitamin-responsive disorders.

  1. **Vitamin B$_{12}$** (hydroxycobalamin or cyanocobalamin) for methylmalonic acidemia, 1–2 mg/day.

  2. **Biotin** for propionic acidemia and pyruvic acidemia (hyperalaninemia), 5–10 mg/day.

V. Clinical aspects of common metabolic diseases

 A. **Phenylketonuria (PKU)**

  1. **Etiology.** PKU results from insufficient activity of the enzyme phenylalanine hydroxylase, which converts phenylalanine to tyrosine.

   a. Affected persons have elevated levels of phenylalanine, depressed levels of tyrosine, and increased excretion of abnormal metabolites of phenylalanine (phenylketones).

b. Several variants of PKU are recognized.

(1) "Classic" PKU is associated with phenylalanine levels above 20 mg/ 100 ml and a clinical syndrome characterized by mental retardation and seizures.

(2) "Atypical" PKU and mild hyperphenylalaninemia (MHP) are associated with lower levels of phenylalanine and do not cause severe clinical morbidity.

(3) Elevated blood phenylalanine can also be caused by metabolic disorders involving synthesis of tetrahydrobiopterin. These disorders cause severe mental retardation and do not respond to conventional therapy.

2. The **incidence** of PKU is 1 in 11,000 and the incidence of MHP is 1 in 16,000 (Massachusetts). Disorders of biopterin metabolism affect 1% of children with elevated phenylalanine levels.

3. Evaluation and diagnosis

a. The diagnosis is routinely made by newborn screening of blood phenylalanine levels. The peak blood phenylalanine levels are as follows: PKU, >20 mg/100 ml; "atypical PKU," 12–20 mg/100 ml; MHP, 4–12 mg/ 100 ml; and normal, < 2 mg/100 ml. Phenylalanine loading tests may aid in distinguishing PKU from MHP.

b. Urine from patients with PKU who are at least 6 months old contains phenylketones that are detectable using a ferric chloride test, Phenistix, or paper chromatography for organic acids.

c. **All infants with PKU or MHP,** especially those who continue to show neurologic deterioration despite adequate dietary control, should be tested to rule out defects of biopterin metabolism.

4. Treatment of PKU or MHP requires a multidisciplinary approach.

a. Dietary therapy is aimed at maintaining blood phenylalanine levels between 4 and 8 mg/100 ml. The diet consists of protein (phenylalanine) restriction and nutritional supplementation with Lofenalac or Phenyl-Free.

b. Termination of a diet is no longer recommended. Significant losses in intellectual performance have been found in children whose diets were terminated at ages 4–6 years.

c. Other measures include psychosocial, developmental, and educational support, genetic counseling, and pregnancy planning.

d. There is no effective treatment for disorders of biopterin metabolism.

5. Prognosis. Persons with PKU or MHP who are treated have normal growth and development and a normal life expectancy.

6. Maternal PKU. Mothers who have PKU and have high phenylalanine levels during pregnancy are at risk for bearing children with microcephaly, congenital malformations, and mental retardation. Preliminary data suggest that controlling maternal phenylalanine levels **prior to conception** may be effective in preventing these problems.

B. Galactosemia

1. Etiology. Galactosemia is due to a failure of galactose utilization due to a deficiency of galactose-1-phosphate uridyl transferase. Affected persons have elevated levels of galactose in the blood, urine, and tissues. If not treated promptly, galactosemia may cause neonatal death, mental retardation, cataracts, and cirrhosis. The **incidence** is 1 in 65,000 (Massachusetts).

2. Evaluation and diagnosis

a. The disease presents in the newborn period with **lethargy, jaundice, vomiting, hepatomegaly, aminoaciduria,** and frequently **gram-negative sepsis.**

b. Galactosemia can be diagnosed by routine newborn screening.

c. The diagnosis can be made by demonstrating urine-reducing substances using Clinitest (Benedict's reagent) and the absence of glucose using Clinistix (glucose oxidase reaction). False-positives with this method may be due to urinary lactose or fructose.

 d. Enzyme activity can be readily measured in erythrocytes. Enzyme assays should be done to rule out variants of galactosemia due to galactokinase deficiency.

3. Treatment

 a. The acutely ill newborn should be treated with glucose, fluids, and electrolytes and aggressive supportive therapy for hepatic failure and sepsis.

 b. Long-term therapy involves rigorous dietary avoidance of milk and milk-containing products (containing lactose or galactose).

4. Prognosis

 a. Galactosemia may be fatal in infancy unless promptly diagnosed and treated.

 b. In treated persons the hepatic failure, cataracts, and aminoaciduria resolve, and normal growth and development may be expected. Some treated children have residual learning disabilities and speech defects.

C. MSUD

1. Etiology. MSUD results from the inability to break down the alpha keto analogues of the branched-chain amino acids leucine, isoleucine, and valine because of deficient decarboxylase activity. The accumulation of the branched-chain alpha keto acids and amino acids causes severe acidosis and neurologic damage. The disorder is often fatal in the newborn period and can cause severe mental retardation and failure to thrive in surviving infants. The severity of the disease depends upon the degree of the metabolic block. The **incidence** is 1 in 175,000.

2. Evaluation and diagnosis

 a. MSUD can be diagnosed by routine newborn screening of blood leucine levels.

 b. Increased concentrations of leucine, isoleucine, and valine are present in the blood.

 c. Large quantities of alpha keto acids can be demonstrated in the urine by Ketostix, ferric chloride, or paper chromatography.

 d. Urine has the characteristic odor of maple syrup. This odor may not be present until the second week of life **after** the onset of clinical symptoms.

 e. Enzyme activity should be measured in leukocytes or cultured skin fibroblasts.

3. Treatment

 a. The acutely ill newborn should be treated with protein restriction, caloric support, and supportive care.

 b. Long-term management involves a synthetic diet, deficient in the branched-chain amino acids. In severely affected persons it may be difficult to provide essential nutrients for growth without precipitating ketoacidosis.

4. The **prognosis** depends on the severity of the metabolic block and the degree of neurologic damage sustained in the newborn period before treatment. Most patients are subject to recurrent episodes of ketoacidosis that can be lethal. Early diagnosis and careful clinical monitoring may enable normal growth and development.

D. Homocystinuria causes a characteristic clinical syndrome of skeletal abnormalities including tall, Marfan-like stature, myopia, dislocation of the lens, hypercoagulopathy, and, often, mental retardation.

1. Etiology. The classic form of the disease is due to deficiency of the enzyme cystathionine β-synthetase. The incidence is 1 in 200,000; up to 5% of persons with atraumatic lens dislocation have homocystinuria.

2. Evaluation and diagnosis

 a. The condition should be suspected in persons with atraumatic lens dislocation or children with thrombotic episodes.

 b. Increased homocystine is present in the urine and can be demonstrated using paper chromatography for amino acids or the nitroprusside test.

 c. The diagnosis in newborn screening can be made by screening for elevated blood methionine levels.

    d. Increased urinary homocystine with low methionine levels may be due to defects in methylcobalamin (methyl–vitamin B_{12}) synthesis or folate metabolism.

    e. Enzyme activity should be measured in skin fibroblast cultures or liver.

3. Treatment

    a. Approximately half of patients with cystathionine β-synthetase deficiency respond to **pyridoxine** (vitamin B_6) at doses of 50–250 mg/day.

    b. Pyridoxine-unresponsive patients can be treated with a low-methionine diet supplemented with cystine.

    c. Thrombotic episodes are not prevented by aspirin and dipyridamole.

4. Prognosis. Diagnosis and therapy prior to the onset of clinical symptoms may prevent significant clinical sequelae. Therapy has little effect on pre-existing clinical abnormalities.

E. Disorders of the urea cycle cause clinical syndromes characterized by protein intolerance and hyperammonemia. These disorders can present in the newborn period, with feeding intolerance, vomiting, lethargy, convulsions, coma, and death. In older patients the disorder may cause chronic food intolerance, failure to thrive, developmental delay, and episodic hyperammonemia. The **incidence** of arginosuccinic acidemia (arginosuccinase deficiency, AS) is 1 in 75,000 (Massachusetts). Other disorders are less common.

1. Evaluation and diagnosis

    a. The diagnosis should be suspected in any child with hyperammonemia.

    b. Specific enzyme disorders can be distinguished by analysis of blood amino acids.

      (1) Low blood citrulline and arginine are found in carbamyl phosphate synthetase deficiency.

      (2) Ornithine transcarbamylase deficiency is X-linked (only males are clinically affected). Orotic aciduria and low blood citrulline and arginine increase glutamine and glutamic acid in the urine.

      (3) Arginosuccinate synthetase deficiency produces citrullinemia.

      (4) Arginosuccinase deficiency produces arginosuccinic acidemia(uria).

      (5) Arginase deficiency is manifested by elevated blood arginine and elevated urine arginine, cystine, ornithine, and lysine. It may give a positive nitroprusside reaction.

    c. A definitive diagnosis requires an assay of enzyme activity. All enzymes can be assayed in liver; AS (arginosuccinase), ASS (arginosuccinate synthetase), and arginase can all be assayed in leukocytes. AS and ASS can also be assayed in fibroblasts, and AS and arginase can be assayed in erythrocytes.

2. Treatment

    a. Acute episodes of hyperammonemia should be managed as outlined in sec. **IV.** Arginine should be administered for each disease, except for arginase deficiency.

    b. Subacute or chronic forms of urea cycle disorders can be treated with a protein-restricted diet. Essential amino acids may be supplemented using alpha keto analogues. Sodium benzoate (250–500 mg/kg/day) may be administered chronically to enhance ammonia excretion.

3. The **prognosis** depends on the severity of the metabolic block. Complete block at any stage in the urea cycle is generally fatal in the first year of life. Milder deficiencies may respond well to dietary management, though recurrent bouts of hyperammonemia are common.

F. Tyrosinemia is a hepatic disease characterized by increased blood levels of tyrosine and methionine. No specific enzyme abnormality is known. Affected infants present in the first months of life with failure to thrive, progressive hepatic failure, and vitamin D–resistant rickets. The disease is generally fatal in the second or third year of life. The disease is rare, with an **incidence** of 1 in 12,000 in persons of French-Canadian ancestry. There is no known treatment. Several cases of successful liver transplantation have been described.

G. Cystinosis is a disorder characterized by intracellular accumulation of cystine. Clinically, the disorder is manifested by renal dysfunction, including Fanconi syndrome, vitamin D–resistant rickets, and progressive renal failure.

   1. The **diagnosis** should be suspected in any child with Fanconi syndrome or renal dysfunction.

   a. Increased concentrations of cystine are found in leukocytes and fibroblasts of affected persons and heterozygotes (carriers).

   b. Pathognomonic deposits of cystine are found in the cornea.

   2. Treatment

   a. Supportive therapy for acidosis, renal failure, and hypophosphatemic rickets (see Chap. 8).

   b. Renal transplantation corrects the metabolic abnormalities. Cystinosis does not recur in the donor organ.

   c. Ascorbic acid should **not** be used, since it may increase the risk of renal failure. Cysteamine is currently an investigational drug for this disorder.

   3. Prognosis. Cystinosis causes uremia and death before puberty unless successful renal transplantation is performed.

H. Organic acid disorders

   1. Etiology. Methylmalonic acidemia and **propionic acidemia** result from an inability to metabolize the amino acids valine, isoleucine, methionine, and threonine. The accumulation of **propionate** or **methylmalonate** causes a clinical syndrome characterized by metabolic acidosis, protein intolerance, mental retardation, failure to thrive, and, occasionally, hyperammonemia, pancytopenia, and hypoglycemia. **Pyruvic acidemia** results from failure of pyruvic acid degradation and causes lactic acidosis, hyperalaninemia, and a similar clinical syndrome. These disorders can be fatal in the newborn period or can result in varying degrees of retardation and developmental delay. The **incidence** of methylmalonic acidemia is 1 in 95,000 (Massachusetts) and of propionic acidemia, 1 in 300,000 (Massachusetts).

   2. Diagnosis

   a. The diagnosis should be suspected in any child with severe neonatal or recurrent acidosis.

   b. Increased concentrations of organic acids are found in the urine. Propionate can be found in analyses of serum for fatty acids. Propionic acidemia is associated with elevated glycine. Pyruvic acidemia is associated with elevations of alanine.

   c. The activity of enzymes of the organic acid pathways can be measured in liver tissue or cultured skin fibroblasts.

   3. Treatment

   a. Approximately 50% of patients with methylmalonic acidemia respond to vitamin B_{12} (1–2 mg/day). Rare patients with pyruvic acidemia and propionic acidemia respond to biotin (5–10 mg/day).

   b. Dietary management involves restriction of protein.

   4. Prognosis. Patients who respond to vitamin therapy may be expected to grow and develop normally. Those who present with severe acidosis in the newborn period or who are not well controlled on vitamin and diet therapy may have developmental delay, mental retardation, and recurrent, life-threatening episodes of acidosis.

I. Glycogen storage diseases. There is a diverse set of syndromes associated with deficiencies of enzymes required for glycogenolysis. The clinical manifestations are determined by the tissue distribution of the deficient enzyme. Most of the glycogen storage diseases present with hepatomegaly, variable hypoglycemia, and failure to thrive. Pompe's disease (type II) causes severe cardiomyopathy. Types V and VII present with striated myopathy.

   1. The **diagnosis** must be suspected from the clinical presentation. Glucagon stimulation tests and galactose loading tests may distinguish among the various disorders. Definitive diagnosis requires assay of the deficient enzyme from the affected tissue.

2. Treatment. Continuous alimentation with glucose is effective in type I glycogen storage disease in reducing glycogen stores and preventing secondary manifestations of the disorder.

J. Mucopolysaccharidoses are disorders of lysosomal enzymes required for degradation of mucopolysaccharides. The clinical syndromes are characterized by coarse facial features, failure to thrive, mental retardation, hepatosplenomegaly, and skeletal abnormalities.

  1. The **incidence** of Hurler's syndrome is 1 in 100,000; others are less common.
  2. The **diagnosis** is usually suggested by the clinical presentation.
    a. Mucopolysaccharides are detectable in the urine by a Berry spot test in most of the mucopolysaccharidoses.
    b. Diagnosis of the specific disorder requires an assay of enzyme activity in leukocytes or fibroblasts.
  3. Treatment. There is no specific treatment.

K. Disorders of amino acid transport include **cystinuria, Hartnup disease,** and **iminoglycinuria.** These disorders are relatively common, though only cystinuria is associated with any clinical problems.

  1. In cystinuria, a defect in the transport of cystine, lysine, arginine, and ornithine results in increased urinary excretion and impaired intestinal absorption of these amino acids. The clinical symptoms are due to the formation of cystine stones in the renal collecting system. The **incidence** of cystinuria is 1 in 13,000; of Hartnup disease, 1 in 20,000; and of iminoglycinuria, 1 in 14,000.
  2. Evaluation and diagnosis
    a. The diagnosis of cystinuria should be suspected in any person with renal calculi. Analysis of stones for cystine will confirm the diagnosis.
    b. In cystinuria, cystine and the dibasic amino acids can be detected on urine screening for amino acids. The nitroprusside test gives a positive reaction for cystine.
  3. Treatment. Maintaining a dilute urine prevents stone formation in some patients. Penicillamine also lowers the incidence of calculi.

L. Lipid storage diseases result from the failure of degradation of various lipids. Degeneration of the CNS, organomegaly, and failure to thrive constitute the common denominators of many of the lipidoses. Accumulation of lipid in the bone marrow, neurons, and blood vessels provides a means for histologic diagnosis in many of these disorders. The cherry red spot is characteristic of several disorders, including Tay-Sachs and Niemann-Pick diseases. A definitive diagnosis requires an assay of enzyme activity in fibroblast cultures or leukocytes. There is no treatment for any of these disorders.

  Tay-Sachs disease is common among Ashkenazi Jews of eastern European ancestry; 1 in 25 are carriers for this disease. **Carrier testing should be performed on all Jews of eastern European ancestry.**

M. Wilson's disease. See Chap. 20, p. 501.

15

Antibiotics and Infectious Diseases

I. Principles of antimicrobial therapy. Whenever possible, a single antimicrobial agent should be used, and the antimicrobial spectrum should be kept as narrow as possible. The use of multiple antimicrobials is associated with an increased likelihood of colonization and superinfection by drug-resistant organisms. However, when severely ill patients or those whose defenses are impaired are suspected of being infected, they should be given broad-spectrum therapy pending the definitive results of cultures.

A. Identification of the infecting pathogen. The most probable infecting pathogen(s) can often be determined from various host factors, the site of infection, the results of rapid diagnostic procedures, the patient's underlying illness, and local epidemiologic factors.

  1. Host factors

   a. Age. In the neonatal period the most common pathogens are *Escherichia coli,* other gram-negative enteric bacilli, group B streptococci, and staphylococci. *Haemophilus influenzae* type B, pneumococci, and meningococci are common and serious pathogens between the ages of 2 months–5 years.

   b. Defects of humoral immunity (see also Chap. 18, pp. 474ff). Patients with congenital or acquired hypogammaglobulinemia or defects of certain complement components, particularly C3, have an increased incidence of infections with encapsulated pyogenic organisms such as pneumococci, meningococci, *H. influenzae,* and *S. aureus.*
   Isolated deficiencies of C5, C6, C7, and C8 have been specifically associated with meningococcal and gonococcal infections.

   c. Defects in cellular immunity. The T lymphocytes and their effector cells are probably important in the defense against intracellular bacteria, *Listeria, Nocardia,* fungi, certain viruses, and *Pneumocystis carinii.*

   d. Granulocytopenia and granulocyte disorders. See Chap. 17, pp. 453ff.

   e. Miscellaneous defects conferring increased risk

    (1) Patients with **splenic hypofunction** may have fulminant infections, most commonly due to the pneumococcus, meningococcus, and *H. influenzae* type B.

    (2) Patients with severe **hepatic dysfunction** have an increased frequency of bacteremias with *E. coli,* other enteric gram-negative bacilli, and occasionally the pneumococcus.

    (3) Patients with **nephrotic syndrome** have an increased incidence of infections (especially peritonitis) caused by pneumococci, gram-negative bacilli, and *H. influenzae* type B.

    (4) Primary peritonitis occurs almost exclusively in patients with ascites associated with cirrhosis or nephrosis.

  2. Site of infection. Table 15-1 lists the bacterial and fungal pathogens that cause acute infections at various sites. The common pathogens are those responsible for the majority of infections at a given site. The uncommon pathogens are rare or associated only with specific clinical situations, which are indicated. The list is not exhaustive.
  Further discussion of specific sites of infection is found in sec. **IV.**

Table 15-1. Bacterial and fungal etiologies of acute infections in various sites

Site	Common organisms	Less common organisms	Comments
Skin (primary)	Group A streptococcus S. aureus	H. influenzae type B Gram-negative enteric bacilli Candida	Face, periorbital Impaired host Paronychia, intertriginous skin, diaper dermatitis
Skin (trauma)	S. aureus	Group A streptococcus Pseudomonas aeruginosa Anaerobes Clostridium spp. Gram-negative enteric bacilli Erysipelothrix Pasteurella multocida	Burns and surgical wounds (early) Burns (late), puncture wounds of foot Severe trauma and abdominal wounds Severe trauma and abdominal wounds Severe trauma and abdominal wounds Animal products Animal bites
Conjunctiva	Pneumococcus Haemophilus species S. aureus	Gonococcus Chlamydia trachomatis P. aeruginosa	Neonates, sexual history Neonates
Middle ear	Pneumococcus H. influenzae (nontypable and type B) Group A streptococcus Branhamella catarrhalis	Gram-negative enteric bacilli Mycobacterium tuberculosis	Neonates Chronic drainage
Sinuses	H. influenzae (nontypable) Pneumococcus Oral anaerobes	S. aureus Group A streptococcus Aspergillus Phycomycetes	Chronic infection Impaired hosts Impaired hosts, diabetics
Cervical adenitis	Group A streptococcus S. aureus Oral anaerobes	Toxoplasma Nontuberculous mycobacteria M. tuberculosis	Cats Children <4 years Contact history, abnormal chest x-ray
Mouth and pharynx	Group A streptococcus	Gonococcus Candida Oral anaerobes Corynebacterium diphtheriae	Sexual history Antibiotic therapy, impaired host Vincent's infection Sore throat, ...

Site			
Epiglottis	H. influenzae type B	C. diphtheriae	Gray membrane
		Pneumococcus	
Lower respiratory tract	Pneumococcus	H. influenzae type B	Children < 8 years
	Mycoplasma pneumoniae	S. aureus	Influenza, impaired host, neonate
		Group A streptococcus	Pharyngitis, large pleural effusions
		Group B streptococcus	Respiratory distress in neonates
		Klebsiella and other gram-negative bacilli	Impaired hosts
		Oral anaerobes	Aspiration, lung abscess
		Bordetella pertussis	Characteristic cough
		M. tuberculosis	Exposure history
		Chlamydia trachomatis	Infants < 12 weeks
Endocardium	Viridans streptococci	Staphylococcus epidermidis, diphtheroids, etc.	Prosthetic valves
	S. aureus	P. aeruginosa	Addicts
	Enterococcus	Candida and other fungi	Large emboli
GI tract	Shigella	Yersinia enterocolitica	Symptoms of appendicitis
	Salmonella	Vibrio parahaemolyticus	Shellfish ingestion
		Campylobacter	
		Vibrio cholerae	
		E. coli	Foreign travel
		Entamoeba histolytica	Foreign travel
		Giardia lamblia	Foreign travel
		Clostridium difficile	Foreign travel, day care center
			Antibiotic therapy
Urinary tract	E. coli and other enteric gram-negative bacilli	Enterococcus	Chronic recurrent infections
		P. aeruginosa	Chronic recurrent infections
		Staphylococcus saprophyticus	
		S. aureus	Bacteremia, kidney abscess
Bone	S. aureus	Salmonella	Sickle cell disease
		Pseudomonas	Foot puncture
		Streptococcus Groups A and B	
		H. influenzae type B	
		M. tuberculosis	

Table 15-1 (continued)

Site	Common organisms	Less common organisms	Comments
Joints	*S. aureus*	Gram-negative bacilli	Neonates
	H. influenzae type B	Gonococcus	Neonates, sexually active adolescents
	Group A streptococcus	Pneumococcus	
		Staphylococcus epidermidis	Prostheses
		M. tuberculosis	
Meninges	*H. influenzae* type B	Enteric gram-negative bacilli	Neonates, surgery
	Meningococcus	Group B streptococcus	Neonates
	Pneumococcus	*S. aureus*	Surgery and shunts
		Staphylococcus epidermidis	Shunts
		Listeria monocytogenes	Impaired hosts, neonates
		Cryptococcus	Impaired host
		M. tuberculosis	

3. Rapid diagnostic procedures
   a. A **Gram stain** should be performed on all body fluids and exudates from suspected sites of infection. Two common pitfalls include:
   (1) Underdecolorization. This problem is recognized by the blue staining of cell nuclei and can be avoided by repeating the decolorization step of the Gram stain.
   (2) Gram-stained artifacts most commonly resemble "sheets of gram-positive cocci." This problem is avoided by the use of fresh stains and gentle heat fixing.
   b. Methylene blue will demonstrate fecal leukocytes in diarrheal stools. All bacteria will stain dark blue, which can be helpful in detecting small numbers of pleomorphic gram-negative bacteria that have been phagocytosed or are associated with gram-negative debris.
   c. Microbial antigen detection. Rapid immunologic techniques for the detection of microbial antigens in serum, urine, cerebrospinal fluid (CSF), and other body fluids may allow early etiologic diagnosis of hepatitis type B, cryptococcal meningitis, and infections with *H. influenzae* type B, meningococci, pneumococci, K-1 *E. coli*, group B streptococci, and other organisms.
   d. Serology. In general, two serum samples are required to demonstrate a rise (fourfold titer rise or two-tube dilution difference) in antibody titer in the diagnosis of acute viral infection. One sample is taken during the acute phase of the illness and a second is drawn 10–21 days later. However, the following two serologic tests can be performed on a single serum specimen.
   (1) Tests for **heterophil antibody**, which become positive during the second week of infectious mononucleosis.
   (2) Cold agglutinins, which are found in 75 percent of patients with *Mycoplasma* pneumonia during the second week of illness. A simple bedside test will detect a significant titer ($\geq 1:64$): add 2 or 3 drops of whole blood to an oxalate tube (blue top) and place on ice for 2 min. Tilt the tube against the light and observe for agglutination, which disappears on warming to $37°$ C. Various other infectious agents also produce elevations in the titer of cold agglutinins.
   e. All microbiologic specimens should be plated on appropriate media as promptly as possible. Urine specimens may, however, be refrigerated overnight, if necessary.
   (1) Specimens containing cold-labile organisms, such as the meningococcus or gonococcus, should be aspirated into a syringe, sealed, and promptly taken to the laboratory. Many organisms, especially anaerobes, **will not survive on swabs that are allowed to dry.** On the other hand, group A β-hemolytic streptococci will survive at least 24 hr on a dry swab. If this organism is specifically sought, the swab need not be placed in a liquid medium. Thus, irrelevant organisms may not survive, permitting a better yield of streptococci.
   (2) *Shigella* and many *Salmonella* species do not survive cooling and storage of stool specimens. Therefore, the stool must be cultured promptly, or a buffered transport medium should be used. *Salmonella* (but not *Shigella*) survive drying on rectal swabs.

B. Choice and dosage of antimicrobial agents
   1. Antibiotic susceptibility. The recommended choice and dosage of antimicrobials for specific pathogens are outlined in Tables 15-2 and 15-3.
   a. Frequently, the likely pathogen(s) is (are) susceptible to several antimicrobials. A rational choice is then based on drug toxicity, pharmacologic factors relating to the patient (age, renal and hepatic function), and pharmacologic factors relating to the infection (antimicrobial penetration and activity at the site of infection).
   b. Agents with potentially serious side effects should be used only when they offer a definite advantage over less toxic agents.

Table 15-2. Choice of antimicrobial agents for specific pathogens[a]

Organism	Infection	Drug of choice	Pediatric dose[a]
A. *Gram-positive cocci*			
1. Group A streptococcus	Pharyngitis,[b] impetigo	Penicillin G	25,000 U/kg/day PO or IM
	Cellulitis	(Alt.: erythromycin, cephalosporin, vancomycin)	50,000–100,000 U/kg/day PO, IM, or IV
	Pneumonia, empyema, bacteremia		100,000 U/kg/day IV or IM
	Meningitis		300,000 U/kg/day IV
2. Viridans streptococci	Subacute bacterial endocarditis	Penicillin G	250,000 U/kg/day IV
		(Alt.: cephalothin, vancomycin)	
3. Enterococcus	Urinary tract	Ampicillin (or amoxicillin)	50–100 mg/kg/day PO (20–40 mg/kg/day PO)
		(Alt.: nitrofurantoin)	
	Subacute bacterial endocarditis	Ampicillin or penicillin G plus gentamicin	300 mg/kg/day (ampicillin) IV 250,000 U/kg/day (penicillin G) IV
		(Alt.: vancomycin and gentamicin)	180 mg/M² or 4.5–7.5 mg/kg/day (gentamicin) IV
4. Pneumococcus	Pneumonia	Penicillin G	50,000 U/kg/day (penicillin G) PO, IM, or IV
		(Alt.: erythromycin, cephalosporin, chloramphenicol, vancomycin)	
	Meningitis, complications (empyema)		300,000 U/kg/day IV
5. *S. aureus* (penicillin-resistant)[c]	Mild infection	Semisynthetic penicillin	50–100 mg/kg/day PO or IM
	Systemic infection	(Alt.: cephalothin,[d] clindamycin, vancomycin)	200 mg/kg/day IV
6. *S. epidermidis*[e]	Endocarditis	Semisynthetic penicillin	200 mg/kg/day IV
	Shunt infection	(Alt.: cephalothin,[d] vancomycin)	
B. *Gram-positive bacilli*			
7. *Clostridium perfringens*	Gas gangrene	Penicillin G	200,000 U/kg/day IV
		(Alt.: chloramphenicol)	

Organism	Condition	Drug of choice (Alternatives)	Dosage
8. *Clostridium tetani*	Tetanus	Penicillin G (Alt.: tetracycline) Human antitoxin (see Table 15-8)	100,000 U/kg/day IV
9. *Listeria monocytogenes*	Meningitis	Ampicillin ± gentamicin (Alt.: trimethoprim-sulfamethoxazole, erythromycin, tetracycline, chloramphenicol)	300–400 mg/kg/day IV For newborn dosages, see Table 6-1
10. *Corynebacterium diphtheriae*	Diphtheria	Procaine penicillin G (Alt.: erythromycin) Horse antitoxin (see Table 15-8)	25,000–50,000 U/kg/day IM
C. *Gram-negative cocci* 11. Meningococcus	Meningitis Meningococcemia	Penicillin G (Alt.: chloramphenicol, cefuroxime, cefotaxime, sulfonamide)	300,000 U/kg/day IV 150,000 U/kg/day IV
12. Gonococcus (see Table 15-11)	Gonorrhea	See Table 15-11	
D. *Gram-negative bacilli*[g] 13. *E. coli*	Urinary tract	Sulfisoxazole (Alt.: ampicillin, trimethoprim-sulfamethoxazole, cephalexin)	100 mg/kg/day PO
	Surgical wound, pneumonia, sepsis	Gentamicin (Alt.: ampicillin, cephalosporins, chloramphenicol, amikacin)	180 mg/M^2 or 4.5–7.5 mg/kg/day IV
	Meningitis	Ampicillin and gentamicin (Alt.: chloramphenicol, amikacin)	For newborn dosages, see Table 6-1
14. *Klebsiella*	Urinary tract	Trimethoprim-sulfamethoxazole (Alt.: cephalexin, tetracycline, chloramphenicol)	8 mg/kg/day trimethoprim 40 mg/kg/day sulfamethoxazole PO
	Pneumonia, sepsis	Gentamicin (Alt.: cephalosporin, amikacin)	180 mg/M^2 or 4.5–7.5 mg/kg/day IV

Table 15-2 (continued)

Organism	Infection	Drug of choice	Pediatric dose[a]
15. *Proteus mirabilis*	Urinary tract	Ampicillin (or amoxicillin) (Alt.: cephalexin, trimethoprim-sulfamethoxazole, chloramphenicol)	50–100 mg/kg/day PO (20–40 mg/kg/day PO)
	Systemic	Gentamicin (Alt.: ampicillin, cephalosporins, amikacin, chloramphenicol)	180 mg/M² *or* 4.5–7.5 mg/kg/day IV
16. *Proteus*, indole-positive	Urinary tract	Trimethoprim-sulfamethoxazole (Alt.: chloramphenicol, carbenicillin,[f] tetracycline)	8 mg/kg/day trimethoprim 40 mg/kg/day sulfamethoxazole PO
	Systemic	Gentamicin (Alt.: carbenicillin,[f] cefoxitin, amikacin)	180 mg/M² *or* 4.5–7.5 mg/kg/day IV
17. *Pseudomonas aeruginosa*	Urinary tract	Carbenicillin (indanyl) (Alt.: tetracycline with acidification)	50–65 mg/kg/day PO
	Systemic	Gentamicin (Alt.: tobramycin, amikacin) *plus* Carbenicillin[f]	180 mg/M² *or* 4.5–7.5 mg/kg/day IV 400–600 mg/kg/day IV
18. *Salmonella*	Systemic	Chloramphenicol (Alt.: ampicillin, trimethoprim-sulfamethoxazole)	50–100 mg/kg/day PO, IV

Organism	Infection	Drug	Dosage
19. *Serratia*		Gentamicin (Alt.: cefoxitin, trimethoprim-sulfamethoxazole, carbenicillin,[f] amikacin)	180 mg/M^2 *or* 4.5–7.5 mg/kg/day IV
20. *Shigella*		Trimethoprim-sulfamethoxazole (Alt.: ampicillin, chloramphenicol, tetracycline)	10 mg/kg/day trimethoprim 50 mg/kg/day sulfamethoxazole PO
21. *Bacteroides*	Respiratory infections Abdominal abscess, bacteremia	Penicillin G Clindamycin (Alt.: chloramphenicol, cefoxitin, metronidazole)	100,000 U/kg/day IV 25 mg/kg/day IV
22. *Pasteurella multocida*		Penicillin G (Alt.: tetracycline, cephalosporin)	50,000 U/kg/day PO
23. *H. influenzae*	Otitis media	Ampicillin or amoxicillin (Alt.: erythromycin plus sulfonamide, trimethoprim-sulfamethoxazole, cefaclor)	50–100 mg/kg/day PO *or* IM (20–40 mg/kg/day PO)
	Bacteremia Epiglottitis Pneumonia Meningitis	Chloramphenicol *plus* ampicillin initially	100 mg/kg/day IV 200 mg/kg/day IV

[a]See Table 15-3 for maximum doses and Chap. 6, Appendix Table 6-1 for doses in neonates.

[b]Always treat for 10 days to prevent postinfection sequelae.

[c]In life-threatening staphylococcal infections gentamicin may be added for initial therapy.

[d]Cephalosporins are not predictably active in vivo against penicillin-resistant staphylococci, regardless of the results of in vitro susceptibility tests.

[e]May be resistant to semisynthetic penicillins. Usually sensitive to vancomycin, aminoglycosides, and rifampin.

[f]Ticarcillin may be used interchangeably with carbenicillin at two-thirds the dosage.

[g]Since sensitivity patterns vary, antibiotic choice should be based on specific sensitivity determination whenever possible.

Table 15-3. Doses of antimicrobial agents[a]

Antimicrobial	Daily dose	Frequency	Route	Usual maximum adult dose
A. Penicillins				
1. Oral penicillin G[b,c]	25,000–100,000 U/kg	q6h	PO	6.4 MU
Phenoxymethyl penicillin (V)[c]			PO	6.4 MU
2. Parenteral				
a. Aqueous penicillin G[a]	25,000–300,000 U/kg	q2–4h	IV	24 MU
b. Procaine penicillin G[a]	25,000–50,000 U/kg	q12–24h	IM	4.8 MU
c. Benthazine penicillin G[c]	600,000–1,200,000 U	single dose	IM	1.2 MU
3. Penicillinase-resistant				
Methicillin,[a] oxacillin,[a] nafcillin[a]	100–200 mg/kg	q4–6h	IM or IV	12 gm
b. Cloxacillin[c]	50–100 mg/kg	q6h	PO	4 gm
c. Dicloxacillin	12.5–25 mg/kg	q6h	PO	4 gm
4. Broad spectrum				
a. Ampicillin[a]	50–100 mg/kg	q6h	PO	4 gm
	50–400 mg/kg	q4h	IM or IV	12 gm
Amoxicillin	20–40 mg/kg	q8h	PO	3 gm
b. Carbenicillin[a]	50–65 mg/kg	q6h	PO	40 gm
	400–600 mg/kg	q2–4h	IM or IV	
c. Ticarcillin	200–300 mg/kg	q4h	IM or IV	30 gm
B. Cephalosporins				
1. Cephalothin[a]	80–160 mg/kg	q4–6h	IV	12 gm
2. Cefazolin[c]	25–100 mg/kg	q6–8h	IM or IV	6 gm
3. Cephalexin[c]	25–50 mg/kg	q6h	PO	4 gm
4. Cefamandole	50–150 mg/kg	q4h	IM or IV	12 gm
5. Cefuroxime	75–150 mg/kg	q8h	IM or IV	
6. Cefoxitin	80–160 mg/kg	q4–6h	IM or IV	12 gm
7. Cefaclor	40 mg/kg	q8h	PO	4 gm
8. Moxalactam	150–200 mg/kg	q6–8h	IV	
9. Cefotaxime	100–200 mg/kg	q4–6h	IM or IV	

Drug	Dose	Route	Interval	Maximum
C. Erythromycins[c]	30–50 mg/kg	PO	q6h	4 gm
	15–50 mg/kg	IV[d]	q6h	4 gm
D. Clindamycin[c]	10–25 mg/kg	PO	q6h	4.8 gm
	10–40 mg/kg	IM or IV	q6h	4.8 gm
E. Sulfonamides[c]	150 mg/kg	PO	q6h	8 gm
	100 mg/kg	IV	q6h	960 mg TMP
Trimethoprim-sulfamethoxazole	8–20 mg TMP/kg	PO	q12h	4.8 gm SMZ
	40–100 mg SMZ/kg	IV	> 10 yr: q12h	
	150 mg TMP/M² dose[e]		< 10 yr: q8h	
F. Aminoglycosides				
1. Streptomycin[c]	20–30 mg/kg	IM	q12h	2 gm
2. Kanamycin	600 mg/M² or 15–22.5 mg/kg	IM	q8h	1.5 gm
3. Gentamicin[a]	180 mg/M² or 3–7.5 mg/kg	IM or IV	q8h	5 mg/kg/day
4. Tobramycin	150 mg/M² or 3–5 mg/kg	IM or IV	q8h	5 mg/kg/day
5. Amikacin	600 mg/M² or 15–22.5 mg/kg	IM or IV	q8h	1.5 gm
G. Nitrofurantoin[c]	5–7 mg/kg	PO	q6h	400 mg
H. Chloramphenicol[a]	50–100 mg/kg	PO or IV	q6h	4 gm
I. Tetracycline,[c,f] Chlortetracycline,[c,f] Oxytetracycline[c,f]	20–40 mg/kg	PO	q6h	2 gm
	10–20 mg/kg	IV or IM	q12h	2 gm
1. Doxycycline[c,f]	5 mg/kg	PO	q12h	200 mg
2. Minocycline[c,f]	4 mg/kg	PO	q12h	200 mg
J. Vancomycin	50 mg/kg	PO	q6h	2 gm
	40 mg/kg	IV	q6h	2 gm

[a] For newborn doses see Appendix Table 6-1.
[b] 1 mg = 1600 units.
[c] Not recommended for newborns.
[d] May be given in continuous drip.
[e] Loading dose is 250 mg TMP/M² if no trimethoprim-sulfamethoxazole has been given in the past 24 hrs.
[f] Not recommended for children < 8 years of age.

Table 15-4. Therapeutic and toxic serum levels of antimicrobials with a narrow toxic-therapeutic ratio

Antimicrobial	Therapeutic peak levels (μg/ml)	Probably toxic peak levels (μg/ml)	Probably toxic trough levels (μg/ml)
Gentamicin	4–8	>12	>2
Tobramycin	4–8	>12	>2
Kanamycin	15–35	>35	>10
Amikacin	15–35	>35	>10
Streptomycin	15–35	>35	>10
Chloramphenicol	5–25	>25[a]	
(free)		>50[b]	
Vancomycin	25–40	>40	
5-Fluorocytosine	50–100	>100	
Trimethoprim	5–10	>10	

[a] Reversible marrow suppression.
[b] Gray syndrome.

2. **Combinations of antimicrobial agents.** Although a single antimicrobial agent should provide adequate therapy for the majority of infections, combination therapy is recommended for specific organisms or certain clinical situations. These include **endocarditis** (see p. 405) caused by enterococci or by viridans streptococci relatively resistant to penicillin, **severe *Pseudomonas* infection** (an aminoglycoside [gentamicin or tobramycin] and a penicillin [carbenicillin or ticarcillin]), **active tuberculosis** (see p. 409), **cryptococcal** meningitis and disseminated infections caused by other yeasts (amphotericin B and 5-fluorocytosine, **provided** the organism is sensitive to 5-fluorocytosine), and **empirical antibiotic therapy** for severely ill patients. Widely used regimens for suspected bacterial sepsis are ampicillin and gentamicin in neonates, ampicillin and chloramphenicol in older infants and children, and carbenicillin and gentamicin in immunosuppressed patients.

3. **Monitoring antimicrobial dosage.** Treatment with antibiotics with a narrow toxic-therapeutic ratio should be monitored by measuring serum peak and trough levels. Table 15-4 gives the recommended therapeutic levels of such antimicrobials.

   a. **Peak levels** should be measured 1 hr after an IM dose, ½ hr after the end of a ½-hr IV infusion, or immediately after a 1-hr infusion. **Trough levels** should be measured just before a dose. Peak and trough levels should be checked shortly after the initiation of and at least once per week during therapy. More frequent monitoring is recommended in neonates and in patients who are seriously ill or who have renal or hepatic dysfunction.

   b. In certain infections such as **endocarditis** and **osteomyelitis, bactericidal** rather than bacteriostatic antibiotics are used, and the effectiveness of the patient's serum in killing the pathogen is monitored during therapy. The peak bactericidal level should be at least 1:8 and the trough at least 1:2.

4. **Antimicrobial activity at the site of infection.** The levels of most antimicrobial agents in well-perfused tissues and serous spaces are adequate for treating infections at these sites. On the other hand, subtherapeutic levels are often attained in sequestered sites such as abscess cavities and in the obstructed urinary or biliary tract. Hence, surgery is vital in the management of these infections.

- **a. Antimicrobial penetration into the CNS**
  - **(1)** Chloramphenicol, the sulfonamides, and most antituberculous agents penetrate normal meninges well.
  - **(2)** The penicillins penetrate effectively, but only in the presence of inflamed meninges. Large doses must be given **parenterally and maintained throughout therapy.**
  - **(3)** The cephalosporins, including cephalothin, cefazolin, cefaclor, cefamandole, and cefoxitin, do not penetrate the CSF in therapeutic amounts. As a result, meningitis due to sensitive organisms may develop during parenteral treatment of bacteremic infections with cephalosporins of poor penetration.
  - **(4)** The levels of aminoglycoside antibiotics in the CSF after parenteral therapy are unpredictable and are often inadequate for the therapy of gram-negative meningitis. Therefore, it may be necessary to monitor CSF levels of these antibiotics and to administer them directly into the ventricular system.
- **b. Antimicrobial activity in the urinary tract** (see Sec. **IV**). In patients with normal renal function, many antimicrobials reach much higher concentrations in urine than in serum. As a result, routine sensitivity tests based on achievable serum concentrations are not always reliable predictors of antibiotic efficacy. **Therefore, a report of antibiotic resistance should prompt a repeat urine culture** rather than a change in regimen, unless the patient's symptoms have failed to respond. An effective regimen should sterilize the urine within 12–24 hr.
  - **(1) Acidification** enhances the activity of the tetracyclines, nitrofurantoin, and the penicillins and cephalosporins. **Alkalinization** markedly enhances the activity of the aminoglycosides and erythromycin and extends the spectrum of the latter to include many gram-negative rods.
  - **(2)** Because of ionic partitioning into acid secretions, **trimethoprim** may be particularly useful in treating recurrent urinary tract infections in females (anterior urethra) and prostatitis in males.
- **5. Failure of therapy.** There is variation in the rate of resolution of infections. Causes for failure of treatment should be considered when fever and signs of infection are prolonged. These include inadequate antibiotic therapy, complication of original infection, complications of treatment, and host factors (immune deficiency, anatomic defect, presence of a foreign body).
- **6. Pharmacologic considerations**
  - **a. Use of antimicrobial agents in infants and young children**
    - **(1)** In **neonates,** antibiotic dosage must be individualized, and serum levels should be monitored, particularly when using toxic drugs. Guidelines for initial antibiotic dosage in neonates may be found in Chap. 6, Appendix Table 6-1.
    - **(2)** In general, dosage intervals are **longer** in younger infants than in older infants. Drug half-lives in premature infants are longer than in full-term infants. Similarly, decreases in renal function are associated with long half-lives of aminoglycoside antibiotics. Therefore, doses and intervals near the lower limits of the ranges given in Chap. 6 should be chosen in these groups.
    - **(3)** To achieve a given blood level, older infants and children less than 10 years of age usually require higher doses of antimicrobials (based on weight) than older children and adults require.
    - **(4)** Dosage of toxic antibiotics should be adjusted according to the age of the patient. For **gentamicin** the usually recommended dosage is 2.5 mg/kg q8h in children under 5 years of age, 2.0 mg/kg in children 5–10 years old, and 1.5 mg/kg in children over 10. However, these recommendations rarely produce levels above the therapeutic range, and levels may be subtherapeutic, particularly in cachectic patients. A

Table 15-5. Metabolism and excretion of commonly used antimicrobial agents

Mainly renal	Renal and nonrenal	Nonrenal
ANTIBACTERIAL AGENTS—SYSTEMIC		

Aminoglycosides
  Streptomycin
  Kanamycin
  Gentamicin
  Tobramycin
  Amikacin
	Penicillins
	
	Cephalosporins
	
	Tetracycline[b]
	Clindamycin
		Chloramphenicol
		
		Erythromycin[a]

Vancomycin		Doxycycline Minocycline

Polymyxins
  Polymyxin B
  Colistin
		Metronidazole

ANTIBACTERIAL AGENTS—URINARY TRACT		
Methenamine[b]	Nitrofurantoin[a,b] Sulfonamides[b] Trimethoprim	Nalidixic acid[b]
ANTITUBERCULOUS AGENTS		
Ethambutol	PAS[a,b]	Rifampin INH
ANTIFUNGAL AGENTS		
5-Fluorocytosine		Amphotericin B Ketoconazole

[a] Should be avoided in severe hepatic failure.
[b] Should be avoided in severe renal failure.

single gentamicin dosage of 60 mg/M^2 q8h produces reproducible peak levels in all age groups regardless of body habitus.

b. Use of antimicrobial agents in renal failure. The routes of metabolism and excretion of antimicrobials are summarized in Table 15-5.

  (1) Antimicrobials handled mainly by the kidneys

  (a) Antibiotics excreted primarily by renal mechanisms are best avoided in patients with severe renal failure.

  (b) Adjustment in dosage is based on estimates of renal function as described for the aminoglycosides (see below). Analogous calculations can be made for other drugs handled mainly by the kidneys (Table 15-6).

   (i) Interval extension. The standard dose of the antibiotic is given, and the dosage interval is prolonged in direct proportion to the increase in serum creatinine concentration as in the following equation.

$$\text{New interval} = \text{standard interval (q8h)} \times \frac{\text{patient's creatinine}}{\text{normal creatinine}}$$

Peak and trough levels with this method are similar to those obtained in patients with normal renal function. However,

Table 15-6. Adjustment of dosage for antimicrobials excreted mainly by the kidney

Antibiotic	Standard dose	Normal renal function		Moderate to severe impairment in renal function	Anuria[a]	
		Half-life (hr)	Dosage interval (hr)		Half-life (days)	Dosage interval (days)
Streptomycin	10–15 mg/kg/dose; maximum, 500 mg/dose	1–3	8–12	Increase dosage interval or decrease dose according to text	2–4	6
Kanamycin[b]	15 mg/kg/dose; maximum, 500 mg/dose	1–3	8	Same as above	2–4	6
Gentamicin[c]	2.5 mg/kg if < 5 years 2.0 mg/kg if 5–10 years 1.5 mg/kg if > 10 years *or* 60 mg/M² all ages	1–3	8	Same as above	2–4	6
Vancomycin	10–20 mg/kg/dose; maximum, 1 gm/dose	6	6–12		9	7–14
5-Fluorocytosine	35 mg/kg/dose	3–6	6		3	Not recommended

[a]The half-life in anuria depends on the rate of extrarenal clearance of the antibiotic. Individual variation is great, and antibiotic levels must be measured.
[b]Amikacin closely resembles kanamycin in its pharmacology.
[c]Tobramycin closely resembles gentamicin in its pharmacology.

this approach may lead to relatively long periods of sub-therapeutic levels prior to the next dose.

(ii) **Dosage adjustment.** The standard dose is given (loading dose), and the standard interval is maintained. Subsequent doses (maintenance doses) are reduced in proportion to increases in the serum creatinine as in the following equation.

$$\text{Maintenance dose} = \text{standard dose} \div \frac{\text{patient's creatinine}}{\text{normal creatinine}}$$

Levels can be maintained within a narrower range with less chance of subtherapeutic levels. However, this method may result in higher peak and trough levels than in (i) and may predispose to greater toxicity.

(c) **The serum creatinine is unreliable in acute or unstable renal disease, in severe uremia, and in intermittent dialysis.** Thus, serum antibiotic levels should be measured frequently and directly to ensure therapeutic levels (Table 15-4).

(2) **Antimicrobials handled by both the kidney and extrarenal mechanisms** may be used in standard doses in patients with mild or moderate renal failure (creatinine clearance > 30 ml/1.74 M^2 or serum creatinine < 3 mg/100 ml). The dosage interval should be increased, as outlined in Table 15-7, if renal failure is moderate or severe. **Nitrofurantoin and all tetracyclines except doxycycline are contraindicated in severe renal failure.** In addition, sulfonamides and para-aminosalicylic acid (PAS) should be avoided in severe renal failure.

(3) **Antimicrobials handled by nonrenal mechanisms.** When these agents are used in patients with renal failure, the dosage need not be adjusted. When possible, amphotericin B should be avoided in such patients, but, if indicated, full doses should be given.

c. **Use of antimicrobials in hepatic failure.** Among antimicrobials metabolized by the liver (see Table 15-5), metabolic and excretory pathways differ. Specific guidelines for dosage modifications in liver failure therefore cannot be formulated. Antimicrobials with a narrow toxic-therapeutic ratio (e.g., **nitrofurantoin**) or with a high risk of hepatotoxicity (e.g., **PAS**) are **contraindicated** in cases of severe liver failure. When possible, **clindamycin, erythromycin, chloramphenicol, tetracyclines, isoniazid (INH)**, and **rifampin** should be avoided in patients with severe liver failure. If any of these agents is used, serum levels should be monitored.

II. **Other aspects of therapy and prevention**

A. **Treatment of fever.** See Chap. 2, pp. 24ff.

B. **Surgery.** The need for adequate drainage of loculated pus, removal of necrotic tissue, relief of obstruction, and removal of foreign bodies should always be considered.

C. **Immune globulin.** Passive immunization is useful in the prevention and treatment of certain infections (Table 15-8). The use of immunoglobulin preparations for hepatitis B is covered in Table 15-14. Additional considerations for hepatitis A and varicella prevention follow.

1. **Immune globulin (IG)** is recommended for prophylaxis of **hepatitis A** for all household and sexual (heterosexual or homosexual) contacts of persons with hepatitis A; for staff, attendees, and, if there is epidemiologic evidence of hepatitis A transmission in a day-care center, all members of households whose diapered children attend; for close contacts if there is a school- or classroom-centered outbreak; for residents and staff in certain institutions for custodial care when outbreaks occur; and for common-source exposure. The dose of IG is 0.02 ml/kg once. For travelers to high-risk areas outside the usual tourist routes, IG may be beneficial for preexposure prophylaxis of hepatitis A. For such travelers, a single dose of IG (0.02 ml/kg) is recom-

Table 15-7. Adjustment of dosage for antibiotics excreted by renal and other routes when given in high dosage

Antibiotic	Standard dose	Normal (50–100%) Half-life (hr)	Normal Standard dose interval (hr)	Moderate impairment[a] (10–30%) Half-life (hr)	Moderate impairment[a] Dose interval (hr)	Anuria[a] (0%) Half-life (hr)	Anuria[a] Dose interval (hr)
Penicillin G	50,000 U/kg/dose	0.5	4	2	6	4	12–24
Ampicillin	50 mg/kg/dose	1	4	No modification		8	12
Carbenicillin	100 mg/kg/dose	1	4	3–6	6–12	16	24
Methicillin	30–35 mg/kg/dose	0.5	4	No modification			12
Oxacillin, nafcillin	30–35 mg/kg/dose	0.5	4	No modification		1–2	8
Cephalothin	25 mg/kg/dose	0.5	4	2	6	6	12
Cefazolin	25 mg/kg/dose	2.0	6	6–12	12–24	36	48
Cephalexin	10 mg/kg/dose	1	6	4	12	24	
Cefamandole	25 mg/kg/dose	1	4		6–8[b]		12[b]
Cefoxitin	25 mg/kg/dose	1	4		8–12[b]		12–24[b]
Moxalactam	50 mg/kg/dose	2	8				
Clindamycin	10 mg/kg/dose	4	6	No modification		12	24
Trimethoprim-sulfamethoxazole	10 mg trimethoprim/kg/dose; 50 mg sulfamethoxazole/kg/dose. Maximum dose, 480 mg trimethoprim/dose, 2.4 gm sulfamethoxazole/dose	12	12	24–36	24	Use not recommended	

[a] Further prolongation of the half-life occurs when hepatic failure is present concurrently.
[b] Reduce dosage concomitantly.

Table 15-8. Immune globulin prophylaxis and therapy

Disorder	Value	Purpose	Dose (IM)	Comment
STANDARD HUMAN IMMUNE GLOBULINS				
Measles	Proved	Modification	0.05 ml/kg	Rarely indicated
		Prevention	0.25 ml/kg	Given immediately after exposure to unvaccinated children
			0.50 ml/kg (maximum, 15 ml)	For immunosuppressed patients
Varicella[a]	Limited	Modification	0.6–1.2 ml/kg	Give immediately after exposure if VZIG is not available. See indications for use in the text
Rubella	Limited	Prevention	20 ml	For pregnant women in the first trimester who will not consider abortion
SPECIAL HUMAN IMMUNE GLOBULINS[b]				
Tetanus (TIG)	Proved	Prevention Treatment	250–500 U 3000–6000 U	See p. 384 for indications
Rabies (RIG)	Proved	Prevention	20 IU/kg	See p. 383 for indications
Varicella-zoster (VZIG)	Proved	Prevention	1 complete vial/10 kg (maximum 5 vials)	See p. 369 for indications Give within 96 hr after exposure
Pertussis	Unproved	Prevention Treatment		Protection not reliable. See Table 15-9 for antimicrobial prophylaxis
Mumps	Unproved	Prevention		No evidence that orchitis is prevented
SPECIAL ANIMAL IMMUNE SERUMS[b]				
Botulism (trivalent ABE)	Proved	Treatment		As soon as possible after testing for sensitivity to serum
Diphtheria	Proved	Treatment	20,000–120,000 U	As soon as clinical diagnosis is made; higher doses for more extensive disease
Gas gangrene (polyvalent clostridial antitoxin)	Unproved	Treatment		No longer commercially available

[a] Zoster immune plasma (ZIP) from patients convalescing from herpes zoster may also modify illness, but carries the risk of hepatitis. The dose is 10 ml/kg IV.
[b] Detailed information about indications, source of supply, and dosage can be obtained from the Centers for Disease Control (404) 329-3311 (8:00 A.M.-5:00 P.M. weekdays) and (404) 329-3644 (off-duty hours).

mended for up to 3 months of travel; for more prolonged stays, 0.06 ml/kg should be given every 5 months. (From *M.M.W.R.* 30:423, 1981).

2. **Varicella-zoster immune globulin (VZIG)** is indicated after significant exposure to **chickenpox** or **zoster** for susceptible children with primary immunodeficiency disorders or neoplastic disease (leukemia or lymphoma), recipients of immunosuppressive therapy, and newborns of mothers who develop varicella within 5 days before or 48 hr after delivery. Premature infants should be evaluated on an individual basis. For distribution centers and detailed recommendations for use of VZIG, see *M.M.W.R.* 33:84, 1984.

D. **Isolation procedures.** Guidelines for hospital precautions and periods of contagiousness of common communicable diseases of childhood can be found in *Pediatrics* 53:663, 1974 and updated in *Infection Control* 4:249, 1983 (CDC Guideline for Isolation Precautions in Hospitals).

E. **Antimicrobial prophylaxis.** Indications for antimicrobial prophylaxis are summarized in Table 15-9.

III. **Specific antimicrobial agents.** Table 15-2 summarizes the drugs of choice and dosages for specific bacterial pathogens. Modification of drug dosage for neonates is discussed on p. 363 and in Chap. 6, and modifications in renal failure on p. 364. Penetration of antimicrobial agents in the tissues and CSF is discussed on pp. 362–363. The antituberculous agents are summarized in Table 15-10. Antifungal agents are discussed on p. 380 and antiviral therapy and agents p. 412.

A. **Antimicrobial agents**

1. **The penicillins** inhibit cell wall synthesis and kill growing bacteria by lysis.

a. **Penicillin**

(1) **Spectrum and indications.** Penicillin is the drug of choice for infections due to pneumococci, streptococci (except enterococci), *Clostridia, Neisseria,* oral anaerobes, and spirochetes. It is also used in anthrax, diphtheria, actinomycosis, leptospirosis, and rat-bite fever. Penicillin G is more active than penicillin V.

(2) **Pharmacology**

(a) **Oral preparations** are penicillin G and penicillin V (phenoxymethyl penicillin). Because it is acid labile, the absorption of penicillin G is **variable.** Penicillin V is well absorbed, especially when given 1 hr before meals.

(b) **Parenteral preparations** differ in their peak serum level and half-life.

(i) **Aqueous penicillin G** results in rapid attainment of high blood levels after IM or IV administration. Its rapid excretion in patients (except newborns) with normal renal function requires that it be administered frequently (usually q4h) for optimal therapy. It is prepared as a potassium or sodium salt ($1.7 \ \text{mEq}/10^6$ units).

(ii) **Procaine penicillin G** is absorbed slowly from IM injections and so produces relatively low but prolonged serum concentrations. It should thus be used only in infections due to highly susceptible organisms or in large dosage.

(iii) **Benzathine penicillin G** produces even lower blood levels, which last for as long as 3–4 weeks. It is used primarily against group A streptococci and *Treponema pallidum,* prophylactically in patients with rheumatic heart disease, and therapeutically when adherence to a program of oral penicillin is questionable.

b. **Penicillinase-resistant penicillins**

(1) **Spectrum and indications.** These agents are resistant to hydrolysis by the β-lactamase produced by staphylococci and are therefore the drugs of choice for penicillin-resistant staphylococcal infections. They are approximately 10 times *less* active than penicillin G against penicillin-sensitive organisms.

Table 15-9. Antimicrobial prophylaxis

Disease	Indication	Antimicrobial and dosage
Preexposure		
Rheumatic fever[a]	History of acute rheumatic fever; lifetime for patients with heart disease; to age 21 in patients without heart disease	*Parenteral* Benzathine penicillin G, 1.2 mg IM monthly *Oral* Sulfadiazine, 500 mg PO qd (< 30 kg), 1 gm PO qd (> 30 kg) Penicillin G or V, 200,000–250,000 U PO qd–bid Erythromycin 250 mg PO bid in patients sensitive to both sulfonamides and penicillin
Endocarditis[b]	*Dental and upper respiratory procedures* in patients with valvular heart disease, prosthetic heart valves, congenital heart disease (but not uncomplicated secundum atrial septal defect), idiopathic hypertrophic subaortic stenosis, and mitral valve prolapse	*Oral* Penicillin V > 60 lb: 2 gm 1 hr before procedure and 1 gm 6 hr later < 60 lb: half adult dose at each time Penicillin allergy: Erythromycin, 20 mg/kg 1 hr before procedure and 10 mg/kg 6 hr later *Parenteral*[c] Ampicillin, 50 mg/kg IM or IV 30 min to 1 hr before procedure and repeat once 8 hr later *or* Aqueous penicillin G, 50,000 U/kg IM or IV 30 min to 1 hr before procedure and repeat once 8 hr later *plus* Gentamicin, 2 mg/kg IM or IV 30 min to 1 hr before procedure and repeat once 8 hr later Penicillin allergy: Vancomycin, 20 mg/kg IV infused over 1 hr, beginning 1 hr before procedure and repeat once 8 hr later
	Gastrointestinal and genitourinary procedures in patients with valvular heart disease, prosthetic heart valves, congenital heart disease (but not uncomplicated secundum atrial septal defect), idiopathic hypertrophic subaortic stenosis, and mitral valve prolapse	*Parenteral*[c] Ampicillin, 50 mg/kg IM or IV 30 min to 1 hr before procedure and repeat once 8 hr later *plus* Gentamicin, 2 mg/kg IM or IV 30 min to 1 hr before procedure and repeat once 8 hr later Penicillin allergy: Vancomycin, 20 mg/kg IV infused over 1 hr, beginning 1 hr before procedure and repeat 8 hr later

Table 15-9 (continued)

Disease	Indication	Antimicrobial and dosage
		plus Gentamicin, 2 mg/kg IM or IV 30 min to 1 hr before procedure and repeat once 8 hr later
		Oral[d]
		Amoxicillin
		> 60 lb: 3 gm 1 hr before procedure and 1.5 gm 6 hr later
		< 60 lb: half adult dosage at each time
Postexposure		
Tuberculosis	Household exposure to active disease[e]	Isoniazid, 10 mg/kg/day to 300 mg/day for 1 year
	Recent or prior tuberculin conversion not previously treated	
	Tuberculin-positive child or adolescent in circumstances favorable to reactivation[f]	
Meningococcal disease[g]	Persons in intimate contact with index case, including household members, day care center contacts, medical personnel	Rifampin
		< 1 mo: 5 mg/kg PO bid × 2 days
		≥ 1 mo: 10 mg/kg PO bid × 2 days (max. 600 mg/dose)
		Sulfadiazine (if strain susceptible)
		< 1 yr: 500 mg PO qd × 2 days
		1–12 yr: 500 mg PO bid × 2 days
		≥ 12 yr: 1 gm PO bid × 2 days
Haemophilus influenzae type B disease	Household contacts if child ≤ 4 yr lives in the home; possibly day-care center contacts	Rifampin, 20 mg/kg/day PO once/day × 4 days
Pertussis	Contacts not previously immunized	Erythromycin, 50 mg/kg/day PO × 10 days
Gonorrhea	Neonates	Erythromycin ophthalmic ointment
	Contact of known case	See Table 15-11
Syphilis	Contact of known case	Benzathine penicillin G, 2.4 mg IM

[a] Modified from M. Markowitz, Rheumatic Fever. In R. E. Behrman and V. C. Vaughn, *Nelson Textbook of Pediatrics*. Philadelphia: Saunders, 1983. P. 593.

[b] *Med. Lett. Drugs Ther.* 26:3, 1984.

[c] Oral regimen is safer and preferred for most patients. Parenteral regimens are recommended for those with prior endocarditis and those on continuous oral penicillin prophylaxis.

[d] Parenteral regimens are more likely to be effective.

[e] A PPD test should be performed after 3 months; if negative, prophylaxis may be discontinued if no further contact takes place.

[f] Circumstances include corticosteroid or immunosuppressive therapy (INH for the duration of therapy); measles vaccine administration (1 month); illness with measles, pertussis, or influenza (1 month); and surgery with general anesthesia (1 month).

[g] If serogroup A or C, immunization with meningococcal A or C vaccine may be helpful, since half the secondary cases occur more than 5 days after the index case. *M.M.W.R.* 30:113, 1981.

Table 15-10. Drug therapy in tuberculosis

Drugs	Daily dose per kilogram of body weight[a]	Route and mode of administration of daily dose	Major adverse reactions
Isoniazid	10–20 mg (max. 600 mg)	PO in 1–2 divided doses	Hepatotoxicity,[b] peripheral neuropathy[c] Rash, fever
Rifampin	10–20 mg (max. 600 mg)	PO in 1–2 divided doses	Hepatotoxicity,[b] GI disturbance, thrombocytopenia (rarely)
Streptomycin	20–40 mg (max. 1 gm)	IM in 1–2 divided doses	Eighth cranial nerve toxicity (primarily vestibular), rash, fever, nephrotoxicity
Para-aminosalicylic acid	200–300 mg (max. 12 gm)	PO in 2–4 divided doses	GI irritation (10%) Rash, fever
Ethambutol[d]	10–15 mg (max. 1500 mg)	PO in 1 dose	Optic neuritis (especially with higher doses—ophthalmologic monitoring recommended) Rash, fever

[a]The high dose is recommended for critically ill patients and the low dose for prophylaxis and long-term therapy after improvement.
[b]Hepatotoxicity is rare in children. Therapy should not be stopped because of mild abnormalities in liver function tests unless the patient has clinical symptoms.
[c]Pyridoxine is unnecessary in most children, but is important in adolescents, whose diets may be inadequate, or in malnourished children.
[d]Not recommended by manufacturer for children under 13.

(2) Pharmacology. The only clinically significant difference between preparations is in their routes of administration. Because **methicillin, oxacillin,** and **nafcillin** are not well absorbed after oral administration, they are used only parenterally. **Cloxacillin** and **dicloxacillin** are well absorbed orally.

c. Ampicillin and amoxicillin

(1) Spectrum and indications

(a) Ampicillin has the gram-positive spectrum of penicillin and is more active against enterococci and *Listeria*. Like penicillin, **it is inactive against penicillinase-producing staphylococci.** It is also active against many gram-negative organisms, including most *H. influenzae* strains, *Shigella, Salmonella, Proteus mirabilis,* and some *E. coli.*

(b) The spectrum of **amoxicillin** is similar to that of ampicillin, except that it is less effective against *Shigella* infections.

(2) Pharmacology. The major difference between ampicillin and amoxicillin is that the latter is better absorbed after oral administration, even when given with meals. Amoxicillin is therefore given in lower dosage and may produce fewer GI side effects and result in a lower incidence of maculopapular rash than ampicillin. Since amoxicillin may be given q8h rather than q6h as with ampicillin, compliance may be improved.

d. Carbenicillin and ticarcillin

(1) Spectrum and indications. These agents extend the spectrum of ampicillin to include *Pseudomonas aeruginosa* and some *Proteus* species. Some strains of *Enterobacter* and *Serratia* may also be sensitive. Carbenicillin may also be effective against *Bacteroides fragilis*. Ticarcillin is more potent than carbenicillin against *P. aeruginosa* and is therefore used in lower dosage. **Carbenicillin (and other penicillins and cephalosporins) should not be mixed with aminoglycosides for simultaneous administration because they react at high concentrations to form an inactive complex.**

(2) Pharmacology. Oral indanyl carbenicillin attains therapeutic levels only in urine and is indicated only for UTIs caused by gram-negative organisms resistant to ampicillin and other oral agents.

e. Ureidopenicillins. Three newer semisynthetic penicillins, namely, azlocillin, mezlocillin, and pipericillin, also extend the spectrum of the penicillins to include *P. aeruginosa.*

f. Side effects of the penicillins

(1) Immediate allergic reactions include anaphylaxis, angioneurotic edema, and urticaria. **A previous maculopapular rash due to ampicillin does not signify an increased risk of immediate reactions.** Because penicillins share the same chemical structure, patients allergic to one preparation may react to others and occasionally may react to the cephalosporins.

(a) Patients suspected of having a penicillin allergy may be skin tested with two types of materials: penicilloyl-polylysine (PPL, available commercially as Pre-Pen) and a "minor determinant" mixture (not commercially available, but aqueous penicillin G may be substituted). Patients with a positive reaction to PPL are likely to have an allergic reaction to therapeutic doses of penicillin. Patients with a positive reaction to minor determinants are likely to have an immediate reaction such as anaphylaxis.

(b) Intradermal skin testing with aqueous penicillin G may cause severe reactions in the highly allergic patient. Therefore, a scratch test with a dilute solution (5 units/ml in saline) should first be performed (together with a saline control). If no local reaction occurs within 20 min, a second scratch test is performed with a more concentrated solution (10,000 units/ml). If this is negative, a small skin bleb is raised by intradermal injection of the concentrated solution. A negative intradermal test suggests that an anaphylactic reaction to therapeutic penicillin G is unlikely **but does not absolutely exclude this possibility. Appropriate drugs and equipment for respiratory and circulatory assistance should be at the bedside during the skin-testing procedure and the first doses of penicillin.**

(2) **Aqueous procaine penicillin G** may produce a **nonallergic immediate reaction** simulating anaphylaxis, especially when mistakenly injected into the intravascular space.

(3) **Delayed reactions** include fever, eosinophilia, hemolytic anemia, serum sickness, and urticaria. Interstitial nephritis may occur with all penicillins but has been most often described with methicillin. Neutropenia and anicteric hepatitis occur rarely. The most common delayed reactions are maculopapular rashes, which occur during 8% of all treatment courses with ampicillin (50–100% in the presence of infectious mononucleosis); they are less common with other penicillins. When indications are clear, antibiotic therapy can be continued because the rash usually disappears. Very rarely, it may progress to erythroderma and exfoliative dermatitis.

(4) Dose-related effects include CNS toxicity, hypokalemia, and coagulation disorders. The last of these is most typical with carbenicillin, but may also occur with penicillin, especially in patients with renal failure. Diarrhea from oral preparations may also be dose related. The sodium or potassium contained in aqueous penicillin preparations can produce congestive heart failure or hyperkalemia.

2. **Cephalosporins.** Mechanism of action is similar to that of the penicillins.

a. **Cephalothin and its analogues**

(1) **Spectrum and indications. Cephalothin** and its analogues **cefazolin, cephalexin, cefadroxil, cephapirin, cephacetrile,** and **cephradine** have similar antimicrobial spectra. They are active against gram-positive cocci, including penicillinase-producing *S. aureus,* and against gram-negative rods, including many strains of *E. coli, Klebsiella,* and *Proteus mirabilis.* Generally, they have poor activity against enterococci, and despite disk sensitivity tests indicating activity against methicillin-resistant staphylococci, the cephalosporins are usually ineffective against these organisms. Cephalothin and cefazolin are more resistant to staphylococcal penicillinase than other cephalosporins (including the newer cephalosporins to be discussed) and are therefore the cephalosporins of choice for serious staphylococcal infections.

(2) **Pharmacology.** Cephalothin and its analogues differ in their pharmacologic properties, especially with respect to routes of administration. Cephalothin, cefazolin, cephapirin, and cephacetrile are available only for IM or IV administration. Cephalothin is painful when administered IM and should be given IV. Cephradine may be given parenterally or orally; cephalexin and cefadroxil are given PO only. The half-life in blood of most of these agents is very short (30–60 min), and parenteral therapy should therefore be given at 4-hr intervals except for cefazolin (q6-8h). **The cephalosporins (except cefuroxime and the third-generation agents) penetrate poorly into the CNS and should therefore not be used when meningitis may ensue as a complication of a bacteremic condition.**

b. **Second-generation cephalosporins**

(1) **Spectrum and indications.** Cefamandole, cefuroxime, and cefoxitin extend the spectrum of the older cephalosporins to many strains of resistant gram-negative bacteria. Cefamandole and cefuroxime are more active against *H. influenzae* type B (including ampicillin-resistant strains). Cefaclor is 2–8 times more active than cephalexin

against *H. influenzae* type B and is used for acute otitis media. However, some strains, including some β-lactamase–producing strains, are resistant to cefaclor. In general, aerobic gram-negative enteric organisms are more likely to be sensitive to gentamicin or tobramycin, anaerobes to clindamycin or chloramphenicol.

   (2) Pharmacology. Cefamandole, cefuroxime, and cefoxitin are given IV q4–8h. Since they are excreted unchanged into the urine, the dosage should be reduced in patients with renal insufficiency (see Table 15-7). Cefuroxime, but not the others in this group, has good penetration into CSF through inflamed meninges. Cefaclor is given PO q8h.

c. Third-generation cephalosporins

   (1) Spectrum and indications. Cefotaxime, moxalactam, and cefoperazone have broad-spectrum activity against gram-negative bacteria, many of which are resistant to the older cephalosporins and aminoglycosides. These agents are active against *H. influenzae* type B (including β-lactamase–producing strains) and against most anaerobes except *Clostridium difficile*. These drugs penetrate well into the CNS and are under evaluation for the treatment of neonatal gram-negative and childhood *H. influenzae* meningitis.

   (2) Pharmacology

   (a) Cefotaxime has a pharmacokinetic profile similar to that of cephalothin; the drug is primarily excreted into the urine, and the dosage is similar to that for cephalothin.

   (b) Moxalactam has a longer half-life (2–3 hr) and higher peak serum levels than cefotaxime and may be given q6–8h. Most of the drug is excreted unchanged in the urine.

   (c) Cefoperazone is unique among the cephalosporins in that it is primarily excreted in the bile; thus, a dosage adjustment may be necessary for biliary obstruction, but not for renal insufficiency.

d. Side effects of the cephalosporins. These include the following:

   (1) Allergic reactions, nephrotoxicity, thrombocytopenia, granulocytopenia, dose-related encephalopathy, and anicteric hepatitis. Moxalactam and cefoperazone may cause bleeding, due to an increase in prothrombin time, reversible with vitamin K; moxalactam may induce platelet dysfunction.

   (2) Local irritation after IM injections and phlebitis from IV administration are common, particularly with cephalothin. Severe irritation may occur when cephalothin is added to wound irrigation fluids.

3. Aminoglycosides inhibit protein synthesis at the ribosome.

a. Spectrum and indications. The aminoglycosides are bactericidal against a broad range of enteric gram-negative bacilli and *S. aureus,* but the various analogues differ in their antimicrobial spectra.

   (1) They are not effective against streptococci and pneumococci, anaerobes, and spirochetes.

   (2) Many gram-negative bacilli, especially in hospitals, have become resistant to **streptomycin** and **kanamycin.** In addition, neither agent is active against *P. aeruginosa.* **Streptomycin** is now used mainly as an antituberculosis agent. **Kanamycin** may be used for gram-negative infections after sensitivity has been established.

   (3) Gentamicin is active against most gram-negative rods, including *P. aeruginosa,* and is the aminoglycoside of choice for the empirical treatment of gram-negative infections, in which resistant gram-negative bacilli are common.

   (4) Tobramycin is more active than gentamicin against *P. aeruginosa* (including isolates resistant to gentamicin).

   (5) Amikacin is active against many enteric gram-negative bacilli that are resistant to gentamicin. Unless such organisms are common, this agent should be reserved for infections proved resistant to the other aminoglycosides.

   b. Pharmacology
      (1) The aminoglycosides are poorly absorbed from the GI tract. However, they may reach toxic levels after oral administration in patients with a damaged gut or with renal failure.
      (2) Because the aminoglycosides have a narrow toxic-therapeutic ratio, dosage must be carefully adjusted to obtain safe, effective serum levels (see Table 15-4).
      (3) Aminoglycosides are excreted almost entirely by the kidneys. The dosage must be adjusted when there is even a minor degree of renal impairment (see Table 15-6).
   c. Side effects
      (1) Nephrotoxicity due to renal tubular damage is enhanced by the concurrent use of cephalosporins and diuretics (especially when sodium depletion occurs) and by preexisting renal disease. It is usually reversible. **The serum creatinine should be monitored in all patients on aminoglycoside therapy.**
      (2) Ototoxicity (both vestibular and auditory) is enhanced by preexisting ear disease (e.g., otitis media), concurrent administration of diuretics, and preexisting renal disease. **It may be irreversible** unless recognized early. Patients should be examined daily for symptoms of "fullness" in the ears, tinnitus, or vertigo. Ability to hear a watch tick provides a simple but sensitive bedside screening test for the high-tone hearing loss characteristic of aminoglycoside toxicity. Head shaking elicits symptoms of vertigo in patients confined to bed.
      (3) Neuromuscular blockade with respiratory paralysis has been described, usually after peritoneal irrigation with high concentrations of aminoglycoside.
4. Erythromycin inhibits bacterial protein synthesis by binding to ribosomes.
   a. Spectrum and indications. Erythromycin is bacteriostatic at low concentrations against *Mycoplasma pneumoniae,* spirochetes, and most gram-positive organisms. It is commonly used as an alternative drug in penicillin-allergic patients with group A streptococcal and pneumococcal infections. Some staphylococci may be resistant de novo, or resistance may emerge during therapy. It is moderately active against *H. influenzae* and may be used with a sulfonamide in treating otitis media. **Erythromycin** is the drug of choice for *Legionella and M. pneumoniae* infections, pertussis, the diphtheria carrier state, and conjunctivitis and pneumonia due to *Chlamydia.*
   b. Pharmacology. Erythromycin base is acid labile and poorly absorbed. Erythromycin estolate is well absorbed, even in the presence of food, but must be hydrolyzed to the active base by the liver. A variety of parenteral preparations are also available. Active erythromycin is excreted in low concentrations in urine and in higher concentrations in bile.
   c. Side effects include nausea, vomiting, and diarrhea. Erythromycin estolate occasionally causes a cholestatic jaundice, probably on a hypersensitivity basis.
5. Clindamycin inhibits bacterial protein synthesis.
   a. Spectrum and indications
      (1) Clindamycin has a spectrum similar to that of erythromycin, except that it is inactive against *M. pneumoniae, Neisseria gonorrhoeae, Neisseria meningitidis,* and *H. influenzae.* It is quite active against nonenterococcal gram-positive organisms and most anaerobes.
      (2) Clindamycin is the drug of choice for serious anaerobic infections due to *B. fragilis.* It is an alternative to penicillin for infections due to group A streptococci and pneumococci and to penicillinase-resistant penicillins for staphylococcal infections. However, resistance to clindamycin may emerge during therapy, and staphylococcal endocarditis may relapse after clindamycin treatment.

    b. Pharmacology. Absorption is not decreased by the presence of food. Metabolism is by the liver.

    c. Side effects

        (1) GI side effects (nausea, vomiting, abdominal cramps, diarrhea) are common. **Pseudomembranous colitis** may develop and become severe if treatment is continued. Assays for the enterotoxin of *C. difficile* in the stool may confirm the diagnosis; oral vancomycin is the treatment of choice.

        (2) Uncommon side effects include rash, anaphylaxis, and hepatitis. **Rapid IV infusion may produce syncope or cardiopulmonary arrest.**

6. Chloramphenicol inhibits bacterial protein synthesis at the ribosomal level.

    a. Spectrum and indications

        (1) Chloramphenicol is active against most gram-positive organisms, most gram-negative bacilli (except *P. aeruginosa*), anaerobes, (including *B. fragilis*), and *Rickettsia*. At low concentrations it is bacteriostatic for most organisms and bactericidal for highly sensitive organisms such as *H. influenzae*; at high concentrations it is bactericidal for sensitive organisms.

        (2) It is the drug of choice for serious infections caused by *H. influenzae,* systemic *Salmonella* infections (including typhoid fever), and serious rickettsial infections (including Rocky Mountain spotted fever).

    b. Pharmacology. Chloramphenicol is well absorbed from the GI tract and diffuses well into tissues and the CSF. Most of the drug is conjugated in the liver and excreted in the urine.

    c. Side effects

        (1) Aplastic anemia is a rare (1 in 50,000 courses of treatment) but serious side effect unrelated to either dose or plasma concentration. There are inadequate data to suggest that the oral preparation is more likely to cause this side effect than is parenteral administration.

        (2) Dose-related bone marrow suppression is common and reversible, occurring regularly when plasma-free chloramphenicol levels exceed 25 μg/ml. Manifestations include increased serum iron, decreasing reticulocyte counts, and a falling hematocrit. Thrombocytopenia and leukopenia also occur. The bone marrow shows the characteristic vacuolation of erythroblasts. Free erythrocyte protoporphyrin may be elevated.

        (3) In neonates in whom high serum levels of chloramphenicol (> 50 μg/ml) develop, a shocklike syndrome ("gray syndrome") may occur. Dosage should be reduced and serum levels monitored (see Table 15-4).

        (4) Chloramphenicol may delay the metabolism of tolbutamide, dicumarol, and phenytoin and may enhance the metabolism of phenobarbital.

        (5) Rare side effects include optic neuritis, peripheral neuritis with prolonged therapy, and allergic reactions.

7. The tetracyclines inhibit bacterial protein synthesis and are not used commonly in childhood because of their side effects.

    a. Spectrum and indications

        (1) The tetracyclines have broad-spectrum bacteriostatic activity against gram-positive organisms, enteric gram-negative bacilli, anaerobes, mycoplasmas, spirochetes, and rickettsiae. However, an increasing number of strains have become resistant. *Serratia, Proteus,* and *P. aeruginosa* are almost always resistant.

        (2) Tetracyclines are the drugs of choice for brucellosis, cholera, Q fever, relapsing fever, Rocky Mountain spotted fever (in children older than 8 years), psittacosis, lymphogranuloma venereum, and nonspecific urethritis. They are second-line drugs for *Mycoplasma* pneumonia, tularemia, gonorrhea, syphilis, meliodosis, granuloma inguinale, and eradication of the meningococcal carrier state (minocycline).

   b. Pharmacology. The absorption of tetracycline is impaired by concurrent food intake and the presence of divalent cations (calcium, iron). The serum half-life is relatively short (6 hr). Doxycycline and minocycline are absorbed more completely than tetracycline, and the half-life is long (14–20 hr). Most tetracyclines are excreted mainly by the kidney, but also reach high concentrations in bile. **Doxycycline,** which is eliminated mainly by nonrenal mechanisms, **is the only tetracycline that can be safely used in renal failure.**
   c. Side effects
   (1) Tetracyclines may produce **permanent yellow discoloration of the deciduous teeth** (when given during the second and third trimester of pregnancy and the first 3 months of life) and of permanent teeth (when given to children 3 months–6 years of age). Tetracyclines should therefore be avoided during these periods. Other side effects include upper and lower **GI symptoms,** candidal superinfection, and dose-related **hepatitis.**
   (2) Preexisting renal dysfunction is exacerbated by all the tetracyclines except doxycycline.
   (3) Rare side effects include allergy, photosensitivity (dimethyl chlortetracycline), benign intracranial hypertension, and reversible vestibular disturbance (minocycline).
8. Vancomycin inhibits bacterial cell wall synthesis.
   a. Spectrum and indications. Vancomycin is bactericidal for most gram-positive organisms but only bacteriostatic for enterococci. It is active against staphylococci, β-hemolytic streptococci, viridans streptococci, pneumococci, *Corynebacterium,* and *Clostridium.*
   (1) Vancomycin is useful in the treatment of serious infection caused by methicillin-resistant staphylococci.
   (2) Vancomycin and gentamicin combined are the treatment of choice for enterococcal endocarditis in patients who have an allergy to penicillin.
   (3) Oral vancomycin is effective treatment for staphylococcal enterocolitis and antibiotic-induced colitis associated with enterotoxin-producing *Clostridium.*
   b. Pharmacology. Vancomycin is not absorbed after oral administration. After parenteral administration it enters tissues well, but diffuses poorly across uninflamed meninges. It is excreted primarily by the kidneys, and dosage must be adjusted in renal failure and serum levels must be followed (see Table 15-4). **It is not eliminated by hemodialysis** (see Table 15-6).
   c. Side effects include:
   (1) Fever, phlebitis, and maculopapular and urticarial rashes. Anaphylaxis is rare.
   (2) Ototoxicity and **nephrotoxicity** may occur with high serum levels and may be enhanced when aminoglycosides are used concurrently. Renal and auditory function should be monitored with aminoglycosides (see p. 376).
9. The sulfonamides block the synthesis of dihydrofolic acid from para-aminobenzoic acid in bacterial cells.
   a. Spectrum and indications
   (1) Sulfonamides have a broad bacteriostatic spectrum, including most gram-positive cocci (but not enterococci), gram-positive bacilli, most gram-negative organisms including *H. influenzae, Chlamydia, Actinomyces, Nocardia,* and protozoa (malaria, *Toxoplasma* and *Pneumocystis*). Unfortunately, sulfonamide resistance has become common with most of the bacterial groups mentioned.
   (2) The **major indications** for sulfonamides include uncomplicated urinary tract infection, *Nocardia* infections, and, together with other drugs, toxoplasmosis and *P. carinii* pneumonia.

(3) Erythromycin with a sulfonamide remains an effective regimen for otitis media.

(4) Sulfonamides provide effective rheumatic fever prophylaxis, but cannot be relied on for the treatment of group A streptococcal infections.

   b. Pharmacology (e.g., sulfisoxazole). Most sulfonamides are well absorbed orally. They are metabolized by the liver, and both active drug and metabolites are excreted primarily by the kidney. Products of tissue necrosis inhibit the action of sulfonamides. Therefore, these agents should not be used for severe suppurative infections.

   c. Side effects

      (1) Allergic reactions include fever, rash (usually maculopapular, occasionally urticarial, rarely exfoliative or the rash of Stevens-Johnson syndrome), systemic vasculitis, myocarditis, and pulmonary eosinophilia.

      (2) Rare **hematologic effects** include reversible agranulocytosis and fatal aplastic anemia. Acute hemolytic anemia may occur in patients with glucose 6-phosphate dehydrogenase deficiency.

      (3) Sulfonamides compete with bilirubin for albumin-binding sites, thereby increasing the risk of **kernicterus** in neonates. **They are contraindicated in pregnancy near term and during the first 2 months of life.**

10. Trimethoprim-sulfamethoxazole. Both drugs inhibit folic acid synthesis.

   a. Spectrum and indications

      (1) The antimicrobial spectrum includes most gram-positive cocci, enteric gram-negative bacilli, *H. influenzae,* and *P. carinii.*

      (2) The **major indications** include treatment and prophylaxis of urinary tract infections, prostatitis, and *P. carinii* pneumonia. It is an alternate drug in the treatment of acute otitis media and may also be useful in the treatment of shigellosis, resistant *Salmonella* infections, and infections caused by gram-negative bacilli resistant to other antimicrobials.

   b. Pharmacology. The dosage should be decreased in patients with severe renal dysfunction (see Table 15-7). IV usage for *P. carinii* is discussed in Chap. 16.

   c. Side effects. (See also **9**).

      (1) High oral doses may produce GI irritation. Rash, nausea, vomiting, and thrombocytopenia are the most common side effects. Hematologic suppression due to weak inhibition of folic acid metabolism may be reversible with folinic acid. **The drug should be used with caution in patients with preexisting hematologic disease and in patients receiving immunosuppressive therapy.**

      (2) Mild, reversible renal impairment may occur.

11. Nitrofurantoin may inhibit bacterial carbohydrate metabolism.

   a. Spectrum and indications

      (1) Nitrofurantoin is active against most gram-positive cocci (including enterococci) and gram-negative bacilli that cause urinary tract infections. Sensitive organisms usually do not become resistant during therapy.

      (2) The **only indications** for nitrofurantoin are the treatment and prophylaxis of urinary tract infections.

   b. Pharmacology. The drug reaches therapeutically effective levels only in the urine, which is its major route of excretion.

   c. Side effects

      (1) GI side effects (nausea, vomiting, abdominal cramps) occur frequently and are dose-related. They are less common with the macrocrystalline form, which is more slowly absorbed but equally effective. Serious systemic toxicity may occur in renal failure.

      (2) Other adverse reactions include allergy (rashes, fever, eosinophilia, hepatitis, asthma, and acute pneumonitis), dose-related peripheral neuritis, pulmonary fibrosis, and hemolytic anemia in patients with glucose 6-phosphate dehydrogenase deficiency.

12. Metronidazole is reduced by enzymes in anaerobic bacteria. These reduction products disrupt DNA and inhibit nucleic acid synthesis.

a. Spectrum and indications

(1) Most aerobic organisms are resistant, but metronidazole is bactericidal for most gram-negative anaerobic organisms, including *B. fragilis* and *Clostridium.*

(2) Metronidazole is probably the drug of choice only for endocarditis due to *B. fragilis* (because of its bactericidal activity) and for *B. fragilis* infections resistant to other drugs. Metronidazole is also useful in the treatment of trichomoniasis and amebiasis (see Chap. 16, p. 430) and is an alternative drug when therapy is indicated for giardiasis, although it is not yet approved by the FDA for this purpose.

b. Pharmacology

(1) Metronidazole is well absorbed from the GI tract and enters into all tissues, including the CSF. Serum concentrations after oral dosage are similar to those achieved with equal IV doses.

(2) The drug is largely metabolized in the liver and excreted by the kidney. No alteration in dosage is necessary for renal insufficiency; however, the dosage in patients with hepatic disease should be decreased and serum levels monitored.

c. Side effects

(1) Nausea, dry mouth, and metallic taste are most frequent.

(2) Uncommon neurologic reactions include reversible peripheral neuropathy, vertigo, ataxia, and convulsions. Reversible neutropenia and rash have also been reported.

(3) Metronidazole should be considered **potentially carcinogenic** and **potentially teratogenic.** It is contraindicated in pregnancy.

B. Antifungal agents

1. Amphotericin B and nystatin. Both bind to a sterol constituent in the fungal cell membrane, thereby increasing its permeability.

a. Spectrum and indications

(1) Both drugs are active against *Candida* species, *Cryptococcus neoformans, Sporotrichum schenckii, Blastomyces dermatitidis, Histoplasma capsulatum, Coccidioides immitis, Aspergillus* species, and *Phycomycetes.*

(2) These drugs are the antimicrobials of choice for fungal infections on the skin and mucosal surfaces (nystatin) (see Chap. 22, p. 534) or disseminated to other organs (amphotericin B). Severe mucosal infections may require systemic amphotericin B.

b. Pharmacology. Both drugs are poorly absorbed after oral administration.

(1) Nystatin is available only for topical use on the skin, mucosal surfaces, and in the GI tract. **Amphotericin** is given by slow (2- 6-hr) IV infusion in 5% dextrose. Premedication with an antihistamine, antipyretic, and meperidine and the addition of 10–50 mg of hydrocortisone to each 500 ml of 5% D/W of the infusate may minimize systemic reactions. Dosage should be increased gradually, beginning with a dose of 1 mg on the first day. Nonetheless, in serious sytemic fungal infections, it is important to increase dosage quickly to full therapeutic levels.

(2) Amphotericin B has a half-life of approximately 20 hr and may therefore be given in increased dosage every other day when prolonged treatment is necessary, especially on an outpatient basis.

c. Side effects

(1) Immediate side effects during infusion of amphotericin B are very common and include fever, chills, headache, nausea, vomiting, and rarely, hypotension. Reversible **nephrotoxicity** and **normochromic normocytic anemia** also occur.

(2) Rare adverse reactions include allergic reactions, peripheral neuropathy (with intrathecal administration), and cardiotoxicity with rapid infusion.

2. **5-Fluorocytosine (5-FC)** may be converted to the antimetabolite 5-fluorouracil within the fungal cell and thereby interfere with nucleic acid synthesis.

a. **Spectrum and indications**

(1) 5-FC is active against *C. neoformans,* most species of *C. albicans,* and *Torulopsis glabrata.* All these organisms may become resistant during therapy, particularly when 5-FC is used alone in low dosage. Sensitivity must be confirmed before this agent is used alone for *Candida* infections.

(2) The **major indication** for 5-FC is its use together with amphotericin B for cryptococcal meningitis. This combination may also be useful for severe disseminated infections with sensitive *Candida* species and possibly *Aspergillus.*

b. **Pharmacology.** 5-FC is well absorbed orally, is not metabolized significantly, and is excreted almost entirely by glomerular filtration. In patients with renal dysfunction, the dosage should be adjusted and serum levels monitored (see Tables 15-4 and 15-6).

c. **Side effects include** bone marrow suppression and, rarely, hepatitis, GI side effects, and skin rashes.

3. **Clotrimazole** interferes with synthesis of the fungal cell wall. It is active against dermatophytes, most species of *Candida, C. neoformans,* and most filamentous fungi.

Only topical forms of clotrimazole are currently available as an effective alternative for cutaneous dermatophyte and candidal infections and for vaginal candidiasis.

4. **Ketoconazole** impairs the synthesis of ergosterol, thus affecting fungal cell-membrane permeability.

a. **Spectrum and indications**

(1) Ketoconazole is active against *Candida* species, *Coccidioides immitis, Histoplasma capsulatum, Blastomyces dermatitidis, Paracoccidioides brasiliensis,* and the dermatophytes.

(2) The drug is approved for the **oral** treatment of certain systemic fungal infections, including candidiasis, candiduria, chronic mucocutaneous candidiasis, oral thrush, histoplasmosis, coccidiodomycosis, chromomycosis, and paracoccidioidomycosis. Since it penetrates poorly into the CSF, it should not be used for fungal meningitis. Few controlled studies of the efficacy of ketoconazole have been done in infants and children, and there are limited toxicity data for children under 2 years of age.

b. **Pharmacology.** Ketoconazole has the advantage of oral administration. It is metabolized by the liver and excreted in bile.

c. **Side effects.** The frequently reported adverse effects have been nausea and vomiting, and these symptoms may be minimized by taking the drug with meals. Liver dysfunction is a possible serious adverse effect.

IV. **Treatment of infectious diseases**

A. **Skin infections**

1. **Impetigo.** See Chap. 22, p. 537.

2. **Scaled skin syndrome, bullous impetigo,** and **staphylococcal scarlet fever** represent a spectrum of dermatologic manifestations of staphylococcal infection resulting from release of soluble toxins by *S. aureus.*

a. **Etiology.** The infecting organism is *S. aureus* (usually bacteriophage group II).

b. **Evaluation**

(1) Cultures of the skin, nose, throat, and blood should be made (exceptions include children with only localized bullous impetigo and older children who are afebrile and nontoxic.

(2) Gram stain of the denuded skin or bullous fluid, or both, will differentiate direct staphylococcal skin invasion from the more common toxin-mediated skin changes. The fluid aspirated from intact bullae will be sterile in scalded skin syndrome but may contain *S. aureus* in bullous impetigo.

c. The **diagnosis** is established by the clinical picture in association with recovery of *S. aureus* from the patient. Nikolsky's sign (gentle rubbing of the skin results in sloughing of the epidermis) is usually indicative of the scalded skin syndrome; its absence does not exclude the diagnosis.

d. Therapy

(1) A 7 to 10-day course of a penicillinase-resistant penicillin usually is sufficient. Except in mild bullous impetigo, the antibiotic is usually given parenterally (e.g., oxacillin, 100–200 mg/kg/day q4h IV).

(2) After a good clinical response has been achieved, therapy may be completed with oral dicloxacillin, 25 mg/kg/day qid.

(3) Contact precautions are indicated until the lesions have resolved.

(4) Corticosteroids have not been demonstrated to be beneficial.

(5) In patients with extensive skin losses, hydration and maintenance of normal body temperature are important. Avoid unnecessary skin trauma (e.g., adhesive from tape).

3. Cellulitis (including erysipelas)

a. Etiology. *S. aureus,* group A streptococci, and, in children under age 5, *H. influenzae* type B

b. Evaluation

(1) Needle aspiration of the advancing border of an active lesion should be carried out for Gram stain and culture.

(2) A blood culture and antigen detection studies (e.g., counterimmunoelectrophoresis or latex agglutination) should be done in patients with severe cellulitis, fever, generalized toxicity, or impaired host defenses.

(3) Sinus x-rays should be done in patients with periorbital cellulitis.

c. The **diagnosis** is usually established by the characteristic warm, erythematous, tender, and indurated skin.

(1) Streptococcal cellulitis (erysipelas) is suggested by advancing, well-demarcated, heaped-up borders; facial involvement may assume a butterfly distribution.

(2) *H. influenzae* type B is suggested by a fever higher than 38.9°C (102° F) and the characteristic purple discoloration of the skin. Most patients with *H. influenzae* type B cellulitis are bacteremic, and the disease often presents as unilateral cheek cellulitis, sometimes associated with ipsilateral otitis media.

d. Therapy

(1) Application of local heat, e.g., warm compresses, 10–20 min qid or more

(2) If feasible, immobilization and elevation of the affected extremity

(3) Incision and drainage of any primary suppurative focus

(4) Antibiotics

(a) Localized cellulitis without fever may be treated with oral antibiotics. However, if evidence of systemic toxicity is present, parenteral antibiotics should be given until sustained clinical improvement has occurred.

(b) Initial therapy for the child over 5 years of age with extremity cellulitis includes a penicillinase-resistant penicillin if *H. influenzae* type B is not suspected, or an agent like cefuroxime, which provides broad coverage for the possible infecting organisms.

(c) For the younger child with cheek cellulitis, chloramphenicol should be used in the initial treatment regimen.

(d) For therapy in immunocompromised patients, an antibiotic effective against gram-negative enteric organisms and *Pseudomonas* should be included.

(e) Streptococcal disease or erysipelas usually responds to benzathine penicillin G, 0.6–1.2 MU IM in 1 dose, or oral penicillin V, 125–250 mg qid. More severely ill patients may initially require procaine penicillin G, 600,000–900,000 units IM q12h, or even IV penicillin, 100,000 units/kg/day q4h. Treatment should be continued for 7–10 days.

(f) Staphylococcal cellulitis is usually treated with a penicillinase-resistant penicillin, depending on the organisms' in vitro sensitivity; e.g., nafcillin or oxacillin (100–200 mg/kg/day IV q4h) for severe infections or dicloxacillin (25–50 mg/kg/day qid PO) for milder infections.

(g) *H. influenzae* cellulitis, in view of the high incidence of positive blood cultures in this disease, is treated initially with ampicillin, 200 mg/kg/day q4h, and with chloramphenicol, 100 mg/kg/day q6h, pending ampicillin sensitivity testing.

(h) Orbital cellulitis. Hospitalization and high doses of antibiotics given IV are indicated (see Chap. 23, p. 551). The initial choice should include a penicillinase-resistant penicillin and, in children, an antimicrobial effective against *H. influenzae*.

B. Bites

1. Animal bites

a. Etiology. Potential pathogens include *S. aureus,* anaerobic and microaerophilic streptococci, other anaerobic cocci, *Clostridium* species (including *C. tetani*), *Pasteurella multocida, Streptobacillus moniliformis,* and *Spirillum minus* (the latter two cause the two types of rat-bite fever).

b. Evaluation includes an assessment of the patient's immunity to tetanus as well as the extent of the wound.

c. The **diagnosis** of a bacterial complication of an animal bite is suggested by the finding of cellulitis.

d. Therapy. Besides cleansing, local antisepsis and surgical care of the bite, including irrigation and debridement if necessary, prophylactic measures for rabies and/or tetanus should be considered.

2. Human bites, especially those occurring on the palmar surface of the hand, may result in extensive, rapidly developing infection.

a. Etiology. Infections are usually mixed and are caused by a variety of organisms, including staphylococci, gram-negative anaerobes and spirochetes from the mouth, and aerobic streptococci.

b. Evaluation. The principles of management are similar to those for management of animal bites, but irrigation, debridement, and provision for drainage assume much greater importance. Because of the potential for anaerobic infection, these wounds are usually not sutured.

c. Therapy with a penicillinase-resistant penicillin or a cephalosporin, begun prophylactically at the time of the bite, will cover the usual etiologic organisms.

3. Rabies prophylaxis. The recommendations are based on those of the Public Health Service Advisory Committee (*M.M.W.R.* 29:265, 1980).

a. Evaluation. Consider the following before administering antirabies treatment:

(1) Species of biting animal

(a) Carnivorous wild animals (especially skunks, racoons, foxes, coyotes, and bobcats) and bats are more likely to be infective than other animals. Postexposure prophylaxis should be initiated after the bite of one of these animals unless the animal is tested and shown not to be rabid.

(b) Domestic dog or cat bites sometimes require prophylaxis, depending on local epidemiology, but bites of rodents and lagomorphs rarely do. The state or local health department should be consulted in questionable cases.

(2) **Vaccination status of the biting animal.** An adult animal immunized properly with 1 or more doses of rabies vaccine has only a minimal chance of having rabies and transmitting the virus.

(3) **Circumstances of the biting incident.** An unprovoked attack is more likely to indicate that the animal is rabid than is a provoked attack. Bites sustained during attempts to feed or handle an apparently healthy animal should generally be regarded as provoked.

(4) **Type of exposure.** The likelihood that rabies infection will result from a bite varies with its extent and location. A nonbite exposure (scratches, abrasions, open wounds, or mucous membrane contamination with saliva or other potentially infectious material from a rabid animal) may also result in rabies virus transmission. Casual contact, such as petting a rabid animal without sustaining a bite, may not be an indication for prophylaxis.

b. **Postexposure prophylaxis**

(1) **Local wound treatment** includes thorough cleansing with soap and water along with measures to prevent bacterial infection (see Chap. 22, p. 537) and tetanus (see **4**).

(2) **Immunization.** If prophylaxis is indicated, both rabies immune globulin (RIG), 1 dose of 20 IU/kg (up to half a dose infiltrated in the wound and the rest given IM), and human diploid cell rabies vaccine (HDCV) should be given. Five doses of HDCV, 1 ml IM, are given on days 0, 3, 7, 14, and 28. Routine serologic testing of persons who have received this series of HDCV is unnecessary.

4. **Tetanus immunization**

a. **Tetanus toxoid,** 0.5 ml IM (DT in children < 6 years old; Td in those > 6 years old) is indicated in the following:

(1) Clean, minor wounds if the fully immunized child (3 or more previous doses) has not received a booster dose in the last 10 years, or if the child is incompletely immunized (< 3 previous doses of toxoid)

(2) Contaminated wounds (tetanus-prone wounds) if the fully immunized child has not received a booster dose in the last 5 years, or if the child is incompletely immunized

(3) All wounds neglected for more than 24 hr

b. Human tetanus immunoglobulin (TIG), 250–500 units IM in a separate injection site, should also be given in the following situations:

(1) Contaminated wounds if the child is incompletely immunized

(2) All wounds neglected more than 24 hr

c. If tetanus immunization is incomplete at the time prophylaxis for a wound is given, the recommended series should be completed.

C. **Otitis media.** Eustachian tube dysfunction causes inadequate ventilation of the middle ear, resulting in a negative middle ear pressure. Persistent negative pressure produces a sterile transudate within the middle ear. Concurrent or subsequent contamination of the middle ear with infected nasopharyngeal contents occurs by aspiration and insufflation during crying and nose blowing.

1. **Acute otitis media**

a. **Etiology**

(1) *Streptococcus pneumoniae, H. influenzae,* group A streptococcus, and *Branhamella catarrhalis; S. aureus* and enteric gram-negative bacilli (in neonates) are less frequent causes.

(2) Viruses and *Mycoplasma pneumoniae* have been isolated from middle ear fluid infrequently; their significance is uncertain.

(3) *H. influenzae* type B is usually isolated from children less than 5 years of age and is frequently associated with invasive disease. Nontypable *H. influenzae* (nonencapsulated) comprise the majority of middle ear isolates, are not associated with invasive infection, and are responsi-

ble for a small but significant proportion of infections in older children and adults.

b. Evaluation

(1) Pneumotoscopy

(2) Tympanometry

(3) Tympanocentesis. Middle ear aspiration should be performed on children who are seriously ill, have a poor response to antibiotics, or have a complication of acute otitis media. It should also be done in newborns.

Diagnostic tympanocentesis should be performed under semisterile conditions with the aid of an operating microscope or otoscope with operating head; an 18-gauge spinal needle is inserted through the anterior inferior segment of the tympanic membrane.

c. Diagnosis. A bulging, opacified, discolored eardrum through which the landmarks are poorly visualized, together with decreased mobility of the drum, defines acute otitis media. Perforation and a pulsatile discharge may be seen in the anterior inferior segment of the membrane.

d. Treatment

(1) Antibiotics PO are prescribed for all symptomatic patients.

    (a) Amoxicillin, 40 mg/kg/day q8h for 10 days, *or*

    (b) Erythromycin, 30–50 mg/kg/day, plus sulfisoxazole, 100–200 mg/kg/day q6h for 10 days *or*

    (c) Trimethoprim, 8–10 mg/kg/day, and sulfamethoxazole in combination (TMP, 40 mg/5 ml, and SMX, 200 mg/5 ml) q12h for 10 days *or*

    (d) Cefaclor, 40 mg/kg/day q8h PO for 10 days

(2) Analgesics (acetaminophen, codeine) may be indicated.

(3) Antihistamines and **decongestants** are not indicated in otitis media except to relieve coryza symptoms.

(4) The patient should be reevaluated within 30 days after starting therapy to determine whether effusion persists. If complete resolution has occurred, the patient is discharged. Periodic monitoring is required for patients with repeated episodes of otitis media. If effusion persists after 4 weeks, treatment is the same as that for chronic otitis media.

(5) Repeated episodes of otitis media with clearing of middle ear effusion between attacks may be managed by the use of prophylactic antibiotics, including trimethoprim-sulfamethoxazole (4 mg and 20 mg, respectively/kg/day) or sulfisoxazole (50 mg/kg/day) in a single daily dose.

2. Subacute and chronic otitis media

a. Etiology. Persistent negative intratympanic pressure results in a sterile transudate within the middle ear. Persistence of fluid within the middle ear space for 4–8 weeks after acute otitis media defines subacute otitis media, and thereafter the condition is referrred to as chronic otitis media. A low-grade inflammatory reaction may lead to an exudative "glue" secretion. Bacteria are present in up to 50 percent of "glue" effusions; their exact role is unclear.

b. Evaluation

(1) Pneumotoscopy is essential.

    (a) The tympanic membrane is classically thickened with a gray or amber fluid in the middle ear. Sometimes, a fluid meniscus, air bubbles, or bluish fluid may appear in the middle ear.

    (b) The mobility of the tympanic membrane is always impaired.

    (c) Protracted eustachian tube dysfunction may lead to the development of a cholesteatoma if it is not reversed by restoring normal middle ear ventilation.

(2) Tympanometry can be performed when the findings are equivocal.

      (3) Audiometry may be performed on children over 3 years of age.

      (4) Anatomic defects may be present.

  c. Diagnosis. An immobile tympanic membrane with diminished mobility and fluid can be seen on pneumotoscopy.

  d. Treatment

      (1) Attempts can be made to improve ventilation of the middle ear by the Valsalva maneuver, blowing up a balloon, etc.

      (2) The efficacy of decongestants, antihistamines, and adenoidectomy has not been proved.

      (3) An effusion present for longer than 12 weeks may be removed by myringotomy with insertion of ventilation tubes, especially if it is associated with a hearing deficit.

3. Chronic suppurative otitis media with perforation or cholesteatoma is a sequela of acute suppurative infection and should be referred to an otolaryngologist for evaluation and management.

D. Oropharyngeal infections

  1. Streptococcal pharyngitis (tonsillitis)

    a. Etiology. Group A β-hemolytic streptococci

    b. Evaluation must include a properly obtained throat culture (vigorous swabbing of both tonsillar areas and the posterior pharynx, which, if done properly, usually induces a gag reflex).

      (1) The disease should be suspected in any patient with a sore throat and fever. In infants, streptococcal infection is more likely to present as persistent nasopharyngeal discharge, with fever and excoriation of the nares.

      (2) Any history in the patient or family of recent streptococcal pharyngitis, scarlet fever, rheumatic fever, or penicillin allergy should be noted.

    c. The **diagnosis** is supported by a positive throat culture and confirmed by a rising antistreptolysin O titer (500 Todd units as an absolute value on a single specimen, or a two-tube rise in serial specimens analyzed simultaneously). Other causes of exudative pharyngitis include viruses, gonococci, and groups C and G streptococci. *Corynebacterium diphtheriae* may produce a gray-to-black fibrinous exudate (membrane) in the posterior pharynx. Oral anaerobes sometimes cause painful, deep, punched-out ulcerations on an erythematous base that is covered by a poorly adherent pseudomembrane.

    d. Therapy

      (1) Penicillin. Prevention of rheumatic fever requires either benzathine penicillin G given IM, or a 10-day course of oral penicillin. The parenteral route ensures treatment for a sufficient length of time, while oral therapy is dependent on the cooperation of the patient. Treatment schedules are as follows:

        (a) Intramuscular penicillin (benzathine). Children should be given a single injection of 600,000–1,200,000 units. The larger dose is preferable for children over 60 lbs.

        (b) Oral penicillin. Children and adults are given 125 or 250 mg* tid–qid for a full 10 days. Therapy must be **continued for the entire 10 days,** even though the temperature returns to normal and the patient is asymptomatic.

      (2) For patients with documented penicillin allergy, oral erythromycin, 40 mg/kg/day in 4 divided doses, or clindamycin, 10–20 mg/kg/day in 4 divided doses for 10 days, is recommended. Sulfonamides, while

---

*Of the various oral forms available, buffered penicillin G is satisfactory and least expensive. Although higher blood levels may be achieved with α-phenoxymethyl penicillin (penicillin V) or α-phenoxyethyl penicillin (phenethicillin), especially when taken near mealtime, their superiority in the prevention of rheumatic fever has not been documented.

effective in the prophylaxis of streptococcal infection, are ineffective in their treatment.

(3) Bed rest is not necessary. Children can return to school as soon as the symptoms subside.

(4) Throat cultures are indicated for symptomatic family members but are not necessary for others unless recurrent streptococcal pharyngitis occurs in the family. Such recurrences may necessitate antibiotic treatment of the entire family.

2. Vincent's angina

a. Etiology. Mixed oral anaerobic bacteria are the causative organisms.

b. Evaluation. Culture of the ulcerated lesion is necessary to rule out diphtheria and group A streptococcus.

c. Diagnosis. Painful, deep, punched-out ulcerations on a red edematous base are present, covered by a poorly adherent gray pseudomembrane. Involvement may include the tonsillar fossa, soft palate, and pharynx; inflammatory neck nodes are present. Culture and microscopic examination may confirm the diagnosis.

d. Treatment

(1) Antibiotics. Penicillin V, 50 mg/kg/24 hr in 4 divided doses, is given for 10 days.

(2) Local hygiene. 3% Hydrogen peroxide mouthwash and gargles q2h, with normal saline gargles at alternate hours. Cēpacol or Chloraseptic mouthwashes may be soothing.

(3) Analgesics are given as necessary: acetaminophen and/or codeine, viscous lidocaine, or diclonine HCl mouthwashes and gargles q2–3h.

3. Abscesses involving the peritonsillar, retropharyngeal, or parapharyngeal spaces may complicate infections in and around the oropharynx.

a. Peritonsillar abscesses commonly occur in children over 10 years of age.

(1) Etiology. Group A streptococci and oral anaerobes

(2) Evaluation. The soft palate and uvula may be swollen and displaced toward the unaffected side. The patient complains of severe throat pain and may speak with a muffled, "hot-potato" voice.

(3) Diagnosis. Surgical drainage of the abscess usually yields the organism.

(4) Therapy

(a) Surgical drainage is the cornerstone of effective therapy and should be performed under general anaesthesia using a cuffed endotracheal tube to minimize the chances of aspiration and/or mediastinitis.

(b) After effective surgical drainage, the antibiotic treatment of choice is a 10-day course of penicillin, initially IV until acute manifestations have subsided and then continued PO.

b. Retropharyngeal or parapharyngeal abscesses commonly occur in children younger than 3 years.

(1) Etiology. Group A streptococci, *S. aureus,* and oral anaerobes

(2) Evaluation. Abscesses in these locations should be suspected with displacement of structures or a mass in the posterior pharynx. A lateral neck x-ray will corroborate the former, but a submental vertex view may be required to demonstrate the latter. The possibility of an embedded foreign body should never be overlooked.

(3) Diagnosis. Culture of aspirated surgical drainage may yield the organisms.

(4) Therapy. Because of the high incidence of mixed infections at these sites, a pencillinase-resistant penicillin should be given in addition to penicillin G. Clindamycin is an alternative drug for the penicillin-allergic patient. Surgical drainage is the mainstay of treatment.

E. Cervical adenitis. Lymph nodes often enlarge in response to localized or systemic infection. Marked enlargement (3 cm or more) associated with tenderness and erythema indicates progressive infection within the node.

1. The **etiology** varies with the location of the infected neck glands:
   a. **Tonsillar nodes** (at the angle of the jaw) are likely to be infected by throat pathogens.
   b. **Submandibular node infection** follows oral or facial disease. Unilateral "cold" submandibular nodes, in the absence of orofacial infection, suggest infection with atypical (nontuberculous) mycobacteria.
   c. **Posterior cervical node infection** suggests an adjacent skin infection.
   d. **Bilateral cervical node enlargement** of marked degree indicates infectious mononucleosis, acute toxoplasmosis, secondary syphilis, a phenytoin reaction, or infiltrative node disease.
   e. **Recurrent** episodes of adenitis should raise the suspicion of chronic granulomatous disease or immunoglobulin deficiency.
2. **Evaluation and diagnosis.** The history, examination of the area drained by affected lymph nodes, and laboratory data (including antistreptolysin O, monospot, CBC and differential, and VDRL as indicated) may reveal the likely cause of adenitis.
   a. Needle aspiration of the node offers a simple, safe means of diagnosis. Gram and acid-fast stains of aspirates may provide immediately helpful information. Aspirates should be cultured for aerobes, anaerobes, and mycobacteria.
   b. Although *M. tuberculosis* adenitis is now uncommon, tuberculin testing is prudent. A positive tuberculin skin test mandates a chest x-ray.
   c. Surgical drainage or excisional biopsy is appropriate for infected nodes that are fluctuant ("pointing") or refractory to broad-spectrum antibiotic therapy.
3. **Therapy**
   a. Unless stains of the node aspirate suggest another organism, a penicillinase-resistant penicillin should be given as initial therapy, since the most likely organisms are *S. aureus* and group A streptococci.
   b. **Streptococcal adenitis.** Penicillin G, either IM (procaine, 600,000 units–1.2 million U/day) or IV (aqueous, 100,000–250,000 units/kg/day) in severe cases, is given until the fever and localized inflammation have subsided. This response should occur within 2–3 days, after which a 10-day course of oral penicillin (penicillin G, 50,000 units/kg/day, or penicillin V, 50 mg/kg/day) can be completed. Hot compresses and antipyretics also are prescribed.
   c. **Staphylococcal adenitis.** Since the organism is often penicillin-resistant, one of the penicillinase-resistant semisynthetic penicillins is given initially and continued if the infecting pathogen is resistant to penicillin. Severity of the illness determines whether or not the IV route and hospitalization are necessary.
      (1) Recommended preparations are as follows:
         (a) **IV.** Nafcillin, oxacillin, or methicillin, 100–200 mg/kg/day q4h
         (b) **PO.** Dicloxacillin, 25 mg/kg/day qid
      (2) The duration of treatment is determined by the patient's response, but a 10–14 day course is usually sufficient.
   d. **Tuberculous adenitis.** Antituberculous drugs are given (Table 15-10).
   e. **Nontuberculous mycobacterial adenitis.** Although the natural history of this disease is variable, the adenopathy will often resolve spontaneously. The nontuberculous mycobacteria are not communicable from human to human, and the patient presents no danger to siblings or classmates.
      (1) Since nontuberculous strains are frequently resistant in vitro to the usual antituberculous drugs, observation is usually the preferred management.
      (2) When increasing adenopathy or related symptoms indicate more aggressive management, complete surgical excision of the involved

nodes is recommended. Antituberculous therapy should be given post-operatively until culture reports demonstrate that *M. tuberculosis* is not present.

F. Infections of the respiratory tract

  1. Epiglottitis is a rapidly progressive bacterial cellulitis of the supraglottic tissues resulting in narrowing of the airway inlet, with risk of total airway obstruction. **It is a medical emergency.**

   a. Etiology. The causative organism is *H. influenzae* type B in virtually all cases.

   b. Evaluation and diagnosis. To prevent death, skillful handling of patients with a tentative diagnosis of epiglottitis is essential. The onset of respiratory difficulty is usually acute, with rapid progression, most often in children 3–6 years old. Bacteremia is present in over 90% and is associated with fever and toxicity, dysphagia, drooling, inspiratory stridor, muffled voice, and extended neck.

   (1) Unnecessary stress, including examination of the epiglottis, must be avoided in the child with marked respiratory distress.

   (2) The swollen, cherry-red tip of the epiglottis may be readily visible in the throat of a cooperative child, but examination must not be forced, lest sudden, complete obstruction occur.

   (3) Radiographs should be done only under controlled conditions with skilled personnel and equipment to evaluate the patient's ventilation and to secure the airway swiftly if necessary. Lateral radiographs of the neck delineate the epiglottis and aryepiglottic folds well and are helpful in puzzling cases.

   c. Therapy

   (1) Conservative management of epiglottitis includes prophylactic naso-tracheal intubation to prevent sudden death. Skillful intubation has generally replaced the need for tracheostomy in patients with obstructed airways. Intubation is well tolerated and briefly required (1–3 days).

   (2) Antibiotic therapy directed against *H. influenzae* is begun immediately with ampicillin, 200 mg/kg/day, and chloramphenicol, 100 mg/kg/day, given IV. Later, treatment may be changed to ampicillin alone if the isolate is susceptible. Treatment is continued for 7–10 days.

   (3) Early in convalescence, patients should be carefully evaluated for metastatic *Haemophilus* infection, such as pneumonia, pericarditis, meningitis, or septic arthritis.

  2. Croup. Viral laryngotracheobronchitis is complicated by subglottic edema, resulting in a characteristic barking cough and a hoarse voice.

   a. Etiology. Parainfluenza viruses, respiratory syncytial virus, adenoviruses, and influenza viruses are the most common causes. Bacterial infection is rare.

   b. Evaluation

   (1) History. A mild upper respiratory prodrome is common, with sudden onset of barking cough and hoarseness, often at night and typically in a child under 3 years of age.

   (2) Physical examination. High fever or toxicity is unusual. Examination is directed toward the extent of airway narrowing: inspiratory stridor at rest, tachypnea (40/min), retractions, and diminished breath sounds indicate critical narrowing. Restlessness, tachycardia, altered mental status, and pallor or cyanosis suggest hypoxia.

   (3) Laboratory data. A CBC and arterial blood gas estimation are indicated if they can be done by skilled personnel. A lateral neck radiogram will clarify the clinical presentation.

   c. The **diagnosis** of croup is confirmed by neck radiographs showing subglottic narrowing.

d. Therapy
   (1) Hydration and **moisturized air.** Cool, moist air with O_2 is provided as necessary.
   (2) Sedation. A quiet room where a parent may stay with the child and elimination of unnecessary procedures help to reduce the associated anxiety. In patients in whom excessive apprehension aggravates the respiratory distress, mild sedation (chloral hydrate, 10–15 mg/kg q6–8h) may be beneficial (see Chap. 1, p. 6).
   (3) Aerosolized racemic epinephrine (2.25% solution, 0.5 ml in 4 ml normal saline) may produce transient relief of symptoms. Frequent treatments are often necessary, and rebound may occur.
   (4) Corticosteroids. A short course of high-dose corticosteroids (1–3 doses of dexamethasone, 1 mg/kg q6h) in severe croup has become commonplace, although current studies have not yet shown a clear-cut benefit.
   (5) Intubation is indicated for respiratory failure.
   (6) Home care. Most cases of croup are mild and can be managed at home. Therapeutic measures include a humidifier, a steamed-up bathroom, and, occasionally, outdoor air. Parents should be instructed to call a physician if the child's respiratory distress increases.
3. Bronchiolitis is a syndrome of acute small airway obstruction in young infants, with the risk of respiratory failure.
   a. Etiology. Usually viral (most commonly, respiratory syncytial virus)
   b. Evaluation should include assessment of hydration and respiratory exchange.
   c. The **diagnosis** is suggested by the onset of coryza, cough, and dyspnea in an infant and by prominent wheezing, hyperinflation of the lungs, and retractions. Fever may not be present.
   d. Therapy
      (1) Humidified O_2 (30% or more). In severe cases, arterial blood gases should be monitored.
      (2) Adequate hydration of the patient is important. Whether fluids are administered PO or IV depends on the severity of the respiratory distress. **In severe respiratory distress, administration of oral fluids may induce vomiting and aspiration pneumonia and is contraindicated.**
      (3) In severe cases, assisted ventilation may be required.
      (4) Congestive heart failure can develop in severely ill patients, necessitating digitalis (see Chap. 9, pp. 248ff).
      (5) Antibiotics are not routinely given, but are indicated if associated otitis media or pneumonia is present.
      (6) Corticosteroids have **not** been shown to be beneficial.
      (7) Bronchodilators given parenterally or by inhalation may be worth trying, but are not reliably effective (see Chap. 19, pp. 481ff).
      (8) Patients with bronchiolitis may continue to excrete respiratory syncytial virus for several weeks and should be placed on precautions in the hospital to prevent cross-infection of other infants.
4. Pneumonia
   a. Etiology
      (1) Neonates. Gram-positive cocci, particularly group B streptococcus and occasionally *S. aureus,* and gram-negative enteric bacilli cause most neonatal bacterial pneumonias.
      (2) Children 1 month–5 years of age. Respiratory viruses cause the majority of pediatric pneumonias. *Chlamydia trachomatis* causes an afebrile pneumonia in infants under 16 weeks of age, in which conjunctivitis is present in 50% of infants, eosinophilia is common, and the chest x-ray shows hyperinflation and diffuse interstitial or patchy infiltrates. The major bacterial pathogens in this age group are *Streptococcus pneumoniae* and *H. influenzae* type B. Pneumococci commonly cause lobar or segmental consolidation, but bronchopneumonia

is not infrequent. *H. influenzae* type B can mimic pneumonia caused by a number of organisms and is not infrequently associated with extrapulmonary infection. *S. aureus* is suggested by rapidly evolving respiratory distress, empyema, and the characteristic radiologic features of rapid progression, lobular ectasia, and pneumatoceles in a child less than 3 years old. Even in an extremely ill child, however, the initial x-ray film may demonstrate only faint local mottling.

- **(3) Children 5 years of age and older.** The pneumococcus is the major cause of bacterial pneumonia in this age group. *Mycoplasma pneumoniae* is a common cause of pneumonia in school-age children, adolescents, and young adults.
- **(4) Immunocompromised hosts** are subject to pneumonia caused by any organism, but gram-negative organisms, *Pneumocystis carinii,* and fungi are frequently found in pneumonia in these patients.
- **(5) Anaerobic bacteria,** especially penicillin-sensitive oral anaerobes, may cause pneumonia and lung abscess in patients who aspirate.
- **(6)** After viral infections, *S. aureus,* group A streptococcus, and *S. pneumoniae* may cause bacterial pneumonia. Group A streptococcal pneumonia may occur in children without prior illness and usually has a sudden onset, with high fever, chills, dyspnea, and pleuritic pain. Bacteremia and a serosanguineous pleural effusion are often associated.
- **(7) Tuberculosis** should always be considered as a possible cause of infectious pneumonia, especially in the child who responds slowly or not at all to antibiotic therapy.

  b. Evaluation
  - **(1)** Chest x-ray (posterioanterior and lateral)
  - **(2)** Tuberculin skin test
  - **(3)** Sputum or deep tracheal aspirate for Gram stain and culture. Cultures for bacteria from the nasopharynx should be interpreted with great caution.
  - **(4)** Cultures for respiratory viruses (which are rarely found in asymptomatic persons) and fluorescent antibody techniques for rapid diagnosis of certain viruses (e.g., influenza and respiratory syncytial virus) are now more widely available.
  - **(5)** Blood culture(s) in the patient who appears toxic
  - **(6)** A diagnostic thoracentesis if pleural fluid is present
  - **(7)** Serologic titers (acute and convalescent) are not very satisfactory for most pathogens, but for mycoplasma (cold agglutinin titer $\geq$ 1:64), group A streptococcus (antistreptolysin O titer), *Chlamydia, Legionella,* and *Rickettsia* (Q fever) may be the most useful means to make a presumptive diagnosis.
  - **(8)** Rapid diagnostic techniques for detecting bacterial antigens in body fluids
  - **(9)** Lung puncture (*Pediatrics* 44:486, 1969) or open lung biosy in critically ill children to establish the etiologic diagnosis to guide antimicrobial therapy
  - **(10)** Leukocyte and differential counts are occasionally helpful, but, in general, should not be relied upon to distinguish bacterial from other causes.

  c. The **diagnosis** is usually established by the chest x-ray and physical signs of consolidation. An etiologic diagnosis is usually made from the clinical features described, the cultures, antigen detection studies, and, in the case of a few organisms, by serology.

  d. Therapy
  - **(1) Antibiotics**
    - **(a)** Children who are mildly ill with features suggestive of viral disease can be managed without antibiotics, provided the patient can be followed closely.

(b) Infants and hospitalized patients should receive antibiotics when pneumonia is diagnosed.

(c) The choice of specific antibiotics is based on interpretation of available gram-stained specimens, the patient's age, and other suggestive clinical features.

(d) Specific recommendations prior to etiologic diagnosis

    (i) Neonates should receive both a penicillinase-resistant penicillin and an aminoglycoside IV.

    (ii) The toxic, hospitalized child aged 1 month–5 years should be treated with both a penicillinase-resistant penicillin (200 mg/kg/day q4h) and chloramphenicol (75 mg/kg/day q6h).

    (iii) The nontoxic child aged 1 month–5 years should be given an antibiotic effective against both *S. pneumoniae* and *H. influenzae* type B, such as ampicillin or amoxicillin. Cefuroxime (75 mg/kg/day q8h) is an alternative and also provides staphylococcal and ampicillin-resistant *H. influenzae* coverage. If the clinical syndrome clearly suggests *Chlamydia,* erythromycin (30–50 mg/kg/day q6h) should be administered.

    (iv) In the older child, suspected *Mycoplasma* pneumonia is treated with oral erythromycin (30–50 mg/kg/day in 4 daily doses for 10 days).

    (v) Identification of the pathogen or failure to respond to these regimens necessitates reevaluation of the choice of antibiotics.

    (vi) The **duration** of antimicrobial therapy is based on the individual patient's clinical response, but, in general, staphylococcal pneumonia requires 3 weeks of parenteral therapy followed by 1–3 weeks of oral therapy, *H. influenzae* and streptococcal pneumonia usually respond to 2–3 weeks of therapy, and pneumococcal pneumonia responds to 7 days of therapy.

(2) Indications for hospitalization include the following: significant respiratory distress or toxicity, cyanosis, age under 6 months, empyema or pleural effusion, possible staphylococcal pneumonia, and inadequate home care.

(3) In the case of empyema, **drainage** by repeated aspiration or insertion of a chest tube is necessary (see Chap. 3, pp. 54ff). (Loculated pleural fluid may explain persistent fever in the face of seemingly adequate antibiotic therapy.)

(4) Symptomatic care should include O_2 if necessary, maintenance of adequate hydration, high humidity (such as the use of a humidifier in the home), bronchodilators if bronchospasm is present, and deep tracheal suction in patients with an ineffectual cough.

(5) Postural drainage and **physiotherapy** may be helpful, particularly with underlying bronchiectasis.

(6) Initial follow-up of the ambulatory patient should be on a day-to-day basis until definite clinical improvement has occurred.

(7) Although radiologic resolution may lag behind clinical improvement, persistence of radiologic abnormalities without improvement for more than 4–6 weeks should alert the physician to possible underlying pulmonary disease (e.g., tuberculosis, foreign body, cystic fibrosis).

G. Infections of the central nervous system

  1. Meningitis

    a. Etiology. Meningitis is a complication of bacteremia. *H. influenzae* type B (60–65 percent), meningococci, and pneumococci account for most cases of acute bacterial meningitis in children over 2 months of age. Infrequently involved organisms are streptococci, *S. aureus,* and gram-negative enteric bacteria, except in neonatal meningitis.

b. Evaluation

    (1) In infants, the **presenting symptoms and signs** are nonspecific and include a high-pitched cry, irritability, anorexia, vomiting, lethargy, and/or a full fontanelle. Meningeal signs are uncommon, and fever is not invariably present. The closest attention must be paid to alterations in consciousness if an early diagnosis is to be made. Convulsions may be an early manifestation of meningitis. Thus convulsions associated with fever in infancy are generally an indication for CSF examination.

    (2) In older children, meningeal signs are more reliable. Brudzinski's sign (flexion of the neck with the patient supine causes involuntary flexion of the hips) can be helpful in determining the need for lumbar puncture (LP).

    (3) Patients with evidence of bacteremia should be carefully assessed for meningitis.

    (4) An **LP** should be performed as soon as the diagnosis is suspected. **Before** the LP is performed, a blood glucose should be obtained for comparison with the CSF glucose.

    (5) **Papilledema is a relative contraindication to LP,** and, if it is present, a neurosurgical consultation should be considered before proceeding. (Papilledema is rare in **acute** bacterial meningitis, and its presence may suggest other diagnostic possibilities, e.g., brain abscess.)

    (6) Other diagnostic procedures include blood culture, smears and cultures from any purpuric lesions, cultures of other body fluids (e.g., stool, urine, joint, abscess, middle ear), BUN, serum and urine electrolytes and osmolarity, chest x-ray, and tuberculin test. In infants, transillumination should be performed and the head circumference carefully measured.

c. The **diagnosis** can be established only by LP.

    (1) In bacterial meningitis the CSF is characteristically cloudy and under increased pressure, with > 100 WBC/mm^3, predominantly neutrophils, elevated total protein, low glucose (less than one-half of the pre-LP blood glucose concentration), and organisms in the CSF gram-stained smear. However, some of these findings may often be absent, and any of these abnormalities must be viewed with suspicion, particularly the presence of **any** neutrophils. The CSF culture usually confirms the diagnosis.

    (2) Rapid etiologic diagnosis of bacterial meningitis may be possible by using methods to detect capsular polysaccharide antigens (see Sec. **I.A.3.c**).

d. Therapy. IV antibiotic therapy should be initiated immediately after bacteriologic specimens have been obtained. The initial choice of antibiotics usually is based on the CSF gram-stained smear and the patient's age.

    (1) **In children over 2 months of age** in whom there is no reason to suspect an unusual organism, chloramphenicol is the drug of choice (100 mg/kg/day q6h), in combination with ampicillin (200–400 mg/kg/day q4h). Since ampicillin-resistant *H. influenzae* type B has now been isolated in all areas of the United States, anticipatory use of chloramphenicol is advisable. If *H. influenzae* is recovered, and sensitivity is confirmed in vitro, ampicillin is used to complete therapy. If the culture discloses meningococci or pneumococci, penicillin G is the drug of choice.

    (2) **Infants less than 2 months old.** See Chap. 6, p. 174.

    (3) The duration of therapy depends on the infant's clinical course, but antibiotics should be given for a minimum of 10 days.

    (4) **Other aspects of management**

        (a) All patients should be carefully evaluated for evidence of hypotension, abnormal bleeding, and the syndrome of inappropriate secretion of antidiuretic hormone (SIADH), which usually occurs within the first 72 hr of therapy. Fluids should be restricted to two-thirds maintenance until it is documented that SIADH is absent.

(b) During treatment, frequent observation of vital signs and daily neurologic examinations, measurement of head circumference, and transillumination of the head (if the fontanelle is open) should be performed.

(c) LP should be repeated after 24–48 hr of therapy in patients whose disease is severe or who respond poorly to treatment. Cultures and stains are usually negative after 48 hr if treatment is effective.

(d) Fever during therapy most commonly results from phlebitis, drugs, nosocomial infection, subdural effusion (which may occur in up to 50% of infants and children during the acute illness, usually without producing symptoms or fever), or coexisting viral infection. Unless an obvious cause is found, prolonged or secondary fever during therapy should prompt a repeat CSF examination and a search for localized infection in the subdural space, bones, joints, pericardium, or pleural spaces.

(e) At the completion of antibiotic therapy, children may be observed for recurrence of fever for 24–48 hr before discharge from the hospital. However, a recent review indicates that the earliest relapse of bacterial meningitis occurred on the third day after completion of antibiotic therapy. In addition, a routine LP at the end of adequate therapy may not be necessary if the patient has had a satisfactory clinical response and an uneventful hospital course (*Pediatrics* 67:188, 1981).

(f) Close household and day-care center contacts of children with meningitis are at increased risk of secondary disease caused by *H. influenzae* type B (for household contacts < 6 years, the risk is about 0.5%) and *N. meningitidis* (for all persons, the risk is about 0.5%). Close observation is mandatory, and prophylaxis should be considered for persons at risk.

(g) Currently it is recommended that all children with invasive disease due to *H. influenzae* type B receive rifampin therapy (once daily for 4 days in a 20 mg/kg dose; maximum dose, 600 mg/day) prior to discharge to eradicate carriage from the nasopharynx (*Red Book,* American Academy of Pediatrics, 1982).

2. For a discussion of **neonatal meningitis,** see Chap. 6, p. 173.

3. Brain abscess. Normal brain tissue is resistant to bacterial infection. However, ischemic brain injury (e.g., cyanotic heart disease), parameningeal infection (sinusitis, mastoiditis, skull osteomyelitis), and skull trauma increase the risk of brain abscess.

   a. Etiology. Causative bacteria are usually derived from the upper airway or mouth. Mixtures of aerobes (α-streptococci, *S. aureus,* diphtheroids, *Haemophilus*) and anaerobes (*Peptococcus, Bacteroides*) are common. Unusual agents are occasionally responsible, especially in immunocompromised patients.

   b. Evaluation. Brain abscess must be considered in patients with evidence of a rapidly progressive intracranial mass.

   (1) The **history** should focus on possible predisposing causes. Headache and seizures are common. Fever is seldom prominent.

   (2) In the **physical examination,** attempts should be made to uncover extracranial infection and localize the neurologic lesion. An assessment should be made for elevated intracranial pressure.

   (3) Laboratory examination includes blood cultures and a CT scan and may require skull x-rays and an electroencephalogram. **CSF exami-**

nation should be avoided in patients with increased intracranial pressure. It seldom adds to the evaluation (CSF changes are not universally present nor pathognomonic for brain abscess). Leukocytosis may or may not be present.

    c. The **diagnosis** is made by confirmation of an intracranial mass by CT scan. Even small abscesses may be localized by skilled personnel and generally make an arteriogram unnecessary. When CT scan facilities are unavailable, other radiologic techniques are required.

    d. Therapy

        (1) Surgical excision or drainage of the abscess is usually necessary for cure. Antibiotics may be started prior to operation **but will not likely cure (or halt the progression of) an established abscess.** Mortality and CNS sequelae are closely proportional to the depth of coma at the time of drainage.

        (2) Initial empiric antibiotic therapy usually includes chloramphenicol (100 mg/kg/day IV q6h) and penicillin (300,000 U/kg/day IV q4h). This can be modified after bacteriologic evaluation of the abscess contents.

        (3) To reduce brain swelling, fluids should be restricted moderately to keep the patient "dry." Hyperosmotic agents, such as mannitol, and dexamethasone may also help to reduce cerebral edema (see Chap. 3, p. 62).

        (4) Follow-up radionuclide or CT scans are used to monitor resolution of the abscess and to determine the duration of antibiotic therapy.

        (5) Parameningeal foci of infection responsible for brain abscess may also require surgical drainage (sinus, mastoid).

H. Gastrointestinal Infections: bacterial gastroenteritis. See Chap. 10 for viral and Chap. 16 for parasitic infections.

    1. Etiology

        a. Bacterial agents cause diarrhea infrequently. The principal agents in the United States are *Salmonella, Shigella,* and in some areas, *Campylobacter fetus* subspecies *jejuni.* Other agents include *Yersinia enterocolitica,* and *Vibrio parahemolyticus* (which causes shellfish poisoning). Enteropathogenic *E. coli* (EPEC) organisms are uncommon in the United States.

        b. Traveler's diarrhea, a self-limited disease lasting several days, is usually caused by enterotoxigenic *E. coli* (ETEC), although *Shigella* and *Salmonella,* other bacteria, viruses, and *Giardia* have been implicated.

        c. Pseudomembranous colitis (antibiotic-associated colitis) is caused by *Clostridium difficile* toxin, produced as the organism overgrows the residual gut flora of antibiotic-treated patients.

        d. Food poisoning can be caused by several bacteria (usually toxin-producing), including staphylococci, *Clostridium perfringens; C. botulinum* (botulism), *Vibrio parahemolyticus,* and *Bacillus cereus.*

    2. Evaluation includes an epidemiologic history, assessment of the character and duration of the abnormal stools, and careful assessment of the patient's state of hydration.

        a. The demonstration of sheets of fecal leukocytes in diarrheal stoools is well correlated with inflammatory (usually bacterial) disease.

        b. Indications for stool cultures are bloody stools, toxicity, severe diarrhea, chronic disease or impaired host defenses, and epidemic diarrhea (see Chap. 10, p. 264, for culture methods).

        c. Hospitalized patients with fever and diarrhea should have one or more blood cultures.

    3. Diagnosis

        a. Stool cultures handled routinely will identify only *Salmonella* and *Shigella.* If *Campylobacter, Yersinia,* or *Vibrio* is suspected, the laboratory should be alerted. Toxin-producing *E. coli* (EPEC) are reliably identified only by special assay for enterotoxin. The toxin of *C. difficile* can be identified directly in stool samples from patients with pseudomembranous colitis.

b. For *Yersinia,* a fourfold rise in serologic titer is diagnostic.

c. In **food poisoning** the contaminating organism can be inferred from the incubation period (time from ingestion to onset of symptoms)—for *S. aureus,* 3–6 hr, but as early as 30 min; for *C. perfringens,* 1–25 hr, usually 8–12 hr; and for *Salmonella,* 12–18 hr, up to 72 hr; or from careful epidemiologic history and the physical signs as with botulism.

4. Therapy and prevention. Therapy is directed primarily toward fluid and electrolyte management.

a. *Salmonella.* Since antibiotics may prolong the carrier state, most patients with *Salmonella* in the stool are not treated.

    (1) Indications for treatment are infection in young infants, impaired host defenses, sickle cell anemia, chronic inflammatory bowel disease, severe toxicity, and enteritis with bacteremia if fever and toxicity persist by the time the positive blood culture is obtained.

    (2) *Salmonella* infections may be treated with ampicillin (100 mg/kg/day), amoxicillin (50 mg/kg/day), or chloramphenicol (50–100 mg/kg/day). Trimethoprim (TMP)-sulfamethoxazole (10 mg TMP/kg/day) may be effective for multiply resistant organisms.

b. *Shigella sonnei* are likely to be resistant to ampicillin. Thus, trimethoprim-sulfamethoxazole (10 mg TMP/kg/day q12h for 5 days) should be given when *Shigella* is isolated before susceptibility is known. Susceptible strains may be treated with ampicillin (100 mg/kg/day q6h for 5 days). Amoxicillin is ineffective, and antidiarrheal drugs may prolong the course of disease.

c. Enteritis caused by *Campylobacter* may be successfully treated with erythromycin (40 mg/kg/day PO q6h for 5–7 days) if symptoms have not resolved by the time the culture result is available.

d. Traveler's diarrhea

    (1) Drinking only boiled or carbonated water or other processed beverages and avoiding unpeeled fruits, salads, and ice may prevent infection.

    (2) Several drugs, including doxycycline, bismuth subsalicylate, and trimethoprim-sulfamethoxazole may help prevent infection. Since the disease is generally self-limited, no specific prophylactic therapy is recommended.

e. Pseudomembranous colitis is treated by withdrawal of the implicated antibiotic (may be a penicillin or cephalosporin if clindamycin has not been used) and institution of oral vancomycin (40 mg/kg/day in 4 divided doses) when the presence of *C. difficile* toxin in the stool has been confirmed. Vancomycin therapy should be continued for 7 days or until follow-up stools are negative for toxin.

I. Genitourinary infections

  1. Urinary tract infections (UTIs)

    a. Etiology. First infections are most commonly caused by *E. coli.* Other pathogens include *Proteus, Klebsiella, Pseudomonas, Streptococcus faecalis, S. epidermidis,* and, rarely, *S. aureus.*

    b. Evaluation and diagnosis. Clinical manifestations of urinary tract infection (UTI) vary with age. UTI must be considered in any acutely ill or nonthriving infant.

        (1) Pyelonephritis is suggested by high fever ($\geq$39° C [$\geq$102° F]), toxicity, flank pain, and costovertebral angle tenderness and is commonly associated with ureteral reflux. **Cystitis** is associated with suprapubic pain, dysuria, frequency, urgency, and enuresis. Localization of the site of infection may be very difficult, especially in young children.

        (2) At any age, UTI may be asymptomatic (asymptomatic bacteriuria) and persist without treatment, seldom becoming overtly symptomatic.

Up to two-thirds of preschool and school-age girls may be symptom-free with their first UTI.

(3) Physical examination should include blood pressure measurement, a search for congenital malformations, and a careful examination of the abdomen, genitalia, and perineum.

(4) Laboratory studies

(a) Urine microscopy can provide an accurate provisional diagnosis of UTI if used to quantitate the concentration of bacteria in a fresh, clean sample: One or more bacteria per oil field in gram-stained, **uncentrifuged** urine = $\geqslant 10^5$ colonies/ml. The presence of numerous bacteria per high-power field does not necessarily indicate infection.

(b) Pyuria is not specific for infection. Proteinuria and hematuria are uncommon with UTI.

(c) Urine culture provides proof of infection, but its value in young children is reduced by frequent sampling errors.

(i) Infected urine will contain $>10^5$ colonies/ml (except in some neonates, in whom $>10^4$ colonies may indicate infection). Negative cultures of voided samples are of value in ruling out infection.

(ii) Repetition of cultures increases diagnostic precision in all age groups. A single midstream, clean-catch specimen will accurately predict the presence of UTI 80% of the time; two consecutive positive cultures increase the accuracy to 95%.

(iii) Diagnostic precision is greatest with urine obtained by suprapubic bladder aspiration, for which any growth of bacteria should be considered significant, or sterile catheterization, for which 10^3 colonies/ml are probably significant. In skilled hands, both procedures are safe. They are most appropriately used to resolve urgent or difficult diagnostic problems in younger children.

(iv) Note that contamination of samples may provide $\geqslant 10^5$ colonies/ml of a single species. More typically, contaminated cultures contain several species in concentrations $<10^5$ colonies/ml. Urine specimens should be refrigerated at 4°C and cultured promptly to avoid growth of contaminants.

(d) A **blood culture** should be obtained in patients with pyelonephritis and in neonates with UTI.

(e) Indications for an intravenous pyelogram and a voiding cystourethrogram are as follows: age less than 6 years; toxicity or sepsis (suggestive of pyelonephritis); and first infection in a male and second infection in a female (unless the history, physical findings, and/or clinical response to the first infection suggests an early workup). In these circumstances, a serum BUN, creatinine, and creatinine clearance are also indicated.

(f) Contributing factors to recurrent infections include poor perineal hygiene, vulvovaginitis, pinworm infestations, and constipation.

c. Therapy

(1) Most initial and uncomplicated UTIs respond to oral sulfonamides such as sulfisoxazole (120–150 mg/kg/day PO qid). Effective alternatives are ampicillin (50 mg/kg/day PO qid), amoxicillin (25 mg/kg/day PO tid), and nitrofurantoin (5 mg/kg/day qid). The usual duration of therapy is 10 days. In children the efficacy of single-dose therapy remains to be proved.

(2) Children with **pyelonephritis** require parenteral antibiotics, hydration, and hospitalization. Ampicillin (100–200 mg/kg/day q4h IV) is effective against many urinary tract pathogens. A previous history of pyelonephritis or infection with a resistant organism indicates the need for broad-spectrum coverage with gentamicin (3.0–7.5 mg/kg/

day q8–12h IM or IV) in addition to ampicillin. The recommended duration of therapy is usually 10–14 days, but clinical improvement should be evident within 48–72 hr.

(3) Infants, especially newborns, with UTI should have prompt urologic evaluation as well as aggressive antibiotic treatment.

(4) Ongoing antimicrobial therapy is based on the clinical response of the patient and the results of subsequent urine cultures.

(a) A culture should be obtained 24–48 hr after therapy has been initiated, and at this time the urine should be sterile (or have $<$ 10^4 bacteria/ml).

(b) A Gram stain of the unspun specimen should not show organisms, and the sediment should be clear of leukocytes 24–48 hr after therapy.

(c) Adequate clinical responses may be seen despite in vitro resistance of the organism isolated, because of the high concentrations of certain antimicrobials in the urine (see **I.B.4.b**).

(d) Failure to respond should increase suspicion of an underlying anatomic abnormality.

(5) Adequate **hydration** of the patient is important.

(6) Continuous bladder drainage by an indwelling catheter should be done only when absolutely necessary and discontinued at the earliest possible time; a **closed drainage system is mandatory.** On removal of the catheter, a urine culture should be obtained.

d. Follow-up of a UTI should be carefully organized, since infection tends to recur, often in asymptomatic form. Recurrence is most likely during the first 6–12 months after an infection.

(1) After therapy is discontinued, urine cultures are indicated 1 week later, every month during the subsequent 3 months, every 3 months during the next 6 months, and then twice yearly. There is increased risk of recurrences with marriage and pregnancy.

(2) Among patients with **significant reflux,** recurrent infection is prevented by prophylactic antibiotic therapy, which is continued until reflux resolves or is repaired.

(3) Some normal girls experience **multiple recurrences** of UTI. They should be carefully assessed for correctable contributing factors. When infections are are frequent, socially distressing, or associated with renal scarring, prophylactic antibiotic therapy is often prescribed for 6–12 months. Trimethoprim-sulfamethoxazole (2 mg TMP/kg/day PO in 1 dose) or nitrofurantoin (2 mg/kg/day in 1 dose) may be used.

(4) Home screening can improve the follow-up of UTI, using simple, inexpensive tests such as the nitrate chemical test for bacteria and agar-coated dip slides.

2. Gonorrhea. The infecting organism is *N. gonorrhoeae*. The disease is seen with increasing frequency in children **under** 12 years of age.

a. Evaluation

(1) In males, urethral specimens can be obtained by "stripping" the penis.

(2) In females, pelvic examination allows the physician to evaluate cervical and adnexal tenderness as well as obtain culture material from the cervix. In prepubertal females, gonococcal infection may present as purulent vulvovaginitis rather than cervicitis.

(3) The rectum and pharynx should be cultured in both males and females for *N. gonorrhoeae*.

(4) *N. gonorrhoeae* is relatively fastidious, and specimens should be cultured promptly and placed in a high CO_2 atmosphere (e.g., candlejar). Transgrow medium is an excellent transport medium for *N. gonorrhoeae* and should be used when direct cultures are not practical.

(5) **A serologic test for syphilis should be performed in all patients with gonorrhea** (see **4.a**) and repeated 2 months after treatment if an agent other than penicillin is used. Coexisting sexually transmitted diseases should be considered.

   b. Diagnosis. *N. gonorrhoeae* is identified by demonstration of gram-negative diplococci on gram-stained smears of urethral discharge or by culture of appropriate specimens on Thayer-Martin media. Smears of cervical mucus are not reliable.

   c. Treatment. Treatment is outlined in Table 15-11. Case contact finding, as well as sex education and counseling, is as important as the drug therapy. Child abuse must be investigated in cases involving young children.

   (1) Patients should abstain from sexual relations for 7 days and return for repeat cultures 7–14 days after treatment.

   (2) Contacts of the patient should be cultured and treated.

3. Pelvic inflammatory disease

   a. Etiology. *N. gonorrhoeae* can be cultured from the cervix in about 50% of cases of pelvic inflammatory disease (PID). Pathogens causing nongonococcal PID include *Chlamydia trachomatis,* gram-positive and gram-negative anaerobes, gram-negative aerobic bacilli, *Mycoplasma hominis,* and *Actinomyces israelii.*

   b. Evaluation

   (1) A **history** of acute lower abdominal pain with vaginal discharge, fever, and chills suggests the diagnosis. The menstrual period is often a precipitating factor.

   (2) Pelvic findings include pain on cervical motion, adnexal tenderness, and sometimes a mass.

   (3) Laboratory abnormalities include a normal to elevated WBC count and an elevated erythrocyte sedimentation rate (ESR) (75–85%). Culture of the endocervix and rectum or pharynx for *N. gonorrhoeae*—and intraoperative cultures if surgical drainage is required—should be obtained.

   (4) Ultrasound examination may help to delineate the extent and foci of infection within the pelvis.

   (5) Laparoscopy is occasionally necessary to establish the diagnosis.

   c. Diagnosis

   (1) Gram stain of cervical drainage may or may not reveal gram-negative intracellular diplococci; nevertheless, the diagnosis must be confirmed by culture.

   (2) When cultures for *N. gonorrhoeae* are negative and the response to therapy for gonococcal PID is poor, the diagnosis of nongonococcal PID becomes more likely.

   (3) Differential considerations include: acute appendicitis, ectopic pregnancy, ruptured ovarian cyst, ovarian abscess, and endometriosis.

   d. Therapy (*Med. Lett. Drugs Ther.* 26:5, 1984; *M.M.W.R.* 31:35S, 1982.)

   (1) Indications for admission to the hospital include toxicity, uncertain diagnosis, suspected pelvic abscess, signs of peritonitis, pregnancy, inability to take oral medications, failure of response to outpatient therapy, and poor follow-up arrangements.

   (2) Inpatient therapy must be individualized, and surgical drainage may be necessary. Some regimens for gonococcal PID follow.

   (a) Cefoxitin (2 g IV qid) plus doxycycline (100 mg IV bid) are given until improvement. This is followed by doxycycline (100 mg PO bid) to complete 10 days.

   (b) An alternative is to give doxycycline (100 mg IV bid) plus metronidazole (1 gm IV bid) until improvement. This is followed by doxycycline (100 mg PO bid) plus metronidazole (1 gm PO bid) to complete 10 days. This regimen is favored when the infection is associated with a tubo-ovarian abscess or an intrauterine device.

   (3) Outpatient therapy

   (a) Cefoxitin (2 gm IM once) plus probenecid (1 gm PO once) are

Table 15-11. Recommended treatment schedules for gonococcal infections

Type	Drugs of choice	Dosage	Alternatives
Urethritis/cervicitis or anal—women	Amoxicillin plus probenecid, followed by tetracycline HCl	3 gm PO once 1 gm PO once 500 mg PO × 7 days	Penicillin G procaine, 4.8 million U IM[a] once plus probenecid 1 gm PO once Spectinomycin, 2 gm IM once Cefoxitin, 2 gm, or cefuroxime, 1.5 gm, IM once Cefotaxime, 1 gm IM once
Anal—men	Penicillin G procaine plus probenecid	As for urethritis	Spectinomycin, 2 gm IM once
Pharyngeal	Tetracycline HCl[b] or Penicillin G procaine plus probenecid	As for urethritis	Trimethoprim-sulfamethoxazole, 9 tablets[c] PO qd for 5 days
Pelvic inflammatory disease	See text, p. 399.	As for urethritis	
Ophthalmia (adults)	Penicillin G crystalline plus saline irrigation	10 million U IV daily for 5 days	Cefoxitin, 1 gm, or cefotaxime, 500 mg, IV qid for 5 days plus saline irrigation
Bacteremia and arthritis	Penicillin G crystalline followed by amoxicillin	10 million U IV daily for 3 days 500 mg/PO qid for 4 days	Tetracycline, 500 mg PO qid[b] for 7 days Spectinomycin, 2 gm IM bid for 3 days Erythromycin, 500 mg PO qid for 7 days Cefotaxime, 500 mg, or cefoxitin, 1 gm, IV qid for 7 days

Condition	Drug	Dose	Alternative
Meningitis	Penicillin G crystalline	At least 10 million U IV daily for at least 10 days	Cefotaxime, 2 gm IV q4h for at least 10 days; Chloramphenicol, 4–6 gm/day for at least 10 days
Endocarditis	Penicillin G crystalline	At least 10 million U IV daily for at least 3 to 4 weeks	
Neonatal			
Ophthalmia	Penicillin G crystalline *plus* saline irrigation	50,000 U/kg/day IV in 2 doses for 7 days	
Arthritis and septicemia	Penicillin G crystalline	75,000–100,000 U/kg/day IV in 4 doses for 7 days	
Meningitis	Penicillin G crystalline	100,000 U/kg/day IV in 3 or 4 doses for at least 10 days	
Children (< 45 kg)			
Urogenital, anal, and pharyngeal	Amoxicillin *plus* probenecid, *or* Penicillin G procaine *plus* probenecid	50 mg/kg PO once; 25 mg/kg (max. 1 gm) once; 100,000 U/kg IM once; 25 mg/kg (max. 1 gm) once	Spectinomycin, 40 mg/kg IM once *or* Tetracycline (> 8 yr), 10 mg/kg/day in 4 divided doses for 7 days
Arthritis	Penicillin G crystalline	150,000 U/kg/day IV for 7 days	Cefoxitin, 100 mg/kg/day *or* Cefotaxime, 50 mg/kg/day IV in divided doses for 7 days; Tetracycline (> 8 yr), 10 mg/kg/day in 4 divided doses for 7 days; Erythromycin 50 mg/kg/day PO in 4 divided doses for 7 days
Meningitis	Penicillin G crystalline	250,000 U/kg/day IV in 6 divided doses for at least 10 days	Cefotaxime 200 mg/kg/day IV for at least 10 days; Chloramphenicol, 100 mg/kg/day IV for at least 10 days

Source: Modified from *Med. Lett. Drugs Ther.* 26:5, 1984.

[a] Divided into two injections at one visit.

[b] Or doxycycline, 100 mg PO bid.

[c] Each tablet contains trimethoprim, 80 mg, and sulfamethoxazole, 400 mg.

followed by doxycycline (100 mg PO bid) for 10 days. An alternative is tetracycline HCl (500 mg PO qid) for 10 days.

(b) Patients should be reevaluated in 48–72 hr; those not responding favorably should be hospitalized.

4. Syphilis The infecting organism is *Treponema pallidum*.

a. Evaluation and diagnosis. See also Chap. 6.

(1) Dark-field examination of skin lesions (chancre or rash). The material is infectious and should be handled with care.

(2) Serologic tests for syphilis are usually nonreactive when the chancre first appears, but become reactive during the following 1–4 weeks. Biologic false-positive test with nonspecific antigens (VDRL, RPRCT, Wasserman, Hinton, Kolmer) may be caused by a variety of other illnesses and should be confirmed by tests specific for *T. pallidum* (FTA-ABS, TPI).

(3) Congenital syphilis. Although a positive serological test for syphilis in the neonate may represent passively acquired maternal antibody, these infants should be treated if a definite history of adequate maternal treatment cannot be obtained.

b. Therapy for syphilis is outlined in Table 15-12. Case contact finding, as well as sex education and counseling, is as important as the drug therapy. Child abuse must be investigated in cases involving younger children.

5. Toxic shock syndrome

a. Etiology. Toxic shock syndrome (TSS) is a multisystem illness caused by a toxin produced by *S. aureus*.

b. Evaluation. The illness most often occurs in menstruating women, especially in women using tampons, but it has been seen in children of both sexes who have nonvaginal foci of infection.

(1) TSS typically begins suddenly with high fever, vomiting, and watery diarrhea and sometimes with sore throat, headache, and myalgias. Within 48 hr the disease may progress to hypotensive shock with the appearance of a diffuse scarlatiniform rash and nonpurulent conjunctivitis. The rash later desquamates. Alterations in consciousness may be present, and renal, cardiac, and pulmonary dysfunction may develop.

(2) Laboratory findings may include elevated BUN, creatinine, bilirubin, SGOT, and CPK. There is usually a leukocytosis with a left shift and a low to normal platelet count. The urinalysis may reveal pyuria and proteinuria.

(3) Cultures of the blood (although bacteremia is not part of this syndrome), vagina, nasopharynx, anus, and any wound should be obtained in suspected cases.

c. The presumptive **diagnosis** can be established by recovery of *Staphylococcus aureus* from a mucosal site in a patient with a clinically compatible illness.

d. Therapy

(1) Adequate volume repletion with colloid-containing fluids and blood pressure support with pressors may be required.

(2) Penicillinase-resistant penicillin therapy should be given parenterally (e.g., oxacillin, 200 mg/kg/day in divided doses q4h).

(3) Menstruating patients should be advised about the possible recurrence of TSS if tampons are used.

J. Infections of the bones and joints

1. Septic arthritis

a. Etiology. Usually *S. aureus, H. influenzae* type b, or β-hemolytic streptococci. Penetrating injuries or skin infections are associated with S. aureus infections. Suppurative arthritis, sterile inflammatory arthritis, and tenosynovitis may be associated with gonococcal disease in sexually active adolescents, sometimes with characteristic skin lesions. Gram-

Table 15-12. Recommended treatment schedules for syphilis*

Stage	Choice	Dosage	Alternatives
Early (primary, secondary, or latent less than 1 year)	Penicillin G benzathine	2.4 million U IM once	Tetracycline HCl, 500 mg PO qid for 15 days Erythromycin, 500 mg PO qid for 15 days
Late (more than 1 year's duration, cardiovascular)	Penicillin G benzathine	2.4 million U IM weekly for 3 doses	Tetracycline HCl, 500 mg PO qid for 30 days Erythromycin, 500 mg PO qid for 30 days
Neurosyphilis	Penicillin G crystalline or Penicillin G procaine or Penicillin G benzathine	2 to 4 million U IV q4h for 10 days 2.4 million U IM qd *plus* probenecid, 500 mg PO qid, both for 10 days 2.4 million U IM weekly for 3 doses	Tetracycline HCl, 500 mg PO qid for 30 days Erythromycin, 500 mg PO qid for 30 days
Congenital CSF normal CSF abnormal	Penicillin G benzathine Penicillin G crystalline or Penicillin G procaine	50,000 U/kg IM once 25,000 U/kg IM or IV bid for at least 10 days 50,000 U/kg IM daily for at least 10 days	

*Modified from *Med. Lett. Drugs Ther.* 26:5, 1984.

negative enteric bacteria, pneumococci, and *N. meningitidis* are less commonly involved. Tuberculous arthritis is uncommon.

b. Evaluation

(1) Careful **examination** of the patient for other foci of infection

(2) **X-ray films** of the joint(s) and adjacent bones

(3) Multiple **blood cultures** and examination of blood and joint fluid by rapid immunologic techniques for microbial antigen detection (see **I.A.3.c**).

(4) **Arthrocentesis.** To avoid introducing bacteria, joint aspiration is performed with full surgical asepsis. Analysis of the joint fluid includes Gram stain, culture (including plating on prewarmed chocolate agar if *H. influenzae* or *Neisseria* is suspected), WBC and differential, total protein, and joint/blood glucose ratio.

(5) Joint infection may be overlooked in the toxic, prostrate patient with bacteremia. **Delayed diagnosis may result in extensive damage to growth cartilages.**

(6) Hip involvement is common in children, and this joint is difficult to assess. **Repeated examinations of the hips and all other joints** is an important aspect of managing bacteremic patients.

c. Diagnosis. The presence of bacteria in the synovial fluid establishes the diagnosis. Joint or blood cultures, or both, are positive in most patients with septic arthritis.

d. Therapy

(1) **Drainage.** Prompt aspiration of the affected joint is both diagnostic and therapeutic, since adequate drainage is critical to the prevention of sequelae. Whether or not open surgical drainage or repeated needle aspiration is chosen depends on the **joint involved** (e.g., the hip and shoulder usually require surgical drainage); **age** (infants and young children usually require surgical drainage); **viscosity** of the synovial exudate; the offending **pathogen** (staphylococcal disease usually necessitates surgical drainage, while meningococcal or gonococcal arthritis may require only needle aspiration); and the **response** of the patient to antibiotics.

(2) **Antibiotics.** The initial choice of antibiotics is based on the gram-stained smear of the synovial fluid and the patient's age.

(a) In the absence of a diagnostic Gram stain, the initial choice should include a penicillinase-resistant penicillin (e.g., oxacillin, 200 mg/kg/day q4h IV, up to 12 gm/day). For children 2 months–5 years of age, an agent effective against *H. influenzae* should be added (chloramphenicol, 75 mg/kg/day q6h, IV).

(b) Once the pathogen is identified, therapy may require modification to provide the most effective drug with the least toxicity.

(c) Because antibiotics diffuse well into synovial fluid, local instillation is not necessary.

(d) Antibiotic therapy for 2–3 weeks is usually sufficient.

(3) Other therapeutic measures include early immobilization of the joint and physical therapy when the inflammation subsides.

2. Acute osteomyelitis

a. Etiology

(1) *S. aureus* is the organism responsible in 75–80% of cases.

(2) Other organisms include group A streptococci, pneumococci, and *H. influenzae*. Special associations include *Salmonella* in sickle cell anemia, gram-negative enteric pathogens and group B streptococci in neonates, and *P. aeruginosa* following a penetrating injury of the foot or in drug addicts. Mycobacteria are rare causes.

b. Evaluation

(1) **A careful search for metastatic infection in other bones and soft tissues is indicated.**

(2) Multiple blood cultures, cultures of other sites, x-ray films, and radionuclide scans of suspected bony sites.

(3) In the presence of localized bony tenderness and a positive bone scan, needle aspiration of the bone for Gram stain and culture is indicated.

c. The **diagnosis** is based on the characteristic clinical picture and results of needle aspiration or bone biopsy. Although the classic radiologic findings of disease may not appear until 10 or more days, deep soft tissue swelling **in conjunction with local bone tenderness** is good evidence of osteomyelitis. Bone scans may provide early confirmation.

d. Therapy. Prevention of chronic osteomyelitis and other sequelae depends on early diagnosis and treatment.

(1) Administration of a penicillinase-resistant penicillin (e.g., oxacillin, 200 mg/kg/day q4h IV, up to 12 gm/day) is started as soon as the appropriate cultures have been obtained.

(2) A second antibiotic is chosen if an organism other than *S. aureus* is suspected (e.g., chloramphenicol in the child < 5 years of age or when *H. influenzae* is a possibility).

(3) Patients with sickle cell anemia should also receive ampicillin, 200 mg/kg/day q4h IV; neonates should be given gentamicin, 5.0–7.5 mg/kg/day q8–12h IV.

(4) *Pseudomonas* osteomyelitis usually requires surgical drainage as well as antibiotic therapy with gentamicin and carbenicillin.

(5) Surgical drainage should be considered for most long-bone infections unless the history prior to diagnosis is short and the response to antibiotic therapy is prompt.

(6) Antibiotic therapy is usually given for 4–6 weeks. In patients responding promptly, therapy may be completed with oral antibiotics (e.g., dicloxacillin, 100 mg/kg/day q6h PO), provided the organism is known, compliance is certain (e.g., the child remains in the hospital), and serum inhibitory and bactericidal titers are monitored (*J. Pediatr.* 92:485, 1978).

(7) Initial immobilization of the affected limb helps to relieve pain.

K. Infections of the cardiovascular system

1. Infective endocarditis

a. Etiology. In children, congenital heart disease is present in most cases of bacterial endocarditis. Predisposing lesions include tetralogy of Fallot, ventricular septal defect, patent ductus arteriosus, aortic stenosis, and coarctation. Cyanotic children with shunts (Blalock, Waterston, Potts) are also at risk.

(1) A prior event leading to bacteremia (e.g., dental manipulation or infection or manipulation of the GI or genitourinary tracts) or prior cardiac surgery (e.g., prosthetic valve implantation or creation of an aortopulmonic shunt) is not infrequently implicated as a precipitating factor.

(2) Viridans streptococci and *S. aureus* are most commonly involved.

(3) *Haemophilus* species, *S. pneumoniae,* group A streptococci, and anaerobes rarely cause endocarditis in children; enterococci cause it infrequently. When infection complicates cardiac surgery, *S. epidermidis,* gram-negatives, and fungi should be considered.

b. Evaluation includes the following:

(1) A **history,** with special attention to fever (particularly its duration, height, and time of onset), malaise, and symptoms of embolism (to the brain, kidneys, or spleen).

(2) **Physical examination,** with attention to cardiac auscultation for new or changing murmurs; cutaneous manifestations such as petechiae, splinter hemorrhages, Osler's nodes, Janeway lesions; splenomegaly; and, if indicated, needle marks from ilicit drug use.

(3) **Laboratory studies,** including a CBC, erythrocyte sedimentation rate

(ESR), and urinalysis, should be obtained. Urine culture, multiple microscopic examinations of fresh urine sediment for red blood cells and red cell casts, cultures of possible noncardiac foci, chest x-ray, serum complement, serum protein analysis, and rheumatoid factor are recommended.

(4) Cultures of blood (six sets over a 48-hour period) from different sites should be obtained before starting therapy in subacute bacterial endocarditis. In the seriously ill child who requires immediate therapy, at least three sets of blood cultures should be obtained.

(5) Since bacteremia is continuous in endocarditis, there is no advantage to culturing only with temperature spikes or to drawing blood for culture from arteries rather than veins. If antibiotics have recently been given, the drug(s) should be discontinued before blood culture is obtained.

(6) Once isolated, the causative organism should be saved. After appropriate antibiotics have been started, serum bactericidal levels should be determined [see **d.(4)**].

(7) **Echocardiographic evaluation** can be helpful in establishing a presumptive diagnosis and in following the course of the infection.

c. The **diagnosis** is established by positive blood cultures in association with a compatible clinical picture:

(1) Typically the bacteremia is low grade and continuous. Consequently, the majority (85–90%) of blood cultures are positive.

(2) Splenomegaly is common.

(3) The development of a new regurgitant murmur and extracardiac findings indicating systemic emboli or vasculitis are significant.

(4) **Laboratory abnormalities** include anemia, leukocytosis with a shift to the left, elevated ESR, microscopic hematuria, and hyperglobulinemia.

(5) When the blood cultures are negative, a presumptive diagnosis is based on the typical clinical syndrome.

d. Therapy

(1) If the diagnosis is clinically evident, initiation of antibiotics is reasonable while the results of the blood cultures are still pending.

(2) In acute bacterial endocarditis, therapy with penicillinase-resistant penicillin and gentamicin **should be initiated within several hours of the patient's admission to the hospital.**

(3) Once the pathogen has been identified, recommended antibiotics are as follows (see Table 15-2):

(a) **Viridans streptococci.** Aqueous penicillin G, 250,000 units/kg/day q4h IV, up to 20 MU daily.

(b) **S. aureus.** A penicillinase-resistant penicillin (e.g., oxacillin, 200 mg/kg/day q4h IV) should be given. In severely ill patients, gentamicin (4.5–7.5 mg/kg/day q8h IV) may be added for the first 7–10 days. Vancomycin (40 mg/kg/day q6h IV) is an alternative in penicillin-allergic patients.

(c) **Enterococci.** Give ampicillin, 300 mg/kg/day q4h IV, and gentamicin, 3.0–7.5 mg/kg/day q8h IV.

(4) Drug therapy is individualized on the basis of the organism's in vitro sensitivities and the results of serum bactericidal tests. A serum bactericidal level of 1:8 or greater at the time of peak antibiotic concentration is desirable. Although subjective improvement (e.g., in appetite) may be prompt, fever can remain elevated for several days after initiation of antibiotic therapy.

(5) In general, the duration of antibiotic therapy is 4–6 weeks.

(6) In addition to a daily physical examination, the erythrocyte sedimentation rate and urinalyses are useful variables to follow.

(7) Recurrent manifestations attributed to embolization and associated vasculitis do not necessarily indicate failure of antibiotic therapy.

(8) **Surgical replacement** of the infected valve, when indicated, may be lifesaving. The indications for surgery in endocarditis include congestive heart failure refractory to medical therapy, more than one major embolic episode, worsening valve function, ineffective therapy (as in fungal endocarditis), mycotic aneurysm, and most cases of prosthetic valve endocarditis.

e. Prevention of endocarditis. Prophylactic antibiotic regimens are outlined in Table 15-9. The choice of regimen should be individualized according to the risk of the underlying heart disease and the risk of the procedure. The regimens requiring parenteral administration of potentially toxic antibiotics should be reserved for high-risk situations.

(1) Patients with prosthetic heart valves or grafts are at highest risk; patients with rheumatic heart disease are also at high risk. Patients with congenital heart diseases, such as ventricular septal defect, atrial septal defect, patent ductus arteriosus, and the "click-murmur" syndrome, are at lower risk.

(2) High-risk procedures are dental manipulations, especially surgery and tooth extractions in patients with poor oral hygiene, and manipulations of the infected genitourinary tract, especially when enterococci are present. Procedures such as bronchoscopy, endoscopy, proctosigmoidoscopy, barium enemas, and liver biopsies may be associated with bacteremia but have a lower risk.

2. Acute rheumatic fever

a. Etiology. Acute rheumatic fever (ARF) is a sequel of pharyngeal infection with a group A streptococcus, but the exact pathogenesis is still unknown. It has been proposed that the disease may be (1) a direct reaction to streptococcal extracellular or cellular substances; or (2) an immunologic process stimulated by *Streptococcus;* or (3) a persistent infection by *Streptococcus* or one of its variants.

b. Evaluation should include the following:

(1) A **history,** with emphasis on antecedent infections, fever, arthralgia, and previous RF, as well as a familial and social history.

(2) **Physical examination,** with attention to joints, skin (rashes and subcutaneous nodules), and the cardiovascular system.

(3) **Laboratory studies** should include ESR, C-reactive protein, CBC, ECG, chest x-ray, streptococcal antibodies (antistreptolysin O, anti-DNase B, anti-NADase, antihyaluronidase), and throat culture.

c. Diagnosis

(1) No single laboratory test, symptom, or sign is pathognomonic, although several combinations are suggestive of ARF.

(2) According to the revised Jones criteria, RF is likely in the presence of one major and two minor criteria [see **(4)** and **(5)**], or two major criteria plus evidence of a preceding streptococcal infection. Chorea alone may be sufficient for a diagnosis, **but**

(3) **ARF may not fulfill the revised Jones criteria,** especially early in the disease. Conversely, other diseases, such as rheumatoid arthritis, systemic lupus erythematosus, Schönlein-Henoch purpura, serum sickness, sickle cell hemoglobinopathy, and septic or postinfectious arthritis may occasionally fulfill the criteria at certain points in their natural history.

(4) **Major criteria**

(a) **Carditis**

(b) **Polyarthritis.** Tenderness, usually with heat, swelling, and redness, involving more than one joint especially, but not exclusively, and involving the larger joints, especially the knee, ankle, elbow, wrist, and hip.

(c) **Subcutaneous nodules** usually occur only in children with severe carditis of several weeks' duration.

    (d) Erythema marginatum is an uncommon finding in RF and is not specific to the disease.

    (e) Chorea is often associated with emotional instability.

  (5) Minor criteria

    (a) Fever. Rarely, above 40°C (104°F) or associated with shaking chills.

    (b) Arthralgias. Joint pain without objective findings

    (c) Prolonged P-R interval on the ECG (not in and of itself diagnostic of carditis)

    (d) Increased ESR, C-reactive protein, leukocytosis

    (e) Previous history of ARF or rheumatic heart disease

  (6) Other criteria include epistaxis, abdominal pain, and rheumatic pneumonia.

d. Treatment

  (1) Eradication of streptococci. See Table 15-2.

  (2) Antiinflammatory agents

    (a) Aspirin is indicated for arthritis without carditis and possibly in children with mild cardiac involvement. The dosage of acetylsalicylic acid is 100 mg/kg/day in 4–6 divided doses for 3–4 weeks. The optimal serum level is about 20–25 mg/100 ml. Although salicylates undoubtedly give symptomatic relief, there is no proof that they alter the course of the myocardial damage.

    (b) Corticosteroids have been controversial in the therapy of ARF since their introduction.

      (i) Corticosteroids are almost mandatory in patients with severe carditis and CHF. Prednisone, 2 mg/kg/day for 4–6 weeks, is given, with tapering over the next 2 weeks. Corticosteroids reduce inflammation promptly, but there is no conclusive evidence that they prevent residual valvular damage.

      (ii) In patients with carditis without cardiomegaly or CHF, the use of corticosteroids instead of salicylates remains controversial and more a matter of personal preference.

  (3) Anticongestive measures, including digitalis (see Chap. 9, pp. 248ff), should be used in patients with ARF in the same fashion as in other patients with CHF, despite possible increased sensitivity in the inflamed myocardium.

  (4) Bed rest is accepted during the acute phase when CHF is present. In the absence of objective data, we think it is prudent to keep children on limited activity, if not on bed rest, until the ESR returns to normal.

  (5) Children with chorea should be moved to a quiet environment with understanding nurses and should be protected against self-inflicted injury due to uncontrollable movements. Drug treatment with phenobarbital, chlorpromazine, diazepam, and haloperidol has been tried, with varying success.

  (6) Prevention of rheumatic recurrences

    (a) All children with documented RF with or without carditis—and all those with rheumatic heart disease—should receive prophylaxis against a second attack (see Table 15-9).

    (b) Any of the following approaches is acceptable, provided compliance is assured. If severe residual heart disease is present or the patient is unreliable, the first alternative is preferable.

      (i) Benzathine penicillin, 1.2 million U every 28 days

      (ii) Penicillin G or V, 200,000–250,000 U PO qd-bid

      (iii) Sulfadiazine, 0.5 mg/day for those weighing under 30 kg; 1 gm/day for those weighing over 30 kg

      (iv) Erythromycin, 250 mg PO bid, in patients sensitive to both sulfonamides and penicillin

3. Myocarditis. See Chap. 9, p. 254.

L. Tuberculosis

1. Etiology. *M. tuberculosis* is the infecting organism.

2. Evaluation

  a. Clinical manifestations of childhood tuberculosis (TB) include:

    (1) Persistent cough, pulmonary infiltrates, and pleural effusion or enlarged hilar nodes

    (2) Chronic draining otitis media, cervical adenopathy

    (3) Aseptic meningitis

    (4) Occult fever, failure to thrive, weight loss, and anemia or hepatosplenomegaly

    (5) Aseptic pyuria

    (6) Monoarticular arthritis, dactylitis, back pain, or bony tenderness

  b. Screening. The tuberculin skin test is the best means of identifying infected children. Serious tuberculous disease (e.g., meningitis, miliary disease) will almost never develop in the child with primary tuberculosis who receives isoniazid prophylaxis for a year. An annual or biennial tuberculin test is recommended by the American Academy of Pediatrics for the office or outpatient clinic, unless local circumstances necessitate more frequent testing. For screening, the tine test is adequate, but an intermediate-strength PPD (5-TU) is indicated for patients whose tine tests are positive or who are suspected of having TB.

  c. When TB is suspected, a detailed inquiry into possible contacts with persons with active TB, an intermediate strength PPD (5 U) and a chest x-ray are essential.

  d. Atypical (nontuberculous) mycobacteria can cause cervical adenitis or (uncommonly) pulmonary infection. These strains are often resistant to conventional TB therapy. Nontuberculous strains may cross-react with intermediate strength PPD, but the reaction is usually less than 10 mm unless infection is recent.

  e. In the presence of a positive skin test and chest x-ray, the following should be done:

    (1) Obtain and culture three **gastric** aspirates in the morning, immediately on the patient's awakening.

    (2) Culture three **first-voided** morning urine collections.

    (3) Liver function tests. A liver biopsy, or bone marrow biopsy, may be necessary if miliary disease is suspected. A pleural biopsy may be diagnostic in patients with pleural effusions.

  f. In the presence of neurologic abnormalities, **CSF examination,** including culture and acid-fast stain, is necessary.

  g. In proved cases of TB, **skin tests and chest x-rays of family members and contacts** are indicated.

3. Diagnosis

  a. The demonstration of acid-fast bacilli in exudate or tissue is the most direct method of diagnosis. The judicious use of needle biopsy specimens of pleura, liver, or bone marrow often yields the diagnosis.

  b. The culture may not become positive for 3–6 weeks, but a presumptive diagnosis of TB is often made on the basis of the clinical presentation, epidemiologic history, and skin test reactivity to tuberculin antigen. Induration greater than or equal to 10 mm from an intermediate strength PPD generally indicates prior infection with the tuberculosis bacillus (symptomatic or asymptomatic).

4. Therapy. See also Table 15-10.

  a. Asymptomatic converter (positive skin test with a negative chest x-ray). Oral isoniazid, 10 mg/kg (maximum of 300 mg) once daily for 1 year. Follow-up chest x-rays are obtained at 3- to 6-month intervals and again on completion of therapy.

  ʰ Primary nonprogressive pulmonary TB (including an effusion) and

cervical adenitis. Oral isoniazid, 10 mg/kg/day q24hr, plus rifampin, 10 mg/kg/day q24hr, or para-aminosalicylic acid (PAS), 0.2–0.3 gm/day. Ethambutol, 15 mg/kg/day, is given in place of PAS for patients over 13 years of age. The major side effect of ethambutol is optic neuritis (blurred vision, color blindness, visual field alteration), which is difficult to monitor in younger children.

   c. **Tuberculous meningitis, progressive pulmonary disease, and miliary TB.** Isoniazid (20 mg/kg/day) and rifampim (10 mg/kg/day) for 12–24 months plus streptomycin (20–40 mg/kg/day to 1 gm/day) for the first 4 weeks of therapy.

   d. **Nonpulmonary primary disease, skeletal TB, and urinary tract TB.** Treatment is as described in **b** for 12–24 months.

   e. If the isolated *M. tuberculosis* is resistant in vitro to isoniazid, a number of other agents are available. When possible, in vitro susceptibility testing should guide their selection. In patients from areas where resistance is endemic, initial therapy for most forms of TB should include three first-line agents.

   f. **Household contacts**

      (1) Household exposure to an adolescent or adult with active TB requires isoniazid prophylaxis (10 mg/kg/day). If the child's PPD is still negative at 3 months, and if the person with active TB is under regular treatment or has left the home, the child's treatment may be discontinued. Periodic tuberculin tests should be followed.

      (2) The infant born to a woman with active tuberculosis should be separated from the mother until she is considered noncontagious. BCG may be helpful when close medical supervision of the infant in the first year of life cannot be guaranteed. Isoniazid for 1 year is probably effective prophylaxis, but its potential neurotoxicity must be considered.

   g. **Pyridoxine,** 25–50 mg once daily, is unnecessary in children under 10 years of age unless nutrition is inadequate.

   h. Corticosteroids given in conjunction with antimicrobial therapy may lessen the inflammatory complications of tuberculous pericarditis and pleuritis. They may also be indicated when large hilar lymph nodes are obstructing the passage of air and when severe respiratory distress complicates diffuse pulmonary tuberculosis. In meningitis, corticosteroids may reduce increased intracranial pressure.

   i. Isoniazid treatment commonly causes a transient asymptomatic elevation of liver enzymes during the first 3 months of therapy. Routine monitoring for hepatotoxicity is unnecessary, but if overt hepatotoxicity occurs, the drug should be discontinued.

M. Fungal diseases

   1. Candidiasis

   a. **Etiology.** *C. albicans* is the most common pathogen, but other species, including *C. tropicalis, C. krusei, C. parapsilosis,* and *C. guillermondii* may also cause invasive disease.

   b. **Evaluation**

      (1) **Cultures** of the blood, urine, oropharynx, and stool

      (2) **Gram stain** and KOH prep of mucosal lesions.

      (3) If esophageal involvement is suspected, a **barium swallow** and **esophagoscopy** (with biopsy and culture of lesions) are most helpful.

      (4) If disseminated disease is suspected, the ocular fundi and skin should be carefully examined. Cardiac ultrasound and lumbar puncture may be indicated.

   c. **Diagnosis.** The demonstration of yeasts and pseudohyphae in scrapings of skin or mucosal lesions or tissue specimens is diagnostic. Repeated isolation of *Candida* from the blood suggests endocarditis, an infected intravascular device (e.g., a hyperalimentation line), or disseminated candidiasis. Recovery of $> 10^3$ organisms/ml suggests urinary tract infection.

   d. **Treatment.** The duration of therapy depends on severity of disease and speed of response.

   (1) Esophagitis in immunocompromised hosts can be treated with amphotericin B (to 1 mg/kg/day) for 7–10 days.

   (2) Disseminated infection, endocarditis, and meningitis should be treated with full doses of amphotericin B (1 mg/kg/day). 5-Fluorocytosine (150 mg/kg/day q6h) may be added in seriously ill patients, but only if the organism is sensitive to this agent.

   (3) Candidal infection restricted to the bladder may respond to continuous irrigation with amphotericin B (50 mg/1000 ml) (maximum dose, 1 mg/kg/day in sterile **distilled water**). Infection restricted to the bladder or kidney may also be treated with 5-fluorocytosine alone, 50–100 mg/kg/day PO q6h for 7 days.

   (4) Chronic mucocutaneous candidiasis has been successfully treated with oral ketoconazole.

2. **Cryptococcosis**

   a. **Etiology.** The causative organism is *C. neoformans*.

   b. **Evaluation**

   (1) History. Respiratory symptoms and subtle neurologic symptoms, including headache and diplopia

   (2) CSF examination, including India ink preparation, culture for fungus, and cryptococcal antigen test. Culture yields are improved by culturing a large volume of CSF.

   (3) Sputum and urine culture for fungus

   (4) Cryptococcal antigen test on the serum and urine

   (5) Chest x-ray; occasionally, a lung biopsy is necessary.

   c. **Diagnosis.** The presence of cryptococcal antigen in the CSF, serum, or urine or a "positive" India ink smear strongly suggests the diagnosis. The diagnosis is established by the growth of cryptococci from CSF or lung tissue.

   d. **Treatment**

   (1) Cryptococcal meningitis may be treated with a combination of amphotericin B, 0.3 mg/kg/day, and 5-fluorocytosine, 150 mg/kg/day PO divided q6h for at least 6 weeks. Patients with severe marrow impairment in whom further marrow suppression from 5-fluorocytosine may develop may be treated with amphotericin B alone (1 mg/kg/day) to a total dose of 2 or 3 gm.

   (2) Treatment should be monitored with weekly examination of the CSF by culture and India ink smear and for cryptococcal antigen concentration. Cultures should become sterile promptly. Microscopy should show a decrease in the number of organisms, and antigen testing should show at least a fourfold decrease in level during treatment.

   (3) After completion of treatment, the CSF should be examined q2–3 months for 1 year to detect relapses.

   e. **Cryptococcal pneumonia,** in the absence of dissemination to the CNS, may not require therapy unless it is progressive. Close observation for at least 1–2 months is necessary if treament is not given.

3. **Invasive aspergillosis**

   a. **Etiology.** A variety of *Aspergillus* species are pathogenic in humans, the most common being *A. fumigatus*.

   b. **Evaluation**

   (1) Careful examination for sinusitis, necrotic nasal lesions, pneumonia, pleuritic pain, and necrotizing skin lesions

   (2) X-rays of the sinuses and chest

   (3) Direct microscopic examination and **culture of sputum** and **biopsy specimens from suspected sites.** Early diagnosis is essential, and biopsies should be performed promptly.

    c. Diagnosis
       (1) Demonstration of septate hyphae 3–4 μ in diameter with an acute (45-degree) angle branching in tissues is diagnostic of invasive aspergillosis.
       (2) A chest x-ray showing a ball within a cavity is suggestive of aspergilloma.
    d. The **treatment** for invasive aspergillosis is amphotericin B, 0.75–1 mg/kg/day (for total dosage 30–35 mg/kg over a period of 6 weeks or longer) and surgical débridement of cutaneous and sinus lesions. In severely ill patients, rifampin may be added.

V. Antiviral therapy
  A. Principles
    1. Viruses are obligate intracellular parasites that depend on the host cell for growth and replication. Clinically useful antiviral agents must act at stages of infection or replication involving virus-specific metabolic activities.
    2. The **toxicity** of antiviral drugs depends on the degree to which the metabolic apparatus of the host cell is able to utilize the drug. Most new antiviral agents have little or no toxicity.
  B. Antiviral agents in clinical use
    1. Amantadine has a mechanism of action that is not fully understood. It may interfere with penetration and uncoating of virus.
      a. Antiviral spectrum. Active against all influenza A strains but not against influenza B.
      b. Pharmacology. Rapidly absorbed from the GI tract, with peak blood levels 2–4 hr after an oral dose. Of an orally administered dose of amantadine, 90% is excreted unchanged in the urine and has a serum half-life of 20 hr.
      c. Adverse effects. Amantadine is well tolerated in children. In 3–7% of healthy adults there are CNS symptoms such as difficulty in thinking, confusion, light-headedness, hallucinations, anxiety, and insomnia.
      d. Clinical indications. Amantadine is useful in chemoprophylaxis of influenza A in unvaccinated persons at high risk and provides 60% protection against clinical illness. It is also useful in chemotherapy of infection, if begun in the first 24–48 hr of illness, and results in a diminution of fever and a reduction in the duration of illness.
    2. Adenine-arabinoside (vidarabine, Ara-A, Vira-A) blocks DNA synthesis by inhibiting the activity of the virus-specific DNA polymerase.
      a. Antiviral spectrum. Ara-A has activity against the herpesviruses, pox viruses, vaccinia, and possibly hepatitis B.
      b. Pharmacology. Ara-A is rapidly deaminated to arabinosyl hypoxanthine and excreted in the urine. The plasma half-life is 4 hr. The drug is poorly soluble and must be given parenterally in large volumes of fluid. The 3% ophthalmic ointment has poor ocular penetration.
      c. Adverse effects. In small numbers of patients, nausea, vomiting, and diarrhea develop at doses less than 15 mg/kg/day. At 20 mg/kg/day, tremors, weight loss, and bone marrow megaloblastosis are seen. Doses of 30 mg/kg/day produce thrombocytopenia and leukopenia. There is occasional neurologic toxicity consisting of tremors, ataxia, painful paresthesias, encephalopathy, or abnormal EEG findings.
      d. Clinical indications. Ara-A is currently approved for use in herpes simplex encephalitis, neonatal herpes, and topically in acute herpetic keratoconjunctivitis and recurrent epithelial keratitis.
    3. Acyclovir (acycloguanosine) acts as an inhibitor of the virus-specific DNA polymerase after being converted to the phosphorylated active form by a virus-specific thymidine kinase.
      a. Antiviral spectrum. Acyclovir is active against herpes simplex types 1 and 2, varicella-zoster, and Epstein-Barr virus.
      b. Pharmacology. The pharmacology of acyclovir is not yet fully detailed. It

Table 15-13. Common childhood viral exanthams

Disease	Prodrome	Rash	Other diagnostic signs
Measles	3–4 days of fever, conjunctivitis, coryza, and cough	Reddish-brown maculopapular rash appears first on face and neck, then spreads to trunk and extremities. Brawny desquamation last 5–6 days (*no* desquamation of hands and feet).	Koplik's spots
Rubella	No prodrome in children	Discrete pink maculopapular rash appears first on face and neck, then spreads to trunk and extremities. Rash disappears in 3 days in same order as it appeared. No desquamation.	Lymphadenopathy
Varicella	Mild or absent	Clear vesicles on an erythematous base, small pustules, and small crusted ulcers. Lesions appear in crops. Several stages of lesions are usually present at one time. Very pruritic crops appear over 3–5 days. More lesions on trunk than extremities.	Lesions may appear on mucous membranes

is well absorbed both topically and orally and may also be given parenterally.

    c. Adverse effects. Toxicity has thus far proved to be minimal.

    d. Clinical indications. Acyclovir is currently being evaluated in experimental trials.

  4. Interferon acts by binding to specific cell-surface receptors and inducing the production of cellular enzymes that subsequently block viral reproduction by inhibiting the translation of viral messenger RNA into viral protein.

    a. Antiviral spectrum. Interferon is not virus specific and can interfere with a wide variety of DNA and RNA viruses.

    b. Pharmacology. Interferon is usually administered IM and has a half-life of 4–6 hr. Little is known about its metabolism.

    c. Adverse effects. Most adverse effects seem to relate to the purity of the preparation. Fever, nausea, vomiting, local erythema and pain, leukopenia, and thrombocytopenia are seen.

    d. Clinical indications. Interferon is currently undergoing clinical trials and has not yet been released for use.

 C. Treatment of specific viral diseases. (For evaluation and clinical features of childhood viral exanthams, see Table 15-13.)

  1. Hepatitis

    a. Etiology. Hepatitis can be caused by a wide range of viruses. The most common agents are hepatitis A (infectious hepatitis), hepatitis B (serum hepatitis), and hepatitis non-A, non-B (which is probably more than one virus and is now a diagnosis of exclusion). Other viruses that can cause hepatitis include Epstein-Barr virus, cytomegalovirus and coxsackievirus A and B. Neonatal hepatitis may be the result of infection with herpesvirus, cytomegalovirus, echoviruses, or toxoplasmosis.

b. Diagnosis. The common hepatitis viruses cannot be cultured, and diagnosis is made primarily by serology. Tests include the following:

(1) **Hepatitis A antibody.** An IgM antibody rise to hepatitis A indicates acute hepatitis.

(2) Hepatitis B surface antigen (HBsAg), formerly called Australia antigen (HAA) can be present both in acute disease and in the carrier state.

(3) Antibody to HBsAg (anti-HBs) develops after an infection and is indicative of immunity.

(4) Hepatitis B e antigen (HBeAg) is a soluble antigen that correlates with a high titer of hepatitis B virus in the serum and a high degree of infectivity.

(5) The presence of antibody to HBeAg (anti-HBe) indicates a low rate of infectivity in a HBsAg carrier.

(6) Heterophil or Monospot

(7) Serology for toxoplasmosis

(8) Viral cultures if cytomegalovirus or enteroviruses are suspected

c. Treatment

(1) There is no specific therapy for viral hepatitis.

(2) Prophylactic immune globulin should be given to contacts. (See p. 366 for IG for hepatitis A immunization.)

(a) **Hepatitis A** immune globulin in a dose of 0.02 ml/kg should be given to household, sexual, and day care contacts as soon as possible after exposure.

(b) **Hepatitis B.** Percutaneous inoculation by needlestick or transfusion or exposure of contact's mucous membranes or newborn exposure to infectious material requires prophylaxis with either immune globulin or high-titer hepatitis B immune globulin and may require vaccine according to Table 15-14.

2. Herpes simplex infections

a. Genital herpes

(1) **Etiology.** Usually involves herpesvirus (HSV) type 2; HSV type 1 occurs less frequently.

(2) **Evaluation** may include a Tzanck preparation of vesicles to look for multinucleated giant cells and/or tissue culture recovery of the virus.

(3) **Therapy.** Many agents have been tried, but none has proved efficacious to date. Symptomatic therapy is indicated, with treatment of superinfection with antibiotics.

b. Herpes simplex encephalitis

(1) **Etiology.** Usually, HSV type 1; rarely, HSV type 2.

(2) **Evaluation**

(a) The **history** often includes olfactory hallucinations, headache, and confusion.

(b) **Physical examination** may reveal focal neurologic signs.

(c) A brain scan, EEG, and CT will usually reveal a focal defect, most often in the temporal lobe(s).

(d) An accurate **diagnosis** requires isolation of virus from a brain biopsy specimen, since several often treatable diseases may mimic HSV encephalitis.

(e) **Immunofluorescence assays** for HSV antigen on frozen brain sections are less sensitive than viral cultures, but can result in an earlier diagnosis.

(f) Orofacial HSV infection or rising antibody titers are not diagnostic.

Table 15-14. Hepatitis B immune globulin and vaccine prophylaxis

Exposure	HBsAg testing	Recommended prophylaxis*
HBsAg-positive person	—	HBIG (0.06 ml/kg IM) within 24 hr and 1 month later*

HBsAg status unknown
  High risk for positivity
    Acute hepatitis
    Institutionalized Down syndrome patients
    Hemodialysis
    IV drug user
    Male homosexual
    Person of Asian origin
	Yes (if results can be obtained within 7 days of exposure)	IG (0.06 ml/kg) immediately, and, if HBsAg is positive: HBIG (0.06 ml/kg) immediately *and* 1 month thereafter*; if HBsAg is negative, no further therapy needed.

Low risk for positivity Average hospital patients	No	Nothing or IG (0.06 ml/kg)
Source unknown	No	Nothing or IG (0.06 ml/kg)
Exposure of a newborn to an HBsAg-positive mother (especially those mothers who are also HBeAg positive)		HBIG (0.5 ml IM) within 12 hr of birth and hepatitis B vaccine*

Source: Adapted from the recommendations of the Immunization Practices Advisory Committee. *M.M.W.R.* 30:423, 1981 and 33:285, 1984.
*For use of hepatitis B vaccine, see *M.M.W.R.* 33:285, 1984.

   (3) Therapy
      (a) Careful management of increased intracranial pressure (ICP)
      (b) Adenine arabinoside is now the drug of choice. The dosage is 15 mg/kg/day given by slow IV infusion over 12 hr for 10 days.
         (i) A brain biopsy prior to initiation of therapy is considered optimal medical management.
         (ii) Adenine arabinoside is discontinued after 5 days if the viral culture is negative.
         (iii) The drug is poorly soluble and requires 2 ml of IV solution per mg for suspension. Fluid overload should be avoided. The WBC, platelet, and reticulocyte counts should be followed.
      (c) Acyclovir may become the drug of choice in the future.
  c. Disseminated herpes simplex
    (1) Etiology. Usually HSV type 1 in older children and HSV type 2 in neonates
    (2) Evaluation
      (a) The **history** will usually include evidence of immunosuppression as the result of immunodeficiency or chemotherapy.
      (b) The **physical examination** should include careful inspection for evidence of complications such as bacterial superinfection, tenderness of the liver, or pneumonia.
    (3) Adenine arabinoside in a dose of 30 mg/kg/day is the drug of choice in neonatal herpes. Immunocompromised children should receive 5 mg/kg of acyclovir IV q8h for 7 days.
3. Infectious mononucleosis syndromes are most commonly the result of infection with Epstein-Barr virus but can also be due to cytomegalovirus or toxoplasmosis.

- **a. Epstein-Barr Virus (EBV)**
  - **(1) Evaluation**
    - **(a)** The **history** includes sore throat, malaise, and fever.
    - **(b)** The **physical examination** may reveal fever, lymphadenopathy, splenomegaly, hepatomegaly, jaundice, periorbital edema, and/or rash, with or without an exudative pharyngitis.
    - **(c) Laboratory findings** include lymphocytosis with 10% or more atypical lymphocytes, a positive Monospot after the second week of illness, and/or a heterophil titer of over 1:32. Children under 3 may not have a positive Monospot but will have positive serology for EBV (antibody to viral capsid antigen).
  - **(2) Treatment**
    - **(a)** Primarily supportive. The illness usually lasts 5–20 days, with a prolonged convalescence.
    - **(b)** For airway compromise or marked splenomegaly, prednisone, 1–2 mg/kg/day for 5–7 days, is recommended.
    - **(c)** Avoid ampicillin, since it may cause rashes.
    - **(d)** To avoid splenic rupture, strenuous activity should be prohibited while the spleen is enlarged.
- **b. Cytomegalovirus**
  - **(1) Evaluation**
    - **(a)** The physical findings and history are similar to those for EBV.
    - **(b)** Monospot or EBV serology is negative.
    - **(c)** Diagnose by a rise in antibody to CMV or by culture of the virus.
  - **(2) Treatment** is supportive.
- **c. Toxoplasmosis.** See Chap. 16, pp. 434ff.
- **4. Varicella-zoster**
  - **a. Etiology.** Herpes zoster and varicella (chickenpox) are caused by varicella zoster virus (VZV). The reactivation of VZV months or years after chickenpox occurs in a dorsal spinal or cranial nerve ganglion, with spread to the appropriate cutaneous dermatome and occasionally to distant sites. The spread of infection to visceral organs (disseminated zoster or chickenpox) is usually due to underlying immunodeficiency.
  - **b. Evaluation and diagnosis**
    - **(1)** In zoster patients, the **history** should exclude other causes of localized vesicular disease.
    - **(2)** The **physical examination** should include careful inspection for the number and character of vesicles and for evidence of complications such as bacterial superinfection, cutaneous dissemination, tenderness in the abdomen or liver, and paresis of the muscles in the involved area (e.g., urinary retention). When cranial nerve V is involved, vesicles on the tip of the nose (innervated by the nasociliary branch) suggest the possibility of keratoconjunctivitis and/or uveitis.
    - **(3)** A Tzanck preparation is done to look for multinucleated giant cells. Without a viral culture the diagnosis of herpes zoster is not completely reliable, since herpes simplex virus can also cause dermatomal involvement.
    - **(4)** In immunosuppressed persons, the tempo of disease and extent of viral spread should be determined by periodic pox counts, serial chest x-rays, serum liver enzyme analyses, and CNS examinations.
  - **c. Treatment**
    - **(1)** Wet-to-dry soaks are applied to involved dermatomes tid, using Burow's solution to facilitate debridement. Superinfection is treated with a penicillinase-resistant oral penicillin and topical antibiotics.
    - **(2)** Pain symptoms are treated appropriately. Since postherpetic neuralgia is not a problem in children, there is no indication for systemic corticosteroids.
    - **(3)** When **cranial nerve V** is involved, referral to an ophthalmologist is indicated.

(4) Scopolamine eyedrops (0.3%) are used to produce **mydriasis** and **cycloplegia.** Corticosteroid drops are indicated when **interstitial keratitis** or **uveitis** is present (in the absence of dendritic keratitis).

(5) Disseminated skin vesicles may occur in 10% of previously healthy persons. This does not indicate an adverse prognosis, and they need not be treated.

(6) In the immunosuppressed person the presence of fever, rapidly increasing numbers of new vesicles, failure of vesicle maturation, elevation of serum liver parenchymal enzymes, and onset of respiratory or CNS symptoms are indications for treatment with adenine arabinoside (10 mg/kg/day). **There is no indication for the use of zoster immune globulin or plasma. Acyclovir** may become the drug of choice in the future.

(7) Broad-spectrum antibiotics are indicated in the febrile neutropenic patient.

(8) Hospital contacts of patients with zoster or chickenpox who have no history of prior chickenpox or whose VZV immunofluorescent antibody tests are negative must be isolated in the hospital, discharged, or kept away from work from the eighth to twenty-first day after exposure.

(9) **Immunosuppressed** children who have not had chickenpox should receive varicella-zoster immune globulin or zoster immune plasma (10 ml/kg) following close exposure to zoster or chickenpox.

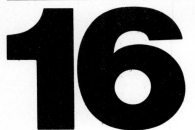

Parasitic Infections

Infections with protozoa and helminths are subject to rational principles of diagnosis and therapy. Most parasitic infections occur in temperate as well as tropical environments. Their incidence varies with climate, sanitation, and socioeconomic conditions. The frequency with which the clinician in temperate areas encounters parasitic infections is increasing, both as a result of intercontinental travel and the use of immunosuppressive agents.

This chapter is limited in scope to the parasitic diseases most commonly encountered by pediatricians in the United States. Diseases not discussed include schistosomiasis, filariasis, trypanosomiasis, and leishmaniasis, despite their impact as major world health problems. Standard parasitology or tropical medicine texts should be consulted.

I. **Principles of diagnosis.** The diagnostic features of common parasitic infections are summarized in Table 16-1.

A. **General**

1. **The diagnosis of parasitic infection can rarely be made on clinical grounds alone.** The clinical picture in many parasitic infections may be identical, and different clinical presentations may be produced by a single parasite. In addition, parasitic infections are often asymptomatic or produce only mild symptoms. Commonly, a diagnosis of parasitic infection is suspected only because of an abnormal, unexpected laboratory finding.

2. **The diagnosis of most helminthic or protozoal infections requires the demonstration of the parasite in body excreta, fluids, or tissue.**

3. Many parasites have an intricate route of migration through the human host and affect several organs successively or simultaneously. The choice of appropriate diagnostic techniques and materials thus rests on some understanding of the life cycles of the possible infecting agents.

4. Knowledge of the **geographic distribution** of parasitic infections and their **mode of acquisition** and **means of spread** often aids diagnosis and therapy. Detailed information is available from standard parasitology texts.

5. **Patients commonly harbor several parasites.** A complete evaluation must be made to avoid overlooking the most important infecting species in each clinical setting.

B. **Hematologic changes in parasitic infections**

1. **Erythrocytes.** Anemia is an inconstant and nonspecific finding in most parasitic infections. It reflects the general nutritional status of the patient rather than any direct effect of the infecting parasite. Iron deficiency anemia in hookworm disease and hemolytic anemia in malaria and babesiosis are exceptions.

2. **Eosinophils**

a. Eosinophilia is often the first clue to the presence of a **helminth** infection. **Protozoa,** conversely, do *not* evoke an eosinophilia. The finding of eosinophilia in amebiasis, malaria, toxoplasmosis, or giardiasis suggests an additional helminth infection.

b. **The level of eosinophilia is of diagnostic aid.** In general, tissue-living helminths evoke a profound eosinophilia, and those that exist within the lumen of the bowel evoke a mild eosinophilia or none at all (Table 16-1).

Table 16-1. Diagnostic features of commonly encountered parasitic infections

Disease	Mode of spread	Location in humans	Clinical features	Laboratory diagnosis	Eosinophilia*	Remarks
Roundworms (nematodes)						
Ascariasis	Fecal-oral	Adult: small intestine; Larvae: lung	Vague abdominal distress; cough and pneumonia during lung migration	Eggs in feces	Usually mild; moderate to marked during migration	Aberrant wanderings may cause clinical disease
Hookworm	Larvae in soil; skin penetration	Small intestine	Vague abdominal distress; anemia in severe infections	Eggs in feces	Mild to moderate	Distinguish infection from disease
Whipworm	Fecal-oral	Large intestine	Rarely symptomatic	Eggs in feces	Absent to mild	
Strongyloidiasis	Larvae in soil; skin penetration	Upper small intestine	Duodenitis; hyperinfection syndrome rarely	Larvae in *fresh stool*; duodenal aspirate	Moderate to marked	
Pinworm	Fecal-oral	Large intestine, perianal area	Perianal pruritus	Scotch-tape swab for eggs; gross examination of area for worms	Absent	Very common; usually asymptomatic
Creeping eruption (cutaneous larva migrans)	Larvae in soil; skin penetration (larvae from dog, cat feces)	Skin	Intensely pruritic, serpiginous skin lesions	Physical examination	Variable	
Visceral larva migrans	Fecal-oral, via pica (eggs from dog, cat feces)	Liver, lung, muscle, eye	Fever, hepatosplenomegaly	Clinical diagnosis	Marked	
Trichinosis	Ingestion of undercooked pork	Striated muscle	Fever, diarrhea, periorbital edema, muscle pain	Biopsy of muscle, skin; serologic tests	Marked	

	Transmission	Location	Symptoms	Diagnosis	Eosinophilia	Distribution
Tapeworms (cestodes)						
Beef tapeworm	Ingestion of undercooked beef	Small intestine	Asymptomatic	Proglottid segments passed with feces	Absent	
Pork tapeworm	Ingestion of undercooked pork	Small intestine	Asymptomatic; rare autoinfection with CNS symptoms (cysticercosis)	Proglottid segments passed with feces	Absent	
Fish tapeworm	Ingestion of raw or undercooked fish	Small intestine	Asymptomatic; rarely, vitamin B_{12} deficiency	Eggs in feces	Absent	
Hydatid disease	Fecal-oral (eggs from carnivore feces)	Liver, lung, bone, brain	Usually asymptomatic; occasionally, pressure symptoms in affected organ	Removal of cyst; skin and serologic tests	Variable	
Flukes (trematodes)						
Schistosoma mansoni	Cercarial in streams; skin penetration	Venules of large intestine	Fever, colitis, hepatomegaly, portal hypertension	Eggs in feces; rectal biopsy	Moderate to marked	Africa, S. America; common in Puerto Ricans
Schistosoma haematobium	Same	Venules of urinary bladder	Fever, malaise, hematuria	Eggs in urine; bladder or rectal biopsy	Moderate to marked	Africa
Schistosoma japonicum	Same	Venules of small intestine	Fever, malaise, abdominal pain, diarrhea, hepatomegaly	Eggs in feces; rectal biopsy	Moderate to marked	S.E. Asia
Protozoa						
Intestinal amebiasis	Fecal-oral	Lumen and wall of large intestine	Bloody diarrhea, fever, abdominal pain; mild, intermittent GI symptoms	Trophozoites in *fresh stool* or proctoscopic material, cysts in stool	Absent	

Table 16-1 (continued)

Disease	Mode of spread	Location in humans	Clinical features	Laboratory diagnosis	Eosinophilia*	Remarks
Extraintestinal amebiasis	Hematogenous dissemination from intestinal sites	Liver, lung	Hepatomegaly, fever	Trophozoites from abscess or sputum; serologic tests	Absent	
Giardiasis	Fecal-oral	Upper small intestine	Diarrhea, abdominal pain, malabsorption	Cysts and trophozoites in *fresh stool*; duodenal aspirate	Absent	
Toxoplasmosis	Congenital, raw meat, cat feces (?)	CNS, eye, reticuloendothelial system—potentially any organ	Congenital; acute mononucleosis-like illness; asymptomatic; disseminated in immunosuppressed	Biopsy; serologic tests	Absent	
Malaria	Bite of infected *Anopheles* mosquito; transfusion or congenital acquisition rarely	Erythrocytes, hepatocytes	Fever, splenomegaly, anemia, thrombocytopenia; shock, encephalopathy with *P. falciparum*	Repeated blood smears	Absent	Important to distinguish *P. falciparum* from relapsing malarias
Pneumocytosis	Unknown	Lungs	Fever, cough, hypoxia, lung infiltrates in compromised host	Sputum; bronchial brushings; lung biopsy	Absent	Compromised host
Babesiosis	Bite of tick; transfusion	Erythrocytes, reticuloendothelial system	Resemble malaria	Repeated blood smears	Absent	Severe in asplenics; certain areas in U.S.

*Mild, 5–10%; moderate, 10–20%; marked, > 20%.

C. Direct identification of parasites. Many techniques are available to identify parasites in excreta, fluids, and tissue. Examination of specimens is usually done by hospital, public health, or private laboratories. However, there are several simple procedures, requiring little equipment, that the physician can perform when the patient is seen. It is helpful to have charts of diagnostic stages of helminths and protozoa available for accurate interpretation. If more sophisticated procedures are needed, standard texts of parasitology can be consulted.

   1. Blood

   a. The **thin dry smear** is useful in detecting malarial or babesial parasites. The technique is identical to routine blood smears used for hematologic studies. Wright's or Giemsa stain is used in the usual fashion, and parasites are seen within red blood cells. Species differentiation is of therapeutic importance once malaria parasites have been identified.

   b. The **thick dry smear** for the detection of malaria parasites yields a much higher concentration of parasites than the thin smear and thus is useful when the parasites are few and thin smears are negative. However, the thick smear is harder to interpret, since the erythrocytes are lysed, and the parasites are seen on a background of stained proteinaceous debris. The technique is as follows:

   (1) Spread a drop of blood on a clean microscope slide, using an applicator or corner of another slide. (The smear should be about the diameter of a dime and of a thickness sufficient to allow for transparency when the hemoglobin is removed.)

   (2) Allow the smear to dry for 1–2 hr at 37°C.

   (3) Cover the slide with distilled water until the color of the hemoglobin has disappeared.

   (4) Dry the slide and cover it with Wright's stain as for routine blood smears, or with dilute Giemsa stain for 45 min.

   (5) Examine for parasites under the oil immersion lens.

   2. Stool. Examine feces as soon after passage as possible and before barium or cathartics are given. Helminth ova and protozoal cysts can be identified in older specimens, but the identification of free-living, motile forms requires the examination of **freshly passed, warm stool.**

   a. Direct examination of stool enables the rapid identification of intestinal parasites. Free-living, motile forms and ova and cysts can be identified, particularly if there is a heavy infestation. The procedure takes a few minutes and makes use of supplies found in all laboratories.

   (1) Examine the specimen grossly for flecks of blood and mucus. If present, take a sample from these areas.

   (2) Place a match-head-size sample on each of two microscope slides with a wooden applicator.

   (3) Mix one sample with 2 drops of saline and cover with coverslip.

   (4) Add 2 drops of dilute iodine solution to the other sample, mix, and cover similarly.

   (5) Observe for the presence of erythrocytes and leukocytes. **Erythrocytes** suggest amebic colitis, and **leukocytes,** bacterial infection or inflammatory bowel disease and *not* parasitic infection. A Gram and/or Wright's stain may be indicated.

   (6) Examine the stained slide for the presence of helminth eggs under low power and for protozoal cysts under high power and oil immersion.

   (7) Examine the unstained slide under low and high power for the presence of motile organisms (ameba, trophozoites, larvae).

   b. Concentration. A number of techniques are available for examination of larger quantities of feces for parasites. A useful reference is D. M. Melvin and M. M. Brooke, *Laboratory Procedures for the Diagnosis of Intestinal Parasites* (2nd ed.), U. S. Dept. of Health, Education, and Welfare, Public Health Service, publication # CDC 76-8282, 1975, pp. 95–108.

   c. Quantitation. In certain helminthic infections, estimation of the **worm burden** by quantitation of egg excretion is of great importance. The method of Stoll is commonly employed (D. L. Belding, *Textbook of Parasitology* [3rd ed.], New York, Appleton-Century-Crofts, 1965).

   d. Scotch-tape examination is a useful and simple technique for the demonstration of pinworm eggs.

     (1) Evert a strip of Scotch tape, gummed side outward, on the edge of a tongue blade.

     (2) Dab the perianal area first thing in the morning.

     (3) Place on a microscope slide, sticky side down, on a drop of toluene.

     (4) Examine under low power for characteristic eggs.

D. Serologic tests in parasitic diseases

   1. Immunodiagnostic tests are helpful in several parasitic infections. They are to be used and interpreted **in conjunction with** clinical and laboratory evaluation and should not be solely relied on for diagnosis.

   2. The tests are specifically helpful in invasive amebiasis, trichinosis, toxoplasmosis, and echinococcosis.

   3. The serologic tests referred to in Table 16-1 are performed at the Centers for Disease Control, Atlanta, Georgia, and by some local health departments.

II. Principles of treatment

A. Protozoal infections are always treated. The principles of treatment consist of the identification of the responsible parasite and the selection of an appropriate therapeutic agent, administered in appropriate dosage. For specific treatment regimens, see **III,** where the drug of choice is listed, followed by alternatives. All regimens are to be administered PO unless otherwise indicated.

B. Helminthic infections are not always treated. After identifying the causative parasite, the clinician must weigh several additional factors before initiating treatment. These include:

   1. The number of worms harbored by the patient and the life span of the infecting worm(s)

   2. The likelihood and seriousness of personal and public health complications resulting from infection

   3. The availability and efficacy of therapeutic agents and their expected side effects and toxicity (Table 16-2)

C. Treatment must be individualized and arbitrary rules avoided.

D. Follow-up clinical and laboratory assessment is always indicated to determine if treatment has been efficacious. Stools should be examined several weeks after the treatment of intestinal parasites is completed, and retreatment given if cure has not been achieved. In general, re-treatment with the same drug is more desirable than proceeding to an alternate agent that is more toxic, less efficacious, or both.

E. Patient education. The physician should always combine treatment with patient education aimed at **prevention** of future parasitic infection. Attention should be given to the environmental circumstances that resulted in the child's acquisition of infection.

III. Specific parasites

A. Roundworms (nematodes)

   1. Ascaris

     a. Etiology. Fecal-oral passage of infective ova of *Ascaris lumbricoides*. The human is the only susceptible host. The infection is worldwide in distribution.

     b. Evaluation and diagnosis. Two distinct clinical phases occur:

       (1) Transient blood-lung migration phase of the larvae. Pneumonia occurs, with cough, blood-tinged sputum, patchy pulmonary infiltrates, and fever. A marked peripheral eosinophilia is typical. Characteristic larvae may be found in the sputum.

       (2) Prolonged intestinal phase of the adults. The patient is usually asymptomatic, although vague abdominal discomfort may occur. On rare occasions, more serious manifestations may occur, including intestinal obstruction, appendicitis, and regurgitation and aspiration of wandering adult worms.

Table 16-2. Adverse effects of antiparasitic drugs

Drug	Frequent	Infrequent
Chloroquine phosphate (Aralen Phosphate)	Anorexia, nausea, visual disturbances	Retinopathy—only with prolonged, high dosage
Dehydroemetine	Diarrhea, nausea, vomiting, myalgias, ECG changes	Hypotension
Diiodohydroxyquine, U.S.P.		Rash, acne, slight thyroid enlargement, nausea, diarrhea, cramps, anal pruritus, optic atrophy and vision loss in children after prolonged use in high dosage for months
Diloxamide furoate (Furamide)	Flatulence	Nausea, vomiting, diarrhea, urticaria, pruritus
Furazolidone (Furoxone)		Anorexia, nausea, hypersensitivity reactions*
Mebendazole (Vermox) **contraindicated in pregnancy**		Diarrhea, abdominal pain
Metronidazole* (Flagyl) **contraindicated in first trimester**	Anorexia, nausea, vomiting, metallic taste	Peripheral neuropathy, ataxia, neutropenia
Niclosamide (Yomesan)		Nausea
Paromomycin (Humatin)	Anorexia, nausea, vomiting	Nephrotoxicity
Pentamidine isethionate	Dizziness, tachycardia, headache, vomiting, hypotension	Nephrotoxicity, hepatotoxicity
Piperazine citrate (Antepar)		Anorexia, rash, ataxia
Primaquine phosphate	Anorexia, nausea	Hemolytic anemia in G-6-PD deficiency, methemoglobinemia
Pyrantel pamoate (Antiminth)	Anorexia, nausea	
Pyrimethamine (Daraprim) **contraindicated in pregnancy**		Folate-deficient macrocytic anemia
Pyrvinium pamoate (Povan)	Anorexia, nausea, red-colored stool	
Quinacrine HCl (Atabrine Hydrochloride)	Nausea, vomiting, dizziness	Psychoses, exfoliative dermatitis, hepatic necrosis, yellowing of skin
Quinine sulfate	Tinnitus, nausea, vomiting, vertigo	Hypotension, hemolytic anemia
Thiabendazole (Mintezol)	Anorexia, nausea, vomiting, dizziness	Tinnitus, drowsiness, shock
Trimethoprim-sulfamethoxazole (Bactrim, Septra)		Rash, hemolytic anemia, bone marrow suppression

*Carcinogenic in rats and mutagenic in bacteria (see *Med. Lett. Drugs Ther.* 17:53, 1975). Significance for humans not known.

(3) The **diagnosis** is confirmed by:
   (a) Characteristic ova in feces by direct examination or concentration techniques
   (b) Regurgitation or stool passage of adult worms
   (c) Occasionally, demonstration of adult worms on abdominal x-ray films

c. Treatment. The occasional aberrant wanderings of individual worms and subsequent serious consequences require that **all** ascaris infections be treated. Tetrachlorethylene, used in the treatment of hookworm infection, may provoke ascaris wandering. Ascaris intestinal infections should thus be treated first if a combined infection is present and this agent is used.
   (1) Ascaris pneumonitis. Symptomatic treatment
   (2) Intestinal ascariasis.
      Pyrantel pamoate, 11 mg/kg in 1 dose (maximum 1 gm)
      Mebendazole, 100 mg bid for 3 days for children 2 years old or older
      Piperazine citrate, 75 mg/kg/day for 2 days (maximum 3.5 gm/day)

d. Prevention. Sanitary disposal of feces

2. Hookworm
a. Etiology
   (1) Human hookworms belong to two genera, *Necator* and *Ancylostoma*. The former are prevalent in the southern United States, South and Central America, Asia, and Africa. The latter are rarely seen in the United States.
   (2) Infections spread by skin penetration of soil-living larvae hatched from eggs passed in infected feces.

b. Evaluation and diagnosis. Three clinical phases of hookworm infection are recognized:
   (1) Penetration of the skin by larvae. A local papulovesicular dermatitis and a history of walking barefoot in feces-contaminated soil suggest the diagnosis.
   (2) Transient blood-lung migration by larvae. A mild pneumonitis with peripheral eosinophilia is suggestive. Hookworm larvae may be found in the sputum.
   (3) The **prolonged intestinal phase** results from the attachment of blood-feeding adult worms to the small intestinal mucosa of the host.
      (a) In **hookworm infection** the number of infecting worms is small, and diarrhea and abdominal cramps may be the only clinical findings. Infection is confirmed by demonstrating hookworm ova in feces.
      (b) In **hookworm disease** large numbers of worms are present, and significant blood loss occurs. The disease is confimed by
         (i) Signs and symptoms of anemia.
         (ii) Documentation of iron deficiency.
         (iii) The finding of occult blood in the feces.
         (iv) The demonstration of large numbers of hookworm ova in the feces by the method of Stoll (see reference in sec. **I.C.2.c,** or other standard text, for details).

c. Treatment
   (1) Drugs
      Mebendazole, 100 mg bid for 3 days for children 2 years old or older
      Pyrantel pamoate, 11 mg/kg in 1 dose (maximum 1 gm)
      Thiabendazole, 50 mg/kg/day in divided doses bid for 2 days (maximum 3 gm/day)
   (2) Differentiation between *Necator* and *Ancylostoma* infections is difficult. Infections acquired in the Western Hemisphere should be assumed to be due to *Necator* and treated accordingly.
   (3) Moderate to very heavy infections should always be treated with

antihelminthics, as should hookworm disease. Light infections need not be specifically treated if the patient is adequately nourished.

(4) Iron supplementation should be given to patients with hookworm disease.

d. Prevention. Sanitary disposal of feces and wearing of shoes to prevent contact of bare feet with contaminated soil

3. Whipworm

a. Etiology. Fecal-oral spread of *Trichuris trichiura.* The infection is worldwide, and the human is the natural reservoir and only susceptible host.

b. Evaluation and diagnosis

(1) Diarrhea and abdominal pain have been associated with trichuriasis, but the vast majority of infections are asymptomatic.

(2) The presence of typical ova in feces by direct fecal smear or concentration techniques is diagnostic.

(3) Eosinophilia is not associated with trichuriasis, and its presence should suggest another parasitic infection.

c. Treatment should be limited to patients who are symptomatic or who have heavy infestations. Give mebendazole, 100 mg bid for 3 days, to children 2 years old or older.

d. Prevention. Sanitary fecal disposal and wearing of shoes to prevent skin penetration by the larvae.

4. Pinworm

a. Etiology. Fecal-oral spread of *Enterobius vermicularis,* a 4-mm worm just visible to the naked eye and the most common helminth found in humans in the United States. The infection often affects entire households. Autoinfection is also common. Humans are the only known hosts.

b. Evaluation and diagnosis

(1) Perianal itching, vulvitis, and vaginitis in young children suggest the presence of pinworms. Symptoms may be intense enough to cause insomnia, restlessness, hyperactivity, and nocturnal enuresis.

(2) Adult worms may be seen in the perianal area and on the surface of freshly passed feces, particularly in the early morning.

(3) Characteristic ova are demonstrated by Scotch-tape swab (see sec. **d,** p. 424). Examination should be made first thing in the morning and repeated on consecutive days if necessary. A single swabbing reveals only about 50 percent of infections; three swabbings will uncover 90 percent; and five examinations are required before the patient is considered free from infection. Scrapings from beneath the fingernails may show eggs in 30 percent of infected children.

(4) If diagnostic procedures fail to reveal pinworms, a therapeutic trial is reasonable in markedly symptomatic children.

c. Treatment

Mebendazole, 100 mg in 1 dose for children 2 years or older
Pyrantel pamoate, 11 mg/kg in 1 dose (maximum 1 gm)
Pyrvinium pamoate, 5 mg/kg in 1 dose (maximum 250 mg)
Piperazine citrate, 65 mg/kg daily for 7 days (maximum 2.5 gm/day)

All members of a household should be treated simultaneously.

d. Prevention. Boiling of sheets, undergarments, pajamas, and the like is of little or no value. Hand washing and fingernail cleanliness may reduce transmission and autoinfection.

5. *Strongyloides*

a. Etiology. Skin penetration of *Strongyloides stercoralis* larvae passed in infected feces. Autoinfection may occur.

b. Evaluation and diagnosis. Children may be asymptomatic or complain of upper GI distress, since the adult worms live within the duodenal submucosa. Larvae (not ova) are found in freshly passed feces or by aspiration of duodenal contents. Infections are associated with a moderate to marked eosinophilia. Fatal, overwhelming infection may occur in children who harbor this parasite and who are undergoing immunosuppression.

   c. Treatment. Thiabendazole, 50 mg/kg/day in divided doses bid for 2 days (maximum 3 gm/day)
   d. Prevention. Sanitary disposal of feces and wearing of shoes

6. Visceral larva migrans
   a. Etiology. Ingestion of the ova of dog and cat ascarids, *Toxocara canis* and *Toxocara cati*. Larvae emerge in the intestine and migrate extensively throughout the body.
   b. Evaluation and diagnosis
      (1) The presumptive diagnosis is based on the clinical manifestations in a child with pica. These include fever, cough, hepatosplenomegaly, and transient pneumonia. Ocular involvement can occur with or without systemic symptoms.
      (2) Hypergammaglobulinemia, marked elevation of isohemagglutinins, marked eosinophilia (20% or more), and leukocytosis are present.
      (3) The parasite is rarely demonstrated; stool examination and tissue biopsy are useless.
   c. Treatment
      (1) The disease is often mild and self-limited, lasting several weeks. Specific treatment is usually unnecessary.
      (2) In severe cases, or in patients with ocular involvement, antihelminthic therapy may be beneficial.

      Thiabendazole, 50 mg/kg/day in divided doses bid for 5 days (maximum 3 gm/day), *or*
      Diethylcarbamazine, 6–12 mg/kg/day in divided doses tid for 3 weeks

      (3) Antiinflammatory therapy with corticosteroids or antihistamines, or both, may offer relief of severe symptoms. Corticosteroids should be used in conjunction with antihelminthics in treating ocular disease.
      (4) Thiabendazole (for 2 days) can be used for treating cutaneous larva migrans.
   d. Prevention. Avoidance of contamination of play and work areas by dog and cat feces.

7. Trichinosis
   a. Etiology. Ingestion of raw meat containing encysted larvae of *Trichinella spiralis* (pork is the principal source of human infection). The infection is more common in temperate than in tropical environments.
   b. Evaluation and diagnosis
      (1) A history of ingestion of uncooked pork
      (2) The clinical picture may suggest the diagnosis, but is often unclear until the second or third week of infection. At this time the full-blown picture of fever, facial and periorbital edema, headache, photophobia, conjunctivitis, and severe muscle pain and tenderness may develop. Signs of encephalitis, meningitis, and myocarditis may appear.
      (3) A muscle biopsy specimen showing the characteristic larvae. Histologic examination of tissue for the presence of an inflammatory reaction is essential to confirm **recent** infection. A negative biopsy does not rule out the diagnosis.
      (4) Marked peripheral eosinophilia (in 20–80%) after the third week of infection, which may persist for months.
      (5) A positive intracutaneous skin test with *Trichinella* larval antigen (85–100% sensitivity). An immediate wheal and flare reaction occurs after injection of 0.1 ml of antigen. The test becomes positive about 3 weeks after infection and remains positive for 5–7 years.
      (6) Agglutination or flocculation reactions with rising titer demonstrated on paired samples (tests turn positive in the third week of infection and may remain positive for months to years).

- **c. Treatment**
    - **(1)** The efficacy of specific antihelminthic therapy is in question. In severe cases, thiabendazole may be tried in a dose of 50 mg/kg/day in divided doses bid for 5 days (maximum 3 gm/day).
    - **(2)** Corticosteroids may ameliorate severe symptoms, but they are not universally considered beneficial.
- **d. Prevention.** Consumption of only well-cooked pork. Pork is *not* inspected for trichinosis in the United States.

B. Tapeworms (cestodes)

1. Beef tapeworm

- **a. Etiology.** The disease is transmitted by the ingestion of undercooked beef containing *Taenia saginata* larval cysts. The infection is worldwide in distribution; the human is the definitive host, and cattle are the intermediate host.
- **b. Evaluation and diagnosis.** Most patients are asymptomatic, and the infection is noted only when migrating proglottids pass through the anus. Observation of gravid proglottids is diagnostic.
- **c. Treatment**
    - **(1) Niclosamide** achieves a 90% cure rate.
        - **(a)** No prior bowel preparation is required, but tablets should be chewed thoroughly. The dosage is as follows:

            11–34 kg, 1 gm in 1 dose
            34–50 kg, 1.5 gm in 1 dose
            > 50 kg, 2 gm in 1 dose

        - **(b)** The worm will be macerated, and search for the scolex (head) is thus unprofitable.
        - **(c)** Re-treat if proglottids reappear in subsequent months.
    - **(2) Quinacrine** achieves a 75% cure rate. The total dose is 25 mg/kg. Treatment is as follows:
        - **(a)** Give a cathartic the evening before treatment and a cleansing enema (Fleet's) in morning.
        - **(b)** Quinacrine on an empty stomach is given in 4–5 divided doses every 10 min until the total dose is given. Each dose is given with 250 mg sodium bicarbonate.
        - **(c)** Give a saline purge several hours later and follow by a stool examination for scolex for the next 24 hr.
        - **(d)** Re-treat if proglottids reappear in subsequent months.
- **d. Prevention.** Thorough cooking of beef

2. Pork tapeworm

- **a. Etiology.** Ingestion of uncooked pork containing larval cysts of *Taenia solium*
- **b. Evaluation and diagnosis.** Adult worms rarely produce symptoms. The passage of gravid motile proglottids through the anus raises the suspicion of infection. Confirmation is obtained by laboratory examination of the proglottid.
- **c. Treatment. Quinacrine** is the drug of choice [see **1.c.(2)**].
- **d. Prevention.** Thorough cooking of pork.

3. Hydatid disease

- **a. Etiology.** Humans acquire the infection by ingesting the eggs of *Echinococcus granulosus* passed in the feces of carnivores.
- **b. Evaluation and diagnosis**
    - **(1)** A slowly growing, usually asymptomatic cyst in the proper epidemiologic setting suggests the diagnosis. Two-thirds occur in the liver; one-fourth in the lung; and the remainder are widely scattered.
    - **(2)** The **x-ray** appearance is typical but not pathognomonic.
    - **(3) Casoni's intradermal skin test.** An immediate wheal and flare constitute a positive test specific for *E. granulosus* and 75% sensitive.

(4) Hemagglutination and bentonite flocculation tests are positive in the majority of cases.

(5) Demonstration of the characteristic gross and histologic appearance on removal of the cyst. **(Aspiration is dangerous and should not be done.)**

  c. Treatment. Easily accessible cysts are removed surgically. Most cysts are asymptomatic and may, in fact, be left untreated. Freezing of the cyst and subsequent surgical removal have given favorable results (*N. Engl. J. Med.* 284:1346, 1971). When surgery is contraindicated or if cysts rupture spontaneously during surgery, mebendazole can be tried (*Am. J. Trop. Med. Hyg.* 29:1340, 1980).

  d. *Echinococcus multilocularis* has a life cycle similar to that of *E. granulosus,* but adult worms reside in foxes. The larvae reside in small wild rodents. Infected dogs and other sources of egg contamination represent the link to occasional human infection. *E. multilocularis* is found mainly in Alaska, Canada, Siberia, and central Europe. In humans, larvae form irregular, alveolar cysts. The germinative tissues spread rapidly to produce neoplasmlike growths that are difficult or impossible to manage surgically. The prognosis is especially poor, even with medical treatment.

4. Fish tapeworm

  a. Etiology. The disease is transmitted by the ingestion of undercooked or raw fish containing *Diphyllobothrium latum* larvae. The infection is worldwide, but it is concentrated in the cool lake regions of the major continents (e.g., in the Great Lake region).

  b. Evaluation and diagnosis. Most patients are asymptomatic, although, rarely, a vitamin B_{12} deficiency state may occur, caused by the adult worms' capacity of taking up vitamin B_{12} in the upper small intestine. Mild abdominal symptoms may occur. Characteristic eggs are passed in the stool.

  c. Treatment. Give Niclosamide as in **B.1.c.(1).**

  d. Precaution. The fish should be cooked properly.

C. Protozoa

  1. Amebiasis

    a. Etiology. Fecal-oral passage of cysts of *Entamoeba histolytica.* Amebiasis is worldwide in distribution, and the human is the only known host. Sporadic localized epidemics occur in the United States, and the disease is endemic in many institutionalized populations.

    b. Evaluation and diagnosis

      (1) Intestinal amebiasis

        (a) Intestinal amebiasis varies in presentation from the asymptomatic carrier state (by far the most common) to fulminant colonic disease.

          (i) Mild colonic infection is characterized by alternating diarrhea and constipation.

          (ii) Amebic dysentery presents most frequently as subacute illness. Mild tenderness, bloody diarrhea, low-grade fever, weakness, and malaise are characteristic. The tempo of the illness may clinically distinguish it from more acute, bacillary dysentery. Abdominal tenderness is common, particularly over the sigmoid and cecal areas; appendicitis is sometimes erroneously diagnosed.

        (b) Confirmation in acute cases is obtained by demonstrating motile amebic trophozoites in **fresh stool,** or cysts in the carrier state. Proctoscopy may be useful if multiple stool samples are negative.

        (c) Erythrocytes are plentiful and leukocytes are minimal in the stool, which is helpful in distinguishing between amebic and bacillary dysentery.

        (d) Eosinophilia is *not* found.

(2) Extraintestinal amebiasis most commonly affects the liver.

   (a) Disease may occur without the signs or symptoms of intestinal infection. Fever, chills, an enlarged, tender liver, elevated right diaphragm, minimal liver function abnormalities, and the finding of a filling defect on liver scan are highly suggestive. Of all amebic abscesses, 95% are single and situated in the upper part of the right lobe of the liver.

   (b) Serologic tests for invasive amebiasis (indirect hemagglutination, complement fixation) are extremely accurate.

   (c) Percutaneous liver aspiration is recommended in large abscesses only. Aspirated material may show amebas. However, their absence does not rule out hepatic infection, since organisms tend to be located at the margins of the abscess.

   (d) A therapeutic trial is an accepted diagnostic measure **in a severely ill patient.**

c. Treatment

   (1) All stages of amebiasis are treated.

   (a) Asymptomatic carrier state

   Diloxanide furoate, 20 mg/kg/day in divided doses tid for 10 days (maximum 1.5 gm/day), **or**

   Diiodohydroxyquin, 30–40 mg/kg/day in divided doses tid for 20 days (maximum 2 gm/day)

   (b) Intestinal infection

   Metronidazole, 35–50 mg/kg/day in divided doses tid for 10 days (maximum 2.25 gm/day)

   As a second choice, paromomycin, 25–30 mg/kg/day in divided doses tid for 5–10 days, can be used alone.

   In severe cases, use dehydroemetine HCl, 1.0–1.5 mg/kg/day IM for 5 days (maximum 90 mg/day), **and**

   Diiodohydroxyquin as above.

   (c) Hepatic infection

   Metronidazole, as in **(b), and**

   Diiodohydroxyquin, as in **(a), or**

   Dehydroemetine, as in **(b),** followed by

   Chloroquine phosphate, 10 mg base/kg/day for 21 days (maximum 300 mg base/day), **and**

   Diiodohydroxyquin, as in **(a)**

   (2) In addition to specific amebicidal therapy, **supportive care** is important in invasive amebiasis. Hospitalization, bed rest, and good nutritional intake may contribute to rapid recovery.

   (3) Follow-up stool examinations should be done at 1 and 2 months to ensure that a cure has been achieved.

d. Prevention. Sanitary disposal of feces and treatment of asymptomatic cyst passers.

2. Giardiasis

   a. Etiology. Fecal-oral spread of *Giardia lamblia.* Infection is world-wide and is common in institutionalized populations.

   b. Evaluation and diagnosis

   (1) There are often no symptoms. Abdominal pain, chronic and recurrent diarrhea, and weight loss may occur. The diarrhea is not bloody; stools may be bulky and offensive. Steatorrhea and malabsorption, including lactose intolerance, may occur.

   (2) The diagnosis is confirmed by the demonstration of characteristic motile trophozoites in **fresh diarrheal stool** or **duodenal aspirate** by direct examination. Cysts may be seen in formed stools by direct or concentration methods.

Table 16-3. Differentiation of malarial parasites

Falciparum	Relapsing
Small ring forms	Large ring forms
Ring forms and pathognomonic, crescent-shaped gametocytes	Intermediate forms also
Rings frequently with two chromatin dots	Rings rarely with two chromatin dots
No Schüffner's dots	Schüffner's dots (*Plasmodium vivax* and *P. ovale*)
Parasites at margins of red blood cells	Parasites usually central
More than one parasite per red blood cell	Usually only one parasite per red blood cell

    c. Treatment
      (1) Specific therapy is highly effective.

        Furazolidone suspension, 5 mg/kg/day in divided doses qid for 7–10 days
        Metronidazole, 15 mg/kg/day in divided doses tid for 5–10 days (maximum 750 mg/day)
        Quinacrine, 6–9 mg/kg/day in divided doses tid for 5–7 days (maximum 300 mg/day)

      (2) Supportive measures and restoration of nutritional status are important in patients with malabsorption.
    d. Prevention. Sanitary disposal of feces.
  3. Malaria
    a. Etiology. Malaria, among the most common worldwide human infections, is transmitted by the bite of an *Anopheles* mosquito infected with *Plasmodium.* Four species of *Plasmodium* infect man: *P. falciparum, P. vivax, P. ovale,* and *P. malariae.* Transfusion-induced malaria occurs infrequently, as does perinatally acquired malaria.
    b. Evaluation and diagnosis
      (1) The clinical manifestations of malaria infection are nonspecific. Fever, rigors, malaise, headaches, myalgias, and arthralgias commonly occur in acute infections. **Splenomegaly** is the most consistent physical finding. In children, GI complaints, including loss of appetite, vomiting, or diarrhea, may predominate. In infants, pallor or jaundice is also seen.
      (2) The fever pattern may become periodic after infection is well established: q48 hr in *P. vivax* and *P. ovale* infections; q72 hr in *P. malariae* infections; and q36–48 hr in *P. falciparum* malaria. Typically, the patient appears well between fever paroxysms.
      (3) It is exceedingly important to distinguish between relapsing malaria (*vivax, ovale,* and *malariae*) and falciparum malaria (Table 16-3). The former group usually produces a self-limited illness that may relapse after months or years. The latter species can infect red blood cells of all ages, with resultant heavy parasitemia, serious complications, and possible fatal outcome. *P. falciparum* **infections, even when the level of parasitemia is low, should be treated immediately. The patient should be observed in the hospital until clinical improvement or a decrease in parasitemia is noted.**
      (4) The complications of *P. falciparum* infection include cerebral malaria (presenting as coma, delirium, and convulsions), massive hemolysis, disseminated intravascular coagulation, renal failure, pulmonary edema, and cardiovascular collapse.

(5) A history of residence or travel in an endemic area is almost always elicited.

(6) The diagnosis rests on the demonstration of malaria parasites in the peripheral blood (see **B**, p. 419, and **C**, p. 423).

As previously noted, laboratory differentiation between falciparum malaria and the relapsing malarias is of great importance and will affect the choice of antimalarial agents (see Table 16-3). If there is any doubt, the patient should be treated initially as if the infecting organism is *P. falciparum*. Mixed infections do occur, and one should be aware of this possibility. Textbooks of parasitology should be consulted to aid in species differentiation.

c. Treatment. The choice of antimalarial drugs depends on the infecting species and the geographic area of acquisition of infection.

(1) Falciparum infections acquired in Southeast Asia and localized areas of Central and South America must be assumed to be resistant to chloroquine phosphate. Sporadic chloroquine resistance has been reported in East Africa as well. Alternative drugs should be given, as outlined in **(4)(b).**

(2) In **relapsing malaria,** therapy must be directed against both the erythrocytic and exoerythrocytic parasites to prevent relapse. There is no resistance to chloroquine, but relapse may occur if this agent is used alone. If nonfalciparum malaria is acquired by other than a mosquito bite (e.g., via transfusion or perinatally), then there is no exoerythrocytic cycle, and chloroquine alone is appropriate.

(3) In addition to vigorous antimalarial therapy, the complications of falciparum malaria require intensive supportive measures. Transfusions with packed RBCs are given in severe hemolytic anemia. Mannitol may be used in renal failure, and dialysis may be necessary. Careful attention to fluid and electrolyte balance is essential. Anticonvulsants are often required in cerebral malaria. Splenic rupture is a rare but life-threatening complication.

(4) Recommended treatment regimens

  (a) Relapsing malaria

Chloroquine phosphate, 10 mg/kg PO (or IM if necessary), followed by 5 mg/kg 6 hr later, then 5 mg/kg daily for 2 days, **and**

Primaquine, 0.3 mg/kg/day for 14 days (maximum 15 mg base/day)

Patients deficient in glucose 6-phosphate dehydrogenase may demonstrate a hemolytic anemia with primaquine.

  (b) Falciparum malaria

    (i) Nonchloroquine-resistant area

Chloroquine phosphate, as in **(a)**

    (ii) Chloroquine-resistant area

Quinine sulfate, 25 mg/kg/day in divided doses tid for 3 days (maximum 2 gm/day), **and**

Pyrimethamine

    < 10 kg, 6.25 mg/day for 3 days

    10–20 kg, 12.5 mg/day for 3 days

    20–40 kg, 25 mg/day for 3 days

    > 40 kg, 50 mg/day in divided doses bid for 3 days, **and**

Sulfadiazine, 100–200 mg/kg/day in divided doses qid for 5 days (maximum 2 gm/day)

If the patient is critically ill and unable to take medication PO, use quinine dihydrochloride IV in a dosage of 25 mg/kg/day. Give one-half dose over 1 hr, then one-half dose 6–8 hr later if oral therapy still cannot be started. (Dilute medication to a concentration of 0.5–1.0 mg/ml in normal saline and infuse at a rate of 0.5–1.0 mg/min with ECG and blood pressure monitoring; maximum 1,800 mg/day.)

  (5) Response to therapy is followed by dramatic clinical improvement. Repeated blood smears show disappearance of parasitemia. **Pyrimethamine and primaquine are contraindicated in pregnancy.**

  d. Prevention. Persons traveling through or residing in malarious areas should receive prophylactic suppressive therapy with chloroquine phosphate, 5 mg (base)/kg once a week, to be continued for 6 weeks after the last exposure. To prevent relapsing malaria, a 14-day course of primaquine should be taken concurrently with the final 2 weeks of chloroquine therapy. For travelers to areas of chloroquine resistance, pyrimethamine (maximum 25 mg) and sulfadiazine or sulfadoxine (maximum 500 mg) should be taken once a week in addition to chloroquine. In areas of pyrimethamine-sulfadoxine resistance, quinine may be used prophylactically. Recently, patients have been successfully treated with clindamycin and quinine. Treatment should be restricted to immunocompromised or ill patients with babesiosis (see **6**).

4. Toxoplasmosis

  a. Etiology. *Toxoplasma gondii,* an obligate intracellular parasite, is responsible for this infection. Congenital transmission has been clearly established. The mode of acquisition of postnatally acquired infection remains obscure. Transmission by meat ingestion and spread by cat feces are strong possibilities.

  b. Evaluation and diagnosis

  (1) Infection is largely asymptomatic. Serologic evidence of prior infection is demonstrated in 25–40% of the population of the United States. Several symptomatic forms are recognized:

  (a) Congenital infection is usually the result of acute infection in the mother. Prematurity or spontaneous abortion may occur. Newborns with toxoplasmosis are asymptomatic at birth, and most remain so. In a small number of infants, fulminant disease may appear at birth, as manifested by jaundice, hepatomegaly, chorioretinitis, microcephaly, cerebral calcification, or seizures. A number of subclinically infected infants, asymptomatic at birth, may be found to have chorioretinitis, mental retardation, or learning problems later in life.

  (b) Acquired infection shows clinical variations ranging from a mild viral-like illness with lymphadenopathy to chorioretinitis without systemic illness to fatal pneumonia and encephalitis in the compromised host.

  (2) Demonstration of **rising antibody titers** by complement-fixation (CF), hemagglutination (HA), indirect fluorescent antibody tests (IFA), and the Sabin-Feldman dye test establishes the diagnosis. Newborn infections can be diagnosed by demonstration of IgM *Toxoplasma* antibodies or the persistence of high titers of CF, HA, or IFA beyond 4 months of age.

  (3) Rarely, in special circumstances, the diagnosis may be established by the demonstration of organisms in tissue sections or smears of body fluids. Intraperitoneal mouse inoculation is required for isolation. To determine if an infection is recent, however, rising serologic titers are still required.

  c. Treatment

  (1) There have been no controlled clinical trials to establish the efficacy of drug therapy.

  (2) Infants with active disease should be treated in the hope of preventing further destruction of tissue.

  (3) Treatment of acquired toxoplasmosis depends on the clinical severity of the illness. Patients with underlying severe illness and immunoincompetence should be strongly considered for treatment if infection is clinically apparent.

(4) Specific therapy

(a) The treatment of congenital disease varies with the degree and location of disease. Drugs used include pyrimethamine, sulfadiazine, spiramycin, and, in some cases, corticosteroids. For a concise discussion of therapeutic regimens, see J. S. Remington and G. Desmonts, Toxoplasmosis, in J. S. Remington and J. O. Klein (eds.), *Infectious Diseases of the Fetus and Newborn Infant,* Philadelphia, Saunders, 1976, p. 302.

(b) The drugs for treatment of the immunocompromised host include pyrimethamine and sulfadiazine. An infectious disease consultation should be obtained.

(c) The treatment of ocular disease requires the addition of corticosteroids to the antiprotozoal drugs.

(d) Dosages

Pyrimethamine, 1 mg/kg/day (load with 2 mg/kg/day for 3 days; maximum 25 mg/day)
Sulfadiazine, 100–200 mg/kg/day (maximum 6 gm/day)
Spiramycin 50–100 mg/kg/day (maximum 4 gm/day)

The duration of treatment depends on the site and severity of disease, as well as on the immune status of the host.

(5) With pyrimethamine treatment, supplemental folinic acid should be given. **Pyrimethamine is contraindicated in pregnancy.**

d. Prevention. Since the mode of spread of infection remains unknown, preventive measures are speculative. Avoidance of ingestion of raw meat and areas of cat feces contamination, particularly during pregnancy, may be of benefit.

5. *Pneumocystis* pneumonia

a. Etiology. *Pneumocystis carinii,* an organism of uncertain classification, is the etiologic agent. Little is known of the route of infection or the pathogenesis of disease, but the pulmonary focus suggests a respiratory portal of entry.

b. Evaluation and diagnosis

(1) *P. carinii* produces a bilateral diffuse interstitial pneumonia in immunologically compromised hosts. The pneumonia is perihilar in distribution, and symptoms are usually insidious in onset. The diagnosis must be considered when pneumonia develops in patients with leukemia, lymphoma, hypogammaglobulinemia, and those receiving immunosuppressive therapy. This is an opportunistic infection seen in malignancy in **remission** and in malnutrition states as well. Bacterial pathogens should be ruled out by appropriate sputum studies.

(2) Diagnosis requires the demonstration of the parasite by methenamine silver stains in tissue sections obtained at lung biopsy. Rarely, sputum and bronchial brushings may show organisms.

c. Treatment

(1) *P. carinii* pneumonia is usually present as a terminal event in patients with severe underlying illness. Spontaneous recovery has been documented; the effect of therapy is thus difficult to assess.

(2) Oxygen and other respiratory supportive measures are of great importance.

(3) Trimethoprim-sulfamethoxazole (Bactrim), 20 mg trimethoprim and 100 mg sulfamethoxazole/kg/day in 4 divided doses, IV or PO, is the drug of choice for therapy of *P. carinii* pneumonia. The IV preparation is preferred because higher serum levels can be attained. Vigorous attempts should be made to confirm the diagnosis before instituting therapy. In a desperately ill patient in whom this is impossible, the drug may be started when the disease is suspected.

(4) Pentamidine isethionate, 4 mg/kg IM daily in 1 dose for 12–15 days, is a more toxic alternative. Its IV use is associated with significant side effects. It is rarely justified to give pentamidine empirically. The side effects and toxicity of the drug and the possibility of misdiagnosis strongly favor proof of infection by lung biopsy before institution of therapy. Pentamidine and trimethoprim-sulfamethoxazole should not be used together, since this combination may adversely affect the outcome. (Pentamidine is available from the Parasitic Diseases Branch of the Centers for Disease Control, Atlanta, Georgia 30333. Telephone: 404-329-3311.)

(5) The use of trimethoprim and sulfamethoxazole (Bactrim) for prophylaxis, 5 mg trimethoprim and 20 mg sulfamethoxazole/kg/day in 2 divided doses, has been successful in preventing *P. carinii* pneumonia in immunocompromised patients when the disease is strongly suspected.

(6) The dosage of parenteral trimethoprim-sulfamethoxazole is as follows:

(a) Loading

< 10 years old, 250 mg/M^2 trimethoprim or 12 mg/kg for 1 dose
> 10 years old, 250 mg/M^2 trimethoprim or 8 mg/kg for 1 dose

(b) Maintenance:

< 10 years old, 150 mg/M^2 trimethoprim or 7 mg/kg/dose
> 10 years old, 150 mg/M^2 trimethoprim or 5 mg/kg/dose

Maintenance doses should begin 8 hr (for a child < 10 years old) or 12 hr (for an older child) after loading. These intervals are also appropriate for maintenance therapy. Dosage should be altered for abnormalities of renal function (see Chap. 15, p. 463).

6. Babesiosis

a. Etiology. *Babesia* species are intraerythrocytic protozoan parasites introduced into humans via tick bites. Babesiosis may also be acquired by blood transfusion.

b. Evaluation and diagnosis. Children and healthy adults may be asymptomatic, while older people, especially those who are asplenic, may have a severe disease, characterized by fever and hemolytic anemia. Transfusion-acquired disease may affect all ages. The diagnosis requires the demonstration of parasites in thin or thick blood smears. Inoculation into hamsters or serologic tests can provide confirmation.

c. Treatment. Chloroquine has been used and produces symptomatic improvement without a reduction in parasitemia. Pentamidine isethionate has also been used with unsatisfactory results.

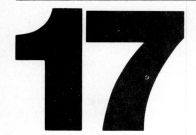

Blood Disorders

I. Microcytic hypochromic anemias
A. Iron deficiency
1. **Etiology**
   a. Inadequate stores provided at birth (prematurity, fetal-maternal bleeding, severely iron-deficient mother).
   b. Failure of dietary iron intake to keep up with increasing requirements of an expanding blood volume as the child grows (usually seen in the first few years of life in children with inordinately high milk intake [> 1 quart/day], and again in menstruating adolescents because of a combination of inadequate iron intake and increased iron loss).
   c. Iron loss (hemorrhage).
2. **Evaluation and diagnosis.** See Table 17-1.
   a. Microcytic hypochromic smear, decreased serum iron, and increased iron-binding capacity; the iron-binding protein (transferrin) is less than 15 percent saturated. A quick and usually reliable bedside test is to look at the patient's serum in a spun hematocrit tube; in iron deficiency it is strikingly pale.
   b. Hemoglobin electrophoresis shows a low hemoglobin A_2 level, but otherwise normal findings.
   c. Bone marrow examination shows absent stainable iron.
3. **Therapy.** The goal of therapy is to replenish marrow iron stores as well as to achieve a normal hemoglobin value. Therefore treatment should be continued at least 6 months after a normal hemoglobin level has been reached. Since dietary iron rarely provides sufficient replacement, a supplement is required. Oral therapy is preferred unless the patient is unable to tolerate it, or the family is not considered sufficiently dependable to administer the dose regularly.
   a. **Oral therapy.** The recommended therapeutic dose is 6 mg/kg/day of elemental iron given in 3 daily doses. Ferrous sulfate is probably the most effective and least expensive iron-containing drug. Since it consists of 20% elemental iron by weight, the usual daily dose is 30 mg/kg. Oral iron must **not** be given with food. The best results are obtained when iron is given 30 min prior to meals.
   b. **Parenteral therapy**
      (1) The calculated total dose should aim at raising the hemoglobin concentration to 12.5 gm/100 ml and to provide 20% of total blood iron to replenish depleted body stores. The dose is calculated by using the formula

      $$\text{mg iron} = \frac{(\text{blood volume}) \times (12.5 - \text{observed hemoglobin}) \times (3.4) \times (1.2)}{100}$$

      where blood volume = 75 ml/kg and 3.4 = iron content in mg/gm hemoglobin.
      (2) Imferon, an iron-dextran complex containing 50 mg of elemental iron per milliliter, is used for deep IM injection in the buttock. Since this

Table 17-1. Findings in iron deficiency anemia and thalassemia trait

Iron deficiency	Thalassemia trait
Smear: hypochromia, microcytosis, pencil forms; no stippling	Hypochromia, microcytosis, target cells, stippling
Decreased serum iron	Normal or increased serum iron
Increased iron-binding capacity	Normal or increased iron-binding capacity
Clear plasma	Yellowish plasma
Increased free erythrocyte protoporphyrin	Normal free erythrocyte protoporphyrin
Decreased serum ferritin	Increased serum ferritin
MCV/RBC $\times$ 10^{-6} > 13	MCV/RBC $\times$ 10^{-6} < 12
Decreased A_2 on hemoglobin electrophoresis	Increased A_2 and/or F on hemoglobin* electrophoresis (in β-thalassemia)
Can occur in any ethnic group	Seen predominantly in groups of Mediterranean (β-thalassemia), black, or Oriental (α-thalassemia) origin
Responds to iron	No response to iron
Iron replacement and maintenance therapy usually necessary	No therapy indicated or necessary; genetic counseling may be appropriate

*Patient must not be concurrently iron deficient.

dark brown solution tends to stain superficial tissues, separate needles should be used for withdrawing it from the vial and for injection, and the Z-tract injection technique should be used. Adverse reactions include local pain, headaches, vomiting, fever, urticaria, angioneurotic edema, arthralgias, and anaphylaxis. **The total dosage should be spaced over 2–3 weeks and should not exceed 0.1 ml/kg/dose, with a maximum of 2.0 ml per dose.**

B. Lead poisoning. See Chap. 4, pp. 110ff, for a detailed description.

C. The thalassemias. The thalassemias are hereditary defects in globin chain synthesis transmitted as autosomal recessive traits.

    1. β-Thalassemia (homozygous condition). Inadequate production of beta chains in β-thalassemia leads to unbalanced production of alpha chains, and the excess alpha chains precipitate as intracellular inclusions. This leads to destruction of RBCs in the bone marrow (ineffective erythropoiesis) and marked shortening of the RBC life span. The RBCs that manage to reach the peripheral blood contain reduced hemoglobin levels and are therefore hypochromic.

      a. Evaluation and diagnosis

        (1) Clinical manifestations vary with the age of the patient and the severity of the anemia. It is clinically undetectable in the early months of life, due to the relatively large amount of fetal hemoglobin present. However, as gamma chain synthesis recedes, normal beta chain production does not occur, and anemia and hepatosplenomegaly develop. The characteristic facies is apparent by 1 year of age.

        (2) The combination of increased oral iron absorption and transfusion therapy leads to increased iron overload, resulting in hemosiderosis of vital organs and a bronzed complexion.

        (3) Congestive heart failure (CHF) due to myocardial hemosiderosis is an important source of morbidity and mortality in these patients.

      b. Treatment

        (1) Transfusion with packed RBCs (10–20 ml/kg) should be given at sufficiently frequent intervals to maintain a hemoglobin level of 10–

12 gm/100 ml to allow for normal growth and development and to decrease the erythropoietic activity of the bone marrow.

(2) **Iron chelating agents** (e.g., deferoxamine and ascorbic acid) have been utilized with varied results in an attempt to mobilize the increased iron stores. At present this is an experimental procedure that should be conducted only under a research protocol.

(3) **Splenectomy.** The indications for this procedure are generally considered to be

(a) Hypersplenism as manifested by increasing transfusion requirements

(b) Symptoms (e.g., "small stomach syndrome") resulting from marked splenic enlargement

(c) After splenectomy, thalassemic patients have a significant increase in the risk of **septicemia,** especially if they are under 4 years old. The procedure should be deferred, if possible, until the child is over 4 because of this increased risk. Patients should receive pneumococcal vaccination prior to splenectomy. Some advocate antibiotic prophylaxis after splenectomy (see Tables 15-2 and 15-11).

(4) **Folic acid** (1 mg/day) is useful in preventing megaloblastic crises induced by the rapid turnover of erythropoietic cells.

(5) These patients should not be treated with iron preparations because they already have increased tissue iron deposition.

2. **β-Thalassemia trait (heterozygous condition).** The major significance of this condition is that its presentation as a mild microcytic hypochromic anemia frequently causes it to be confused with iron deficiency and mistakenly treated with iron. The major differential points are a normal or increased serum iron level and an increased hemoglobin A_2 on hemoglobin electrophoresis in thalassemia trait (see Table 17-1). **Iron therapy is contraindicated** in this condition unless there is concomitant iron deficiency.

3. **α-Thalassemia (heterozygous condition).** Patients with this problem may have a hypochromic anemia similar to, but usually milder than, β-thalassemia trait. Anemia is rare. Clinical, molecular (DNA sequencing), and family studies are the best way to make the diagnosis.

4. **α-Thalassemia (hemoglobin H disease).** In this form of α-thalassemia, the abnormal gene from one parent is combined with a so-called silent carrier gene from the other parent.

a. Affected patients have a moderately severe anemia (8–12 gm/100 ml) and an abnormal band on hemoglobin electrophoresis. The band corresponds to hemoglobin H (beta tetramer) and may total 12–40% of the total hemoglobin.

b. The need for transfusion therapy will depend on the severity of the anemia.

II. **Macrocytic anemias.** The most common causes are vitamin B_{12}, folate deficiency, and drugs that interfere wtih folic acid metabolism such as phenytoin and certain antimetabolites (methotrexate, trimethoprim, pyrimethamine). Less common causes are hereditary orotic aciduria, liver disease, thiamine deficiency, sideroachrestic anemia, and Di Guglielmo syndrome. Establishment of a correct etiologic diagnosis is of primary importance, since incorrect treatment of B_{12} deficiency with folate may result in hematologic improvement but progressive neurologic damage.

A. **Vitamin B_{12} deficiency**

1. **Etiology.** The causes may be intrinsic factor deficiency (congenital or acquired), congenital transcobalamin deficiencies, generalized intestinal malabsorption, selective B_{12} malabsorption, or resection of the distal ileum.

2. **Evaluation and diagnosis**

a. **Physical examination** may demonstrate the neurologic signs associated with subacute combined degeneration of the spinal cord.

b. **Peripheral smear** shows macro-ovalocytes, marked variation in RBC size and shape, and a high mean corpuscular volume (MCV) (> 110). Although nucleated RBCs may be pesent, there is a reticulocytopenia. Neutropenia and thrombocytopenia may also be present, as well as hypersegmentation of the neutrophils.

c. **Bone marrow examination** shows megaloblastic erythroid maturation and giant metamyelocytes and may also show dysplastic erythroid cells.

d. **Nonspecific laboratory findings** may include a positive Coombs test, hyperbilirubinemia, and elevated lactic dehydrogenase. The most specific findings are low serum vitamin B_{12} (except in transcobalamin II deficiency), abnormal Schilling test results, and a successful response to a therapeutic trial of vitamin B_{12}.

3. **Treatment**

a. **Therapeutic trial.** Give 1–3 μg **vitamin B_{12}** daily (IM) for 10 days. If the patient is B_{12}-deficient, the response will be as follows: Within 24–48 hr the marrow will convert from megaloblastic to normoblastic morphology. Reticulocytosis should appear within 3 days and peak around the fifth day. Hemoglobin should return to normal levels within 4–8 weeks. (Although folate-deficient patients may respond to very high doses of B_{12}, they will not respond to this very low dose.)

b. Subsequently, 100 μg/day IM for 2 weeks should be given to replenish body stores; then 100–1000 μg IM once monthly for the rest of the patient's life or until the underlying disorder is cured.

c. **Life-threatening hypokalemia** may occur during early treatment, and serum K^+ values should be carefully monitored.

d. A rise in serum uric acid often accompanies the reticulocytosis, usually reaching its peak at about the fourth day after the start of treatment. This may be prevented by allopurinol.

B. In **folic acid deficiency,** body stores of folate are relatively small. Deficiency may be manifested within 1 month of folate deprivation, and full-blown megaloblastic anemia is seen within 3–4 months.

1. **Etiology.** Causes include dietary inadequacy, congenital and acquired malabsorption syndrome, antimetabolite therapy, and conditions that create a high folate demand because of increased hematopoiesis (chronic hemolysis, pregnancy, leukemia).

2. **Evaluation.** This condition is often seen in infants with a history of poor growth, serious infection, chronic diarrhea, and goat's milk feeding. The neurologic signs associated with vitamin B_{12} deficiency are absent.

3. **Diagnosis.** Hematologic findings are similar to those associated with B_{12} deficiency. The major differences noted in laboratory studies are a normal B_{12} level, low folate level, and normal Schilling test results. Folic acid deficiency can coexist with iron deficiency anemia, in which case macrocytosis will not be seen. (Folic acid levels should be checked in all patients with iron deficiency believed to be on a nutritional basis.)

4. **Treatment**

a. A therapeutic trial of **folate** consists of 20–200 μg folic acid IM daily for 10 days. If malabsorption does not appear to be a problem, this dose can be given PO. B_{12}-deficient patients do not usually respond to this small dose of folate.

b. A dose of 1–5 mg PO daily for 4–5 weeks is usually adequate to replenish body stores even in patients with malabsorption. Patients with simple dietary deficiency can usually stop therapy at this point if they are on a proper diet, while patients with malabsorption or increased need for folate may require therapy indefinitely.

III. **Hemolytic anemias**

A. **Congenital hemolytic anemias**

1. **Hereditary spherocytosis**

a. **Etiology.** This condition results from autosomal dominant inheritance. Erythrocytes are unusually susceptible to splenic sequestration and destruction, and the patient has a chronic hemolytic anemia that may manifest itself as early as the first day of life (neonatal jaundice) or be sufficiently mild to be noticed only on a routine examination.

b. Evaluation

(1) A peripheral smear shows small, round RBCs that lack the normal areas of central pallor.

(2) There is increased osmotic fragility and high mean corpuscular hemoglobin concentration (MCHC > 36).

c. Treatment

(1) In general, the anemia is rarely severe enough to require transfusion, but, following viral infection, there may be a temporary slowdown of erythropoiesis, causing a sudden drop in hematocrit. Such aplastic crises are associated with an increase in pallor, a drop in bilirubin level and reticulocyte count, and, if severe enough, cardiac decompensation. The process is usually self-limited, but the patient must be observed closely until the return of reticulocytosis.

(2) Secondary folate deficiency may lead to a megaloblastic crisis unless prevented by a prophylactic administration of folate (1 mg daily).

(3) Splenectomy is the treatment of choice when there is severe morbidity. It results in a decrease in bilirubin and reticulocyte count and a rise in hematocrit, despite persistence of spherocytes and abnormal osmotic fragility. If possible, splenectomy should be deferred until the patient is over 4 to lessen the risk of sepsis. Antibiotic prophylaxis should be considered after splenectomy (see Table 15-2) and pneumococcal vaccination should be given prior to splenectomy.

2. Congenital nonspherocytic hemolytic anemias

a. Etiology. This is a heterogenous group of hereditary RBC enzyme defects.

(1) Type of defect. In some patients the Embden-Meyerhof pathway (e.g., pyruvate kinase [PK], triose phosphate isomerase) may be involved. In others, involvement is in the hexose monophosphate shunt (e.g., glucose 6-phosphate dehydrogenase [G-6-PD], glutathione reductase).

(2) Pattern of inheritance. This varies with each enzymopathy. PK deficiency has an autosomal recessive pattern, while G-6-PD deficiency follows an X-linked recessive pattern. The latter is most commonly seen in males of Mediterranean origin and black males.

b. Evaluation. These conditions may present with hemolytic jaundice in the neonatal period, hemolytic anemia at any age, or gallstones. Acute hemolytic episodes following infection or exposure to oxidant drugs is characteristic of hexose monophosphate shunt defects (Table 17-2).

c. Diagnosis. PK deficiency may be associated with burr cells, while hexose monophosphate shunt defects may be associated with Heinz bodies in the RBCs (brilliant cresyl blue staining). The precise diagnosis can only be made by assay for the specific enzyme defect.

d. Treatment

(1) Splenectomy may be useful in increasing the hemoglobin level in patients with Embden-Meyerhof defects. It is best deferred **beyond the age of 4 years** to reduce the risk of overwhelming sepsis. No treatment is needed in mild cases.

(2) In hexose monophosphate shunt defects, therapy consists mainly of avoidance of the large number of oxidant drugs that precipitate hemolysis.

(3) Occasionally, during a severe infection or after exposure to an oxidant drug, anemias may be sufficiently severe to warrant transfusion of packed RBCs. More commonly, adequate treatment of infection or discontinuation of the offending drug is sufficient.

3. Sickle cell anemia

a. Etiology. The RBCs contain hemoglobin S, which consists of two normal alpha chains and two abnormal beta chains (α_2^A, β_2^S). Hemoglobin S forms

Table 17-2. Drugs provoking hemolysis in G-6-PD–deficient red cells

Acetanilid	Para-aminosalicylic acid
Acetophenetidin (phenacetin)	Phenacetin
Acetylsalicylic acid (aspirin)	Phenylhydrazine
N^2-Acetylsulfanilamide	Primaquine
Antipyrine	Probenecid
Colamine	Pyramidon
Fava bean	Salicylazosulfapyridine
Furazolidone	Sulfamethoxypyridazine (Kynex)
Isoniazid	Sulfacetamide
Naphthalene (mothballs)	Sulfisoxazole (Gantrisin)
Naphthoate	Sulfoxone
Nitrofurantoin (Furadantin)	Synthetic vitamin K compounds
Pamaquine	Thiazolsulfone

a linear polymer on deoxygenation that produces a sickle-shaped cell. Sickle cell anemia is a hereditary disorder, affecting mainly blacks. (Approximately 10% of black Americans carry the trait, while 0.2% have the homozygous form of the disease.)

b. Evaluation

  (1) There are usually no clinical manifestations of the disease until a high proportion of the RBCs contain hemoglobin S (at about 6 months of age). An exception to this is the increased risk of infection in infants with sickle cell anemia before other manifestations of the disease are apparent.

  (2) The earliest clinical presentation is often painful swelling of the dorsum of the hand or foot due to ischemic necrosis of the metacarpal or metatarsal bones.

  (3) Other manifestations are hepatosplenomegaly, pallor, cardiomegaly, icterus, and isosthenuria. Progressive episodes of infarction and scarring in the spleen cause it to shrink in size as the patient becomes older, and it is usually no longer palpable by adolescence. The patient may, however, be functionally asplenic even before that time, as demonstrated by the absence of a spleen on a technetium scan and the presence of Howell-Jolly bodies on a peripheral smear.

  (4) Laboratory findings. These include severe anemia (hemoglobin 5–9 gm/100 ml), associated with bizarre RBC shapes (0.5 − >20% are in the sickled form), reticulocytosis (usually 10–20%), and variable hyperbilirubinemia. Exposure of the blood to a reducing agent (e.g., sodium metabisulfite) produces the characteristic sickling change. Hemoglobin electrophoresis demonstrates the abnormal band corresponding to hemoglobin S; no hemoglobin A is seen, and there are variable amounts of hemoglobin F. The degree of hemolysis is related to the number of irreversibly sickled cells, but the number and severity of the crises are more often related to the amount of hemoglobin F present.

c. Treatment is palliative and revolves about the various "crises" that afflict these patients.

  (1) Painful crises. The signs and symptoms depend on which organ's microvasculature is involved (e.g., bone, liver, spleen, GI tract) with vaso-occlusion. Among the precipitating causes are infections, dehydration, acidosis, and hypoxia. **Treatment** consists of reversing these factors and providing analgesia.

(a) Adequate **hydration** is the mainstay of therapy. These patients, even when dehydrated, often cannot concentrate their urine. Thus, urine specific gravity should not be used as a guide to fluid therapy.

(b) Parenteral therapy is preferred if pain or dehydration is severe. Use ½ NS containing 5% dextrose infused at 1.5–2.0 times maintenance. Sodium bicarbonate may be added to the IV fluid in sufficient quantity to raise the urine pH to 6.5–7.0. Extra care must be taken to guard against fluid overload in older patients who have cardiac decompensation.

(c) Oxygen should be considered in severe crises, especially if there is concomitant pulmonary infection.

(d) In severe vaso-occlusive episodes (especially if the CNS is involved), dilution of the sickle cells with normal RBCs has been found to be beneficial. This is rapidly achieved by partial exchange transfusion or pheresis with complete exchange. Unless complete removal of hemoglobin is undertaken, the final hematocrit should be less than 40. **Risks** include circulatory overload, isoimmunization, hepatitis, and increasing blood viscosity; if the sickle crisis has not terminated, the latter problem can lead to increased severity.

(e) Long-term transfusion therapy (to turn off production of hemoglobin S) should be considered in children with neurologic foci of thrombotic crises, recurrent severe, painful crises, or recurrent priapism. This is usually done for a period of 1–2 years to try to break the cycles of recurrent crises. Long-term therapy involves the additional risk of sensitization and iron overload. Therefore **any patient with sickle cell anemia should have a complete blood typing,** and, unless it is an emergency, the patient should be transfused with blood as closely matched as possible and should be monitored for signs of iron overload.

(2) **Aplastic crises.** Infections can sometimes result in complete cessation of RBC production for 7–14 days, with disappearance of reticulocytes, a rapid drop in hemoglobin level, and a decrease in serum bilirubin.

(a) These episodes are usually self-limited. However, when anemia is severe or when symptoms of CHF are present, the patient should be slowly transfused with packed RBCs at a rate of 2–3 ml/kg q8h until the hemoglobin level reaches 7–8 gm/100 ml and the cardiac status stabilizes. Partial exchange transfusion with packed RBCs may be better tolerated.

(b) Oxygen should be given to dyspneic patients, but digitalization is usually not necessary.

(c) In severe CHF, transfusion should be monitored by frequent central venous pressure readings.

(3) **Sequestration crises.** Sudden presentation of shock, apnea, and marked hepatosplenomegaly due to pooling of blood in a patient with hemoglobin SS disease requires immediate resuscitation with packed RBCs (use type O Rh − in emergency). **Treatment** is directed at improving hypovolemia and raising the hematocrit while avoiding pulmonary edema (see sec. **IX.C.3**).

(4) **Hyperhemolytic crises** are probably not frequent, but may occur when the patient is coincidentally G-6-PD deficient and has an infection or is exposed to an oxidant drug. If severe anemia is present, packed RBCs should be given slowly.

(5) **Megaloblastic crises** are due to the increased folate requirements of rapid erythropoiesis. Treatment with folic acid, 1 mg/day, is preventive.

(6) Miscellaneous problems

(a) Infection. Patients with sickle cell disease have increased susceptibility to bacterial infections, notably *Streptococcus (Diplococcus) pneumoniae, Salmonella*, and *Haemophilus influenzae* in the young patient. This should be borne in mind when unexplained fever is present. If bacteremia is suspected at all, the patient should be admitted for observation. Although patients with sickle cell disease often have elevated white counts, an increase over their baseline may be significant. Young patients with sickle cell anemia should be treated as if they were asplenic and should be placed on prophylactic penicillin. All patients above the age of 2 should be given pneumococcal vaccination.

(b) Gallstones are common in sickle cell patients after the age of 10. Surgical intervention must be carefully considered in patients with obstructive jaundice, fever, and abdominal pain because this constellation can also be produced by intrahepatic cholestasis secondary to sickling.

(c) In **operations** on patients with sickle cell disease, general anesthesia must be approached with caution and with scrupulous avoidance of hypoventilation, hypoxia, acidosis, and dehydration. It is generally a good idea to increase O_2-carrying capacity and dilute hemoglobin S (to <40%) by slowly transfusing the patient preoperatively with packed RBCs (10 ml/kg). Whole blood exchange by pheresis may be used for emergency surgical situations. A sickle screen should be performed on all black patients prior to general anesthesia.

(d) Interactions with other hemoglobins. Sickle hemoglobin may interact with other hemoglobins (e.g., hemoglobin C [SC] or thalassemias [S-thal]) to produce a hemolytic anemia similar to SS disease. Retinopathy should be carefully watched for in older children with hemoglobin SC, as in patients with homozygous hemoglobin S disease.

4. Other hemoglobinopathies

a. Hemoglobin C

(1) Evaluation. Homozygous hemoglobin C disease is a mild disorder characterized by hemolytic anemia and splenomegaly. Among the symptoms seen are fleeting abdominal pain and cholelithiasis.

(2) Diagnosis. Laboratory findings include mild normocytic normochromic anemia, with many target cells present and a mild reticulocytosis (1–7%). On hemoglobin electrophoresis, a very slow-moving band is seen near the origin.

(3) Treatment is symptomatic. Splenectomy does not appear to influence the clinical course. Retinopathy should be watched for by periodic ophthalmologic examinations.

b. Unstable hemoglobins. These patients have a moderate to severe congenital hemolytic anemia associated with Heinz bodies in the RBCs and abnormal findings on hemoglobin stability tests. Splenectomy is useful in some instances.

B. Acquired hemolytic anemias

1. Autoimmune. Patients with this condition produce antibodies directed against their own erythrocytes that are demonstrable either in their RBCs or in their plasma. In children, this condition is usually idiopathic but may occur secondary to collagen diseases, lymphoma, infections, or drug therapy (e.g., penicillin, methyldopa, quinine).

a. Evaluation and diagnosis

(1) Routine **hematologic studies** show anemia associated with reticulocytosis. The sine qua non for diagnosis is the Coombs, or antiglobulin, reaction. A positive direct Coombs test result indicates antibody coating the erythrocytes; a positive indirect Coombs test result indicates antibody in the patient's plasma.

(2) If the reaction is maximal at about 37°C, a **"warm" antibody** is present, which is usually of the IgG type.

(3) **"Cold" antibodies** are of the IgM type, react best at low temperature, fix complement, and agglutinate RBCs in saline suspension. These are rare in childhood.

(4) This differentiation is important for therapy, since patients with cold antibodies respond poorly to corticosteroid therapy or splenectomy and should avoid exposure to low temperatures.

b. Therapy

(1) If the condition is secondary to a known disease or drug, therapy should be directed at this process.

(2) In addition, corticosteroid therapy is frequently useful in hemolytic anemia associated with warm antibodies. Prednisone may be used (4–6 mg/kg/day) to achieve an initial response and tapered to 2 mg/kg/day within 48 hr when possible. Prednisone dosage should be reduced to the minimal amount necessary to keep the hemoglobin and reticulocyte count within an acceptable range.

(3) If the patient fails to respond to prednisone or requires an unacceptably high dose, **splenectomy** should be considered. If corticosteroids and splenectomy fail to control the process, immunosuppressive drugs should be considered.

(4) Blood transfusion is hazardous in these patients and should be used only if life-threatening anemia develops, since the patient's anti-RBC globulin usually will cross-react with antigens on the donor RBCs and cause a hemolytic transfusion reaction. The unit of blood that is least reactive with the patient's plasma should be used and should be infused extremely slowly, with close monitoring of the patient for evidence of transfusion reaction.

2. Nonautoimmune

a. Etiology. This condition has multiple causes, including mechanical trauma from prosthetic heart valves, chemical agents and drugs, severe burns, and infections (malaria, *Clostridium perfringens*).

b. Diagnosis. The Coombs test is negative. The smear usually contains many fragmented RBCs and spherocytes.

c. Therapy consists of treatment of the primary disease, as well as transfusion with packed RBCs when anemia is severe.

IV. Anemias associated with primary bone marrow disease

A. Aplastic anemia (pancytopenia). There are two general types of aplastic anemia: constitutional and acquired.

1. Constitutional aplastic anemia, or Fanconi's anemia, is commonly associated with skeletal, renal, and pigmentary anomalies and chromosome breaks in lymphocyte culture. Some patients may have the chromosomal anomalies without the phenotypical ones; thus, chromosome studies are mandatory in all patients with aplastic anemia. Although this is an autosomal recessive hereditary condition, the patients commonly do not show signs of hematologic disorder until after infancy. The most common presenting age for boys is 4–7 years and for girls, 6–10 years.

a. Diagnosis. Pancytopenia, reticulocytopenia, and hypoplastic marrow associated with skeletal anomalies and chromosome breaks are diagnostic. Decreased sister chromatid exchange in cultured lymphocytes is found only in this disease.

b. Therapy

(1) In addition to supportive care with RBCs and platelets when necessary, combined administration of **an androgen and a corticosteroid** has been successful in most cases. The usual plan of therapy is to give up to 5 mg/kg/day of oxymetholone and 1 mg/kg/day of prednisone until the hemoglobin is normal.

(2) These medications are then slowly tapered until the hemoglobin falls below 12 mg/100 ml, at which point they are maintained indefinitely. These patients require continued therapy in order to maintain hematologic stability.

(3) Liver function should be monitored in patients being given oral androgen therapy.

c. Prognosis. Despite marked improvement in survival with the use of androgens, leukemia and other malignancies develop in many of these patients. In addition, some become refractory to therapy.

2. Acquired aplastic anemia

a. Etiology. This condition may be secondary to hepatitis, radiation toxicity, drugs (e.g., chloramphenicol), or chemicals (e.g., benzene), or it may be idiopathic.

b. Evaluation and diagnosis. Pancytopenia, reticulocytopenia, and marrow findings that may show varying degrees of hypoplasia or aplasia are characteristic. However, there is generally no family history of anemia nor phenotypical or chromosome anomalies. Fetal hemoglobin is usually elevated.

c. Therapy

(1) Supportive therapy with RBCs and platelets, preferably HLA-matched single donor units

(2) Androgens and corticosteroids are also used as in constitutional aplastic anemia, but the response rate in acquired disease is much lower. However, when a response is obtained, it is often possible to taper and then discontinue drugs completely.

(3) Early bone marrow transplantation is currently the treatment of choice in severe cases (i.e., reticulocyte count < 1%, platelet count < 20,000/mm^3, and a bone marrow that is hypocellular with > 70% lymphoid elements). This procedure is feasible only if an appropriate HLA-matched donor is available and should be performed only in a medical center that has the necessary personnel and equipment. If transplantation is even remotely considered, non-RBC transfusions should be limited, related donors avoided, and washed, frozen RBCs used when RBCs are required.

(4) Current therapeutic trials using antithymocyte globulin are ongoing at some centers and show promise.

B. Hypoplastic anemia (pure red cell anemia, Diamond-Blackfan syndrome)

1. Etiology. The familial incidence suggests hereditary involvement, but no definite inheritance pattern has been established.

2. Diagnosis. Anemia is associated with normal leukocyte and platelet counts. The reticulocyte count is low. Red cell indexes may show slight macrocytosis. Bone marrow examination is diagnostic (an aspirate of normal cellularity containing normal myeloid elements and megakaryocytes, but with a striking paucity of erythroid cells).

3. Therapy

a. Corticosteroid therapy is effective in 75% of cases, especially if begun early in the disease.

(1) The starting dose is 2–3 mg/kg/day of prednisone given qid. A response is usually seen within 2–4 weeks if the regimen is going to be successful.

(2) This dose should be maintained until the hemoglobin concentration attains normal or satisfactory levels, at which time gradual tapering of the dosage should be attempted. Once a normal or satisfactory hemoglobin level is attained, prednisone should be given on alternate days or, if possible, 3 times a week, at the lowest possible dose.

b. Patients who do not respond to prednisone can be supported with periodic transfusion of packed RBCs, although this may lead to hemochromatosis or hepatitis.

V. Acute lymphoblastic leukemia. Acute lymphoblastic leukemia (ALL) is the most common malignant disease of childhood, occurring in approximately 4 children/100,000. Acute lymphoblastic leukemia accounts for 70–80% of childhood leukemias.

  A. Etiology. Although there are many theories involving viruses and immune surveillance, there is no known cause.

  B. Evaluation and diagnosis. The manifestations of ALL are protean, but most of the clinical presentations are related to the lack of normal hematopoietic elements (i.e., pallor of anemia, purpura or bleeding of thrombocytopenia, prolonged or unusual infection of neutropenia). In addition, invasion of organs by leukemic cells can also lead to symptomatology (e.g., bone pain, meningeal irritation, respiratory distress due to mediastinal involvement). The disease is usually suspected when the peripheral blood smear shows unexplained leukoerythroblastic changes such as nucleated red blood cells in the absence of reticulocytosis, teardrop-shaped RBCs, myeloblasts, and other early myeloid elements, without an increase in bands. Whether or not these abnormalities are present, a bone marrow aspiration and often a biopsy must be performed whenever leukemia is suspected; and, if necessary, special stains should be used to determine the nature of the blasts.

  C. Treatment. The goal of all forms of therapy for leukemia is to destroy the leukemic cells while allowing normal cells to grow. Because of the complexity of this task, treatment approaches are guided by protocols in referral centers.

  D. Prognosis. The prognosis for childhood ALL is constantly improving. Protocols used at various cancer centers are projecting a 5-year disease-free survival of 60–80%. Certain prognostic features are associated with a less favorable initial response and final response to therapy. These include (1) an anterior mediastinal mass, (2) a white cell count greater than 50,000/mm^3, (3) massive hepatosplenomegaly, (4) CNS involvement at presentation, (5) T-cell markers on lymphoblasts, (6) a more undifferentiated leukemia, and (7) an age of onset less than 2 years or over 12 years.

VI. Acute nonlymphoblastic leukemias. These disorders include acute myeloblastic leukemia, acute promyelocytic leukemia, acute monomyelocytic leukemia, erythroleukemia, and acute stem cell leukemia. They account for about 25% of all childhood leukemias.

  A. Therapy for these disorders, however, has not had the same success as that for ALL. With current chemotherapy, 75% of patients with these forms of leukemia will go into remission. Cytosine arabinoside and daunorubicin are the mainstays of chemotherapy. CNS prophylaxis is controversial, since in most of the patients the initial relapse is in the bone marrow.

  B. Bone marrow transplantation has been performed in patients with acute myeloblastic leukemia in second remission and has had reasonable success. Many patients still succumb to infection or graft versus host disease. The use of bone marrow transplantation in patients with acute myeloblastic leukemia who are in a first remission and who have an HLA-identical sibling is controversial.

VII. Disorders of coagulation. Bleeding secondary to abnormalities in the coagulation mechanism may be due to a deficiency or abnormality in either clotting factors or platelets. The deficiency may be secondary to decreased production or increased consumption.

  A. Deficiency of clotting factors
    1. Hemorrhagic disease of the newborn
      a. Etiology. Hemorrhage in the first few days of life occurs due to a relative deficiency of factors II, VII, IX, and X (the vitamin K–dependent factors). This follows from the patient's not receiving or being able to utilize vitamin K.
      b. Evaluation
        (1) Check the history for vitamin K administration.
        (2) Evaluate the patient's gestational age.
        (3) Determine the source and extent of bleeding.

    (4) Prothrombin time (PT), partial thromboplastin time (PTT), and platelet count

    (5) Specific factor assays

c. Diagnosis

    (1) The diagnosis is strongly supported by lack of vitamin K administration.

    (2) The condition is more common in prematures than in full-term infants.

    (3) Bleeding may occur from any site and with any degree of severity.

    (4) The platelet count and fibrinogen are normal; PT and PTT are prolonged.

    (5) Factors, II, VII, IX, and X are decreased.

d. Treatment

    (1) Prophylaxis

        (a) Administer 0.5–1.0 mg natural vitamin K_1 IM (Aqua-MEPHYTON) or vitamin K_1 oxide (Konakion) to all newborns at birth.

        (b) The synthetic form of vitamin K_1, menadiol, is felt to have less of a margin of safety than natural vitamin K_1.

    (2) Corrective treatment

        (a) Give 1–2 mg of aqueous colloidal suspension of vitamin K_1 IM. A rise in clotting factors will be noted in 2–4 hr, approaching normal in 24 hr.

        (b) For severe bleeding, transfuse with **fresh frozen plasma** (FFP), 10 ml/kg, and packed red blood cells to correct the anemia.

2. Liver disease

    a. Etiology. Patients with mild destructive liver disease may have bleeding secondary to vitamin K deficiencies in factors I, II, V, VII, IX, and X due to decreased protein synthesis. In addition, they may have decreased factor VIII due to consumption of clotting factors.

    b. Evaluation

        (1) Liver function tests

        (2) PT, PTT, platelet count, fibrinogen, fibrin split products, and factors V and VIII

    c. The **diagnosis** is confirmed by a prolonged PT and PTT. Consumption should be suspected if the platelet count is low, fibrinogen is low, factor VIII is low, and there is marked increase in fibrin split products (these may be slightly elevated in liver disease in the absence of consumption).

    d. Treatment. Vitamin K (1–5 mg) is given slowly IV and the PT and PTT are repeated in 2–4 hr. If there is no response and if bleeding is severe, fresh frozen plasma, 10 ml/kg, should be administered to correct the clotting abnormality. The prophylactic use of FFP is not recommended because of the short half-life of factors V and VII.

3. Hemophilia (hemophilia A; factor VIII deficiency)

    a. Etiology. X-linked recessive deficiency of factor VIII.

    b. Evaluation

        (1) Personal and family history

        (2) Physical examination

        (3) Activated PTT and PT

        (4) Factor assay

        (5) Bleeding time

        (6) Platelet aggregation studies

    c. Diagnosis

        (1) History and physical examination

            (a) In most mild-to-moderate cases there is positive *family* history, but no *personal* history or stigmata, unless the patient has been exposed to trauma or surgery.

            (b) In many severe cases there is no positive family history (de novo mutations), but the patient has a personal bleeding history dating from about 1 year of age or earlier.

(c) Most patients with mild to moderate disease and some with the severe form show no bleeding tendency during the neonatal period and early infancy.

(d) The older patient with severe hemophilia may show chronic joint deformities and contractures secondary to bleeding into joints and muscles.

(2) Laboratory studies

(a) The bleeding time is normal.

(b) The platelet count and platelet aggregation are normal.

(c) The PT is normal.

(d) The activated PTT is prolonged.

(3) Assay for factor VIII

(a) Mild deficiency: 5–30% of normal

(b) Moderate deficiency: 1–5% of normal

(c) Severe deficiency: < 3% of normal

d. Therapy

(1) Factor VIII-containing materials. For each unit per kilogram of factor VIII administered, plasma levels will rise by 2%. The adequacy of therapy should be monitored with activated PTT. This becomes prolonged when factor VIII levels fall below 40% of normal.

(a) Fresh frozen plasma (must be type-specific or compatible)

(i) The amount to be used is limited by volume considerations. Sufficient factor VIII levels to stop closed soft tissue bleeding (10–20% factor VIII) may be obtained, but not enough to stop surface bleeding.

(ii) Dose. Initially, 15 ml/kg and then 10 ml/kg q12h.

(b) Cryoprecipitate. This plasma fraction is obtained by slow thawing of rapidly frozen plasma and dissolving in 10–20 ml supernatant plasma. It contains factor VIII concentrated approximately 20 times. Factor VIII content (expressed as units) in different containers of cryoprecipitate varies, depending on donor and manufacturer.

(c) Lyophilized factor VIII preparations. Concentrations of factor VIII vary from 20- to 100-fold. Preparation from pooled plasma involves a greater risk of hepatitis when compared with cryoprecipitate, which is produced from single units of plasma.

e. Treatment of bleeding. In general, the more severe the bleeding, the higher the dose and the greater the frequency of factor VIII infusion.

(1) Bleeding into joints

(a) For minor bleeding (incipient hemarthrosis not requiring joint aspiration), a single dose of factor VIII concentrate (20 units/kg) will suffice. Immobilization with plaster splints is not usually necessary. If used, early mobilization is essential.

(b) For hemarthrosis with a swollen painful joint, administer 20 units/kg of factor VIII concentrate, followed by one-half this dose q12h for about 2 days. Aspiration of the joint should be avoided if possible. Immobilization for several days with splints may be necessary to prevent contractures. The joint should be slowly rehabilitated with physical therapy, serial splinting to gain full extension, and eventual weight bearing.

(2) Other soft tissue bleeding

(a) Localized or early bleeding into skin or muscle responds to a single dose of factor VIII concentrate (20 units/kg). Ice packs may also be helpful.

(b) Bleeding into more vital areas such as the mediastinum, floor of the mouth, and retroperitoneum may require additional maintenance doses q12h for up to 48 hr.

   (c) The use of traction or splinting must be considered in intramuscular hemorrhage to prevent contracture.
 **(3) Bleeding in surgery. Plasma alone is inadequate to increase factor
   VIII levels to a range safe for operation.**
   (a) Administer **factor VIII concentrate** in a loading dose of 50 units/
   kg, followed by 25–30 units/kg q8h. Factor VIII must be administered for 7–10 days (the duration of wound healing). The dose
   may be decreased by one-third during the second week. Higher
   doses are used in brain surgery or in the presence of infection.
   (b) Epsilon-aminocaproic acid (EACA), in an initial dose of 3 gm/M^2
   PO, is helpful in dental procedures, as is topical thrombin.
   (c) Therapy should be monitored with activated PTT determinations.
 (4) Bleeding from surface wounds
   (a) Small skin wounds and minor epistaxis may respond to ice packs
   and pressure.
   (b) The patient with severe lacerations should be treated like the
   patient with surgical wounds [see **(3)**].
   (c) GI bleeding not involving the mesentery or retroperitoneum usually responds to 3 or 4 doses of factor VIII concentrate in amounts
   used for enclosed soft tissue bleeding. However, consider the need
   for a diagnostic workup to determine the cause of GI bleeding.
   (d) Hematuria, if mild, may stop spontaneously over a few days.
   Severe or persistent hematuria requires replacement therapy for
   1–2 days with high doses of factor VIII sufficient to attain levels
   50% of normal. **EACA is contraindicated in renal bleeding**
   because of the risk of calyceal and ureteral clotting. Prednisone
   has been advocated for renal bleeding, but its efficacy is un-
   proved.
   (e) Bed rest is indicated.
 f. Complications
  (1) Patients with hemophilia should avoid salicylates, antihistamines,
   and other drugs that interfere with platelet function.
  (2) Inhibitors. Antibodies against factor VIII develop in about 8–16 percent of patients receiving factor VIII transfusions.
   **(a) Inhibitors rarely develop in patients who have had more than
   100 days of replacement therapy without their development.**
   (b) The presence of inhibitors is suggested by failure of apparently
   adequate therapy and is documented by demonstrating inhibition
   of coagulation of normal plasma by the patient's plasma.
   (c) Patients with inhibitors should not receive factor VIII. For mild
   bleeding, **local measures** and **rest** are the best treatment. For
   serious bleeding problems and surgery, **activated factors** have
   recently been employed.
  (3) Preparations of Proplex and Konȳne have activated factors that bypass factor VIII and allow coagulation to proceed. The concentration
   of activated factors in these preparations is variable. The initial dosage is usually 50–100 factor IX units/kg. The adequacy of therapy is
   measured by hemostasis and a shortening of the activated PTT to
   about 40 sec. This therapy has been associated with complications
   such as disseminated intravascular coagulation (DIC), and thus the
   patients should be carefully observed. Preparations of activated factors are now being made so that a more uniform dose may be given.
  (4) For serious bleeding or surgery, attempts may be made to overwhelm
   the inhibitor with massive doses of factor VIII. In anecdotal reports,
   the use of pheresis to remove the inhibitor, coupled with the use of
   high doses of factor VIII, has been successful.
 4. Factor IX deficiency (Christmas disease, hemophilia B) is one-fifth as
  common as factor VIII deficiency. Clinically, the two diseases are very similar. Plasma levels can be raised from 0.5–1.5% with 1 unit/kg of factor IX.

Therapy should be monitored with activated PTT. This disease is also transmitted as an X-linked recessive disorder.

    a. Plasma. Regular bank plasma or fresh frozen plasma may be used, but it is adequate only for treatment of enclosed soft tissue bleeding. The dose is 15 ml/kg loading with 10 ml/kg q12h.

    b. Lyophilized factor IX concentrates

        (1) These are made from pooled plasma and thus increase the risk that hepatitis will develop.

        (2) For surgery, administer a loading dose of 40 units/kg, followed by 15 units q12h.

5. von Willebrand's disease (vascular hemophilia). Patients with this autosomal dominant inherited disorder have a mild, lifelong bleeding tendency but may have prolonged epistaxis, gingival and GI bleeding, and easy bruising. Females may be troubled by menorrhagia.

Although there are many forms of the disease and a wide spectrum of severity, most patients with von Willebrand's disease have decreased factor VIII activity, prolonged bleeding time, and a normal platelet count.

    a. The **diagnosis** is suspected when the patient has a prolonged PTT and a normal PT in addition to a prolonged bleeding time and a normal platelet count. The diagnosis is established by a demonstrated decrease in factor VIII (both activity and antigen) and an abnormal ristocetin-induced platelet aggregation.

    b. Treatment is with fresh plasma or cryoprecipitate. Both contain the factor deficient in von Willebrand's disease, and a dose of 10 ml of fresh frozen plasma/kg will correct the factor VIII level and the bleeding time for 24–48 hr to over 50% of the normal level.

B. Disseminated intravascular coagulation (DIC)

    1. Etiology

        a. There is abnormal consumption of clotting elements, leading to their decrease and to thrombosis and bleeding.

        b. Consumption may be initiated by any pathologic state that triggers the cascade of clotting elements at some point in its course.

    2. Evaluation

        a. In the setting of any conditions known to produce DIC, **unexplained bleeding** requires laboratory investigation with the tests listed in Table 17-3.

        b. Physical examination should reveal evidence of bleeding, peripheral thrombosis, or both.

    3. Diagnosis. See Table 17-3.

    4. Therapy

        a. Treat the cause of the consumption, e.g., sepsis, acidosis, hypoxia.

        b. Most patients who succumb to DIC die because of bleeding, not clotting. Fresh frozen plasma, 10 ml/kg, should be administered, together with platelet transfusions, to control bleeding.

Table 17-3. Laboratory evidence of disseminated intravascular coagulation

Platelets decreased
Prothrombin time prolonged
Partial thromboplastin time prolonged
Fibrinogen decreased
Thrombin time prolonged
Fibrin split products: elevated titers
Microangiopathic changes on blood smear
Factor VIII decreased

c. Heparin has not been shown to alter the mortality of DIC. Its use is best reserved for patients with DIC in whom thrombosis rather than bleeding is the major clinical problem. If heparin is given, it is best done as a continuous IV infusion of 12–25 units/kg/hr. The response to therapy is monitored by clinical improvement and fibrinogen levels. Platelet levels can also be followed, but their return toward normal is usually slower than fibrinogen levels.

C. Deficiency in platelets. Most platelet deficiencies are secondary to increased destruction, with the exception of drug-induced aplasia and some congenital thrombocytopenias.

1. Hypersplenism

a. Thrombocytopenia due to hypersplenism is usually mild and does not cause bleeding. The platelet count does not normally fall below 25,000/mm^3. There is often accompanying anemia and neutropenia.

b. If hypersplenism occurs in severe liver disease with depression of clotting factors, abnormal bleeding may be more of a problem.

c. Therapy. Splenectomy is curative but is usually done for symptoms of hypersplenism other than platelet deficiency, such as an increasing transfusion requirement or recurrent infections.

2. Drug-induced thrombocytopenia

a. Etiology. This condition may result from bone marrow depression or increased peripheral destruction due to drug-induced **antibody production.** Drugs most commonly associated with a toxic insult to the bone marrow are diuretics such as the thiazides and furosemide, trimethoprim, tolbutamide, and thioridazine. Drugs that produce thrombocytopenia by an immunologic mechanism include quinidine, phenylbutazone, sulfonamides, penicillins, digitalis, and tricyclic antidepressants.

b. Therapy

(1) The primary treatment for drug-induced thrombocytopenia is to **withdraw the drug.** In addition, drugs that adversely affect platelet function (e.g., aspirin) should be avoided. Cerebral hemorrhage is the major cause of death in drug-related thrombocytopenia, and bed rest is advisable if bleeding is more than mild. Coughing, straining, and other activities that cause increased intracranial pressure should be avoided.

(2) Corticosteroids acutely increase vascular stability and may prevent immunologic destruction of platelets. Prednisone, 1–2 mg/kg/day for 1–2 weeks, is helpful if bleeding is a problem.

(3) Platelet transfusion is helpful in stopping the bleeding from thrombocytopenia secondary to bone marrow suppression. If the platelet count is less than 20,000/mm^3 on the basis of decreased production, significant bleeding is likely, and platelet concentrates (6 units/M^2) may be used. In some cases of severe thrombocytopenia on an immune basis, massive platelet transfusions with high-dose corticosteroids may be indicated.

3. Immune thrombocytopenic purpura (ITP) is an autoimmune thrombocytopenia that in 60% of reported cases follows a viral infection, with about 15% following common exanthems.

a. Etiology. The cause is unknown, but the pathogenesis may be related to immunologic stimulation by a virus.

b. Evaluation

(1) Petechiae and purpura are almost invariably present, and 30% of patients have epistaxis. While hemoglobin, hematocrit, and white blood count may be normal (atypical lymphocytes may be present), the platelet count is less than 50,000/mm^3, and there is a preponderance of large platelets on the peripheral smear.

(2) Antiplatelet antibodies are found in 60% of children with ITP, and if facilities for the test are available, it should be performed.

(3) A **Coombs test** should be done to rule out autoimmune hemolytic anemia. But in childhood, acute ITP is not often associated with other autoimmune disorders.

c. The **diagnosis** of ITP is made by doing a bone marrow aspiration to document the adequacy of megakaryocytes. Often, eosinophilia is present in the marrow. If the clinical history is suggestive and the thrombocytopenia is mild, observations of serial platelet counts to document recovery may be used in place of bone marrow examination. If, however, therapeutic intervention is considered, bone marrow aspiration should be performed to rule out infiltrative diseases.

d. Therapy. Most children with ITP do very well without therapy. In about 70%, platelet counts return to normal within 4 months. Another 10% of cases resolve in the next 8 months; 20% go on to have chronic ITP. Postpubertal children do not do as well, with only 20–30% resolving spontaneously. Mortality in childhood ITP is less than 1%. Death, when it occurs, is due to intracranial, pulmonary, or GI hemorrhage. Of children who die, 90% do so within the first few days of the onset of their disease. Although the risk of significant bleeding is greatest early in the disease, some deaths have been reported among children with chronic ITP.

(1) Drugs that interfere with platelet function **should be avoided.**

(2) Corticosteroids have not increased the number of children achieving a normal platelet count, although they probably affect the rate of rise in platelet count. However, corticosteroids have been shown to acutely enhance the rate at which bleeding disappears in ITP, which is probably related to their effect on vascular stability. Prednisone should be given to patients with ITP who have a platelet count of less than 10,000/mm^3 or who show evidence of mucosal bleeding. The drug may be given at high dosage (4–6 mg/kg/day) and then reduced after 48 hr to 2 mg/kg/day or less. After 2 weeks the drug is tapered over the next week regardless of the platelet count. The use of corticosteroids is to protect against early severe bleeding. Some authorities advocate an additional trial of prednisone for 2–4 weeks for patients who have not spontaneously recovered after 4 months.

(3) Splenectomy. Of the 20% of patients in whom chronic ITP develops, only one-tenth will recover spontaneously. Of patients with chronic ITP who undergo splenectomy, 60–70% are cured, probably because the spleen, in addition to being the organ of platetlet destruction, is a site for production of antiplatelet antibodies.

(a) Before splenectomy, patients should receive **prednisone** or **hydrocortisone,** and, although postoperative bleeding is rare, **platelets** should be available for administration.

(b) The platelet count peaks about 4 days after splenectomy and then reaches a plateau at 2–4 weeks.

(c) Splenectomy is to be avoided in children under 4 years of age.

(d) Most children who undergo splenectomy are placed on prophylactic penicillin (400,000 units bid) for at least 2 years and are given pneumococcal vaccine preoperatively. There are no data, however, to suggest that this affects the risk of sepsis.

(e) About 20–30% of patients will continue to have thrombocytopenia after splenectomy. Some may respond to intermittent corticosteroids. Others require immunosuppressive agents, such as vincristine, azathioprine, or cyclophosphamide. The risk of these drugs should be weighed against risk of bleeding from the thrombocytopenia, which in children is low.

VIII. Neutropenia and defects of neutrophil function

A. *Neutropenia* is defined as less than 1,000 granulocytes/mm^3, while *severe neutropenia* is defined as less than 500 granulocytes/mm^3. If neutropenia is suspected, multiple hand counts should be performed to confirm the granulocyte number.

1. Etiology. Decreased marrow production or accelerated destruction of granulocytes causes neutropenia (see Table 17-4 for specific diagnoses).

Table 17-4. Specific causes of neutropenia

Cause	Characteristics and treatment
Decreased production	
Benign neutropenia	Chronic condition in which neutrophil counts range from $200-1,500/mm^3$; severe infection rare
Chemotherapy (toxin, radiation)	Induced: Removal of offending agent may allow for recovery; severity dependent on agent and dose
Cyclic neutropenia	Oscillation of neutrophil count with associated symptoms occurs at 14- to 24-day intervals; major problem is usually severe stomatitis
	To detect cycling, neutrophil counts must be done twice a week for several weeks
Kostmann syndrome	Severe congenital neutropenia with neutrophil counts $< 200/mm^3$, not raised by corticosteroids or other drugs; prophylactic antibiotics (trimethoprim-sulfamethoxazole bid) may decrease episodes of septicemia but bone marrow transplantation is probably the only chance for long-term survival
	Rarely, the disease may terminate in leukemia
Shwachman-Diamond syndrome	Neutropenia with exocrine pancreatic insufficiency, with major treatment aimed at pancreatic enzyme replacement; may also be a role for prophylactic antibiotics (see Kostmann syndrome)
Marrow failure and infiltrative disease	Neutropenia, usually associated with pancytopenia, as in aplastic anemia or when the marrow is replaced by tumor or fibrosis
	Therapy directed at the primary illness
Nutritional	Folate and vitamin B_{12} deficiency can lead to megaloblastic anemia and neutropenia
Infection	Transient acquired toxic marrow injury, occurring most often in viral infection; neutropenia may be severe and protracted in some cases but is usually self-limiting
	Simultaneous appearance of atypical lymphs clue to diagnosis
	Bacterial infection, especially from *Staphylococcus aureus,* also causes transient marrow injury
Decreased survival	
Isoimmune neonatal neutropenia	Severe neutropenia at birth without other cytopenias, normal myeloid precursors in marrow, and demonstration of anti–white cell antibodies in serum of mother and baby
	Disease abates as maternal anti–white cell antibodies decay in baby's serum
Autoimmune neutropenia	Severe neutropenia without other cytopenias; myeloid precursors present in marrow, often with maturation arrest, positive anti–white cell antibodies

Table 17-4 (continued)

Cause	Characteristics and treatment
	A careful search should be made for any underlying conditions that might be treated, such as collagen vascular disease, juvenile rheumatoid arthritis, and lymphoproliferative disease
	Prednisone, 2 mg/kg/day to start, raises neutrophil count in 50% of cases
	Splenectomy has not been of permanent benefit except for specific disorders (e.g., Felty syndrome); in resistant disease, plasmapheresis to remove antibody might be attempted
Drug-induced neutropenia	Virtually any drug may cause immune neutropenia, but most common in clinical practice are the penicillins (especially oxacillin), sulfonamides, and phenylbutazone-type drugs
	Removal of the drug is the obvious therapy; recovery of the granulocyte count is usually prompt (5–7 days) but may be delayed

2. Evaluation and diagnosis
   a. History, with emphasis on severity, duration or periodicity of the illness, family history, fetal wastage, infections, stomatitis, and exposure to drugs or toxins.
   b. Physical examination, looking specifically for associated phenotypical abnormalities, oral mucosa and gingiva for stomatitis, adenopathy, splenomegaly, and sites of infection. The rectal area should be examined, but formal rectal examination should be avoided unless it is absolutely necessary.
   c. Bone marrow aspirate and **biopsy** should be done.
   d. Specific tests. See Table 17-4.
B. Disorders of neutrophil function. The symptoms relate to the severity of the disorder and are identical to those seen with neutropenia, characterized by severe or repeated infections with a poor response to antibiotics.
   1. Etiology. See Table 17-6.
   2. Evaluation and diagnosis is as in sec. **VII.A.2** (see Table 17-5 for specific tests).
   3. Treatment
   a. General principles. Careful attention must be paid to hygiene and mouth care. The mouth sores that are characteristic of some types of neutropenia or dysfunction are treated with mouthwash ($H_2O_2:H_2O$; 1:1 by volume) after eating and before bed. For prophylaxis of candidal superinfection, use oral nystatin suspension, ½–1 tsp "swish and swallow" qid. The prophylactic use of antibiotics is controversial. (See Tables 17-4 and 17-6 for the therapy of specific syndromes.)
   b. General approach to the therapy of neutropenia with fever (temperature >38°C)
      (1) Careful physical examination
      (2) If the granuloycte count is 500–1,000, and the patient is clinically well, culture and observe.
      (3) If the granulocyte count is 500 or less, or there are signs of serious infection (e.g., rigors, chills) and the trend of bone marrow recovery is

Table 17-5. Some common tests of neutrophil function

Function	Test	Purpose
Bone marrow reserves	Bone marrow aspirate Prednisone stimulation	Measure decreased production versus inability of granulocytes to exit from marrow
Motility	Rebuck skin window	Measure timed appearance of granulocytes and monocytes in abraded skin
Opsonization and recognition	Attachment of particles coated with complement or immunoglobulin membranes	Evaluate functional capacity of granulocyte
Ingestion	Quantitation of ingested particles	Quantitates phagocytic defect
O_2-generation by nitroblue tetrazolium (NBT)	NBT test	Diagnostic of chronic granulomatous disease

not known (i.e., counts are returning rather than dropping), culture, x-ray, and begin broad-spectrum antibiotics, including an aminoglycoside. Patients with neutropenia may not show the usual signs of infection. Physical findings such as rales, erythema, or peritoneal signs may be **absent** despite severe infection. The use of granulocyte transfusions if indicated is controversial (see granulocyte transfusion, sec. **IX.E**).

(4) Antibiotic therapy should not be disconinued until all cultures are negative, the patient is afebrile, and, in those with self-limited neutropenia, neutrophil counts are greater than $300-500/mm^3$ and increasing.

(5) During neutropenia, while the patient is on broad-spectrum antibiotic therapy, repeat the careful physical examination in search of fungal lesions and new sites of infection. Suspicious physically or radiographically observed lesions should be examined by biopsy. The empirical use of amphotericin or other antifungals is controversial.

IX. **Transfusion therapy.** A description of currently available blood products follows, with the indications for their use, as well as recommendations for the treatment of transfusion-induced complications.

A. **Whole blood**

1. **Contents of 1 unit of whole blood**
   a. Total volume 500 ml, hematocrit 40%, and plasma volume 280 ml
   b. Na 25 mEq, K 15 mEq, and plasma acid 80 mEq
   c. Storage longer than 8 hr ablates coagulation factor activity.
   d. Normal immunoglobulins
   e. Fresh whole blood (not collected in heparin) contains clotting factors and active platelets.

2. **Indications**
   a. Treatment of acute blood loss and shock
   b. Replacement of surgical losses
   c. Exchange for removal of toxic substances in centers where pheresis is unavailable
   d. Partial exchange for polycythemia
   e. **Not** the product of choice for chronic anemia

Table 17-6. Specific causes of neutrophil dysfunction

Cause	Characteristics and treatment
Depressed chemotaxis	Seen in chronic illness such as renal failure and diabetes Ameliorating the underlying condition and aggressively treating infection are the therapies of choice
Humoral inhibition of motility	A number of syndromes associated with chronic infection (especially of the skin) with gram-positive bacteria have been identified, with a higher incidence in red headed females and persons with chronic dermatitis; excess IgE and/or IgA often associated Thrust of therapy is to eliminate chronic infection and maintain exquisite skin hygiene. In severe cases, levamisole or plasma therapy may be attempted on an empirical basis
Opsonization disorders	Deficiencies of complement and immunoglobulins
Chédiak-Higashi disease	Repeated, often severe infections with granulocytes that contain large granules; treatment with asorbic acid may be helpful Most patients will succumb to infection, hemorrhage, or to a leukemialike "accelerated phase" At present bone marrow transplantation appears to be only possible therapy
Chronic granulomatous disease	Majority of patients with this predominantly X-linked disorder are males who present with multiple skin abscesses caused by gram-positive bacteria but may go on to have abscesses caused by catalase-producing organisms (both gram-positive and gram-negative) in virtually any organ system Chronic pneumonia may be a serious problem as can gastric antrum narrowing by granulomatous infiltration Major surgery should be avoided if possible Due to the poor clearance of organisms, established infections or granulomatous collections should be treated with appropriate antibiotics for several weeks; prophylactic use of semisynthetic penicillins or trimethoprim-sulfathoxazole may decrease episodes of infection and alter the course of the disease

3. **Amount of infusion**
   a. **Shock or blood loss.** Estimate the amount of blood loss and infuse at the maximum rate (usually 10–20 ml/kg/hr), monitoring vital signs and slowing the infusion when vital signs begin to improve.
   b. For exchange transfusion, assume that blood volume = 80 ml/kg. Usually, one to two volume exchanges are performed.
   c. For partial exchange for lowering hematocrit (Hct), the volume of exchange (ml) = blood volume × (current Hct − desired Hct)/current Hct
   d. Exchange for Rh disease (see Chap. 6, pp. 155ff)
B. **Fresh frozen plasma.** This is collected in acid-citrate-dextrose.
   1. **Contents of one unit**
      a. Volume 250 ml, 50–100 WBCs/mm^3
      b. 40 mEq Na, 1.0–1.5 mEq K, pH 6.6

   c. All clotting factors
   d. Plasma proteins including colloid (e.g., albumin) and antibodies
 2. Indications
   a. Replacement of clotting factors
   b. Volume expander
C. Packed red cells
 1. Contents of one unit
   a. Volume 300 ml, Hct 70%, and plasma volume 80 ml
   b. Na 15 mEq, K 4 mEq, and plasma acid 25 nEq
   c. No immunoglobulin or clotting factors
 2. Indications
   a. Chronic anemia in which there is no expectation that therapy other than transfusion could raise red cell mass before the life-threatening effects of anemia (e.g., CHF) supervene
   b. Hypertransfusion programs (i.e., thalassemia, sickle cell disease)
 3. Amount of infusion
   a. Volume of packed cells = patient's weight (kg) × (Hct desired − Hct observed)
   b. In patients without CHF, the proper rate of infusion = 10 ml/kg/hr maximum
   c. In patients with impending heart failure, **do not exceed 2 ml/kg/hr,** or if vital signs so indicate, IV furosemide should be used during the transfusion to prevent volume overload. In patients with CHF and unstable vital signs, exchange transfusion with packed cells to minimize large volume flux should be performed. In high output CHF due to anemia the aim is to raise the hematocrit above 20–25%, which will return cardiac output toward normal.
 4. Special red cell preparations
   a. Washed packed red cells. 70% Hct in saline with 92% reduction in WBCs and significant dilution of plasma proteins. Used when there is a history of febrile nonhemolytic transfusion reaction (see **F.4**) and other low WBC uses (see **C.4.b**).
   b. Frozen red cells. Volume 200 ml, Hct 70, Na 9 mEq, K 1–2 mEq, and pH 6.8. A 96% reduction in WBCs and no plasma proteins. They are used for febrile nonhemolytic transfusion reactions (see **E.4**), storage of specific-antigen-typed blood for chronic transfusion patients, and low WBC blood for cytomegalovirus avoidance and prevention of sensitization in transplantation candidates.
D. Platelets
 1. Indications
   a. Absolute thrombocytopenia (platelet counts < 50,000) **with bleeding.** The aim should be to raise the platelet count to between 50,000 and 100,000/mm^3.
   b. Prophylactic administration in patients receiving chemotherapy. Many centers routinely transfuse patients with chemotherapy-induced thrombocytopenia with counts less than 10,000–20,000/mm^3 even in the absence of bleeding. This use is controversial.
   c. Qualitative platelet disorders, congenital or acquired (e.g., aspirin) **with bleeding.** When transfusing for this indication, the response to therapy is measured by the clinical effect and the shortening of bleeding time, not by the platelet count.
   d. Massive transfusion. Multiple transfusions with whole blood over 24 hr is often accompanied by thrombocytopenia. Administer platelets for a count less than 50,000.
 2. Amount of infusion
   a. One platelet unit contains approximately 5 × 10^{10} platelets, and 10^7 WBCs, and 35 ml of plasma; pH of 6.0–6.5.
   b. The platelet count is increased to 30,000/mm^3 by 0.1 unit/kg.

   c. In neonatal isoimmune thrombocytopenia, 1 unit of maternal platelets
   should be washed in AB-negative plasma and concentrated immediately
   before infusion to less than 50 ml.
3. A poor response to platelet transfusion is caused by:
   a. Fever alone (even without sepsis)
   b. Infection
   c. Bleeding
   d. Immune mechanisms (antibodies, ITP, posttransfusion purpura)
   e. Consumption (DIC, hemolytic-uremic syndrome)
   f. Splenomegaly
   g. Prolonged storage of platelets (3 days or more)
E. Granulocyte transfusion
   1. The contents of granulocyte transfusion depend on the collection technique. Continuous flow centrifugation (most common) yields a unit containing approximately 2×10^{10} granulocytes/unit with a Hct of 20 and the
   equivalent of 4 units of platelets.
   2. Indications. This is a controversial area.
      a. Severe neutropenia ($<500/mm^3$ absolute granulocyte count) without ex-
      pectation of rapid bone marrow recovery and gram-negative or fungal
      sepsis. (**Note:** Bone marrow examination may be done to document poten-
      tial recovery.) There are no data to suggest that granulocyte transfusion
      lowers mortality if the patient recovers spontaneous bone marrow
      granulocyte function within 5 days.
      b. Gram-positive sepsis probably does **not** respond to granulocyte trans-
      fusion.
      c. Febrile, immunosuppressed patients without evidence of sepsis should
      be evaluated on a case-by-case basis.
   3. Amount of infusion. Often, there is no actual elevation of granulocyte count
   after infusion.
      a. Adults, 1 unit
      b. Children may receive 1 unit, but partial exchange may be necessary to
      prevent volume overload.
      c. Neonates may need partial exchange transfusions with granulocytes, or
      multiple (1–3) 10 ml/kg infusions may be attempted if tolerated. (**Note:**
      Blood collected in CPD and used for exchange transfusion within 4 hr
      may significantly raise the granulocyte count as well as provide platelets,
      clotting factors, and immunoglobulins.)
F. Blood product transfusion reactions
   1. Acute hemolytic transfusion reactions
      a. Caused by blood group incompatibility
      b. Signs and symptoms. These include fever as high as 40.5°C (105°F),
      confusion, vomiting, hypertension, back pain, and hematuria.
      c. Treatment:
         (1) Stop the transfusion and monitor vital signs.
         (2) Volume resuscitation if necessary to stabilize vital signs (see Chap. 3,
         p. 43).
         (3) Establish renal blood flow with furosemide (0.5 mg/kg IV) and/or
         dopamine (1–10 μg/kg/min).
         (4) When urine flow is established, maintain output and alkalinize urine.
         (5) If no urine flow established, treat as in acute renal failure (see Chap.
         8, pp. 209ff).
         (6) Consider pheresis and exchange transfusion.
         (7) Follow blood bank reporting procedures.
   2. Delayed transfusion reactions
      a. These occur 5–10 days after transfusion and are due to an anamnestic
      response to blood group antigens.
      b. Give immediate treatment as in **1.**
      c. Consider plasmapheresis to remove antibodies.

3. **Allergic reactions to any blood product**
   a. **Signs and symptoms.** Urticaria, itching, angioedema, flushing. Anaphylaxis is rare.
   b. **Treatment**
      (1) Diphenhydramine, 1.25 mg/kg IV.
      (2) Also use epinephrine and corticosteroids, depending on the severity of allergic reaction.
      (3) Patients should receive diphenhydramine, hydrocortisone, and acetaminophen prior to further transfusions.
      (4) Special products do not prevent these reactions.
4. **Febrile reactions**
   a. These occur in 0.1% of previously untransfused children and in 4% of those multiply transfused.
   b. Patients may have severe fever with chills.
   c. The reactions are caused by contaminating white cells and white cell fragments.
   d. Patients should be treated with antipyretics and have premedication in the future.
   e. Washed packed RBCs may then be tried if morbid fevers continue.
   f. Frozen washed cells may then be used if washed packed RBCs still induce fever.
5. **Acute pulmonary edema**
   a. This is caused by leukoagglutinin reaction to white cell transfusion.
   b. **Treatment**
      (1) Stop the infusion.
      (2) Maintain vital signs.
      (3) Use whatever respiratory support is necessary until the process reverses itself.
6. **Graft-versus-host disease**
   a. This can occur with any blood product but is proportional to the number of white cells in the product: granulocytes > platelets > red cells > frozen washed red cells > fresh frozen plasma.
   b. This occurs in neonates and in patients who are severely immunosuppressed or those with complete bone marrow ablation for 5 days or more.
   c. Irradiation of blood products prevents graft-versus-host disease.
7. **Sensitization** is defined as antibody formation against blood groups or HLA determinants that leads to a shortened blood-component life span or interference with transplantation.
   a. Patients on chronic red cell transfusion should have complete red cell typing and receive carefully selected blood in order to avoid sensitization. This usually requires frozen cells that have been extensively typed.
   b. Recent studies suggest that the incidence of sensitization in response to chronic platelet infusion is **not** affected by the use of single-donor versus random-donor platelet transfusion. If sensitization to platelets occurs, one should **then** try single-donor or HLA-matched platelets.
   c. Patients who are candidates for bone marrow transplantation should receive frozen washed red cells to decrease their exposure to white cell HLA antigens.
8. **Infection** is the most frequent serious complication of blood transfusion.
   a. **Viral hepatitis**
      (1) Elevated liver function tests in 7–10% of patients receiving chronic transfusion therapy
      (2) Most cases are non-A, non-B, with negative HAA.
      (3) With all-volunteer blood donor programs, the incidence may be falling soon.
      (4) Patients may have elevated liver function tests for months.
      (5) Occasional cases have progressed to chronic active hepatitis.

Table 17-7. Conditions amenable to pheresis

Pheresis as primary treatment
  Renal graft rejection
  Symptomatic paraproteinemia
  Goodpasture's disease
  Myasthenic crisis
  IgM hemolytic anemia
  Raynaud's phenomenon
  Rapid removal of hemoglobin S red cells in sickle cell disease
  Familial hypercholesterolemia
  Thrombotic thrombopenic purpura

Pheresis to relieve acute symptoms
  Systemic lupus erythematosus
  Cryoglobulinemia
  Polyarteritis nodosa
  Wegener's granulomatosis
  Rheumatoid arthritis
  Dermatomyositis
  Hepatic failure
  Thyroid storm
  Acute or delayed transfusion reaction
  IgM cold agglutinin disease

Experimental pheresis indications
  Removal of inhibitors to coagulation factors
  Autoimmune hemolytic anemia
  Idiopathic or immune thrombocytopenic purpura
  Multiple sclerosis

---

  b. Other infections include cytomegalovirus (6–12% of the general popula-
     tion carries this virus), syphilis (all collected units are screened for this),
     malaria (most cases are ruled out by donor travel history, but occasional
     cases are seen with virulent organisms), and AIDS.
X. Plasmapheresis
  A. Indications. See Table 17-7.
  B. Methods
     1. Pheresis should be performed in centers with experience in treating children.
        Volume and temperature regulation are difficult, especially in children
        under the age of 4.
     2. Monitoring must be carefully performed.
     3. The major difference in the morbidity of the pheresis procedure in adults and
        in children is the difficulty in achieving venous access. Careful preparation of
        access in children will significantly increase the ease of treatment.
     4. Most centers use a 1.5–2.0 blood volume pheresis per episode, with one to
        three episodes per week.
     5. Plasma and cell fractions may be isolated.
  C. Adverse effects
     1. Volume shifts can be quickly handled if patients are under close observation.
     2. Bleeding problems may occur, since patients receive heparin during the
        procedure, and clotting factors may be lost. An appropriate amount of prot-
        amine sulfate may be given to reverse the effect of heparin. If bleeding
        occurs, fresh frozen plasma may be infused to restore the temporary deficit of
        clotting factor activity.

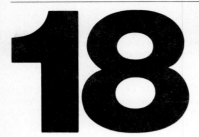

Inflammatory and Immunodeficiency Disorders

I. Inflammatory disorders

A. Juvenile rheumatoid arthritis (JRA) is a generalized systemic inflammatory disease involving the joints, connective tissue, and viscera. The disease may occur at any age, but the peak incidence is at 1–4 years and at puberty.

1. Evaluation. There are three distinct modes of onset: acute febrile or systemic, polyarticular, and pauciarticular. Each may be confused with other diagnoses.

   a. Acute febrile or systemic. This group of children has prominent systemic symptoms with various manifestations of fever, rash, lymphadenopathy, hepatosplenomegaly, abdominal pain, pericarditis, myocarditis, or pleuritis. Joint symptoms may be absent or minimal at presentation, but will eventually develop in most patients.

   b. Polyarticular. The arthritis begins in the large joints, but the small joints of the hands and feet, the cervical spine, and the temporomandibular joint are often involved. The affected joints are swollen, warm, and tender, with limitation of movement and morning stiffness. Low-grade fever, anorexia, and malaise are common.

   c. Pauciarticular. The arthritis is limited to four or fewer joints and usually involves large joints, namely, the knees, ankles, elbows, or hips. The small joints are usually spared. Iridocyclitis occurs in over 25 percent of the patients with this type of presentation and may precede the joint symptoms.

2. Diagnosis. There is no single laboratory test that confirms the diagnosis. Assessment is based on the clinical presentation, laboratory abnormalities, and exclusion of other diseases.

   a. There are no uniformly agreed-on diagnostic criteria. However, the following criteria are useful:

      (1) Polyarticular or monoarticular arthritis persisting for 6 weeks is sufficient for diagnosis if other diseases are excluded. **Arthritis** is defined as swelling of a joint or limitation of motion with heat, pain, or tenderness. The latter two symptoms alone are not sufficient for the diagnosis. Temporomandibular joint involvement, cervical spine involvement, small joint involvement, a nonmigratory pattern, and morning stiffness are suggestive of the diagnosis. The joint involvement may be symmetrical and associated with subcutaneous nodules. The only early x-ray abnormalities are soft tissue swelling and osteoporosis without erosive joint changes. Painless contractions without swelling may occur.

      (2) The acute systemic form will be associated with fever and a characteristic rash consisting of recurrent, evanescent, pale red macules, often with central clearing and found predominantly on the chest, axilla, thighs, and upper arms.

   b. Although there are no diagnostic tests, certain **laboratory findings** may be abnormal in some patients. These include the following:

      (1) An elevated white blood count, anemia, elevated erythrocyte sedimentation rate (ESR), thrombocytosis, and an increase in acute phase reactants.

(2) The assay for anti-gamma globulin (rheumatoid factor) as commonly performed is usually persistently positive in only 10–20% of all patients with JRA. Positive tests are more frequent in older children with polyarticular onset disease. Its presence correlates with a chronic destructive arthritis.

(3) Antinuclear antibody (ANA) may be found in 10–40% of patients with oligoarticular or polyarticular onset disease. An increased percentage of children with chronic iridocyclitis have a positive ANA.

(4) Aspirated joint fluid in JRA is yellow to greenish, cloudy, with low viscosity, and has a poor mucin clot. The white count is 10,000 to 50,000/mm^3, with approximately 75% polymorphonuclears.

(5) There is an increased incidence of the HLA antigen B27 in ankylosing spondylitis, Reiter syndrome, spondylitis with inflamed bowel disease, and arthritis following *Yersinia* or *Salmonella* infection. Laboratory studies to exclude other diseases will often be required.

3. Principles of anti-inflammatory therapy. The treatment of inflammatory diseases depends primarily on the use of anti-inflammatory drugs. The purpose of the drugs is both to reduce the patient's symptoms and, more important, to suppress or eliminate the inflammatory process and thereby preserve function and prevent deformities. With adequate drug therapy and psychological and social service support, at least 75% of children will be left with no significant disability. The basic principle in the management of inflammatory diseases is to use the least amount of therapy that will successfully control the patient's disease. The three principal drugs used are salicylates, corticosteroids, and nonsteroidal agents.

a. Relief of symptoms and control of inflammation. No drug has been specifically approved by the Food and Drug Administration for the treatment of JRA, but aspirin is universally used.

(1) Aspirin is the drug of choice for the relief of acute symptoms and fever. Except during a medical emergency (e.g., myocarditis in JRA, respiratory failure in dermatomyositis) aspirin should be the first anti-inflammatory drug tried.

(a) A dose of 70–100 mg/kg/24 hr in 5 divided doses will give a blood level of approximately 20 mg/100 ml at 2 hr.

(b) If this dose is adequate to control the patient's disease completely, then dose modification is not needed.

(c) If therapy only reduces or does not affect the disease process, then the dose of salicylate should be **increased.** Increasing the dose of aspirin to more than 100 mg/kg/24 hr should be monitored by serum salicylate levels 2 hr after a dose. Salicylate levels as high as 35 mg/100 ml can usually be tolerated without significant side effects. If significant clinical improvement does not occur at 35 mg/100 ml, alternative therapies should be undertaken.

(d) Nonsteroidal agents can be added when patients have a partial but not complete response to aspirin. There is no toxic synergy between nonsteroidals and aspirin. Therefore, no reduction of aspirin dosage is required.

(e) Side effects

(i) Patients and parents should be warned about the symptoms of salicylate toxicity, which include **tinnitus, lethargy, hyperventilation, dizziness, sweating, headaches, nausea,** and **vomiting** (see Chap. 4, pp. 105 ff).

(ii) Aspirin should **not** be taken on an empty stomach. If **gastric irritation** is a problem, antacids may be helpful. However, antacids may decrease the absorption of aspirin and reduce serum levels. **Enteric-coated aspirin should be avoided because of variable absorption.**

(iii) Hepatotoxicity with elevation of serum transaminases occurs in some patients. Enzyme abnormalities occur more commonly with aspirin levels of greater than 25 mg/100 ml but can occur at lower levels. Liver enzyme levels should be checked any time nausea, vomiting, or abdominal discomfort occurs.

(iv) Aspirin should be discontinued if the **prothrombin time** is grossly prolonged, heptatic enzymes are markedly elevated, or clinical evidence of bleeding or liver dysfunction occurs.

(v) GI bleeding should also be looked for if nausea, vomiting, or abdominal discomfort occur even in the absence of hepatotoxicity.

(2) Corticosteroid therapy

(a) The indications for their use are severe pericarditis and myocarditis, iridocyclitis unresponsiveness to topical corticosteroids, and severe, incapacitating systemic symptoms with high fever that are unresponsive to other medication.

(b) If aspirin therapy is unsuccessful, corticosteroids may be utilized in the **acute** treatment of inflammatory diseases. Because of their significant long-term side effects, corticosteroids should not be used for prolonged treatment. They do not alter the long-term course or prevent permanent joint damage. The minimal dose that produces clinical improvement should be used, and attempts should always be made to reduce the corticosteroid dose or, if necessary, to add nonsteroidal agents or aspirin to permit a reduction in the corticosteroid dose. For most inflammatory diseases, prednisone, 1 mg/kg/24 hr, in 2 divided doses is the initial treatment. If this is not adequate to produce clinical improvement, the dose may be rapidly advanced to 2–3 mg/day for 3–5 days and then reduced to 1 mg/kg/day.

(c) Side effects. The sodium and fluid retention that can occur with higher corticosteroid doses have to be closely monitored. Immunosuppression and the occurrence of opportunistic infections are risks. Signs and symptoms of serious intercurrent illnesses may be suppressed. Therefore, patients taking corticosteroids must be carefully monitored. It should be made clear to patients and parents that use of the corticosteroids is only short term. Significant long-term dangers are associated with their use. The response to corticosteroids is so dramatic that it may be difficult for parents to accept its discontinuance.

(3) Nonsteroidal drugs. Patients who are unresponsive to an adequate trial (3–6 months) of aspirin and good physical management or patients with disease progression will require another drug. The choice of this drug will vary at different institutions; controlled trials with these drugs have not been conducted in children. None of the drugs is as benign as aspirin. No clear hierarchy for the use of nonsteroidal drugs has been established in pediatric inflammatory diseases. If no significant change occurs after 2–4 weeks with therapy, another drug should be tried. Most nonsteroidals are not FDA approved for pediatric patients.

(a) Indomethacin, when added to salicylate, has helped certain patients.

(i) The **dosage** is 1–2 mg/kg/day in 2–4 divided doses given after meals

(ii) Side effects include GI intolerance, headaches, and bone marrow suppression. Hemoglobin, WBC, and urinalysis should be evaluated frequently.

(iii) A response to the drug occurs within 2–3 weeks.

(b) Naproxen has not been used extensively in pediatrics.

(c) Hydroxychloroquine (Plaquenil) can be used in patients with JRA or systemic lupus erythematosus.

      (i) The **dosage** is usually 5–7 mg/kg up to 200 mg/day. A therapeutic response usually takes 6–8 weeks.

      (ii) **Side effects** may be severe. Retinitis with irreversible macular degeneration may occur. Patients should be warned to report difficulties with vision, accommodation, photophobia, or field defects and should wear sunglasses in bright light. Patients being treated with hydroxychloroquine should have an ophthalmologic examination every 3 months, and the drug should be discontinued at the first signs of retinal degeneration.

      (iii) Accidental ingestion of the drug is potentially fatal.

      (iv) The duration of treatment should not exceed 1 year.

(d) Gold compounds. If the patient has progressive joint disease despite aspirin administration and can return for regular injections and follow-up, gold may be indicated. Gold can control symptoms and prevent further joint damage, but has little effect on systemic manifestations and will not improve joints deformed from damaged cartilage. This potentially toxic drug is given as a weekly injection over a long period, and a response will not be seen for 2 months.

      (i) The dose is 1 mg/kg (up to 50 mg) IM of gold sodium thiomalate (Myochrysine) as a weekly injection into a buttock. A test dose of 2.5–5.0 mg is given to detect any idiosyncratic reaction. The dose is increased 5 mg weekly until an effective dose is reached.

      (ii) If there is no intolerance, the full dose is instituted once a week for 6 months. This is followed by a reduction to every other week for 2 months, then to every third week for four injections, and then to a monthly injection indefinitely if the patient has shown a response.

      (iii) Toxicity can affect the skin, kidney, bone marrow, and liver. Before initiation of therapy, liver function tests, BUN, creatinine, CBC, platelet count, and urinalysis should be checked. Before each injection, a history of rash, pruritus, and stomatitis should be elicited. In addition, a urinalysis for proteinuria or hematuria, hemoglobin, WBC, differential, and platelet count should be obtained.

      (iv) Gold therapy should be discontinued if rash, albuminuria, hematuria, leukopenia, thrombocytopenia, or eosinophilia occurs. It is sometimes possible to reinstitute therapy at a lower dosage in spite of mild dermatitis.

(4) Exercise, physical therapy, and rest.

    (a) An active program of daily physical therapy is essential to preserve the range of motion, maintain muscle strength, and prevent deformities.

    (b) The most valuable form of therapy is exercise, as long as it does not traumatize an inflamed joint. Even before aspirin has had its full effect, **passive range of motion and mild muscle stretching and strengthening exercises** should be started. The prior application of heat will allow for better results. Passive range of motion therapy should be replaced by active assistive and then active exercises. Moist heat (tub baths and hot packs) will relieve morning stiffness and pain.

(5) Psychological adjustment. Attention to the parents' and child's reaction to JRA is important in interpreting symptoms and judging compliance with the therapeutic regimen. The parents should not be overprotective, and the child should resume an active life with attendance at school as soon as possible.

(6) Orthopedic measures. Early in the disease, acutely painful joints may require intermittent resting splints to prevent flexion contractures and preserve functional alignment. Later, serial splinting may be required to correct contractures. Work splints, skin traction, braces, corrective devices, and intraarticular steroids may be indicated.

(7) Eyes. All patients should be checked by an ophthalmologist with a slit lamp examination to detect **iridocyclitis** when JRA is diagnosed and should be rechecked at least twice a year.

(a) Patients with pauciarticular disease, especially with a high ANA titer, are at an increased risk of the development of eye complications. Patients in whom iridocyclitis develops usually do not have severe joint disease. The onset is insidious, often independent of joint activity, and may occur up to 10 years following the disappearance of joint disease.

(b) Patients should be warned to report a red eye, eye pain, photophobia, or visual difficulties. Topical corticosteroids, mydriatics, and, at times, systemic corticosteroids will be required. A close follow-up is mandatory.

B. Systemic lupus erythematosus (SLE)

1. The **etiology** of this multisystemic inflammatory disorder is unknown, but an interaction of genetic, viral, and immunologic factors has been invoked. Persons with SLE produce autoantibodies, and the deposition of the immune complex of DNA and anti-DNA in the kidney results in a nephritis. Immune complexes may involve other antigens, and it is probable that the type of antibody, its avidity, and the size of the complex determine the symptoms. Autoantibodies to clotting factors and cells account for the circulating anticoagulant, thrombocytopenia, and positive Coombs test seen. The majority of patients (88%) are females, in whom the peak onset is during adolescence; in males, a more uniform age distribution is seen.

In occasional patients the disease can be provoked or exacerbated by sun exposure. In others, SLE or a mild reversible form of the disease can be precipitated by drugs (Table 18-1). Complement deficiency (C1, C2, C4, C5, and C8) may predispose to SLE.

2. Evaluation and diagnosis

a. Clinical

(1) The disease may be highly variable in its manifestations and course, but the most common presenting symptoms are rash (facial butterfly, erythematous blush), fever, malaise, and arthralgia or arthritis. On the initial presentation, only one of these symptoms may be present, or the symptoms may reflect involvement of one organ, such as the kidney.

(2) The American Rheumatism Association has designated preliminary criteria for the classification of SLE (Table 18-2). A diagnosis of SLE can be established if four or more of those symptoms are present. Hepatomegaly and lymphadenopathy may be especially prominent in childhood SLE.

Table 18-1. Drugs precipitating systemic lupus erythematosus

Hydralazine	Sulfonamides
Procainamide	Phenylbutazone
Trimethadione	Para-aminosalicylic acid
Phenytoin	Isoniazid
Penicillin	

Table 18-2. American Rheumatism Association classification criteria for SLE

Facial erythema

Discoid lupus

Raynaud's phenomenon

Alopecia

Photosensitivity

Oral or nasopharyngeal ulceration

Arthritis without deformity

LE cells

Chronic false-positive serologic test for syphilis (STS)

Profuse proteinuria

Cellular casts

Pleuritis, or pericarditis, or both

Psychosis, or convulsions, or both

Hemolytic anemia, leukopenia, or thrombocytopenia

Source: Modified from American Rheumatism Association Handbook.

- b. **Laboratory studies** will be necessary to confirm the clinical impression.
  - (1) Amost all patients with SLE have an **ANA** that is usually directed to native double-stranded DNA. This type of antibody displays a peripheral immunofluorescence pattern of stained nuclei. An ANA may be found in other collagen disorders or chronic inflammatory states, but the titer usually is not as high and the specificity is not usually directed to double-stranded DNA. The titer of anti-DNA antibody may correlate with the presence of clinical symptoms. A rising titer should suggest impending clinical activity.
  - (2) The level of **C3 and C4** may be decreased during active disease secondary to deposition of immune complexes. Circulating immune complexes may be detected, and their levels may also correlate with symptoms.
  - (3) Anemia, a positive Coombs test, leukopenia, abnormal clotting, an elevated ESR, hematuria, and proteinuria may be found.
  - (4) A **renal biopsy** is indicated if renal function is abnormal or urinary abnormalities are present. The biopsy will determine the type of nephritis, which may dictate therapy and the prognosis. Severe (diffuse) proliferate glomerulonephritis is more commonly associated with heavy proteinuria, hypertension, and renal insufficiency and has a worse prognosis than mild (focal) proliferative or minimal (mesangial) lupus nephritis. Membranous lupus nephritis may also present clinically with the nephrotic syndrome and hematuria, but azotemia is less common at onset, and the progression to renal insufficiency is slow when compared with that in diffuse proliferative glomerulonephritis.
- 3. The **goals of therapy** are prevention of progressive tissue damage, relief of incapacitating symptoms, prevention of death from treatment or the disease itself, and restoration of a normal daily routine.
  - a. **General measures**
    - (1) **Adequate rest** and **emotional support** are important. Emotional upsets can trigger an exacerbation.
    - (2) **All unnecessary medications should be discontinued** because of the possibility of drug-induced disease. If sunlight exacerbates the disease, exposure should be limited and a sunscreen containing 10% para-aminobenzoic acid prescribed.

  (3) Cold should be avoided if the patient suffers from Raynaud's phenomenon.

 b. Drugs

  (1) Aspirin is prescribed to control arthralgia and fever.

  (2) Corticosteroids are indicated for patients with active renal, hematologic, or CNS disease. They may also be required for severe skin disease and for fever and arthralgia unresponsive to aspirin or hydroxychloroquine.

  (3) Hydroxychloroquine, used with prednisone, may allow a reduction in the dosage and duration of corticosteroid administration.

  (4) Immunosuppressive agents. The role of these agents in the treatment of childhood SLE has not been clearly defined. Azathioprine, cyclophosphamide, and chlorambucil in conjunction with corticosteroids have been prescribed in patients in whom complications develop with high-dose corticosteroids or who are unresponsive to high doses. They have been used for patients with diffuse proliferative glomerulonephritis and with CNS lupus, in which their effectiveness is under investigation. Abrupt cessation of these agents may precipitate an exacerbation of symptoms. They have potentially serious side effects that should be considered before they are used.

 c. Other measures

  (1) Infections. SLE patients taking corticosteroids or immunosuppressants are highly susceptible to serious infection. At the first sign of infection, cultures should be done and the patient should be treated.

  (2) Hemodialysis and **renal transplantation** should be considered in patients with terminal renal failure.

C. Dermatomyositis

 1. Etiology. The childhood form is a systemic disease with diffuse angiitis involving skeletal muscle, skin, fat, the GI tract, and parts of the CNS. The cause is unknown, but patients have been shown to have lymphocyte sensitization to muscle and deposition of immunoglobulin and complement in skeletal muscle blood vessels.

 2. Evaluation and diagnosis. The characteristic clinical picture of muscle weakness with some pain occurring with constitutional symptoms and the characteristic rash should suggest the diagnosis. The diagnosis will be confirmed by elevated levels of muscle enzymes, an electromyogram, and a muscle biopsy. Myositis may also occur in SLE, JRA, scleroderma, and arteritis, as well as in virus infections.

 3. Therapy

  a. General measures. Active physiotherapy, positioning, and splinting will be necessary to rebuild muscle strength and prevent contractures. Children should sleep in the prone position to prevent hip contractures.

  b. Drugs. Early diagnosis and early initiation of treatment are necessary to prevent further muscle damage and atrophy.

   (1) Aspirin

   (2) Corticosteroids

    (a) High-dose prednisone, $1-2$ mg/kg or $50-75$ mg/M^2/day up to a dosage of 80 mg/day, should be prescribed for $4-6$ weeks or until clinical improvement of constitutional symptoms and skin manifestations and an increase in muscle strength occur. Muscle enzyme levels will usually decrease with clinical improvement.

    (b) The corticosteroid dose should be tapered gradually over $2-3$ months and the patient maintained on 0.25 mg/kg/day or $5-10$ mg/day or the lowest possible dose that keeps the disease quiescent and nonprogressive.

    (c) Maintenance therapy should continue for $1-3$ years. During this period, patients are susceptible to periods of relapse, with exacerbation of symptoms. If this occurs, high-dose corticosteroids must be reinstituted. Rarely, exacerbations may occur several years later.

(3) Immunosuppressants. In a limited number of cases, IV methotrexate and other immunosuppressants have been prescribed to control the disease in patients unresponsive to or requiring continuous high-dose corticosteroids.

  c. Involvement of the palatal-respiratory muscles, as clinically evidenced by dysphagia, regurgitation, or a change in the voice, demands close attention to **suctioning, postural drainage,** and **respiratory function.**

  d. Long-term follow-up is mandatory to treat chronic contractures and atrophy and to attend to the psychological and social needs of the patient.

D. Vasculitis: Polyarteritis nodosa, mucocutaneous lymph node syndrome, Henoch-Schönlein purpura. (For serum sickness and urticaria, see Chap. 19.)

  1. Etiology. Usually, the etiology is unknown. However, it is believed that in many cases the vessel inflammation is secondary to the deposition of immune complexes or antibody or cells directed to antigen existing in the vessel wall. The inciting antigen may be drugs (e.g., amphetamines, sulfonamides), infectious agents (e.g., hepatitis B, streptococcal antigens, or autologous immunoglobulins (cryoglobulinemia).

  2. Evaluation

   a. The **clinical symptoms** reflect the protean manifestations of multisystemic involvement. The symptoms may include the following:

   (1) Fever

   (2) Symptoms of **skin and mucosa involvement** (purpura, livedo reticularis, pyoderma gangrenosum, subcutaneous nodules, conjunctivitis, and enanthemas)

   (3) Kidney involvement (hematuria, proteinuria, renal insufficiency)

   (4) Heart involvement (congestive heart failure, myocardial infarction)

   (5) GI tract involvement (abdominal pain, melena, pancreatitis, hepatitis, cholecystitis)

   (6) Lung involvement (cough, wheezing)

   (7) CNS involvement

   (8) Myositis

   (9) Hypertension

   b. Laboratory investigations

   (1) All **tests for dysfunction of various organ systems,** especially the kidney, GI tract, lungs, and heart, should be performed.

   (2) Studies of cryoglobulins, anti–gamma globulins, circulating immune complexes, levels of C3 and CH_{50}, ANA, and hepatitis B surface antigen should be made.

   (3) Arteriography may demonstrate microaneurysms or irregularities of the vessel wall.

   (4) Biopsies of the skin, muscle, kidney, or testis may be necessary.

  3. Diagnosis

   a. Polyarteritis nodosa may present in an infantile form in children under 1 year of age or in older children and adolescents.

   (1) Clinical symptoms of the **infantile form** include an intermittent or prolonged fever, fleeting erythematous rash, conjunctivitis, cough, cardiomegaly, hypertension, congestive heart failure, abdominal pain, and abnormal findings on urinalysis.

   (2) The **childhood form** is more variable. Arteriography of the coronary arteries may show microaneurysms, and a biopsy may show necrotizing vasculitis of small-sized and medium-sized arteries with fibrinoid necroses and aneurysm formation. Eosinophilia and an elevated IgE level are often found.

   b. Mucocutaneous lymph node syndrome (MCLS, Kawasaki disease)

   (1) Clinical symptoms

    (a) Typically, there is fever lasting over 5 days, which does not respond to antibiotics; reddening and indurative edema of the palms and soles, with membranous desquamation from the fingertips during convalescence; polymorphous exanthem of the trunk; bilateral conjunctivitis; reddening and fissuring of the lips, with a strawberry tongue; reddening of the nasopharyngeal mucosa; and swelling of the cervical lymph nodes.

(b) Other symptoms include tachycardia, gallop rhythm, heart murmurs, abdominal pain, diarrhea, and, rarely, arthralgia, aseptic meningitis, and mild jaundice.

(c) A mortality of 1–2% is secondary to **myocardial infarction** due to coronary thromboarteritis.

(2) Laboratory findings include leukocytosis, thrombocytoses, abnormal acute-phase reactants, elevated IgE level, ECG abnormalities, and a reduction in suppressor T lymphocytes.

(3) Coronary angiography may reveal aneurysms, dilatation, stenosis, and irregularities in a large percentage of patients.

c. Anaphylactoid purpura (Henoch-Schönlein purpura)

(1) Clinical symptoms. The typical clinical picture of involvement of the skin, joints, GI tract, and kidneys secondary to a vasculitis of capillaries and precapillary and postcapillary vessels makes the diagnosis evident.

(a) The **characteristic skin lesions** occur especially on the buttocks and lower extremities, appearing initially as urticarial, with rapid evolution into pink maculopapules that become either small and discrete or enlarged, blotchy, and confluent. The initial red color becomes brownish, and ecchymotic areas may appear. Petechial lesions may be seen.

(b) The **joints,** especially the ankles and knees, **are swollen in the periarticular spaces** and are often painful.

(c) GI symptoms include abdominal pain, melena, vomiting, and hematemesis.

(d) Renal involvement occurs in 20–70% of patients. The spectrum varies from microscopic hematuria to acute, rapidly progressive nephritis or nephrotic syndrome. The renal manifestations usually appear within a month of the other manifestations, but occasionally may present later and sometimes before the skin lesions.

(e) Recurrent attacks of the syndrome are not uncommon.

(2) Laboratory investigations may reveal an abnormal urinalysis, elevated serum IgA level, and a normal C3 level and antistreptolysin O titer. Bleeding times and platelet counts are normal.

4. Therapy

a. Any unnecessary drugs should be discontinued and a careful history taken to determine exposure to infectious agents, insect stings, foreign proteins, and medications. Before any drug is used, a history of previous adverse reactions should be elicited.

b. Rigorous symptomatic treatment of various symptoms (including congestive heart failure, myocardial insufficiency, renal insufficiency, and hypertension) should be undertaken because the clinical course may be self-limited.

c. Specific therapy

(1) Polyarteritis nodosa. High-dose corticosteroids should be started promptly. The clinical condition, including heart involvement, and the laboratory findings should be followed to assess the response. Patients unresponsive to prednisone may require a higher dose, and immunosuppressants should be considered.

(2) Patients with the **mucocutaneous lymph node syndrome** should be treated symptomatically.

(3) Anaphylactoid purpura

(a) Patients with **severe arthralgia** may be helped with aspirin, which may have to be increased to higher levels for relief [see **A.3.a.(1)**].

Table 18-3. Immunodeficiency disorders

Classification	Cellular	Humoral
General	Agranulocytosis Hyposplenia Chronic granulomatous disease Primary granulocyte disorders	Complement disorders
Specific	Severe combined immune deficiency DiGeorge syndrome Mucocutaneous candidiasis Wiskott-Aldrich syndrome Ataxia telangiectasia	Severe combined immune deficiency Transient hypogammaglobulinemia Agammaglobulinemia IgG subtype deficiency Hyper-IgE syndrome

  (b) **Acute renal failure** should be treated vigorously because there
      are a considerable number of spontaneous cures.
  (c) Patients with **GI involvement** should be watched carefully for the
      complications of **severe hemorrhage, intussusception, and per-
      foration.** If melena occurs, patients should be prophylactically
      crossmatched.
  (d) There has been no controlled study of the use of corticosteroids in
      anaphylactoid purpura. They do not affect the total duration of
      the illness, the frequency of recurrences, or the renal disease.
      However, some physicians have used them for patients with se-
      vere, colicky abdominal pain and melena, to provide a more rapid
      relief of symptoms and prevent intussusception. If abdominal
      pain does not respond to corticosteroids, a fixed lesion of the GI
      tract should be suspected.
II. **Immunodeficiency disorders.** Immune defenses can be divided into those that re-
    quire previous exposure to a pathogen (specific) and those that do not (general). They
    can be further subdivided into those that are cellular and those that are humoral.
    Table 18-3 gives a classification of specific disorders of immunodeficiency.
    A. **Etiology and evaluation**
      1. An immunodeficiency should be suspected if a child has an increased fre-
         quency of infection, or infections of unusual severity, of prolonged duration,
         or with unusual complications. Unusual or opportunistic organisms may
         cause the infections. Although the normal child may have up to six respira-
         tory infections in a year, the child with an immunodeficiency will have more
         prolonged infections and may not recover completely between infections.
         Chronic candidiasis or bronchiectasis, chronically draining ears, or chronic
         diarrhea may be the presenting symptom.
      2. Abnormal humoral immunity will predispose to recurrent pyogenic infec-
         tions such as otitis, sinusitis, pneumonia, and meningitis caused by
         Pneumococcus, Haemophilus influenzae, Staphylococcus, or *Streptococcus*
         species. Antibody is necessary for opsonization for phagocytosis of these or-
         ganisms. Maternal IgG protects the infant for the first 3–4 months, and thus
         the child with isolated antibody deficiency will be asymptomatic for the first
         6 months of life (Fig. 18-1).
      3. Immunity to many fungal and viral infections resides in cellular or T cell–
         mediated processes. The infant with a T-cell deficiency has no maternal
         protection, so that symptoms begin during the first 3 months. Chronic can-
         didiasis resistant to treatment in an infant, or a complication after viral
         infection or immunization, may reflect such a deficiency.
      4. Complement is necessary for opsonization and immune adherence, and cir-
         culating white cells and fixed macrophages phagocytize and kill ingested
         organisms. Deficiency of any of these components results in pyogenic infec-
         tions, recurrent abscesses, or recurrent stomatitis.

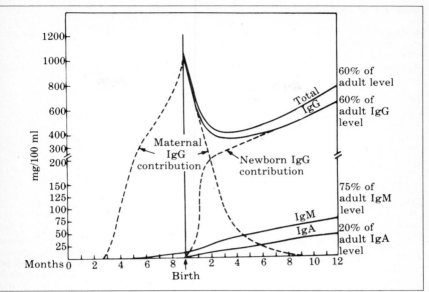

Fig. 18-1. Immunoglobulin (IgG, IgM, and IgA) levels in the fetus and infant in the first year of life. The IgG of the fetus and newborn infant is solely of maternal origin. The maternal IgG disappears by the age of 9 months, by which time the endogenous synthesis of IgG by the infant is well established. The IgM and IgA of the neonate are entirely endogenously synthesized, since maternal IgM and IgA do *not* cross the placenta. (From E. R. Stiehm and V. A. Fulginiti, *Immunologic Disorders in Infants and Children.* Philadelphia: Saunders, 1973.)

5. In the majority of cases, historical information will permit a presumptive diagnosis to be made that can be later substantiated by laboratory tests (Table 18-4).
   a. **Congenital immunodeficiencies** with known inheritance include X-linked disorders (congenital hypogammaglobulinemia, severe combined immunodeficiency, Wiskott-Aldrich syndrome, chronic granulomatous disease) and those inherited in an autosomal manner (combined immunodeficiency, with or without absence of the enzyme adenosine deaminase, and ataxia-telangiectasia).
   b. **Acquired immunodeficiencies** may be associated with congenital rubella, Epstein-Barr virus infection, malnutrition, malignancy, immunosuppression, protein-losing diseases, transcobalamin II deficiency, and use of phenytoin.
6. **Physical examination** should involve a search for the presence of lymphoid tissues (tonsils, lymph nodes, spleen), signs of infection, and incapacitation from chronic infection (hearing loss, failure to thrive, evidence of malabsorption). Skin involvement with eczema, candidiasis, telangiectasia, or petechiae should be noted.
7. The **laboratory evaluation** should be used to confirm a clinical suspicion based on the type of infection, the age of onset, family history, and physical examination.
   a. Antibody deficiency and combined deficiency are more common than isolated T-cell deficiency or phagocytic and complement disorders. If an immunodeficiency is suspected, **certain diagnostic and therapeutic procedures are contraindicated.**
   (1) **Injection of live attenuated virus** may cause a chronic viral disease.

Table 18-4. Laboratory evaluation of immunologic function

Immune compartment	Phenotypic	Function
T lymphocytes	E rosette formation	Blastogenic response to phytohemagglutinin
	Monoclonal antibody staining	Blastogenic response to antigens
B lymphocytes	Surface immunoglobulin Immunoglobulin levels IgG subtype	Specific antibody to tetanus toxoid, specific viral antigens
Complement	C1 through C9 levels	Total hemolytic complement (CH_{50})
Granulocytes	See Table 18-3	
Splenic function	Colloid scan	Colloid scan

       (2) A **transfusion of blood products** may induce the **lethal** complication of graft-versus-host disease from transfused viable allogeneic lymphocytes. Irradiation of whole blood, packed red cells, frozen washed red cells, platelets, or frozen or fresh plasma with 5000 rads will prevent this complication.

    b. The laboratory evaluation should proceed from the simpler to the more complicated tests. Results should be interpreted in relation to age-matched controls. The levels of immunoglobulins vary at different ages, and there is a wide normal range (see Fig. 18-1).

B. Diagnosis and therapy of specific disorders

  1. Antibody deficiency

    a. Pathophysiology

      (1) Specific antibodies are the basis for protection against bacterial infections caused by encapsulated respiratory organisms and viral infections following immunizations. Persons without the capacity to form specific antibodies suffer with recurrent infections from upper respiratory bacteria (*Staphylococcus, Streptococcus, Haemophilus influenzae,* meningococcus, and pneumococcus). These antibodies attach to the capsular polysaccharide antigens of the respiratory bacteria. Early complement components (C1, C4, C2, and C3) sequentially interact with antibody-coated bacteria. The opsonized bacteria are then phagocytized and destroyed by circulating or fixed phagocytic cells. The absence of specific antibody means that the rate of ingestion and destruction of pathogens is markedly reduced.

      (2) At birth, since IgG crosses the placenta, an infant has IgG levels and antibody protection equivalent to that of the mother. There is little or no maternal IgM present (see Fig. 18-1), since it does not cross the placenta. Thus, at birth, children have significant protection against common viral illnesses and many respiratory bacteria but little antibody protection against enteric gram-negative organisms provided by IgM. Initially, there is a decline in transplacentally derived maternal IgG, followed by the onset of de novo IgG and IgM synthesis. By approximately 2 years of age, adult levels of IgG, IgM and IgA are present.

      (3) Circulating IgA has little protective value. Secretory IgA is the primary protective antibody in secretions of the upper respiratory and GI tracts and in breast milk.

    b. Diagnosis

      (1) Transient hypogammaglobulinemia of infancy. In some infants there is a delay in immunoglobulin synthesis, so that the nadir of IgG seen at 3–4 months (approximately 300 gm/100 ml) is prolonged and continues to decrease (see Fig. 18-1). IgG levels remain low (often <200 mg/100 ml), and IgM and IgA may be normal or low. During the time between the elimination of maternal IgG (6 months of age) and the onset of de novo synthesis (18–24 months), these children have little antibody protection and may suffer from recurrent infections caused by upper respiratory bacteria. The severity of these infections is not as great as those of persons who have a lifelong inability to produce specific antibodies. Wheezing, respiratory infections, and diarrhea may be the clinical symptoms.

(2) X-linked agammaglobulinemia. Male children with this severe form of antibody deficiency present at approximately the sixth to twelfth month of life with recurrent infections with respiratory bacteria. Affected children have no significant IgG (<150 mg/100 ml), IgM or IgA. There is an absence of B lymphocytes. This diagnosis can be made at birth by demonstrating the absence of B lymphocytes in the cord blood. Neutropenia, thrombocytopenia, and hemolytic anemia are common.

(3) *Common variable agammaglobulinemia* is a term used to describe a congenital inability to form specific antibody that is not due to X-linked agammaglobulinemia. Children with this condition are characterized by the presence of B lymphocytes that are incapable of the synthesis and/or secretion of normal immunoglobulin and antibody. The time of onset and spectrum of infections is identical to that of males with X-linked agammaglobulinemia. Both males and females can be affected.

(4) In **IgA deficiency,** an IgA level less than 5 mg/100 ml is found, with normal levels of IgG and IgM and normal antibody responses. The lack of serum IgA is accompanied by absence of secretory IgA, and it is the latter that accounts for the sinopulmonary infections, diarrhea, or malabsorption seen. Circulating B cells with IgA are usually present.

(5) IgG subtype deficiency. IgG can be divided into four subtypes. Patients have been described who have normal total IgG levels but a marked reduction in gamma G1 levels, which normally represent 70% of the total IgG. The deficiencies in gamma G1 can be found either alone or in association with defects in gamma G2 and/or gamma G3. These patients suffer from recurrent infections similar to that of individuals with a total absence of IgG.

(6) Hyper-IgE syndrome. These patients have elevated serum IgE levels and recurrent pyogenic infection, particularly skin abscesses due to *Staphylococcus aureus.* The IgE in some individuals contains specific antibody to *Staphylococcus.* The interaction of the specific IgE antibody with the *Staphylococcus* inhibits the opsonization of the bacteria by IgG antibody and blocks the phagocytosis and the destruction of *Staphylococcus* by circulating phagocytic cells.

c. The **therapy** for all forms of immunoglobulin deficiency is replacement with pooled human immunoglobulin, which can be given either IM or IV.

(1) The IM preparation is given as an initial loading dose of 1.8 ml/kg and then a maintenance dose of 0.6 ml/kg every 3–4 weeks. IV gamma globulin, which is commercially available, is given as a loading dose of 200 mg/kg and a maintenance dose of 100 mg/kg/month. Both the IM and IV immunoglobulin preparations contain more than 99% IgG and little IgA or IgM. Some physicians choose IV fresh frozen plasma, 10 mg/kg/month, for replacement, since it contains IgA and IgM in addition to IgG.

(2) If infections are not controlled, the interval between immunoglobulin replacement should be shortened.

(3) Rarely, systemic reactions occur after an injection of gamma globulin. Treatment should include epinephrine, antihistamines, and general support.

(4) Patients with recurrent upper respiratory tract infections caused by viruses will not benefit from the use of pooled immunoglobulin since the IgG that is present does not pass into the mucosal secretions. No treatment is required for patients with absent serum IgA; replacement may produce an anaphylactic reaction since anti-IgA antibodies may be produced.

(5) Aggressive and immediate antibiotic treatment should be instituted for infection. Bronchiectasis should be managed with physical therapy, postural drainage, and antibiotics. Hearing loss should be prevented. Malabsorption and diarrhea should be treated with dietary restriction, and, if *Giardia* infestation is demonstrated on duodenal aspirate, the patient should be treated with metronidazole.

(6) Family members should be screened for immunodeficiencies.

2. T-lymphocyte defects

a. Pathophysiology. T lymphocytes are derived from lymphoid stem cells that differentiate under the influence of the thymus into peripheral T lymphocytes, which are responsible for protection against viruses and fungi and which regulate immunoglobulin synthesis.

b. Diagnosis

(1) **Congenital thymic aplasia (DiGeorge syndrome).** This developmental abnormality of the third and fourth pharyngeal pouches results in absence of the thymus and parathyroid glands, cardiac defects, and a characteristic facies. Neonatal tetany, candidiasis, heart murmurs, and the absence of a thymic shadow should suggest the diagnosis. Decreased T cells and poor in vitro lymphocyte responses will be seen.

(2) **Mucocutaneous candidiasis.** Patients with mucocutaneous candidiasis have recurrent *Candida albicans* infections of the fingernails and toenails, mouth, and vagina. They do not suffer recurrent infections caused by other organisms. They may have associated autoimmune abnormalities affecting their adrenal and thyroid glands, leading to Addison's disease and hypothyroidism.

(3) **Miscellaneous disorders.** Absence of the enzyme nucleoside phosphorylase, malnutrition, drug immunosuppression, and lymphocyte loss will cause T-cell dysfunction.

c. Therapy

(1) **DiGeorge syndrome.** Transplantation of a fetal thymus corrects the immune defect. Children with a partial defect may gradually acquire T-cell function without treatment. Irradiate all transfusions [see **A.7.a.(2)**].

(2) **Mucocutaneous candidiasis.** Prophylaxis with oral ketoconazole is the therapy of choice.

(3) **Associated endocrinopathies** must be treated.

3. Combined (antibody and cellular) immunodeficiency

a. Diagnosis

(1) **Severe combined immunodeficiency** may be inherited as an X-linked or autosomal recessive disorder, and the latter may be associated with absence of the enzyme adenosine deaminase (ADA). Affected infants lack normal lymphoid stem cells and therefore do not have normal T-lymphocyte and B-lymphocyte immunity. Frequently, they are clinically well for the first 2–3 months of life, and then the clinical triad of candidiasis, diarrhea, and pneumonitis develops. The male-female ratio is 3:1.

(a) The **diagnosis** is confirmed by low immunoglobulin levels, absent antibody responses, and low numbers of circulating or cord blood T cells with abnormal in vitro responses. ADA should be assayed in red cells. With ADA deficiency the diagnosis can be made prenatally by the absence of enzyme activity in cultured amniotic fibroblasts.

(b) Bony abnormalities may be seen on x-rays of the rib cage, pelvis, and spine in ADA deficiency.

(c) If the child has inadvertently been given a nonirradiated transfusion or had a maternal-fetal transfusion, a graft-versus-host reaction may complicate the clinical picture with skin rash, diarrhea, hepatosplenomegaly, and failure to thrive.

(2) Wiskott-Aldrich syndrome is an X-linked disorder characterized by eczema and T-lymphocyte abnormalities, including decreased T-lymphocyte function and an inability to make anticarbohydrate antibodies. Affected patients also have thrombocytopenia with platelets of reduced size and function. Patients are at risk of death due to bleeding and/or recurrent viral, fungal, and bacterial infection.

(3) Ataxia-telangiectasia is diagnosed by the occurrence of ataxia, choreoathetosis, dysarthric speech, telangiectasis, sinopulmonary infection, and the frequently found IgA deficiency and abnormal T-cell function. Alpha-fetoprotein is often elevated.

b. Therapy

(1) Severe combined immunodeficiency (SCID) is treated definitively by bone marrow transplantation from a histocompatible donor. The use of hapto (half)-identical donors is currently being evaluated.

(2) Patients with **bleeding and Wiskott-Aldrich syndrome problems** can be treated by splenectomy and placed on prophylactic (Bactrim or ampicillin) antibiotics to protect against bacterial sepsis. Excellent care of eczema is mandatory (see Chap. 22, pp. 531 ff). The only definitive treatment is bone marrow transplantation.

(3) Blood products should be irradiated prior to transfusion [see **A.7.a.(2)**].

(4) Aggressive treatment with antibiotics is necessary. Multiple organisms may be responsible for clinical disease. Lung infiltrates may be secondary to *Pneumocystis*, which is treated with trimethoprim-sulfamethoxazole or, rarely, pentamidine, if the former fails (see Chap. 16, pp. 435 ff). Gamma globulin prophylaxis is indicated for viral exposure.

(5) Siblings of affected children should be isolated at birth and screened for SCID.

4. Phagocytic and complement disorders

a. Granulocyte disorders. See Chap. 17, pp. 453 ff.

b. Complement abnormalities

(1) Deficiency of C1 associated with a lupuslike syndrome and susceptibility to bacterial infection

(2) C2 deficiency associated with anaphylactoid purpura and SLE

(3) C3 deficiency and C3b inactivator deficiency associated with a history of recurrent pyogenic infections that mimic hypogammaglobulinemia. Can be inherited or acquired during nephritis or in disease in which C3 consumption occurs (SLE).

(4) C4 deficiency with SLE

(5) C5 deficiency associated with recurrent infection and SLE

(6) C5 dysfunction with seborrhea, sepsis, and diarrhea

(7) C7 deficiency with Raynaud's phenomenon

(8) C6 and C8 deficiencies associated with recurrent *Neisseria* infections

(9) Therapy consists of appropriate antibiotics. Patients with C5–C9 deficiencies are clinically well.

c. Splenic dysfunction. The spleen is the site of a significant portion of the body's phagocytic capacity. Splenic hypofunction predisposes individuals to significant and overwhelming bacterial infection, particularly with respiratory bacteria.

(1) Pathophysiology
- **(a)** The spleen can be congenitally absent, removed surgically, or hypofunctional as in sickle cell disease.
- **(b)** Patients who undergo splenectomy before the age of 2 have difficulty processing carbohydrate antigens such as the capsular antigens of pneumococcus and *H. influenzae*.

(2) Therapy
- **(a)** **Antibiotics** are indicated for infections. Because of the risk of overwhelming sepsis in patients with splenic absence or dysfunction, IV antibiotic administration should be instituted while awaiting cultures.
- **(b)** **Prevention of infections.** There is no generally accepted practice for the prevention of infections in patients with splenic dysfunction.
  - **(i)** For patients at increased risk, some centers advocate prophylactic oral penicillin, 200,000 units bid, or ampicillin, 125 mg bid and 250 mg bid (for younger and older children respectively).
  - **(ii)** It is important to educate parents about the risk of sepsis and the need to seek immediate medical attention at the first sign of infection. If prompt attention cannot be sought, some advise that the parents should be supplied with oral penicillin, 25,000 units/kg/6 hr, or ampicillin, 25 mg/kg/6 hr, which can be instituted at the first sign of infection.
  - **(iii)** Patients who are hyposplenic before the age of 5 should be immunized prior to splenectomy, if possible, with all available bacteria polysaccharide vaccines.

5. Hereditary angioneurotic edema. This autosomal dominant disorder of dysfunction or deficiency of the inhibitor of the activated first component of complement results in unopposed C1 activation, consumption of C4 and C2, and release of a vasoactive peptide that causes attacks of subcutaneous and submucosal edema by altering the postcapillary venule permeability. Intermittent episodes of nonpruritic edema of the skin of the extremities and face occur after minor trauma, emotional stress, or without a precipitating cause. The swelling may involve the mucous membranes of the hypopharynx and the larynx, causing **laryngeal obstruction and asphyxiation.** Abdominal pain with vomiting or diarrhea secondary to edema of the intestinal wall may occur without skin manifestations, but urticaria does not occur.

a. Diagnosis. In the majority of patients the level of C1 esterase inhibitor is decreased, but about 15% of persons with the disease have a normal level of nonfunctional protein. In both groups, C4 levels are low and fall during attacks.

b. Therapy
- **(1)** The major complications of acute attacks is laryngeal obstruction, and thus patients or parents should be instructed to seek medical attention without delay if hoarseness, voice changes, or difficulty in breathing or swallowing occurs. A tracheotomy will be necessary for laryngeal obstruction. Epinephrine and hydrocortisone are of benefit in controlling swelling in only a rare patient, which contrasts with the relief of urticaria and laryngeal obstruction they afford in anaphylaxis and serum sickness (see Chap. 19, pp. 485 ff).
- **(2)** Fresh frozen plasma has been advocated for acute attacks to provide C1 esterase inhibitor. However, fresh plasma has more substrate for C1 than C1 inhibitor, so that administration may exacerbate the symptoms.
- **(3)** Androgens have been shown to increase the synthesis of C1 esterase, and the use of danazol has been recently approved. The routine use of danazol markedly decreases the frequency and severity of attacks.

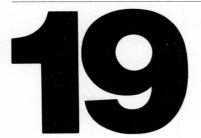

Allergic Disorders

I. Diagnostic procedures

A. Skin tests. Good correlations between the results of skin tests for pollens and inhalants and other in vitro or in vivo tests for immediate hypersensitivity are obtained when **appropriate controls** and **purified allergens** are used.

A small quantity of a suspected allergen is introduced (by scratch, prick, or intradermal method) into the skin. A *wheal and flare reaction* that occurs within 15–20 min and is larger than a control site where the diluent has been injected is interpreted as a positive reaction. A positive **histamine control** should be employed to be certain that the skin can respond properly, especially when all allergen sites are negative. Similarly, a **diluent control site** is important to document dermatographia in a patient who has all positive reactions. Skin testing for foods or drugs is in general less reliable, and the validity of the results must be individualized for each allergen.

B. The **radioallergosorbent test (RAST)** is a semiquantitative assay for allergen-specific IgE. The advantage of this test is that it can be performed in vitro, thus avoiding patient exposure to the allergen. However, the RAST has less sensitivity than skin testing.

The RAST is recommended for patients who have skin conditions precluding accurate skin testing (e.g., urticaria pigmentosa, dermatographia) for patients who must remain on chronic antihistamines; for infants, in whom skin tests are generally unreliable and/or traumatic; and for antigens that may be toxic or may sensitize the subject being tested.

C. IgE levels. Total serum IgE levels are useful in evaluating infants under 18 months of age. In this group, levels greater than 100 IU/ml are strongly associated with asthma or rhinitis in which standard skin tests are negative. The finding of a significantly elevated level should stimulate further investigation for the source of allergen.

D. Challenge. In rare cases it may be necessary to challenge a patient with a suspected allergen either orally or by inhalation to confirm a relationship between exposure and symptomatology. This should be undertaken only with appropriate precautions to treat any undue reactions that may be precipitated by the challenge.

II. Specific entities

A. Asthma. See also Chap. 3, pp. 50 ff.

    1. Evaluation

        a. History. Asthma should be suspected in any child who has a history of frequent or recurrent episodes of cough, dyspnea, wheezing, exercise intolerance, or "bronchitis." These symptoms may be perennial and without an obvious pattern, or they may have a definite seasonal variation. A careful history of inciting factors should be obtained to aid in directing an approach to diagnosis and therapy. A history of rhinitis, conjunctivitis, and atopic dermatitis suggests an atopic predisposition, as does a strong family history of allergic diseases. However, these factors by no means constitute a necessary prerequisite for the development of asthma, since asthma often has no atopic components (Table 19-1).

Table 19-1. Asthma classification

Allergic or extrinsic
Etiology largely on an allergic basis, often seasonal
Animal dander sensitivity often a problem

Idiopathic or intrinsic
No allergic basis identified; mechanism uncertain
Usually, low IgE; modest eosinophilia (<10%) not unusual

Infectious
Episodic wheezing **only** with infectious episodes
Frequent in infants and toddlers
Infections often a component of other types of asthma

Cough variant
Some patients with chronic cough respond to bronchodilator therapy, suggesting under-
lying hyperreactive airway
Auscultation usually reveals no wheezes
Pulmonary function often entirely normal, with reactive airways demonstrated only
by some challenge procedure (e.g., cold air, exercise or methacholine)

Exercise
Bronchospasm occurring usually after vigorous exercise for at least 6 min duration;
often reflects poorly controlled and poorly recognized persistent airway obstruction
or irritability

Aspirin-sensitive
Occurs particularly in patients with nasal polyps, sinus disease, and intrinsic asthma,
but may occur in patients with any type of asthma

Mixed
Most frequently there are many important inciting agents, with one being dominant

b. Physical examination
- **(1)** In an asymptomatic asthmatic patient the physical examination may reveal no abnormalities. In more severe disease, wheezing or rhonchi may be heard even when the patient feels well, suggesting that the child may have persistent bronchospasm and has a poor appreciation of his or her compromised function.
- **(2)** The presence of clubbing, increased anterioposterior diameter of the chest, or failure to thrive should prompt evaluation for other disorders, such as bronchiectasis, cystic fibrosis, or immunodeficiency.
- **(3)** Cough, forced expiration, or exercise may elicit wheezing in an otherwise asymptomatic person.
- **(4)** Edema of the nasal mucosa, allergic shiners, and eczema are often seen in children with allergic asthma.

c. Laboratory data
- **(1) Radiologic studies.** A chest x-ray should be performed during the course of evaluation. In atypical cases with irreversible obstruction or repeated pneumonia or atelectasis, a barium swallow and bronchograms or other studies may be required.
- **(2) CBC. Eosinophilia** is suggestive, though not diagnostic, of an extrinsic cause, since modest eosinophilia is observed even in infectious or idiopathic asthma. An elevated hematocrit suggests chronic hypoxemia.
- **(3) Immunoglobulin levels** are useful, especially in younger children in whom transient hypogammaglobulinemia of infancy or other immunoglobulin defects may present with recurrent wheezing. Total IgE levels are not routinely obtained in a general evaluation.
- **(4) Testing for specific IgE antibodies.** Skin tests for immediate hypersensitivity, together with the clinical history, are useful in iden-

tifying important allergens. When skin testing is contraindicated or difficult to perform, similar information may be obtained from the RAST.

(5) Pulmonary function testing.

   (a) Decreased flow rates (e.g., FEV$_1$ MMFR), reduced vital capacity even in asymptomatic asthma, and increased residual volume may be found.

   (b) Pulmonary function testing is particularly useful in determining the degree of reversibility in severe asthma, in evaluating the cause of chronic cough or dyspnea in a child in whom the physical findings are normal, and in assessing the effect of long-term therapy.

   (c) Reliable results can generally be obtained in children 6 years of age or older by experienced technicians.

   (d) Response to an inhaled beta-adrenergic agent should be evaluated to determine reversibility.

   (e) Normal pulmonary functions do not rule out a diagnosis of asthma, since they may merely reflect a quiescent state. Even when a child is "well," however, underlying airway hyperreactivity may be elicited by some challenge tests, such as inhalation of cold air, exercise, or exposure to a noxious irritant (e.g., histamine or methacholine).

   (f) Other. Special procedures, such as a sweat test, bronchoscopy, or bronchograms, should be performed as indicated.

2. Therapy

  a. General measures

   (1) When allergens that can be eliminated are identified by history, skin testing, or by any method for measuring specific IgE (i.e., RAST), the **best therapy is to remove the allergens from the environment.** They usually include such substances as dust, feathers, molds, and animal danders.

   (a) Dust control can be augmented by the use of airtight mattress and box spring covers, synthetic material for pillows, and removal of rugs and other dust collectors. The use of a fungicide and dehumidification in damp areas aid in mold control. Animals are best kept out of the patient's bedroom and preferably removed from the home.

   (b) In some instances an air purifier can be used to remove particulate matter. Air conditioning is effective in reducing the amount of pollen in the environment during pollinating seasons. Occasionally, foods, food additives, or drugs (especially aspirin) are precipitants of asthma and must be avoided.

   (2) Nonspecific factors. Patients with asthma should not smoke. Furthermore, "passive smoking," i.e., exposure to cigarette smoke from others, is also harmful. In addition to air pollutants, odors (especially perfumes), dust, and other aerosolized particulate matter (e.g., hair spray, insect sprays) can aggravate asthma and should be avoided.

   (3) Physical therapy. For selected patients, chest physical therapy, together with instructions in breathing exercises, may be a useful adjunct to specific therapy.

   (4) Psychiatric support. Since asthma is a chronic, recurring condition, psychological support is often necessary. Depending on the degree of disability, this support may be managed either by a physician or qualified nurse. In more difficult situations, assistance may be required from a social worker, psychologist, or psychiatrist. Programs on chronic asthma offered by local lung associations or hospitals are often helpful in this regard.

  b. Pharmacologic agents. Individual drug therapy allows more flexibility than does the use of the older fixed-combination bronchodilator preparations. Furthermore, the newer beta-adrenergic agents are more effective and less likely to induce tachyphylaxis than is ephedrine, the adrenergic agent used in combination preparations. Intermittent episodes are best treated with occasional doses of a beta-adrenergic agent. Theophylline is generally employed as the primary chronic "maintenance" drug in this country. Although controversial, beta-adrenergic agents are equally effective and may be substituted. If maintenance theophylline, or beta-adrenergic agents, or both are insufficient to control symptoms, a trial of cromolyn sodium is usually added to the regimen.

(1) Xanthines (e.g., aminophylline, theophylline). The efficacy of theophylline preparations is related to the blood levels.

    (a) The best results are observed with blood levels of 10–20 mg/ml; toxicity (abdominal pain, vomiting, diarrhea, headache, seizures, and/or arrhythmias) often results at higher levels. It should be noted that bronchodilation occurs even at lower levels. Since the half-life of this drug is variable in children, the mean is 3.5 hr, with a range of 1.5–9.0), the dose must be individualized. Approximately 90% of theophylline is cleared by liver enzymes. Factors affecting metabolism must be considered when calculating the dose (Table 19-2).

    (b) Therapeutic levels of theophylline can be achieved using a dosage of 12–30 mg/kg/day with therapy initiated at the lower dosages and increased as tolerated or required. A theophylline blood level should be measured 2–3 days after first initiating treatment to adjust the dose and avoid toxicity except when using the lowest dosages. Occasionally, higher dosages are necessary, but this requires careful monitoring of blood levels. Since calculations are made on the basis of anhydrous theophylline, it should be recognized that some preparations are theophylline salts and contain only 60–80% theophylline (Table 19-3).

    (c) For best therapeutic results with **intermittent therapy,** use either a liquid or tablet form with rapid absorption characteristics. Except in very mild attacks, bronchodilators should be continued for several days after symptoms resolve.

    (d) The frequency of attacks may be reduced by employing daily instead of intermittent treatment even if used in reduced doses. With continuous therapy, sustained release preparations offer the advantage of stable blood levels despite less frequent administration. Some may maintain stable levels even when given q12h. Side effects (Table 19-4) such as gastric distress, sleeplessness, and hyperactivity generally decrease with long-term administration.

Table 19-2. Factors affecting theophylline half-life

Prolonged (reduce dose)
    Hepatic dysfunction
    Congestive heart failure
    Viral infections
    Pharmacologic agents (e.g., erythromycin, cimetidine)
Decreased
    Smoking
    Pharmacologic agents (e.g., phenobarbital)
Variable
    Age
    Intrinsic
    Dose related
    Diet

Table 19-3. Theophylline equivalence

Preparation	Percent theophylline	Product
Anhydrous theophylline	100 percent	Accurbron, Bronkodyl, Elixophyllin, Quibron, Slo-Phyllin, Somophyllin-CRT, Slo-bid, Theo-Dur, Theophyl
Theophylline ethylenediamine	80 percent	Aminophyllin, Aminodur, Somophyllin (liquid)
Theophylline calcium salicylate	48 percent	Quadrinal, Verequad
Choline theophyllinate	64 percent	Brondecon, Choledyl
Diphylline	Equivalent to 60 percent	Dilor, Lufyllin

    (e) Routine use of rectally administered theophylline is discouraged because of the unpredictable pattern of absorption, frequent occurrence of proctitis, and the serious risk of overdose.

    (f) Theophylline may be contraindicated in the presence of gastroesophageal reflux as it decreases lower esophageal sphincter tone.

(2) Cromolyn sodium. When maintenance theophylline with or without an adrenergic agent is insufficient to control symptoms, a trial of cromolyn sodium should be added to the regimen. If theophylline or adrenergic agents are poorly tolerated, cromolyn sodium should be considered as the primary agent. This drug is most effective in children with extrinsic or allergic asthma but may be effective even in intrinsic or exercise asthma. Cromolyn is taken as a powder or nebulized solution by inhalation and presumably acts by preventing the release of mediators. However, it also blocks nonspecific irritant responses. The drug must be inhaled properly, since it acts locally in the tracheobronchial tree and is poorly absorbed from the GI tract.

(3) Beta-adrenergic agents. There are two classes of beta receptors: beta-1, affecting cardiac rate and contractility, and beta-2, primarily

Table 19-4. Theophylline side effects and toxicity

Gastrointestinal
  Gastric distress
  Nausea
  Vomiting
  Diarrhea
  Bleeding
Neurologic
  Behavior changes
  Insomnia or somnolence
  Hyperactivity
  Headache
  Seizures
Cardiac
  Tachycardia or bradycardia
  Arrhythmias
Renal
  Diuresis

affecting bronchial smooth muscle tone. Drugs that are partially selective in their affinity for the beta-2 receptors are now available. Currently, there are two oral agents with partial beta-2 selectivity.

  (a) **Metaproterenol and terbutaline.** The usual dose of metaproterenol is approximately 2 mg/kg/day (maximum dose 20 mg) and of terbutaline, 0.05–0.1 mg/kg dose tid (maximum 5 mg). The onset of action is rapid, and tachyphylaxis does not appear to be a problem with long-term administration. The major limiting factors with all beta-adrenergic agents are tremor and tachycardia.

  (b) **Inhalation.** Administration of beta-adrenergic agents by inhalation has the advantage of rapid onset of action and a primary effect at the target organ. This route of therapy has been avoided because of the associated risk of abuse and acute death. The availability of newer beta-selective agents (metaproterenol, albuterol) largely reduces this risk because of less cardiac activity as well as extended duration and slow onset of action, decreasing abuse potential.

  If inhalation agents are prescribed, care must be taken to instruct the patient and/or parent in their proper administration. Metered dose inhalers are most effective when a spacer tube is placed between the inhaler and mouth. The patient should inhale slowly and the breath should be held for a count of 10. Optimal bronchodilation is achieved by inhalation at 5- to 10-min intervals rather than immediately after each other.

(4) Corticosteroids

  (a) When short-term use of systemic corticosteroids is required to control asthma, the equivalent of 1–2 mg/kg/day of prednisone (Table 19-5) may be used initially, divided into 2–4 daily doses until symptoms are relieved. A tapering schedule over 7–10 days can then be arranged.

  (b) If long-term use is necessary, every effort should be made to administer corticosteroids on an every-other-day regimen to minimize side effects. Corticosteroids should be taken every other morning between 7–8 A.M., using the lowest dose that will control the asthma. The only corticosteroids that can be used in this regimen are prednisone or prednisolone, because the long duration of action of other corticosteroids negates the efficacy of the every-other-day regimen.

  (c) **Beclomethasone** is an inhaled corticosteroid with enhanced topical as compared with systemic action. Although early studies suggest no serious long-term side effects, this drug should be reserved for asthmatic patients whose illness is not managed well by standard medication. The major short-term complication is oral candidiasis; this can be avoided by rinsing the mouth after use. Occasionally, irritation from the aerosol can lead to cough or

Table 19-5. Corticosteroid equivalence

Corticosteroid	Equivalent dose (mg)
Cortisone	25
Cortisol	20
Prednisone	5
Methyl prednisolone	4
Dexamethasone	0.75
Betamethasone	0.60

even bronchospasm. If cough is provoked by administration of the aerosol, pretreatment with an inhaled adrenergic agent may be helpful. Pediatric dosages are from 50 gm tid to 200 gm qid. As with other inhaled agents, proper administration is imperative.

(5) Expectorants are of no benefit in the therapy of chronic asthma.

(6) Injection therapy. If an allergen that cannot easily be avoided is implicated in the etiology of extrinsic asthma, injection therapy may be efficacious. This mode of treatment should be used as an adjunct to other types of therapy and should not be looked on as a substitute for either adequate bronchodilator therapy or environmental controls. Documentation of sensitivity by history and **skin testing** should precede institution of a course of injection therapy. In general, before such treatment, a trial of environmental controls with allergens such as molds or dust is advocated. There is no evidence to support the use of bacterial vaccines in infants with infectious asthma.

B. Anaphylaxis

1. Etiology. Systemic anaphylaxis may be a life-threatening allergic reaction. It is caused by the IgE-triggered release of the mediators of immediate hypersensitivity from mast cells. Activated complement components ($C3_a$ and $C3_b$) may also be involved. "Anaphylactoid reactions" clinically resemble anaphylaxis but are caused by direct activation of the mast cell. The most common causes in children are antibiotics, allergy extracts, foods, and stinging-insect hypersensitivity (Table 19-6).

2. Evaluation and diagnosis

a. Anaphylactic reactions generally occur within minutes of exposure to the precipitating agent and may be explosive in onset. When reactions are delayed, a carefully obtained **history** may suggest potential offenders.

b. Laboratory evaluation

(1) When available, RASTs are useful. A CBC may reveal eosinophilia.

(2) Skin testing. In the case of penicillin, foods, insect venoms, and other protein antigens, skin tests for immediate hypersensitivity may be diagnostic.

c. Penicillin test. Penicillin is the major drug implicated in anaphylactic reactions. **Appropriate skin testing** can identify patients at risk of serious reactions. The skin test procedure is, however, complex and should be undertaken only by experienced persons. Penicillin testing should be performed only if the history suggests a previous hypersensitivity reaction in a person who has an acute illness or chronic disease that necessitates the use of penicillin therapy (e.g., congenital heart disease, cystic fibrosis). (See also Table 15-9, p. 370.)

(1) Following administration, penicillin is rapidly degraded into several breakdown products. Since any one of these products could produce an allergic reaction, several different preparations must be used in the

Table 19-6. Major causes of anaphylaxis

Antibiotics
    Penicillin, cephalosporin, tetracycline, streptomycin, and others
Biologicals
    Insect venoms, allergen extracts, gamma globulin, blood transfusions, antitoxins, anti-lymphocyte globulin, hormones, asparaginase, and others
Diagnostic agents
    Iodinated contrast media, BSP dye
Other drugs
    Aspirin, local anesthetics, dextran plasma expanders
Foods
    Especially eggs, milk, fish, shellfish, peanuts, nuts, chocolate

skin test procedure. Furthermore, **dilute** solutions must be used initially to avoid systemic reactions.

(2) The **penicilloyl** moiety is the major degradation product, and a skin test preparation (Penicilloyl-Polylysine, Kremers Urban Pharmaceutical Company, Milwaukee, Wis.) is available commercially. Reactions to this material are most frequently associated with late onset **urticaria** or **serum sickness.**

(3) The multiple degradation products present in smaller amounts and referred to collectively as **minor determinants** are most important in **acute** anaphylactic reactions.

(4) Minor determinant preparations for skin testing are not available commercially, but use of **both** fresh and aged penicillin (a solution that has been kept at room temperature for 1–2 weeks), which are presumed to contain minor determinants, are usually employed as a substitute.

(5) The breakdown products of the **semisynthetic penicillins** may differ from those in benzyl penicillin and, when possible, the specific penicillin product implicated should be incorporated into the test procedure.

(6) A RAST test for the major determinant is currently in use and could be obtained as an adjunct to skin testing. Positive reactions to the major determinant (either RAST or skin test) is the most consistent response with late or delayed sensitivity.

(7) Test procedure. Table 19-7 outlines the sequential skin test procedure.

(a) Initially, a **scratch** test is performed followed by **intradermal** testing using 0.02 ml of increasing concentrations of fresh and aged penicillin. Test sites are read at 15–20 min. A negative diluent and positive histamine control should always be included. A positive reaction with any of these allergens must be viewed as evidence of sensitization.

(b) Entirely negative skin testing when all the solutions are employed suggests that sensitization is unlikely. As discussed in **(4)**, however, since a well-standardized minor determinant mixture is not available, negative skin tests in the presence of a strongly suggestive history must be interpreted with due consideration.

(c) "Desensitization" in a sensitized person should **never** be attempted, **except** when penicillin therapy is an absolute indication in a life-threatening illness, and then only by an **experienced physician** who has appropriate resuscitative equipment available.

d. Anaphylactic symptoms vary in severity. Clinically, one or all of the following may be recognized in an anaphylactic reaction:

(1) Cutaneous. Diffuse flushing may occur as the initial symptom, followed by urticaria, angioedema, or both.

Table 19-7. Penicillin skin test procedure

Type of test	Fresh penicillin (U/ml)	Aged penicillin (U/ml)	Penicilloyl-Polylysine[a]
Scratch or prick[b]	500,000	500,000	6×10^{-5} M
Intradermal	500	500	6×10^{-5} M
Intradermal	5000	5000	
Intradermal	50,000	50,000	

[a] Pre-Pen, Kremers Urban Pharmaceutical, Milwaukee, Wis.
[b] Always include a negative diluent and positive histamine (2.75 mg/ml) control with the initial scratch or prick test.

    (2) Respiratory. Edema of the larynx and upper airway may result in stridor or even complete respiratory obstruction; or bronchospasm may predominate.

    (3) Cardiovascular. Hypotension, tachycardia, or shock may occur.

    (4) Gastrointestinal. Ingested allergens may cause nausea, abdominal pain, vomiting, and diarrhea.

    (5) The diagnosis is made primarily on the basis of the clinical syndrome and a history consistent with exposure to an agent that may be responsible.

3. Therapy (see Chap. 3). It is imperative that therapy be instituted **immediately** on recognition of the process. If the responsible agent is still being administered (e.g., intravenous pyelogram dye, blood products), **it must be discontinued promptly.**

    a. General measures include **epinephrine, fluid therapy, corticosteroids, and tourniquets.**

    b. For treatment of **bronchospasm, laryngeal edema, urticaria,** and **angioedema,** see Chap. 3.

    c. Prophylaxis. To prevent recurrence, cautious avoidance of reexposure to the specific allergen implicated in the original episode is mandatory.

        (1) Stinging-insect allergy. Persons who have had systemic anaphylaxis caused by an insect sting and documented by skin testing should receive injection therapy with stinging-insect venom.

        (2) Ready availability of an **anaphylaxis kit** that contains epinephrine should be emphasized for all persons who have had food or stinging-insect anaphylaxis. Newly available spring-loaded devices for self-administration of epinephrine (Epi Pen, Center Laboratories, Port Washington, N.Y.) may eliminate concerns over the use of a standard syringe. In addition, such patients should wear a Medic Alert necklace or bracelet engraved with the appropriate information.

C. Serum sickness

  1. Etiology. Serum sickness is a condition resulting from the presence of circulating antigen-antibody complexes with resultant complement activation. Tissue-fixed IgE antibodies also participate. At the present time, drugs (e.g., penicillin, streptomycin, phenytoin), antilymphocyte globulin, and stinging-insect venoms are most frequently implicated. This syndrome also occurs in the preicteric phase of viral hepatitis, and possibly in other viral infections.

  2. Evaluation and diagnosis. Symptoms most frequently begin 7–14 days after injection of the offending agent and may persist for weeks. Less frequently, an accelerated reaction may occur, with the onset of symptoms only hours or days after exposure. Fever, adenopathy, urticaria, angioedema, and arthralgias or arthritis, or both, are the most frequent presenting signs and symptoms. Less frequently, vasculitis occurs in other systems, including the GI, pulmonary, cardiovascular, CNS, and rarely renal.

  3. Laboratory findings

    a. CBC. The **differential diagnosis** may reveal a leukocytosis with a shift to the left, leukopenia, or eosinophilia. The finding of circulating plasma cells is very suggestive, since few conditions elicit plasmacytosis. The erythrocyte sedimentation rate is usually elevated.

    b. Serum proteins. With serosal, pleural, or pericardial involvement, there may be a reduction in both total and individual serum protein components. Gamma globulins are generally increased, and serum complement is decreased.

    c. Urinalysis. Rarely, proteinuria or hyaline casts are seen.

    d. Other. Tests for the presence of **immune complexes** (e.g., Clq-binding assays, Raji cell tests) or **activation of complement** (C3, or factor B activation products)

  4. Treatment

    a. Antihistamines. Therapeutic doses of antihistamines should be used throughout the symptomatic period to relieve pruritus. In addition, antihistamines may prevent deposition of immune complexes by particularly diminishing the increased vascular permeability.

b. Corticosteroids. Since serum sickness is usually a benign, self-limited condition, systemic steroid therapy should be reserved for patients with the most severe symptoms who show evidence of organ involvement with vasculitis. If indicated, treatment should be initiated with 1–2 mg/kg/day of prednisone or methylprednisolone in divided doses, with tapering after clinical improvement and discontinuation after a total course of 10–14 days.

c. Aspirin may be used as an antipyretic and for generalized symptoms.

d. Epinephrine, 0.01 ml/kg (maximum dose 0.4 ml) will decrease acute urticaria and angioedema, but the effects are transient.

D. Allergic rhinoconjunctivitis. See also Chaps. 23 and 24.

1. Etiology

    a. Allergic rhinitis may be seasonal or perennial in nature. Onset is usually in childhood or adolescence. It may be characterized by marked paroxysms of sneezing and clear rhinorrhea and associated with conjunctivitis, particularly with the seasonal exacerbations. Polyps are rare. Nasal and peripheral eosinophilia are common.

    b. Nonallergic rhinitis has a variable age of onset. There may be a predominance of nasal eosinophilia but no evidence of allergic etiology by either history or skin testing. The condition is frequently associated with nasal polyps, sinus disease, and aspirin sensitivity in adults.

    c. Vasomotor rhinitis. The onset is in adulthood. The severity is fluctuating, with nonspecific stimulants. The secretions usually contain neutrophils.

2. Evaluation and diagnosis

    a. The **history** is helpful, particularly in the case of seasonal rhinitis or allergic rhinitis due to allergens with intermittent exposure. It is not always useful in perennial allergic rhinitis when continuous exposure masks recognition of the offending allergen.

    b. Eosinophilia, both in a peripheral blood count and nasal smear is consistent with allergic rhinitis, but may be found also in perennial nonallergic rhinitis. Patients with nasal eosinophilia are more likely to respond to topical steroids.

    c. Skin tests are useful in confirming the significance of pollen or mold allergens in seasonal rhinitis. They are most important, however, in suggesting an allergic basis for perennial symptoms where the cause is not obviously allergic in origin.

    d. Serum IgE levels are often elevated in allergic rhinitis.

    e. Physical examination of the nasal mucosa in allergic rhinitis may reveal the following:

        (1) Often, a boggy, pale edema of the turbinates with a clear, watery discharge.

        (2) Nasal polyps may be seen in association with rhinitis. **(Whenever polyps are found in children, a sweat test must be obtained to rule out the possible diagnosis of cystic fibrosis.)** Polyps are commonly seen in children with ciliary dysfunction.

        (3) Conjunctival inflammation is frequently seen in association with seasonal rhinitis. **Periorbital edema** and **infraorbital swelling** ("allergic shiners," or black eyes) are also frequently observed. The upper lids should be everted, to examine for the presence of "cobblestoning," a hallmark of **vernal** conjunctivitis.

3. Treatment

    a. Pharmacologic

        (1) Antihistamines are most effective for rhinorrhea, sneezing, and conjunctivitis and less effective for symptoms of obstruction, which respond better to the addition of a decongestant. Pure antihistamines such as diphenhydramine (Benadryl), 5 mg/kg/day, or chlorphenhydramine (Chlor-Trimeton), 0.35 mg/kg/day, or decongestant-antihistamine combinations (Dimetapp, Actifed) are recommended. For prolonged seasonal or perennial symptoms, continuous therapy is more effective than sporadic use. Continuous use also decreases undesirable side effects such as somnolence but makes tachyphylaxis more likely. In patients in whom somnolence occurs, maintenance can begin with nighttime doses. When tachyphylaxis occurs, rotation of classes of antihistamines is helpful.

   (2) **Local vasoconstrictors** are effective for immediate relief of symptoms, but after use for more than 5–7 days, rebound edema and tachyphylaxis may induce rhinitis medicamentosa.

   (3) **Corticosteroids**

      (a) **Systemic.** A brief course of systemic corticosteroids may be necessary for severe symptoms, particularly for seasonal rhinitis.

      (b) **Topical.** Dexamethasone (Decadron Turbinaire) is useful for short-term (4–6 weeks) management of rhinitis. Absorption occurs, limiting the ability to use the drug for a prolonged period.

      (c) **Beclomethasone (Beconase, Vancenase)** is effective for both allergic and nonallergic rhinitis. No adrenal suppression occurs in recommended doses (one inhalation on each side bid–tid). The major complications include local initiation and epistaxis. There is no evidence of histopathologic changes, and *Candida* infection is rare.

      (d) **Flunisolide (Nasalide).** [See **(c)** beclomethasone].

   (4) Treatment of **allergic conjunctivitis** should be initiated, with frequent instillation of a methylcellulose preparation. Intraocular antihistamines (Vasocon A, Albalon A) can cause rebound conjunctivitis, as with intranasal antihistamines, and they should be used only intermittently for this reason. Because of the potential intraocular complications of steroids (e.g., glaucoma, herpes), they should be used only following consultation with an ophthalmologist.

   b. **Environmental controls.** For persons with allergic rhinitis caused by environmental allergens such as animal dander, dust, or molds, a reduction in exposure may markedly improve symptoms. Avoidance of pollen exposure by the use of an air conditioner is also helpful. Nonspecific irritants, such as noxious odors, rapid temperature change, and cigarette smoke, often constitute a major aggravating factor, both in allergic and nonallergic rhinitis.

   c. **Immunotherapy** is most effective for seasonal allergic rhinitis when symptoms correlate with skin test results. Some benefit can be expected in 75–80% of patients. Immunotherapy is less well studied in perennial rhinitis.

E. **Urticaria.** Approximately 20% of the population experiences at least one acute episode of urticaria or angioedema. Of these cases, only a small percentage progress to the chronic form, defined as recurrence of lesions over a period of 6 weeks. The incidence of **acute urticaria** is slightly higher in an atopic than in a nonatopic population, but the incidence of **chronic urticaria** is unaffected by hereditary background.

The **clinical recognition** of urticaria or angioedema rarely presents a problem. On the other hand, in the chronic form, identification of the precipitating factor or factors is often a perplexing, if not impossible, task.

Urticaria and angioedema frequently coexist. Attacks may last from hours to days. However, it is not unusual for patients with chronic urticaria or angioedema to have recurrent episodes for years. Both because of the long-term morbidity suffered by those whose attacks recur over a prolonged period, as well as the occasional association with a significant underlying disorder (Table 19-8), evaluation of patients with chronic urticaria should be undertaken (Table 19-9).

Table 19-8. Etiology of urticaria and angioedema

Allergic
  Atopic (inhaled allergens)
  Anaphylaxis:
    Ingested allergens (foods, drugs)
    Injected allergenic drugs (e.g., penicillin, biologicals)
Physical
  Dermatographia
  Pressure
  Vibration
  Cold
  Heat
  Solar
  Aquagenic
  Cholinergic
Infections
Agents affecting prostaglandin synthesis
  Nonsteroidal anti-inflammatory agents (aspirin)
  Azodyes and preservatives
Vasculitis
Hereditary angioedema
Drugs (serum products and mast cell–releasing agent)
Neoplasms
Endocrine related
Psychogenic
Idiopathic

Table 19-9. Urticaria and angioedema: Laboratory evaluation

Suspected cause	Procedures
(General screening)	(CBC, urinalysis, chemical profile)
Vasculitis or complement related	Sedimentation rate, immunoglobulin analysis, antinuclear factor, quantitative complement (C3, C4, C$\bar{1}$-inhibitor, CH$_{50}$), skin biopsy
Infections	Culture, stool for ova and parasites, hepatitis-associated antigen, x-rays (sinuses)
Atopic	Eosinophil count, IgE, skin testing and/or RAST for suspected allergen
Physical	
Cholinergic	Mecholyl test/stress induced
Dermatographism	Firm stroking of skin
Cold	Ice-cube application, cryoglobulins, cryofibrinogens, VDRI
Solar	Light exposure
Heat	Warm-water immersion
Hereditary angioedema and acquired angioedema with lymphoma and other neoplasms	C$\bar{1}$-inhibitor, C1, CH$_{50}$, C4, C2

1. **Etiology**
   a. **Mechanism.** Although caused by a number of mechanisms, a final common pathway for urticaria or angioedema is release of the chemical mediators of immediate hypersensitivity.
   b. **Specific agents.** It is difficult to estimate the frequency with which the cause of acute urticaria is identified, since many persons with mild acute episodes may not seek medical assistance. Of those evaluated for chronic forms of the disease, however, it has been estimated that a cause is determined in less than 20% of cases. Because of the diversity of causes and mechanisms involved in this symptom complex, a rational classification is difficult to make. The classification in Table 19-8 lists the known causes without attention to mechanism or frequency.
2. **Evaluation and therapy.** If the urticaria or angioedema is associated with a specific ingested or inhaled substance, avoidance is obviously the preferred approach. Similarly, with physical urticaria, avoidance of the precipitating factor, such as cold or sunlight, is advisable. Sunscreens have been beneficial in solar urticaria.
   a. **Antihistamines.** Urticaria, whether acute or chronic, is best controlled by antihistamine therapy. In general, antihistamine dosages should be increased slowly, either to tolerance or until symptoms are controlled. There is no good evidence that any one antihistamine is more beneficial than another. Though hydroxyzine is often used in the dermic form for urticaria and periactin for the cold-induced type, a combination of H1-type antihistamines from two groups may occasionally be additive in effect. Results with antihistamines of the H2 type have been variable.
   b. **Corticosteroids.** There is no role for topical steroid therapy in this condition, and only rarely should systemic corticosteroid treatment be considered.
   c. In **hereditary angioedema,** androgen therapy, using oxymetholone, 5 mg, has clearly prevented life-threatening attacks. Of major concern in this entity has been the treatment of acute episodes. Recent studies suggest that the use of the purified C1 inhibitor protein would be lifesaving. A more practical approach is the utilization of 5 gm of epsilon-aminocaproic acid, administered q6h in conjunction with oxymetholone, 10 mg q6h, until the reaction is controlled. (See also Chap. 18, p. 478.)
   d. If a more serious underlying entity has been ruled out, reassurance is often the best therapy.

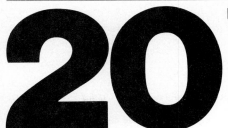

Neurology

I. Disorders of mental status and intracranial hypertension
   A. Coma and acute increased intracranial pressure (ICP). See Chap. 3, p. 61.
   B. Reye syndrome
      1. Etiology. The cause is not understood although it is probably a mitochondrial disease associated with influenza and varicella that primarily involves the liver and brain.
      2. Evaluation and diagnosis
         a. Characteristically, an antecedent viral illness is followed by vomiting and progressive lethargy.
         b. Examination. Tachypnea, fever, lethargy, and stupor or coma are typical. Signs of elevated ICP and, more rarely, seizures may also be noted.
         c. Laboratory findings.
            (1) Elevated serum **hepatocellular enzyme assays** (SGOT, SGPT, LDH) and elevated serum ammonia (arterial) are the laboratory hallmarks; one may also see metabolic acidosis and respiratory alkalosis as well as hypoglycemia and prolongation of the prothrombin time (PT) and partial thromboplastin time (PTT).
            (2) A **CT scan** may be necessary to rule out an intracranial mass.
            (3) Liver biopsy is generally performed when the diagnosis is in question. Features that may indicate the need for biopsy include an unusual age (< 1 year, > 16 years) and recurrent episodes.
      3. Treatment
         a. The primary intent is to maintain **cerebral perfusion pressure** (mean arterial pressure minus ICP) above 50 mm Hg and to avoid the complications of hepatic dysfunction. Both problems are directly related to the severity of the disease. Severity, in turn, is suggested by a number of prognostic variables. These include serum ammonia greater than 300 μg/ 100 ml, rapid clinical evolution through the stages of coma, posturing (decortication or decerebration), and an EEG picture of deeper stages of coma.
         b. Clinical staging and EEG grading of Reye syndrome. See Table 20-1.
         c. For the management of acute hepatic necrosis, see Chap. 10, p. 281.
         d. Cerebral support
            (1) Stage I or II clinically and grade 1, 2, or 3 by EEG
               (a) An EEG is obtained q12h to until EEG, or clinical stabilization, or improved grading is achieved. Progression to higher grades requires additional intervention [see **(2)**].
               (b) Initially, unless the patient is volume depleted, limit fluid to one-half maintenance; fluids should be chosen to prevent hypoglycemia and to avoid reducing serum osmolarity (in 5% or 10% D/W in normal saline), which may exacerbate cerebral edema. The goal is to elevate serum osmolarity to 290–310 mOsm.
               (c) Seizures should be treated with IV phenytoin (Dilantin) to avoid losing the ability to monitor the patient's level of consciousness (see Chap. 3, p. 62). Administer 15–20 mg/kg as a loading dose mixed in normal saline and given no more rapidly than 1 mg/kg/min.

Table 20-1. Clinical staging and EEG grading in Reye syndrome.

Grade	Clinical description	EEG characteristics by age in years		
		10	5–10	< 5
1	Lethargic	Predominantly theta	Theta-delta	Predominantly delta
2	Agitated	Theta-delta	Predominantly delta	Predominantly delta
3	Decorticate	High-voltage delta	High-voltage delta	High-voltage delta
4	Decerebrate	Burst suppression and low voltage, (nearly) isoelectric		
5	Flaccid			

   (d) Electrolytes, osmolarity, blood sugar, and BUN should be monitored q6–12h and an arterial ammonia q12–24h. PT and PTT should also be repeated q12–24h.
   (e) The head should be placed in the midline and upright to 30 degrees to reduce the venous component of ICP.
   (f) Lumbar puncture is contraindicated in patients with Reye syndrome.
   (2) Stage III, IV, or V clinically and grade 4 or 5 by EEG. In addition to the treatment outlines for stages I–II, the patient will require intracranial monitoring and possibly additional therapy, including intubation, hyperventilation, osmotic agents, and barbiturates. (See Chap. 3, p. 61.)
C. Chronic ICP
   1. Etiology. The causes include hydrocephalus, brain tumors, brain abscess, arteriovenous malformations, and chronic subdural hematomas.
   2. Evaluation
      a. Examination. A lateralized examination suggests hemispheric brain tumor, subdural hematoma, abscess, or arteriovenous malformation. Asymmetrical nystagmus, truncal or appendicular ataxia, and brainstem signs suggest a similar posterior fossa process. Nonlateralized and nonfocal signs suggest hydrocephalus and pseudotumor cerebri (see sec. **D** and Chap. 3, p. 65).
      b. Tests
         (1) Cranial CT scan
         (2) Lumbar puncture is contraindicated except in pseudomotor cerebri and simple communicating hydrocephalus.
         (3) Cranial sector scanning ultrasound may be used to evaluate the ventricular system and the cerebral hemispheres when the anterior fontanelle is patent.
   3. Treatment
      a. Treat as in acute increased ICP (see Chap. 3, pp. 61ff).
      b. Posthemorrhagic hydrocephalus in premature newborns may be treated medically by daily lumbar puncture and removal of at least 10 ml of cerebrospinal fluid (CSF). Serial lumbar punctures do **not** prevent the development of hydrocephalus.
      c. Most patients with progressive hydrocephalus will require a shunting procedure.
      d. When surgery is contraindicated, temporization may be achieved with furosemide (0.1–0.5 mg/kg q4–6h), glycerol or mannitol (0.25 gm/kg q6h), or acetazolamide (10 mg/kg q8–12h).
      e. Radiation and/or chemotherapy or surgery are used as indicated for tumors or abscess.
D. Increased ICP without alteration of mental status: pseudotumor cerebri (benign intracranial hypertension)
   1. The **etiology** is unknown.

2. **Evaluation and diagnosis**
   a. **History.** Headache is the rule. There may be complaints of visual loss or diplopia. Occasionally, nausea and vomiting occur.
   b. **Examination.** Papilledema, enlarged blind spot, visual scotoma, and sixth cranial nerve palsy may be seen. Other focal or lateralized neurologic signs, such as other cranial nerve palsies, hemiparesis, ataxia, and sensory deficits, exclude pseudotumor as a diagnostic consideration.
   c. **Tests**
      (1) A **cranial CT scan** must be performed to exclude hydrocephalus or a space-occupying lesion; the ventricles appear either normal in size or slitlike.
      (2) A **lumbar puncture** may be done after establishing the absence of localizing signs and the presence of a normal CT scan.
3. **Therapy.** Untreated, persistent ICP may lead to permanent loss of vision.
   a. A single lumbar puncture, with removal of enough fluid to bring the pressure to approximately 150 mm H_2O or to 50% of the opening pressure is often adequate. Symptoms (headache) are often dramatically alleviated following the lumbar puncture.
   b. Initially, some patients will require a series of lumbar punctures, daily at first, increasing the interval according to exacerbation of symptoms and rate of reaccumulation of CSF.
   c. When repeated lumbar punctures are not successful, acetazolamide (Diamox) may be initiated (10–25 mg/kg in 2–3 divided dosages/day).
   d. **Furosemide (Lasix),** 0.1–0.5 mg/kg q4–6h, may be used if acetazolamide is not successful.
   e. If previous interventions are unsuccessful, then a course of dexamethasone at 0.2–0.5 mg/kg/day is advocated. Corticosteroid dependency may result, however. A response to dexamethasone generally occurs within a few weeks. Improvement can be evaluated by the absence of headache and normalization of eye grounds, as well as by lowered opening pressure on lumbar puncture. With normalization of opening pressure, dexamethasone may be given every other day and then tapered over 2–3 months.
   f. When all other modalities to control increased ICP fail, or when vision is acutely threatened, a lumboperitoneal or ventriculoperitoneal shunt may be necessary.
E. **Attentional deficit disorder with or without hyperactivity.** The principal therapeutic concern is to properly identify the child who has an intrinsic inability to maintain attention, leading to a state of overactivity or inattention with consequent disruption of his or her educational program.
   1. The **etiology** is unknown.
   2. **Evaluation and diagnosis**
      a. **History.** In general, the early years are characterized by excessive activity, inability to sit quietly with a book or to watch a slow-moving television show, and unusual sleeping patterns.
      b. **Examination.** There frequently are "soft neurologic signs," such as synkinesis, stress gait posturing, choreiform movements, and incoordination.
      c. The **differential diagnoses** include hearing loss, petit mal seizures, and psychological responses to stress.
   3. **Therapy.** Stimulant therapy will not be useful for the anxious or depressed child. Its main purpose is to maximize attention. Some children will respond to only one of the three available stimulant medications, and may do so either at very low or very high dosages (Table 20-2). The following principles should be used in administering stimulant medications:
      a. Establish an educator and parental baseline with subjective and objective assessments. A Conner's hyperactivity scale is useful.
      b. Introduce small dosages at first in the morning and at noon for methylphenidate (Ritalin) or dextroamphetamine (Dexedrine) and in the morning only for pemoline (Cylert), Ritalin-SR (slow release), or dextroamphetamine spansules.

Table 20-2. Drugs for attentional deficit disorders[a]

Drug	Dosage (mg)	Dosage interval
Dextroamphetamine (Dexedrine)	2½–15	8 A.M., noon
Dextroamphetamine spansule (Dexedrine)	2½–15	8 A.M.
Methylphenidate (Ritalin, Ritalin-SR)	2½–20 20–40	8 A.M., noon · 8 A.M.
Pemoline[b] (Cylert)	18.75–112.5	8 A.M.

[a] Presence of a tic disorder or appearance of tics while on stimulant medication is a contraindication to its use or continued use.
[b] Liver functions must be monitored with Cylert.

   c. Increase the dosages by ½ tablet/dose every 1–2 weeks until an optimal therapeutic effect is achieved, overdosage is recognized, or an exacerbation of symptoms is identified (see Table 20-2).
   d. Overdosage of medication leads to withdrawal, weepiness, and somnolence.
   e. There is often a "coming down"—or, more appropriately, "going up"—effect as the medication wears off. At this time the child is excessively hyperactive and inattentive, and a very small dose in the late afternoon may ease the transition.
   f. Since the principal intent is to optimize education, in most circumstances, medications may be given on school days or when optimal attention is necessary. It is useful to give the child medication on weekends during the initial weeks, so that parents can also assess drug efficacy. A follow-up educator's assessment is required to establish efficacy.
   g. Often, adjunctive behavior modification and counseling input are important. Many of these children have a poor self-image and have superimposed emotional difficulties. Some have an associated learning disability and will require a modified education plan. A hearing evaluation should be done, and an EEG evaluation is occasionally necessary.
   h. Summer drug holidays may be useful for reassessing the child's continued need for medication.
   i. Serial assessment of height, weight, and blood pressure is recommended.
   j. Some patients, particularly those who are unusually aggressive, will not respond to the "usual" stimulant drugs and may require major tranquilizers. This is most often true for obviously organic or psychiatrically based hyperactivity states.
   k. Rarely, children will respond to elimination of particular food additives as recommended in the Feingold diet.

II. Cranial nerve disorders
  A. Optic neuritis
    1. Etiology. Optic neuritis may occur during or following an infection or may occur unrelated to infection. It involves dymyelination of the optic nerve head (papillitis) or of the area behind the nerve head (retrobulbar neuritis).
    2. Evaluation and diagnosis
      a. History. The critical history is that of lost vision; this may be unilateral or bilateral, and visual acuity may be reduced considerably. There may be associated ocular pain.
      b. Examination. Visual acuity is reduced. With papillitis, papilledema is seen; with retrobulbar neuritis, the funduscopic findings are essentially

normal. A careful neurologic examination may reveal other neurologic deficits to suggest a more disseminated disease.

   c. Laboratory tests

      (1) A **cranial CT scan** may be necessary to rule out raised ICP, which may lead to acute visual loss.

      (2) A **lumbar puncture** is necessary for similar reasons; CSF may be assessed for a more generalized involvement of the nervous system to include basic myelin protein and gamma globulins. (There may be a mild pleocytosis with optic neuritis.)

      (3) Somatosensory, brainstem, visual, and auditory evoked responses may identify more extensive white matter disease.

  3. Therapy. Optic neuritis is often self-limited. When the disease progresses particularly to involve both eyes, **ACTH**, 60–80 units IV, given in 2 divided doses over 4–8h each, should be used; this is changed to IM ACTH gel after 3–7 days and then is slowly tapered over 1–3 months. Patients must be carefully monitored for complications associated with the use of high-dose corticosteroids (see Chap. 11, pp. 307ff). Concurrent antacid therapy is recommended.

B. Bell's palsy and facial palsy

  1. Etiology. Facial nerve palsy may occur as a result of head injury, demyelination, tumor, hypertension, infection, or infarction. Idiopathic cases are termed **Bell's palsy.**

  2. Evaluation and diagnosis

    a. History. Bell's palsy is preceded by an upper respiratory infection in approximately 75% of cases. Patients frequently complain of pain behind or in front of the ear for 1 or 2 days prior to the development of the facial weakness. The evolution of facial weakness occurs over a few hours.

    b. Examination. Mandatory findings in patients with Bell's palsy include weakness of both the lower and upper face, absence of other cranial nerve dysfunction, and normal blood pressure. Findings consistent with the diagnosis of Bell's palsy include hyperacusis of one ear, loss of taste on one side of the tongue, and unilateral overflow of tears or a dry eye.

    c. Tests

      (1) Skull x-rays, with attention to mastoid and petrous bones, are required to rule out infection or tumor.

      (2) A **CBC** and **heterophil antibodies** may also be useful.

  3. Treatment

    a. Supportive. Protection of the involved eye should include the use of a protective eye glass, and a methylcellulose eye lubricant is suggested.

    b. Specific. If begun within 72 hr, a 10-day course of prednisone, starting with 0.75 mg/kg/day and reducing the dosage by 0.25 mg/kg/day every third day, may alleviate the pain associated with Bell's palsy, shorten recovery, and reduce instances of complete, permanent paralysis.

III. Spinal cord and cauda equina compression

  A. Etiology. Spinal cord or cauda equina compression requires emergency intervention. It usually occurs because of trauma, tumor, infection, or hemorrhage. The process may be epidural, subdural, subarachnoid, subpial, or intramedullary.

  B. Traumatic cord compression. (See Chap. 3, p. 64).

  C. Nontraumatic cord or cauda equina compression

    1. History. Note should be made of the following:

      a. Previous history of tumor, bleeding diathesis, fever, or infections

      b. Spinal pain is often the most useful indication of the diagnosis and of localization of the compression. Most often, pain worsens with cough, a Valsalva maneuver, or percussion over the involved area.

      c. Alteration in bowel or bladder control

      d. Change in gait or lower extremity weakness

      e. Perineal loss of sensation

    2. Physical examination

      a. General examination. A stiff neck, particularly for both flexion and rotation, may suggest a lesion at the high cervical area. External evidence of trauma, bruits, or vascular malformations over the spine and vertebral tenderness to percussion may be sensitive localizing signs. Fever suggests epidural or subdural empyema.

    b. Motor level

        (1) Tone and strength. Generally, tone will be increased and strength will be reduced at and below the level of a spinal lesion. Acutely, the tone may be decreased, increased, or normal.

        (2) Deep tendon reflexes. The patient will be normoreflexive above the level of the lesion and hyperreflexive below it. Reflexes may be absent at the level of the lesion. In acute cord compression, one may note spinal shock presenting as total flaccidity and areflexia below the level of the lesion.

        (3) Plantars are usually flagrantly extensor with spinal cord lesions.

    c. Sensory level. One may discern a sensory level to touch, pin, or temperature. Absence of a sensory level, with loss of perianal sensation, suggests a cauda equina lesion.

    d. Lumbrosacral reflexes and signs. A patulous anus and an absent anal, bulbocavernosus, or cremasteric reflex suggest a cauda equina lesion or spinal shock.

    e. Autonomic changes. The presence of Horner syndrome suggests a lesion at the T1 level. Sweating is decreased or absent below the level of the lesion if it is above T10. Urinary retention is common.

  3. Laboratory tests

    a. Plain spine x-rays of the suspected areas should be obtained. If a high cervical lesion is suspected, immobilization of the neck and open mouth views of the odontoid may be necessary.

    b. Clotting studies and **septic workup** should be obtained as indicated. A lumbar puncture is relatively contraindicated and should only be done as part of the myelogram after neurosurgical consultation.

    c. A **myelogram** will usually be necessary and a body **CT scan** is useful in some circumstances to evaluate the limits of a tumor beyond a subarachnoid block and to assess enhancement characteristics.

  4. Treatment

    a. Dexamethasone (Decadron), 0.5–1.0 mg/kg IV as a loading dose and 0.1–0.2 mg/kg q6h, should be administered as soon as a space-occupying lesion is suggested by a previous history of tumor or lytic lesions in bone or when there is evidence for active evolution. Antacid or cimetidine may be given concomitantly.

    b. For **epidural tumors,** radiation therapy has been shown to be as efficacious as decompressive laminectomy in most circumstances. However, hematoma, empyema, and bony impingement on the cord or the cauda equina most often require immediate surgical intervention.

    c. Appropriate antibiotics should be administered for empyema.

    d. Intermittent catheterization is used to treat urinary retention.

D. Transverse myelopathy usually presents as rapidly progressive segmental spinal cord dysfunction.

  1. The **etiology** includes postviral, vascular (involving ischemia in the distribution of the anterior spinal artery), or demyelinating disease.

  2. Evaluation. Proceed as for spinal cord compression; this is a diagnosis of exclusion.

  3. Therapy is controversial and equivocal.

    a. Supportive therapy is the mainstay of treatment, depending on the level.

    b. A trial of **corticosteroids** may be helpful. Prednisone at 1 mg/kg/day is often administered.

    c. Plasmapheresis may be useful.

IV. Neuropathic diseases: Guillain-Barré syndrome (acute infectious polyneuropathy)

  A. Etiology. This acute or subacute symmetric ascending disease of predominantly motor nerves is thought to be immune mediated.

B. Evaluation and diagnosis

1. **History.** There is usually an antecedent viral illness or surgical procedure. Frequently, there are complaints of parathesia and/or weakness of the lower extremities.

2. **Physical examination.** The cranial nerves are usually normal, with bifacial weakness often appearing later in the course. The Fisher variant (descending weakness with ataxia) may present with ophthalmoplegia or facial palsy early in the course of the disease. Distal hypotonia, weakness, and reduced deep tendon reflexes are most often noted. There should be absent extensor plantars, no sensory levels, and no perianal sensory loss.

3. **Laboratory tests.** CSF protein will usually be elevated **following** the first 48 hours of symptoms. Mild pleocytosis (up to 50–100 cells) does not exclude Guillain-Barré syndrome.

C. Treatment. The therapy is largely symptomatic. There are, however, special considerations.

1. **Monitoring of respiratory status.** Compromise of the nerve roots innervating the phrenic nerve, C3, C4, and C5, may cause rapid respiratory embarrassment. Vital capacity must be monitored frequently, and a fall below 15 ml/kg warrants artificial ventilatory support. Compromise of C3, C4, and C5 is usually preceded by weakness of the upper extremities and occurs within the first 2 weeks of the onset of symptoms.

2. **Preparing patient and family.** It is critical that the patient and family be counseled that intubation may be necessary as routine support for the disease **before** urgent measures are required.

3. **Corticosteroids.** The efficacy of corticosteroids in this disease is controversial and considered by some to lead to an increased incidence of relapse.

4. Hypertension, thought to be mediated by the renin-angiotensin system, may occur. Propranolol and, if needed, an alpha-adrenergic blocker are recommended (see Chap. 8, p. 217).

5. **Physical therapy** to prevent contractures is important during the recovery phase.

V. Diseases of the neuromuscular junction and of muscle: myasthenia gravis

A. Etiology and evaluation. Myasthenia gravis is usually an immune-mediated disease involving the neuromuscular junction. It may occur as three clinical syndromes.

1. **Transient neonatal myasthenia gravis** is thought to occur because of passively transferred IgG antibodies. The signs and symptoms of weakness may be severe.

2. **Congenital myasthenia gravis** may present prior to birth with reduced fetal movements, postnatally, or up to several years following birth. The mother does not have myasthenia gravis. The symptoms are milder, though more persistent, than the transient disease.

3. **Juvenile myasthenia gravis** may occur any time during childhood and usually presents with ptosis, diplopia or other bulbar symptoms and signs, and weakness.

B. Diagnosis. The response to anticholinesterase administration is the cornerstone of diagnosis. Repetitive nerve stimulation seeking a decremental response is confirmatory. The response to edrophonium (Tensilon), 0.2 mg/kg with a maximum of 10 mg, is transient, lasting less than 5 min, and may provoke profound cholinergic side effects. Therefore, neostigmine (Prostigmin) is used IM in neonates and occasionally in older children; 0.04 mg/kg of neostigmine will elicit a response within 10 min and peak at 30 min. With either Tensilon or neostigmine, cardiac rhythm and blood pressure must be monitored, and atropine at 0.01 mg/kg/dose, with a maximum of 0.4 mg, must be available for IV injection.

C. Therapy

1. **Transient neonatal myasthenia gravis**

   a. **Supportive therapy** alone will be adequate only in a minority of patients.

   b. With feeding or respiratory difficulty, IM and oral neostigmine are helpful. The IM dosage range is 0.05–0.3 mg/kg; with oral dosages it is 10 times higher. The frequency of administration can be ascertained clinically by respiratory function and force of the cry and may be necessary q1–12h. IM doses may be given 20 min before feedings.

(3) **Plasmapheresis** or **exchange transfusion** may be used for symptoms that are unresponsive to anticholinesterase therapy.

2. **Congenital myasthenia gravis.** In the neonatal period it may be managed as transient myasthenic, although serious problems are not as evident. Plasmapheresis or exchange transfusion would not likely be helpful. Chronic anticholinesterase treatment is often disappointing at any age.

3. **Juvenile myasthenia gravis**
   a. **Anticholinesterase drugs** are the cornerstone of management, both chronically, for cranial nerve dysfunction and weakness, and for acute respiratory embarrassment; Neostigmine or pyridostigmine (Mestinon) are used, starting at 0.3–0.5 mg/kg and 1 mg/kg tid respectively, with increasing dosage and adjustment of frequency of administration according to the response and its duration.
   b. When anticholinesterase medications at higher dosages are not efficacious, prednisone is warranted, starting at 0.5–1.0 mg/kg and increasing by 0.2 mg/kg up to 60 mg/day every other day until an optimal effect is achieved. The prednisone should subsequently be slowly tapered.
   c. **Thymectomy** may be effective therapy when other means of treatment have failed or when requirement for corticosteroids are prolonged, daily, and at high dosages. Thymoma rarely occurs in childhood.
   d. Plasmapheresis has recently shown promise as a means of transiently improving severe symptoms and signs.

4. When using anticholinesterase medications, overmedication may result in weakness, leading to the so-called cholinergic crisis. Systemic cholinergic symptoms and signs suggest the proper diagnosis, and a Tensilon test distinguishes cholinergic crisis from myasthenic crisis. Atropine, 0.4 mg IV, is a treatment of choice for cholinergic crisis.

VI. Movement disorders

A. **Gilles de la Tourette syndrome** is characterized by multiple, complex tics occasionally associated with unusual vocalizations.

1. **Etiology.** This disease is thought to involve an alteration of dopaminergic neurotransmitter systems.

2. **Evaluation and diagnosis.** The diagnosis rests on the clinical identification of multiple, complex tics. Occasionally, this picture can be provoked by stimulant therapy. Children often have an associated attentional deficit disorder, learning disabilities, or emotional problems as well.

3. **Therapy**
   a. Discontinuation of stimulant drugs
   b. Haloperidol (Haldol) is indicated when the frequency of movements has a negative impact on the child's educational, social, or psychological well-being. Dosages will range from 0.25 mg bid to as high as 4 mg tid. Initial dosages should be small, 0.25 mg bid, and increased at weekly intervals until achieving satisfactory control or sedative side effects necessitate discontinuation of the drug.
   c. Clonidine is used as an alternative medication when use of haloperidol is unsuccessful and when clinical dysfunction makes intervention requisite. Initial dosages are 0.05 mg bid. This dose is increased by increments of 0.05 mg/day every 1–2 weeks to final dosages of 0.2–0.5 mg/day. Side effects include dry mouth, transient somnolence, nightmares, emotional lability, gastrointestinal distress and rebound hypertension if the drug is discontinued abruptly. The medicine should be tapered over 4–5 days.
   d. Psychological counseling and modification of the educational program are often indicated.

B. **Sydenham's chorea**
   1. The **etiology** is unknown.

2. **Evaluation** is that of acute rheumatic fever (see Chap. 15, pp. 407ff).
3. The **diagnosis** rests on noting choreiform movements of the arms and fingers, unusual postures of the outstretched arm, facial grimacing, darting of the tongue, and an explosive speech pattern. The patients are frequently restless and emotionally labile. There is hypotonia, and deep tendon reflexes are pendular and may be "hung-up" on repetitive tapping. Signs may be asymmetrical or unilateral.
4. **Therapy**
   a. **Prednisone therapy** (1–2 mg/kg/day) reportedly leads to improvement within a week.
   b. **Haloperidol** (0.02–0.1 mg/kg/day in 2 divided dosages) is reputed to be effective within 2 weeks.
   c. **Phenobarbital** (3–5 mg/kg/day) or chlorpromazine (50–100 mg tid) may be used as a sedative for symptomatic relief from the movements.
C. The **syndrome of opsoclonus-myoclonus (SOMy)** is also known as myoclonic encephalopathy of infancy.
   1. **Etiology.** This syndrome is associated with neuroblastoma and encephalitis or may be idiopathic. It is thought to occur because of inflammation of the brainstem, or cerebellum, or both.
   2. **Evaluation and diagnosis**
      a. Evaluated in the same manner as occult neuroblastoma (see Chap. 8, pp. 233ff).
      b. **Physical examination.** The patients are most often irritable and photophobic. They usually have conjugate, chaotic, quick movements of the eyes in any direction of gaze, often aggravated when they are tired and noted during sleep. Jerking movements of the legs, particularly when attempts are made to place the child on his or her feet, are present. The child may appear markedly ataxic; similar movements may be noted at the upper extremities when reaching.
      c. **Laboratory evaluation.** In addition to tests necessary to evaluate neuroblastoma, these patients should have a CT scan to rule out a posterior fossa mass and a lumbar puncture to evaluate cells and protein and to rule out enteroviral or arboviral infection.
   3. **Therapy**
      Irradiation of neuroblastoma or waiting for a few weeks following a clear infectious etiology may be all that is necessary. However, when SOMy persists, ACTH, given IM, is advocated (60–80 units/M^2 rapidly tapering to every other day and, subsequently, as clinically indicated, over 1–3 months). Some patients become corticosteroid dependent.
D. **Wilson's disease**
   1. **Etiology.** An autosomal recessively inherited inborn error of copper metabolism resulting in accumulation of copper in brain and liver.
   2. **Evaluation**
      a. **History and examination.** May present with basal ganglia signs (tremor, rigidity, dystonia, chorea), psychiatric symptoms, a course of dementia or liver disease (see Chap. 10, p. 284). A neurologic presentation is invariably associated with presence of Kayser-Fleischer rings of the cornea.
      b. **Ancillary evaluations**
         (1) Elevated urinary copper and diminished serum ceruloplasmin concentrations are usual but not invariable features. Liver biopsy is sometimes necessary and demonstrates elevated hepatic copper concentrations.
         (2) Slit lamp examination to evaluate the presence of Kayser-Fleischer rings.
   3. Treatment with penicillamine as outlined in Chap. 4, p. 114.
VII. Paroxysmal disorders
A. **Seizures** represent a symptom complex and not a disease state. The tendency to have recurrent seizures in the absence of acute metabolic alterations or CNS infection loosely defines epilepsy.

1. **Etiology.** In the emergency room setting the most important etiologic considerations include trauma, trauma X, meningitis and encephalitis, space-occupying lesions, metabolic causes, cerebrovascular accidents, and toxic encephalopathies. Poor drug compliance or altered drug metabolism because of intercurrent illness is the most common cause of seizures in a patient with epilepsy.

2. **Evaluation**
   a. The **history** should include questions about previous static or progressive neurologic or developmental dysfunction, symptoms of an infectious illness, or a history of headaches, early morning vomiting, or visual alterations.
      (1) Precise details of the seizure, particularly observing the initial components of the seizures, and observing deviations of the eyes and head is most important. The postictal assessment for eye position or weakness is also useful. The duration of the postictal state should be noted.
      (2) Absence of a return to baseline within 1 hr suggests either ongoing seizures, a response to administered medications, or is due to the underlying disease or a supervening problem.
      (3) A **family history** of febrile and nonfebrile seizures should be noted.
   b. **Physical examination.** A thorough neurologic examination should be performed, with particular attention to evaluation of mental status and the fundi and a search for focal or lateralized signs. The general examination is relevant in particular to meningeal signs, trauma, and diseases of other body systems.
   c. **Specific laboratory assessments** to include serum and CSF evaluation will depend on the clues to the cause provided by the history and physical findings.
      (1) An **awake and asleep EEG** should be done in all patients with seizures. An EEG is particularly useful for confirming the presence of paroxysmal discharges and in helping identify the possible focality of a discharge and space-occupying lesions, helping choose appropriate anticonvulsant medication, and helping determine when anticonvulsants should be discontinued.
      (2) A **cranial CT scan** should be performed in patients with partial seizures, with otherwise unexplained loss of seizure control, with focal or lateralized abnormalities found on the neurologic examination, with focally abnormal EEGs, or with known or suspected specific white or gray matter neurologic diseases. A CT scan is generally not indicated for patients with primary generalized (grand mal) or pure absence (petit mal) seizures in whom the neurologic findings are normal.
   d. The **differential diagnoses** include syncope, breath-holding spells (both may be followed by a brief, clonic seizure), decerebration, narcolepsy, complicated migraine, benign paroxysmal vertigo, and hysteria.

3. **Diagnosis**
   a. **Grand mal (primary generalized, tonic-clonic)** seizures usually start without an aura or focal features. Characteristically, there is a tonic phase, usually lasting less than a minute, often associated with rolling up of the eyes: During this phase there may be little air exchange because of tonic contraction of the respiratory musculature, resulting in cyanosis. The tonic phase is followed by clonic jerking of the extremities, usually lasting 1–5 min, with associated improved air exchange. There may be hypersalivation, tachycardia, and metabolic and respiratory acidosis. There is usually a postictal state lasting less than 1 hr.
   b. **Focal motor seizures (partial seizures with elementary symptomatology).** Characteristically, focal motor seizures start in the hand or face and are associated with head and eye deviation toward the hemisphere opposite the seizure focus. It may start restricted to that area, without loss of consciousness, or it may generalize and quickly and phenotypically resemble grand mal seizures (secondary generalized, tonic-clonic sei-

zures). Following the seizures, a Todd's paralysis or eye and head deviation **toward** the previously discharging hemisphere may be clues to the focality.

   c. **Temporal lobe or psychomotor seizures (partial seizures with complex symptomatology)** are preceded by an aura (e.g., emotional feelings, abdominal or head pain, feeling in the throat) about 50% of the time. These seizures may mimic other seizure types during various ictal episodes. There may be focal, motor, grand mal, or staring seizures; at other times the seizures will appear more complex, with stereotyped, automatic behaviors, including, for example, running, lip smacking, laughing, and unusual movements of the face or hand. In general, there is a postictal state with full or partial amnesia for the seizure.

   d. **Petit mal (primary generalized, absence seizures)** begin in childhood, usually occur after 3 years of age, and are characterized by staring with or without eyelid fluttering or head-nodding movements. The seizures are not preceded by an aura or followed by a postical state and usually last for less than 30 sec. They may occur many times a day and may be provoked by hyperventilation or stroboscopic lights. The associated EEG is specifically a 3/sec spike and wave abnormality. It is important to differentiate these seizures from partial complex seizures because of implications of anticonvulsant treatment, causation, and prognosis. Occasional grand mal seizures occur in 10–20% of patients with petit mal seizures. By puberty the majority (75%) of patients no longer have seizures and have a normal EEG.

   e. **Infantile spasms with hypsarrhythmic EEG.** Infantile spasms begin most often in the first year of life and are characterized by large myoclonic (salaam) spasms. This syndrome may occur as a consequence of various neurologic diseases or may occur without known antecedent problems. Development usually slows with the onset of spasms, and there is a high incidence of subsequent retardation, particularly among patients with antecedent neurologic disease.

   f. **Mixed generalized seizures (atypical petit mal, petit mal variant, minor motor seizures).** This group of seizure disorders is typified by patients with Lennox-Gastaut syndrome, which is characterized by frequent, difficultly controlled seizures to include atonic, myoclonic (sudden muscle jerks), tonic and clonic seizures associated with an EEG pattern of atypical spike and waves (less than 3 per second spike and waves), multifocal spikes, and polyspikes. The age of onset is usually between 18 months and 5 years and often follows infantile spasms. Patients often have developmental delay.

   g. **Febrile seizures** occur between 6 months and 5 years of age in the context of fever, usually above 38.5°C (101.5°F), and most often as the temperature rises or at its peak. The seizures are usually phenotypically grand mal, although they may be tonic, atonic (limp), or clonic.

      (1) They are considered to be simple if they are single, last less than 15 min, and if there are no focal features during or following the fit. Implicit to the definition is an absence of metabolic disarray, absence of nervous system infection, and a normal EEG obtained at least a few weeks following the ictal episodes.

      (2) Complex febrile seizures are multiple, prolonged, or focal.

      (3) All febrile patients with a first seizure under 18 months or over 3 years of age require lumbar puncture and a metabolic screen, as does any patient with complex febrile seizures, altered mental status, neurologic signs, meningeal signs, or uncertain follow-up.

      (4) Risk factors for subsequent development of epilepsy include:
         (a) Antecedent abnormal neurologic or developmental status
         (b) A family history of afebrile seizures
         (c) Complex febrile seizures

      (5) The presence of a single or no risk factor is associated with a less than

Table 20-3. Drugs used for treatment of seizure disorders

Anticonvulsant	Half-Life (hr)	Dosage (mg/kg/day)	Time/ day	Approx. thera- peutic range (μg/ml)	Common side effects
Phenytoin (Dilantin)	24–50	5 5–12[a]	bid	10–20 5–10[b]	Rash, hirsut- ism, gingival hyperplasia, hypertrichosis
Phenobarbital or mephobar- bital (Mebaral)	60–92	3–5 (5–18)	qd	10–45	Lethargy, hy- peractivity
Primidone (Mysoline)	6–14	5–25	tid	5–10	Lethargy, irrita- bility
Carbamazepine (Tegretol)[c]	9–15	15–30	bid– tid	3–11	Lethargy, blurry vision, granulocy- topenia
Ethosuximide (Zarontin)	20–60	20–30	bid	40–120	Nausea, hiccups
Valproic acid (Depakene)[b,c]	8–15	25–60	bid– tid	50–120	GI discomfort, tremor
Clonazepam (Clonopin)	24–48	0.02–0.2	bid– tid	10–60	Lethargy, ataxia, hyper- salivation

[a]Phenytoin is very poorly absorbed in the neonatal period, but absorption gradually improves through the first years of life.
[b]Depakene has interactions with phenytoin and phenobarbital. Total phenytoin will be reduced by approximately one-half and free phenytoin will be doubled. Thus, dosages of phenytoin should not be altered, and the therapeutic range should be considered to be between 5–10 μg/ml. Depakene also tends to increase phenobarbital levels.
[c]Requires weekly CBC and liver functions for 2 weeks, then monthly for 3 months, then every 3–6 months.

2% chance of the development of afebrile seizures. This contrasts with an approximately 6–10% occurrence with two or three risk factors.
4. **Therapy.** See also Table 20-3.
   a. **General principles**
      (1) **Acute seizure management. For management of status epilep- ticus,** see Chap. 3, pp. 59ff.
      (2) **Acute seizure management: after the seizure**
         (a) **A history** and **physical examination** are required and will often help direct further course of therapy, depending on the cause.
            (i) In patients with probable febrile seizures the treatment should be directed at the fever.
            (ii) The patient with serious head trauma or evidence of in- creased ICP and herniation may require mannitol, an im- mediate CT scan, and possible neurosurgical intervention.
            (iii) The febrile patient with meningeal signs will require lumbar puncture and antibiotic treatment.
            (iv) The patient with continued stupor or coma will require con-

Table 20-4. Anticonvulsant choice by seizure type

Seizure type	Principal drug of choice	Adjunctive drugs
Primary generalized (grand mal) seizures	Phenobarbital, mephobarbital (Mebaral) Phenytoin (Dilantin) Carbamazepine (Tegretol)	Valproic acid Acetazolamide (Diamox)
Partial elementary seizures (focal)	Phenobarbital Phenytoin Carbamazepine Primidone (Mysoline)	Valproic acid
Partial complex seizures (temporal lobe epilepsy)	Carbamazepine Phenytoin Primidone	Phenobarbital Valproic acid Acetazolamide Methsuximide
Primary generalized (petit mal, absence) seizures	Ethosuximide (Zarontin) Valproic acid (Depakene) Methsuximide (Celontin)	Acetazolamide Clonazepam (Clonopin) Phenobarbital
Infantile spasms	ACTH Valproic acid Clonazepam	Phenytoin Phenobarbital Acetazolamide
Febrile seizures	Phenobarbital	Valproic acid
Mixed generalized seizures	Phenobarbital Valproic acid Clonazepam	Acetazolamide Diazepam Ethosuximide Phenytoin Clorazepate (Tranxene) Methsuximide Carbamazepine
Neonatal seizures	Phenobarbital Phenytoin	Paraldehyde

sideration of diseases such as Reye syndrome or toxic ingestion.

    (b) A choice and mode of administration of anticonvulsant treatment should depend on

        (i) The need for preservation of an optimal state of consciousness (meningitis, Reye syndrome, head injury, ingestion, stupor or coma of unknown etiology). Phenytoin would be the drug of choice in such a circumstance (see Chap. 3, p. 59).

        (ii) Seizure type (see Table 20-4)

        (iii) Anticonvulsants that the patient is already taking (check Medic Alert tag)

        (iv) Urgency for need to control seizures (increased ICP pressure and respiratory compromise would require IV administration of diazepam) (see Chap. 3, p. 59)

        (v) Recognize allergies (check the patient Medic Alert tag)

(3) Chronic management

    (a) The choice of anticonvulsant should be based on clinical and EEG assessment of the seizure type, with consideration of benefit-risk ratio of the drug.

(b) A single drug at therapeutic level is more likely to be effective than multiple drugs at subtherapeutic levels.

(c) The most effective level of the appropriate drug is established by increasing the dosage until seizures are controlled, side effects are sustained, or the maximum therapeutic level is exceeded.

(d) To alter anticonvulsant regimens, modify one drug at a time, allowing for reequilibration to the new level, which will depend on the drug's half-life. Reequilibration will usually require approximately 5 half-lives.

(e) When substituting a new anticonvulsant for another, it is prudent to add the new anticonvulsant first and attain therapeutic levels before tapering away the previous medication.

(f) Discontinuation of an anticonvulsant, especially phenobarbital and the diazepines, should be done slowly, usually over a period of 1 to 6 months.

(g) When possible, tablets or capsules should be used in preference to liquid formulations. This is more likely to ensure uniformity of dosage.

(h) In general, anticonvulsants may be discontinued when the patient has had no seizures for 4 years and has non-paroxysmal waking and sleeping EEGs.

(i) Patients with febrile seizures may be continued on phenobarbital for 1 year or until 3 years of age, after which the incidence of febrile seizures declines (see **3.g.** for indications). Serum levels of at least 15 µg/ml are required for proper prophylaxis.

b. Specific anticonvulsant therapy. See Table 20-3.

B. Neonatal seizures

1. **Etiology.** The causes may be categorized in the following manner:

   a. Metabolic. Hypoglycemia, hypocalcemia, hypomagnesemia, hyponatremia, and hypoxemia

   b. Toxic. Maternal drug ingestion (withdrawal), inadvertent local anesthetic poisoning

   c. Hemorrhagic. Intraventricular, subdural, and subarachnoid hemorrhage

   d. Infectious. Bacterial, viral (TORCH)

   e. Effects resulting from inborn errors of metabolism. Organic acidemias, errors of amino acid metabolism, pyridoxine dependency, etc.

   f. Effects of asphyxia (hypoxia, ischemia)

   g. Cerebral dysgenesis

   h. Benign familial seizures

2. **Evaluation**

   a. A full **perinatal history** and **neonatal examination** will help differentiate the causes.

   b. Laboratory assessments that are helpful include serum evaluation of blood sugar (Dextrostik), calcium, magnesium, sodium, CBC and cultures, and a toxic screen. A CSF examination, EEG with pyridoxine infusion, cranial ultrasound, and/or cranial CT scan are frequently important for diagnostic, therapeutic, or prognostic purposes.

3. **Diagnosis.** Seizures may be tonic, focal clonic, multifocal clonic, myoclonic, or, most commonly, subtle, which includes eye deviation, nystagmus, apnea, sucking movements, tongue thrusting, and bicycling and swimming movements. Spontaneous clonus and jitteriness should be differentiated from seizures.

4. **Therapy**

   a. As with older children with status epilepticus, attention must first be directed at **vital signs.**

   b. Therapy should subsequently be directed at the cause, in particular, when a metabolic factor such as hypoglycemia is recognized.

   c. Anticonvulsant therapy is required when glucose, calcium, oxygen, and

Table 20-5. Symptomatic treatment of migraine headache

Drug	Dosage and route of administration	Age 3–10 years	Age 11 years and older
Aspirin	Usual analgesic dosages PO or PR	Preferred	Preferred
Acetaminophen	Usual analgesic dosages PO or PR	Preferred	Preferred
Fiorinal (butalbital, 50 mg; caffeine, 40 mg; aspirin, 325 mg)		Under 5 years, ½ tablet; over 5, 1 tablet	1–2 tablets
Ergotamine[a] tartrate (Ergomar)	2 mg, sublingual	Not preferred	Preferred
Cafergot[b] (ergotamine tartrate, 1.8 mg; caffeine, 100 mg)		Not preferred	Preferred; PO: 1–2 tablets at onset of headache; 1 tablet q½h to maximum of 4; PR: ½–1 suppository at onset; ½ tablet q½h to maximum of 2

[a]Medication should not be used in renal or hepatic failure, hypertension, with complicated migraine and should be limited to 3 in 24 hr and 5 in 1 week.
[b]Not to be taken with complicated migraine. Given no more than 6 PO tablets or 2 PR tablets in 24 hr. Limit to 8 PO tablets or 4 suppositories/week.

pyridoxine administration (50–100 mg IV) is unsuccessful, or when the possibility of such a deficiency has been excluded.

d. The cornerstone of therapy is **phenobarbital**; the patient may be loaded with phenobarbital at 10–20 mg/kg administered over 5–10 mins. Phenytoin may be used as a second drug at a loading dose of 20 mg/kg, and phenobarbital may be readministered at 10 mg/kg at hourly intervals for 2 further doses, if necessary, for ongoing seizures. After loading with phenobarbital and phenytoin, rectal paraldehyde is the next drug of choice.

e. The **maintenance dosage** of phenobarbital is 4–5 mg/kg/day in either once or twice a day aliquots. Maintenance dosages for **IV phenytoin** is 5–8 mg/kg/day, usually administered bid.

f. Phenobarbital is well absorbed orally. Phenytoin, however, is very poorly absorbed orally in the first months of life and should, in general, be avoided if possible.

g. Dosages of phenytoin exceeding 10 mg/kg/day are occasionally necessary to maintain therapeutic serum levels.

h. Anticonvulsants may be discontinued at the time of discharge or at 3 months if the patient is no longer having clinical seizures, the EEG is not

Table 20-6. Prophylactic treatment for migraine headache

Drug	Dosage and route of administration	Age 3–10 years	Age 11 years and older
Phenobarbital	3–5 mg/kg/day qhs PO	Preferred	Not preferred
Phenytoin (Dilantin)	5 mg/kg/day bid PO	Preferred	Less commonly used or less effective than others
Propranolol[a]	0.5–3.0 mg/kg/day bid–or tid	Less commonly used or less effective than others	Preferred
Amitriptyline	0.2–0.5 mg/kg/day (in qhs dosages) PO	Not preferred	Preferred
Cyproheptadine	0.25 mg/kg/day bid–tid PO	Less commonly used or less effective than others	Less commonly used or less effective than others
Methysergide[b] (Sansert)	2 mg qd PO	Not preferred	Less commonly used or less effective than others
Biofeedback behavioral modification		Preferred	Preferred

[a]Not to be given to patients with asthma, sinus bradycardia with first-degree block, or congestive heart failure.
[b]May cause retroperitoneal fibrosis and vascular insufficiency. It is to be given only for brief periods (less than 5 months) in adolescence.

paroxysmal, and the neurologic findings are normal. Anticonvulsant levels should be monitored at the time of recurrent seizures, when side effects develop, and 3–4 weeks subsequent to an alteration of the maintenance dosage.

C. **Migraine headache.** The majority of childhood headaches not associated with acute illness are migrainous. Migraine occurs in 5% of children.

    1. **Etiology.** The neurologic symptoms associated with migraine are considered to be a function of cerebrovascular constriction, leading to diminished cerebral blood flow to specific brain areas. The pain is thought to occur because of subsequent vasodilation, leading to stretching of intramural nerves.

    2. **Evaluation and diagnosis.** Migraine headaches are typically periodic. They can be conveniently divided into classic (hemicranial, throbbing and preceded by an aura), complicated (classic and a neurologic deficit), or common (no aura, generalized or bilateral head pain). Rarely, vomiting alone or abdominal pain alone may be the only symptom of a migraine attack.

a. **History and physical examination.** The diagnosis of migraine headache rests on identifying the intermittency of the headache. The majority of children have associated nausea and vomiting, photophobia, and sonophobia. Auras may include visual scotoma or scintillations, vertigo, malaise with associated pallor, perioral numbness, or alterations of perception. Neurologic findings may include confusional state, aphasia, brainstem signs, ataxia, hemiparesis, hemisensory loss, and loss of consciousness. In 90% of the children a family member will have migraine, and many will suffer from motion sickness.

Headache is a symptom complex that may be provoked by many factors. Factors that may alert the clinician to a more serious illness include headaches that frequently occur during sleep, more often occur in the morning on waking, often are associated with vomiting, and are associated with seizures. A focal or lateralized neurologic abnormality interictally, asymmetrical cranial bruits, or evidence of elevated ICP at any time is also a cause for concern and further evaluation. Such evaluation may include an EEG, cranial CT scan, and, occasionally, angiography.

b. **Laboratory evaluation.** The history and physical findings will determine which tests are necessary. The aim of the tests will be to rule out other causes of headache, which, of course, will depend on the clinical setting.

3. **Therapy.** The approach to treatment of migraine headache will depend on headache frequency, the degree of disability, and age.

a. **Migraine-provoking agents** such as chocolates and cheeses should be eliminated.

b. **Other complicating factors,** such as emotional stress and withdrawal from chronic intake of caffeinated beverages, should also be evaluated.

c. **Pharmacologic treatment** may be either symptomatic (Table 20-5) or prophylactic (Table 20-6). Prophylaxis is considered when the frequency is greater than once per week, leading to school absence, when such headaches are unresponsive to symptomatic treatment, or when side effects of the acutely administered medications lead to a similar or worse disability.

21
Behavior

I. **Behavioral treatment program.** The brief program outlined in five steps (see **A–E**) is based on the principle of **operant conditioning** (behavior is determined in part by its consequences). If a behavior is followed by a rewarding event **(positive reinforcement)**, it tends to be strengthened and occur more frequently. If the behavior is followed by no event **(extinction)** or by an aversive event **(punishment)**, it tends to be weakened and occur less frequently. These principles have been applied to a wide range of behaviors (e.g., enuresis, atopic dermatitis scratching, medicine compliance, eating disorders). A good relationship with a motivated or interested family is important for success.

A. **Specify the target behavior.** A detailed history is needed regarding the behavior to be modified, including environmental antecedents and consequences of this behavior (e.g., scratching might be the target, with an important consequence being parent attention).

B. **Measure the target behavior (baseline).** Have the family record the frequency, time, and duration of the behavior. This is an **important step** to allow later determination of the effectiveness of the intervention (e.g., scratching occurs so many times per hour).

C. **Choose the reinforcer(s).** Together with the family, search for a reward or reinforcer that will maintain a new behavior. This is done by looking for what the child likes (e.g., toys, money, stickers) or what the child does a lot (e.g., play computer games).

D. **Arrange the contingency**
   1. An arrangement is made in which access to the reinforcer is contingent on producing the new behavior (e.g., reinforcement is given in response to a specified reduction in scratches per hour).
   2. The reinforcer is maximally effective when it immediately follows the behavior to be strengthened (e.g., stickers might be given for a specified time with no scratching or a reduction in scratching).
   3. In beginning the program the reinforcers must be easily obtainable. Later, the requirements to gain the reinforcer can be increased. A major problem in the failure of programs is making the reinforcement too difficult to obtain at first (e.g., no scratching for 10 min might be required at first; later, 20 min might be required).
   4. The use of stickers, stars, or points that can be posted on a chart or pasted in a book is useful. These can later be turned in for reinforcers (e.g., 10 points may gain a new toy).
   5. Reinforcers definitely include social approval and praise for desired behaviors. Ignoring the nondesired behavior can be used.

E. **Monitor the progress**
   1. The programs usually need repetition to become effective. Recording the child's progress, as in step 4, will allow evaluation of effectiveness.
   2. As the new behavior is established, other reinforcers (e.g., social approval) become important, so that the formal program can be gradually phased out.
   3. In the long run, the use of punishment is not an effective intervention.
   4. These programs can be highly effective with specified behaviors. **However, for difficulties in establishing an effective program, the lack of time re-**

quired to arrange a program, or complex behavior problems, a psychological consultation is indicated.

II. Chronic illness

A. Chronic illness in a child constitutes a major and prolonged stress for the entire family. The psychological reactions of the family, including the child, occur in phases with indistinct transitions. These are as follows:

1. **Shock and disbelief.** Regressive behaviors, unrealistic fears, and, most commonly, denial are prominent (lasting weeks to even months).

2. **Protest and anguish.** Guilt, depression, anger, and sorrow can occur. There is mourning for lost normalcy and dashed hopes. The young child may experience illness as a punishment for being "bad" or may become bitter at illness-related treatments or restrictions. The adolescent may fear "loss of control" or "being different." Blaming parents or physicians is common.

3. **Restitution.** This phase ideally represents awareness of new limitations, development of adequate social patterns, constructive use of strengths, and a denial that is consistent with hope. Families usually adapt well. However, increased emotional problems are found in chronically ill children when compared with control groups.

B. **Evaluation**

1. **History** should emphasize the child's previous adaptive capacities (e.g., school performance problems, poor peer relations, or difficult reactions to loss) or family relationship problems.

2. Maladaptive responses by the child include overdependence, noncompliance, overanxiousness, aggressiveness, and/or withdrawal. Overprotection, indulgence, rejection, and/or blaming may be parental responses.

C. **Treatment**

1. A long-term supportive relationship with the family may allow anxieties and frustrations to be expressed.

2. Clear and honest explanations regarding the diagnosis, prognosis, and management should be given to both parent and child. Repeated explanations, especially at the time of the initial diagnosis, are commonly needed.

3. Siblings often feel guilt, or resentment, or both, about the sick child. Parents should be encouraged to keep the siblings informed, with the physician's assistance if necessary.

4. Parents should be encouraged to minimize as much as possible the "sick child" role. Chronically ill children still need discipline.

5. If available, group meetings for parents and children who have experienced similar problems can be helpful.

6. Compliance is a frequent problem, especially for the adolescent. The following approach is recommended:

a. Early education regarding the illness and clear explanations about the management are preventive. Reassurance and positive verbal feedback regarding compliance are helpful;

b. If compliance becomes a problem, verify the situation (e.g., blood levels). The results then should be discussed directly with the patient. A behavioral treatment program with a positive reinforcement system (e.g., awards, stickers, praise) may then be attempted.

c. If the preceding measures are unsuccessful or time constraints make step 2 difficult, then psychiatric consultation may be necessary.

III. Conduct disorders

A. **Etiology.** Problematic parent-child relationships and child-rearing practices of varying severity are involved in these cases.

B. **Evaluation**

1. The parents or outside agency (e.g., school) usually present complaints of lying, fighting, truancy, bullying, and/or legally defined delinquent acts such as stealing and fire setting. The behaviors, occurring more frequently in boys than in girls, are persistent, troublesome, and socially disapproved.

2. Isolated delinquent acts **without** obvious social or school impairments are common and of little significance. Fire setting between the ages of 4–7 years

may occur out of curiosity rather than pathology. An adolescent's opposi-
tional behavior may reflect a move toward independence and may not violate
major societal rules.
   3. Emotional disorders such as depression may be present, but can be over-
shadowed by the troublesome behavior.
   4. Learning disabilities are frequently associated, along with a history of temperament extremes.
C. Diagnosis. These are conditions in which **repetitive, persistent** behaviors violate either the basic rights of others or major age-appropriate societal norms or
rules.
D. Treatment
   1. Prevention is important. Early prenatal education about the temperamen-
tally difficult infant may be helpful. Counseling and advice should be offered
around firm and consistent discipline techniques. Infant intervention programs or parent-effectiveness training groups may be available.
   2. Supervised recreational experiences, such as organized social clubs (e.g.,
Big Brothers or Sisters) and job placements, can be beneficial. A supportive
relationship (i.e., caring and empathetic with firm age-appropriate limits)
can be established with, for example, a physician, school counselor, or clergyman.
   3. Referral to a child psychiatrist is recommended for the persistently out-of-
control child. Treatment is most helpful when the problems are responses to
emotional difficulties.
   4. For the resistant child it may be necessary for the parents to go to the
juvenile court to obtain court supervision via probation. Frequently, a psychiatric evaluation can be ordered.
   5. A **residential placement** may be needed, either when parents are unable to
provide needed firm structure or when the child's behaviors are extreme.
   6. Assessment of a child's **social attachment** (e.g., friendships in peer group for
more than 6 months; extends to others with no immediate advantage; does
not blame or inform on friends; and/or concern for the welfare of others) can
be helpful in determining responses to intervention. Children with better
attachments have a better prognosis.
IV. Drug and alcohol abuse
A. Etiology. Frequently, the substance abuser grows up in a family environment of
inconsistency and rejection. The needs of the child are met erratically. Low self-
worth, feelings of inferiority, and hostility are often present. Drugs are theorized
to provide relief from this situation. There also may be unclear hereditary components along with contributing sociocultural factors (e.g., peer pressure).
B. Evaluation
   1. A complete **drug and alcohol history** should be obtained, including types,
amounts, and frequency. Include any evidence of physical tolerance or dependence.
   2. School performance is frequently poor, and conduct problems are common.
   3. A **family history** of substance use should be sought.
   4. Evidence of parental inconsistency and rejection may be obtained.
   5. In the drug-abusing child, the substance may be taken for pleasure rather
than for curiosity. Frequently, multiple drugs are used.
C. Diagnosis. A pattern of pathologic substance use that causes impairment in
social or school functioning (for at least 1 month)
D. Treatment. Once abuse is established, treatment is difficult and frustrating, with
only modest success.
   1. Prevention by **early recognition** is important. Significant family or school
problems are indications to pursue a family substance history. Early family
counseling referral can be helpful to the young child.
   2. Efforts should be made to keep school a positive learning experience, including evaluation for a learning disability.
   3. The goal is to establish a supportive relationship with a significant adult,
such as a physician, school counselor, social worker, or clergyman. The sub-

stance abuser will be difficult to engage and may have frequent relapses. The relationship needs to be firm, consistent, and nonrejecting.

4. Additionally, a group treatment program, such as Alcoholics Anonymous, may help to improve peer relationships.

V. Eating disorders

A. Anorexia nervosa

1. **Etiology.** Anorexia nervosa is a symptom complex with different psychiatric diagnoses. It is an increasingly common disorder found in women of the higher and middle socioeconomic class (rarely men) between 10–30 years of age. The clinical course varies greatly and is often frustrating. Mortality ranging from 5–20% has been reported.

2. **Evaluation**
   a. **Early symptoms**
      (1) A self-imposed diet that gradually leads to drastic caloric reduction and marked weight loss
      (2) A preoccupation with food without loss of appetite
      (3) An intense fear of gaining weight and a distorted body image
   b. **Later findings**
      (1) Feelings of incompetence and being out of control
      (2) Eating binges, self-induced vomiting, laxative or diuretic abuse, and/or excessive exercising
   c. Before making the diagnosis, any physical illness that would account for the weight loss, such as inflammatory bowel disease or endocrine disorders, must be excluded. Psychiatric illnesses such as schizophrenic disorders and depressive disorders must be ruled out.
   d. **Physical manifestations** include hypothermia, hypotension, lanugo, and dependent edema. Both primary and secondary amenorrhea occur.
   e. **Laboratory findings** are normal until the later stages of malnutrition. Leukopenia, lymphocytosis, low erythrocyte sedimentation rate, and low fibrinogen levels then occur. Low serum lactic dehydrogenase estrogens, and T_3 have been found, along with incomplete suppression of ACTH and cortisol levels by dexamethasone.

3. **Diagnosis** (adapted from *Diagnostic and Statistical Manual of Mental Disorders* [3rd ed.]* American Psychiatric Association, Washington, D.C. 1980)
   a. Intense fear of becoming fat, which does not decrease as weight loss progresses
   b. Distortion of body image
   c. Refusal to maintain weight over a minimal normal weight for age and height
   d. Body weight is less than 75% of the mean weight for age on pediatric growth charts.

4. **Treatment**
   a. Prior to drastic weight loss, patients may respond to encouragement, kindly firmness, and nutritional education.
   b. If there is no response, psychiatric consultation is indicated. Management requires a collaboration between pediatrics and psychiatry.
   c. Outpatients should be seen medically at least once a week for weight monitoring. Encouragement and support, along with firm and unchanging weight expectations, are indicated.
   d. Although an outpatient program may be attempted and may succeed, hospitalization is often necessary. Indications include severe malnutrition, vital-sign instability, acute dehydration, electrolyte imbalance (e.g., hypokalemic alkalosis), and/or outpatient treatment failure.
   e. **Care during hospitalization**
      (1) Daily morning postvoiding weights should be obtained.
      (2) The diet may start about 500 cal/day **over** the amount required to maintain weight.

*Subsequently abbreviated *DSM III*.

(3) Vomiting or laxative abuse should be monitored by periodic electrolyte determinations. Making the bathroom inaccessible for 2 hr after meals, if necessary, may help to control vomiting.

(4) Constipation is relieved by eating, although stool softeners may be needed.

(5) Behavioral treatment programs with increased environmental structure have been useful.

  (a) Operant conditioning with positive reinforcement, such as visiting privileges, increased physical activities, and social interactions contingent on weight gain are used.

  (b) Negative reinforcers, such as bed rest or tube feeding, have been included.

  (c) Weight gain rather than eating is emphasized, so as to decrease eating anxiety and not teach vomiting. Liquid food supplements are sometimes used to reduce anxiety related to eating food.

  (d) Psychiatric consultation is recommended in establishing this treatment plan.

(6) Neuroleptics and tricyclic antidepressants have been used with limited success.

B. Obesity

  1. Etiology. Social, emotional, learning, genetic, and physical activity factors and/or fat cell size and number have been implicated.

  2. Evaluation

  a. Childhood-onset obesity tends to be severe, with onset more likely at 0–4 and 7–11 years;

  b. Obesity **need not** denote a psychiatric disturbance. However, it is often associated with emotional disorders (often, a body image disturbance). There is no specific personality type.

  c. Weight gain secondary to craniopharyngioma, pituitary tumor, Prader-Willi syndrome, Laurence-Moon-Biedl syndrome, ovarian dysfunction, and Cushing syndrome must be excluded.

  3. Diagnosis. *Obesity* is a marked increase in body fat, resulting in a weight more than 20% above mean weight for age on pediatric growth charts.

  4. Treatment

  a. The **prognosis** for sustained weight loss is poor. Prevention via early recognition and nutritional advice is important. Inappropriate use of food to calm a child's discomfort should be discouraged.

  b. Successful treatment requires high motivation and family involvement. Important components include a balanced low-calorie diet and increased physical activity. Though not ideal, behavioral treatment programs involving positive reinforcement for stepwise weight reduction have been the most effective.

  c. Group support, such as Weight Watchers, may be helpful.

  d. Individual psychiatric treatment may be needed.

C. Bulimia (binge eating)

  1. The etiology is not known. Both psychological and organic theories have been proposed.

  2. Evaluation

  a. This disorder occurs predominantly in late adolescence, with a chronic and intermittent course over years. It is seldom incapacitating. Binges are usually planned and done secretly. Most of the patients are within a normal weight range.

  b. Anorexia nervosa, epileptic equivalent seizures, CNS tumors, Klüver-Buccy-like syndromes, and Kleine-Levin syndrome must be excluded.

  3. Diagnosis (adapted from *DSM III*)

  a. Recurrent episodes of rapid consumption of a large amount of food usually over a 2-hr period

  b. Awareness that the eating pattern is abnormal and fear of not being able to stop voluntarily

      c. A depressed mood following the binges

      d. At least **three** of the following:

         (1) Consumption of a high-calorie, easily ingested food during a binge

         (2) Inconspicuous eating during the binge

         (3) Termination of binges by abdominal pain, sleep, social interruption, or self-induced vomiting

         (4) Weight loss attempts by strict diet, vomiting, cathartics, or diuretics

         (5) Frequent weight changes of over 10 pounds due to binges and fasts.

   4. Treatment

      a. Psychotherapy and **behavioral treatment** may be used with some success. Psychiatric consultation is recommended.

      b. Dehydration and **electrolyte imbalance** (hypokalemia) secondary to the vomiting, cathartics, or diuretics may need correction.

      c. Tricyclic antidepressants are being given clinical trials.

D. Pica

   1. Etiology. A specific nutritional deficit and/or unmet needs from the parental relationship are postulated.

   2. Evaluation

      a. Pica occurs most frequently between the ages of 18 months and 5 years. The normal infant hand-to-mouth reactions are not included. Ingestion ranges from paint to hair to dirt, with no aversion to food.

      b. Developmental disability, mineral deficiencies such as iron deficiency, child neglect, poor parent-child relationships, infantile autism, and schizophrenic disorders may be associated.

      c. Complications depend on the material ingested and include lead poisoning, alopecia, intestinal parasites, and intestinal obstruction (e.g., trichobezoar).

   3. Diagnosis requires evidence of regular eating of a nonnutritive substance.

   4. Treatment

      a. Improved observation and supervision of the child are usually indicated. Improved parental care may occur with direct advice to increase attention to the child. Social service or psychiatric consultation might then be considered if there is no response.

      b. When factors besides inadequate supervision are present, specific therapy should be attempted.

      c. Offending agents, such as paint containing lead, should be removed from the child's environment.

      d. Behavioral treatment using positive reinforcement has had some success.

VI. Emotional disorders

  A. Phobic disorders

   1. Etiology. Psychoanalytic theory assumes displacement of anxiety from an unconscious conflict onto a feared object. **Learning theory** describes learning an irrational response to a benign situation.

   2. Evaluation

      a. Fear of animals, insects, the dark, noise, and death are commonly encountered. Rarely is a phobia the only symptom if an emotional disorder is present. Self-limited phobic fears in the preschool child are well known.

      b. School phobia is common on school entrance and again during early adolescence.

      c. Social phobias (fear of certain social situations) usually begin after puberty.

      d. Agoraphobia can be seen in late adolescence and can be associated with a history of school phobia.

      e. Parental anxiety may play a significant contributing role in the child's anxiety.

   3. Diagnosis (adapted from *DSM III*). A *phobia* is a persistent and irrational fear of a specific object, activity, or situation. The fear and subsequent aversive behavior is a significant source of distress or interferes with social and school functioning.

4. Treatment
    a. Reassurance given to the parents can help alleviate parental anxiety and indirectly reduce the child's anxiety.
    b. Psychiatric consultation is indicated when the phobia becomes disabling. Behavioral treatment is the treatment of choice for simple phobias. More complex phobias often require environmental changes, behavioral treatment, and psychotherapy (individual or group) in various combinations.
    c. Agoraphobia associated with discreet anxiety attacks may respond to antidepressant medications.

B. Depressive disorders
  1. Etiology. Both biologic and psychosocial factors are involved.
  2. Evaluation
    a. Children should be asked about their affective state (e.g., "Do you ever feel really sad or unhappy?" "Do you cry often?"). Severity, frequency, and setting should be assessed. Asking about suicide (e.g., "Do you ever think about hurting yourself?") Will not precipitate the event, but will relieve a child in addition to allowing intervention.
    b. Particular indications for an **affect history** include parental rejection, physical illness, sudden loss, conduct disorders, school refusal and school problems, and sleep disturbances.
    c. Depression in a child is often associated with parental depression.
    d. A history from **different sources** (e.g., child, parent, or school) is helpful. A disparity is not unusual, since the parents may be unaware of their child's depression.
    e. Transitory depressive moods without disabling effects at home or school are common in children.
    f. Infectious diseases (e.g., influenza), hypothyroidism, or medications may cause depressed moods.

  3. Diagnosis (adapted from *DSM III*)
    a. A prominent and persistent depressed mood (e.g., "sad," "blue," "down in the dumps," or "low," or a persistently sad facial expression) or marked lack of interest or pleasure in almost all usual activities
    b. At least three of the following are required for a depressive period:
      (1) Insomnia or hypersomnia
      (2) Appetite changes and significant weight loss or gain
      (3) Low energy level or chronic tiredness
      (4) Feelings of inadequacy or worthlessness
      (5) Decreased effectiveness at school or home
      (6) Decreased attention, concentration, or ability to think clearly
      (7) Social withdrawal; less active or talkative than usual
      (8) Irritability or excessive anger toward parents or caretakers
      (9) Inability to respond with pleasure to praise or rewards
      (10) Pessimistic attitude toward the future or brooding about past events
      (11) Tearfulness or crying
      (12) Negative affect on awakening (e.g., tired, drowsy, sick, or irritable) that improves over the next few minutes or hours
      (13) Recurrent thoughts of death or suicide
    c. Symptoms must be present almost daily for at least 2 weeks.

  4. Treatment
    a. A **supportive relationship** should be established, ranging from environmental manipulations (e.g., school changes or parent education) to individual meetings.
    b. Regular and open **communication** with a physically ill child and family may be preventive.
    c. Psychiatric consultation is recommended for evaluation and treatment of persistent depression.
    d. Antidepressants have been used successfully, but require close monitoring along with ongoing psychological treatment. Sleep disturbances and diurnal affect variations may be clues to a drug-responsive depression.

C. Anxiety disorders
   1. **Etiology.** Excessive states of anxiety may relate to temperamental variation, or chronic environmental stress, or both.
   2. **Evaluation**
      a. The history is elicited by asking what kind of things the patient worries about.
      b. Precipitating stresses include high performance pressure, damage to self-esteem, or feelings of lack of competence.
      c. Accident proneness, hypermaturity, excessive conformity, and difficulty getting to sleep are common symptoms.
      d. Parental anxiety often contributes to the child's worries.
   3. **Diagnosis** (adapted from *DSM III*). The predominant disturbance is generalized and persistent anxiety or worry lasting at least 1 month, as manifested by at least four of the following:
      a. Unrealistic worry about future events
      b. Preoccupation with appropriateness of past behavior
      c. Overconcern about competence (e.g., school, social, athletic)
      d. Somatic complaints, such as headaches or stomach aches, with no established physical basis
      e. Excessive need for reassurance about worries
      f. Marked self-consciousness
      g. Marked feelings of tension or inability to relax; shakiness, trembling, restlessness, or fidgeting
      h. Autonomic hyperactivity (e.g., sweating, heart pounding, dry mouth, diarrhea, high resting pulse and respiration rate)
   4. **Treatment**
      a. Anxiety may be responsive to support, reassurance, and/or advice to the child and the parents. If the child is unresponsive to this supportive relationship and there is interference with school, home, and/or play, psychiatric consultation can be helpful.
      b. **Acute anxiety** may be helped by benzodiazepines, hydroxyzine, or diphenhydramine.
      c. If interested, the child can be instructed in the use of meditative or relaxation techniques. The patient is told to practice twice a day and to use the techniques during acute upsets. The following outlines sample instructions given and demonstrated to the child:
         (1) Arrange a quiet and comfortable place.
         (2) Close your eyes and think about "doing nothing."
         (3) Relax your head, neck, and shoulders slowly.
         (4) Exhale slowly after a medium-deep breath and let "relaxation or calmness" flow through your body down to your hands and feet.
         (5) Repeat a single word (e.g., *calm, relax, one*) after each exhalation and feel "relaxation."
         (6) Continue to focus on the repetition of a single word, and observe the relaxation for about 5–10 min.

D. Conversion disorders
   1. **Etiology.** Psychological theory assumes "conversion" of anxiety into a physical dysfunction to lessen conscious anxiety.
   2. **Evaluation**
      a. Motor or sensory disturbances along with symptoms complicating a physical illness are common presentations.
      b. A **previous history** of undiagnosable physical symptoms, conversion reactions, or both is helpful;
      c. A **coexisting organic illness** does not rule out the diagnosis.
      d. **Emotional stress** prior to the symptom and/or exposure to a person with similar physical symptoms is frequent.
      e. The **differential diagnosis** includes systemic lupus erythematosus and multiple sclerosis, both of which may present with conversionlike symptoms.

3. Diagnosis (adapted from *DSM III*)
 a. The predominant disturbance is a loss or alteration in physical functioning, suggesting a physical disorder.
 b. The symptom cannot be explained by a known pathophysiologic mechanism and is not under voluntary control.
 c. Psychological factors are judged involved, as evidenced by one of the
 following;
  (1) The temporal relationship between an environmental stimulus that is
  related to a psychological conflict or need and the initiation of symptom.
  (2) The symptom enables the patient either to avoid a noxious activity or
  gain support from the environment that otherwise might not be forth-
  coming.
4. Treatment
 a. Psychiatric consultation is indicated. Successful treatment has been obtained with psychotherapy, suggestion, environmental manipulation,
 and direct symptom approach (e.g., hypnosis).
 b. Support of the family is helpful, frequently by reassurance about symptoms that are not medically serious.
 c. In 10–30% of patients with a diagnosis of conversion disorder, organic
 illness will be misdiagnosed. Ongoing pediatric follow-up in conjunction
 with a psychiatric investigation is indicated.

VII. Encopresis
A. Etiology includes:
 1. Chronic constipation with concomitant leakage secondary to the loss of internal sphincter competence
 2. Psychosocial stresses
 3. Hirschsprung's disease (aganglionic megacolon)
 4. Neurologic abnormalities, including spinal cord lesions or autonomic dysfunction
 5. Muscle disorders, including amyotonia congenita and cerebral palsy
B. Evaluation
 1. In most cases a detailed **history and physical examination** will be sufficient
 to rule out pathologic causes. Nighttime accidents are rare and suggest emotional or neurologic abnormalities. Abdominal and rectal examinations are
 helpful in estimating the amount of stool retention. Detailed neurologic or
 motor examinations may be indicated if there is a suspicion of underlying
 neuropathy or myopathy.
 2. Rarely, **laboratory evaluation** may be indicated to rule out underlying abnormalities (e.g., hypothyroidism, hypercalcemia, disaccharidase deficiency,
 malabsorption).
 3. A **plain film of the abdomen** can be helpful in assessing the degree of stool
 retention.
 4. Anal manometry or rectal biopsy may be indicated in the rare case of
 suspected Hirschsprung's disease.
 5. A **urinalysis** and **urine culture** should be done in the initial evaluation of
 girls with encopresis because of the increased incidence of associated urinary
 tract infections.
C. The diagnosis is confirmed by the deposition of stools in a child's underwear,
 occurring after the age of 4 on a regular basis. Primary encopresis applies to cases
 in which bowel continence has never been achieved, and secondary encopresis
 applies to cases in which incontinence occurs in those who were once fully trained
 for at least 6 months.
D. Therapy
 1. Counseling. It should be explained that the lack of control is not the child's
 fault. A physiologic explanation of a distended colon that has lost sensation
 and muscle tone is helpful. Some families may have difficulty dealing with
 stresses and referral for psychiatric or psychological therapy may be necessary, preferably after a period of initial medical intervention.
 2. Conditions to facilitate the development of regular bowel habits should be

established, including easy access to bathrooms, privacy, and toilet seating with foot support for younger children.

3. **Initial catharsis** is aimed at completely disimpacting the bowel. The following is recommended for the average 7-year-old child (appropriate adjustments should be made for larger and for smaller children).

   a. **Home treatment** is practical in most cases.
      (1) **For moderate to severe retention** go through two to four cycles as follows:
         (a) **Day 1.** Hypophosphate enemas (Fleet, adult size) twice
         (b) **Day 2.** Bisacodyl (Dulcolax) suppositories twice
         (c) **Day 3.** Bisacodyl tablet once
      (2) **For mild retention, give senna or danthron,** 1 tablet daily for 1–2 weeks.
      (3) The bathroom should be used for 15 min after each meal.

   b. **Inpatient treatment** for severe retention, when home compliance is poor, or when parental administration of enemas is psychologically stressful.
      (1) High normal saline enemas (750 ml for a 7-year-old) bid for 3–7 days
      (2) Bisacodyl suppositories bid for 3–7 days
      (3) Use of the bathroom for 15 min after each meal

4. The **maintenance phase** is aimed at establishing a consistent bowel pattern. Exacerbations should be expected during this phase and the child should be monitored closely to minimize discouragement. The most common reason for failure of therapy is either too much or too little medication. Doses for individual children should be titrated to a particular end point (e.g., two soft bowel movements/day).

   a. **Mineral oil** (at least 2 tbsp) or other stool softener (docusate sodium) should be used bid, usually for 4–6 months. Light mineral oil is usually better tolerated than regular mineral oil. In most cases, **mineral oil should not be used in children less than 5 years old because of the risk of aspiration.**

   b. In severe cases or during relapses, an oral laxative (senna or danthron) can be added. In severe cases, laxatives can be used daily for 2–3 weeks, then on alternate days for 1 month (given between mineral oil doses). Relapses may require a shorter course.

   c. The child should sit on the toilet for 5 min once or twice a day at the same time each day (usually postprandially). Timing should be consistent.

   d. Multiple vitamins bid between mineral oil doses

   e. High-roughage diet, usually bran cereal

5. **Close long-term follow-up** for support, compliance, and associated symptoms is needed. Visits should take place every 4–8 weeks initially, and a physician should be available by phone to make dosage adjustments when necessary.

6. Parents and patients should be warned of the possibility of relapses. Signs of relapse include large-caliber stools, abdominal pain, decreased frequency of defecation, and soiling. It is important for parents to react to relapses without being punitive or blaming the child.

7. For refractory cases, biofeedback techniques may be useful.

VIII. **Enuresis.** There is a male predominance in enuresis at all ages and an increased familial incidence. By age 5, approximately 92% of children have achieved daytime dryness, 72% nighttime dryness. It is not until age 12 that 90% of children achieve nighttime dryness.

   A. **Etiology.** In the great majority of children, a specific cause is never identified.

      1. **Organic factors** include structural abnormalities of the genitourinary tract, urinary tract infections, neurologic abnormalities, and disorders causing polyuria.

      2. **Congenital delay** of adequate neuromuscular maturation may occur. The spontaneous cure rate from ages 5–20 is approximately 15%/year.

      3. **Psychosocial causes.** Most children with enuresis are emotionally healthy. A sudden onset of wetting may be a response to stress.

4. **Sleep disorders.** In some cases, prolonged nocturnal enuresis is a disorder of sleep arousal.
5. **Seizure disorders** can be associated with enuresis.
6. In some children, diurnal enuresis may merely be a manifestation of a personality style that keeps them from taking the time to void during the day.
7. **Urge syndrome.** In this syndrome there are unpredictable attacks of a sudden urge to void. The child often uses external compression of the urethra to prevent the outflow of urine.
8. **Giggle micturition.** In this syndrome, there is sudden, involuntary, uncontrollable, and complete emptying of the bladder on giggling in a person (usually female) who is otherwise continent.

B. **Evaluation and diagnosis**
1. **History.** A detailed history should be taken to elucidate the following points: the pattern of wetting; the time of day wetting occurs; the number of times per night; the number of nights per week; the number of daytime voidings; periods of dryness; sleeping abnormalities; dysuria; polyuria; description of urinary stream; family history; worsening during periods of personal or family stress; toilet training efforts; parental response to wetting; how the child views the problem; how wetting has affected the child's social relationships and social activities; why the parents have sought help at this time; medications the child is taking.
2. **The physical findings** are normal in the majority of cases. Special attention should be given to the following points: height and weight; blood pressure; genitalia, including locating the urethral meatus; palpation of the abdomen for an enlarged bladder; fecal impaction; abdominal or costovertebral angle tenderness; observation of the urinary stream, including the ability to start and stop it (anatomic and neurologic abnormalities); spine abnormalities; neurologic findings in the lower extremities, including strength, tone, deep tendon reflexes, sensation (may be associated with bladder innervation abnormalities).
3. **Laboratory evaluation** should include:
   a. A urinalysis in all cases. Urine cultures are indicated in females and sometimes in males.
   b. Radiologic studies if anatomic abnormalities, recurrent urinary tract infections, or an abdominal mass is suspected
   c. BUN, creatinine, and creatinine clearance if renal disease is suspected
   d. Cystoscopy and cystometrogram in rare cases
   e. An EEG if a seizure disorder is suspected
   f. Rarely, sleep studies

C. **Treatment**
1. **Organic causes** for enuresis should be treated appropriately.
2. **Therapy for idiopathic enuresis is highly controversial.** In all cases it is important to decrease the blame and guilt feelings of the child as well as the struggle between parents and child. Explain that there are many other children with the same problem. It is helpful to involve the child actively in any therapeutic modalities, and he or she should become involved in caring for himself or herself.
   a. **Reassurance** is sufficient treatment in many cases, especially with younger children, since a large proportion will have spontaneous resolution. Although some recommend restricting drinks in the evening and waking the child at night to void, there is no documentation of success with these techniques.
   b. **Conditions should facilitate dryness,** such as easy access to bathrooms during the school day, privacy, and a light in the bathroom at night.
   c. **Conditioning devices** are commercially available.* Bed mattress devices sensitive to moisture activate an alarm when the child voids in bed.

---

*One such device is the Palco Wet-Stop, available from Palco Laboratories, 5026 Scotts Valley Drive, Scotts Valley, CA 95066.

Relapses are common, and several courses may be needed. Complications include rashes on the perineum or buttocks. Some children fail to awaken with the alarm.

d. Behavior modification (see sec. I) is helpful for a number of children. A system of rewards for dry nights or dry days can be instigated. Regular times for voiding can be helpful.

e. Bladder training exercises to stretch the bladder and increase its capacity may be helpful. Once a day children are asked to hold onto their urine for as long as possible.

f. Medication. Imipramine has been shown in controlled studies to decrease the frequency of enuresis. It can be particularly helpful on a short-term basis for control of nocturnal enuresis when symptoms may prevent visiting friends overnight, going to camp, and so on. In some cases a pattern of dryness can be established that may persist after the medication is tapered.

  (1) The **dose** is approximately 1 mg/kg $\frac{1}{2}$–1 hr before bedtime (15–25 mg for children under 12 years of age, 50 mg for children over 12). If there are no effects after 10–14 days, the dosage can be increased to a maximum of 50 mg for younger children and 75 mg for older children.

  (2) Medication should be given for a maximum of 4 months. The drug should be tapered over 4–6 weeks for best results. Relapses off medication are common.

  (3) Side effects of imipramine include mood, sleep, and GI disturbances. **Life-threatening cardiac arrhythmias may occur with overdosage**, and care must be taken to prevent unsupervised administration.

g. Relapses are common, and parents should be counseled so that they can react to relapses without being punitive or blaming the child.

IX. Infantile autism

A. Etiology. Most likely, it is an organic brain disorder.

B. Evaluation

1. These children manifest a pervasive developmental disorder. Their lack of attachment behavior is marked, although there may be some improvement by age 5. Useful speech may eventually be gained in 50% of the children.

2. **Associated behaviors** include stereotyped movements, tantrums, overactivity, and extreme fears.

3. Mental retardation is present in 75% of cases.

4. Seizures and EEG abnormalities are common.

5. Phenylketonuria, congenital rubella, and hypsarrhythmia have been associated.

6. A similar "childhood-onset pervasive developmental" disorder differing only in age of onset (30 mo–12 yr) and being less severe must be considered.

C. The **diagnosis** includes:

1. Impaired social relationships manifested by lack of eye-to-eye gaze, discriminating people, cuddling, or smiling

2. Language retardation involving decreased comprehension, echolalia, and pronominal reversal

3. Ritualistic phenomena with "an insistence on sameness"

4. Onset before 30 months

D. Treatment

1. A developmental-educational-psychological assessment of the child and the family is indicated. Skilled special education is needed in a structured and supportive environment. This frequently should occur in a residential or day treatment setting. Unmanageability or danger to the child or others is an indication for a residential setting.

2. Behavioral treatment has been a useful adjunct for social responses, communication, self-abusive behavior, and so on.

3. **Neuroleptics** (e.g., chlorpromazine) have been useful in agitation and management, but do not correct global impairment. These drugs may decrease the seizure threshold, resulting in a possible exacerbation of seizures.

4. About 60% remain handicapped and unable to lead an independent life. Good social adjustment is found in 15%, although relationship problems continue, with the other 25% somewhere in between these extremes. An improved prognosis is found with a higher I.Q. and speech by age 5 years. Long-term support is needed from the pediatrician.

X. Nonorganic failure to thrive

A. The **etiology** includes family stress, poverty, and parental emotional illness.

B. Evaluation

1. **Organic causes** should be ruled out by a complete history and physical examination. There is an increase in secondary physiologic disorders in children with nonorganic failure to thrive.

2. To determine growth patterns, the history should include previous weights, heights, and head circumferences. Typically, weight falls off the growth curve before height and head circumference.

3. A detailed **social history** to determine the child's emotional and physical environment is indicated. Risk factors include single-parent families, economic stress, disorganized families, parental depression, hostile parent-child relationships, and a history of chronic or recent maternal loss.

4. Observation of **interactions between parent(s) and child** in an inpatient or outpatient setting is helpful, but artificial settings can lead to unrepresentative behavior.

5. A **rapid weight gain** early during hospitalization is supportive of nonorganic etiology, but failure of weight gain does not rule out the diagnosis.

C. The **diagnosis** is confirmed by evidence of strained parent-child relationships. This does not exclude an organic diagnosis.

D. Therapy

1. The goal of therapy is the improvement of a child's physical and/or emotional environment by the support of parents. Sometimes hospitalization is indicated and should take place in specialized units when possible.

2. Although an interdisciplinary team approach is often helpful, it is important to identify one primary caretaker, particularly for long-term follow-up.

3. Parental self-esteem should be encouraged and feelings of guilt alleviated.

4. Parents should be involved in the investigation and treatment as part of the team.

5. Interactional issues need to be addressed, and parents need support as these are worked through.

6. If a child is hospitalized, conditions should be as conducive as possible to normal parent-child relationships.

7. Parents should be assured of long-term follow-up and support. Children with nonorganic failure to thrive are at risk of subsequent behavior problems, psychological problems, delayed cognitive development, school problems, and continued slow growth.

XI. Poor school performance

A. The **etiology** includes the following:

1. Physical disabilities and illness

2. Developmental disability (overall developmental delay may not be recognized until school demands exceed abilities), neurodevelopmental dysfunction (minimal brain dysfunction, developmental dyslexia, attention deficit disorder, and learning disability)

3. Emotional disorders, including individual or family problems and environmental deprivation

4. Confounding factors include poor school or class environment, unrealistic parental expectations, and excessive absences.

B. Evaluation and diagnosis

1. A full **history** by interview and supplemented by questionnaires should be obtained from the parents. It should include a description of the following:

   a. Gestational and perinatal history

   b. Developmental milestones

   c. Description of early temperament

  d. First hints of difficulties in functional areas

  e. First school experience and subsequent experience

  f. Functioning at home and in neighborhood

  g. Medical problems

  h. Rate of deterioration of performance

  i. Lapses of attention

 2. The **school history** should be obtained from the parents and the school and should include descriptions of current placement, current functioning, and the results of previous evaluations.

 3. A complete **physical examination**, including vision and hearing screens, should be performed.

 4. The following **evaluations** may be performed by the pediatrician, school, or consultant, depending on their areas of expertise:

  a. Neurodevelopmental examination

  b. Educational evaluation, including achievement tests

  c. Psychological testing, including:

   (1) Cognitive testing with standardized tests (e.g., WISC-R WAIS, McCarthy)

   (2) Emotional assessment requiring an interview and, when appropriate, projective testing

  d. **Classroom observation** of the child

C. Treatment

 1. All physical disabilities or illnesses should be treated appropriately.

 2. In conjunction with the parents and school, an educational plan should be formulated. This plan should include the following:

  a. Description of present function and objectives for intervention

  b. Means to provide the intervention should be described, including classroom placement, plans for special help (time, place, student-teacher ratio), type of instruction, and means for evaluating the success of intervention.

  c. The intervention plan should include:

   (1) A plan for remediation in areas of weakness

   (2) A plan to circumvent areas of weakness (e.g., dictating a portion of a written assignment for a child with significant problems in written output)

   (3) A plan to sustain the child's self-concept

 3. Children with significant emotional or family problems should receive psychological intervention.

 4. Medication may be appropriate for a small group of children with attentional problems (see Chap. 20, p. 495).

XII. School refusal

A. The **etiology** includes separation anxiety or fear of school, which may reflect real school problems such as a "class bully," a difficult teacher, or difficulty with new school material. School refusal may be a partial manifestation of a more pervasive social withdrawal in all spheres.

B. Evaluation and diagnosis

 1. A child presenting with vague physical complaints with normal physical and laboratory findings should prompt the physician to ask about school absences.

 2. The **history** should emphasize the following:

  a. Earlier separation problems

  b. Previous undefined illnesses with prolonged school absence

  c. The temporal pattern of symptoms. Children with school refusal often have more symptoms on Sunday night and Monday morning than at other times. They often are without symptoms on holidays and weekends.

  d. Specific school problems that might be contributing to absences

 3. The longer the sustained absence and the older the child, the more serious and urgent the problem.

C. Treatment
1. Reassure the child and parents **after** the physical examination and necessary laboratory tests that the symptoms do not represent serious disease.
2. The family can be told that anxiety can cause physical discomfort and acknowledge that the child is experiencing the symptom.
3. Suggest that school is the child's **job** and that there are few excuses acceptable for absences.
4. Prepare the parents for possible escalation of symptoms when attendance is first enforced.
5. If the child is to be permitted to stay home for illness, the child should be seen that morning for an examination by the physician.
6. Help the family organize a specific plan for getting the child to school. The process may be slow, and desensitization techniques such as shortened school days are helpful.
7. Try to ease the child's way back into school by speaking to the principal, or teacher, or both about decreasing any complicating stresses during the first few days.
8. Many children can be helped by their pediatrician. If, however, problems persist, or it is determined that school avoidance represents a more general social withdrawal, the child should be referred for further psychiatric evaluation and treatment.

XIII. Separation experiences
A. Death of a parent, sibling, or significant other.
As in chronic illness (see sec. II), a child's grief is phasic, with indistinct transitions. The stages are: shock and disbelief, protest and anguish, and detachment and reorientation toward a new relationship. The child's reaction is intimately connected to that of the parents or surviving parent, such that the more distraught child usually has a parent who also has not resolved the loss. The finality of death is not fully understood until approximately age 10 years. Prior to this, reversibility is possible in the child's view. The child frequently attributes the incident to something he or she "has done." Crying, sleep difficulties, anxiety, irritability, regression, depression, preoccupation with the deceased, feeling the presence of the deceased, or somatic concerns can be observed. The duration can be from weeks to a year. Reactions going beyond 1 year denote an unresolved grief reaction. **Treatment** is as follows:
1. The parents can be encouraged to be as open as possible with their explanations and their own individual reactions. It is beneficial and reassuring to the child to be told exactly what has or will take place. Evasive information will only ultimately further confuse the child. Parents should be encouraged to state their genuine beliefs about the type of survival after death when asked by the child.
2. When an impending death is occurring, it is helpful to inform the child about the upcoming loss and allow visitation if possible.
3. Reassurances are important for the child at the time of the death. The child should be informed that he or she will be taken care of, that the child will not die, that he or she does not have the same illness that caused the death, and that no one else is going away. It is important that the child be reassured that no one, in particular the child, is to blame for the loss.
4. It is helpful to the child to attend the funeral. Attendance can provide meaningful information to the child, and he or she can observe the appropriate expression of emotions. A supportive adult relationship should be provided to the child during the ceremonies. For the younger child, attendance at a portion of the funeral may be arranged.
5. The parents should be told that the child will often ask very painful questions. Direct questions about death are frequent and repeated.
6. The child and the family may benefit by referral for counseling. This can be offered routinely to each family when such a loss has occurred. Referral is also indicated when there appears to be a "block" in the mourning process, evidenced by a continued yearning for the lost person over years.

B. **Hospitalization.** Emotional distress during a hospitalization is most marked between the ages of 6 months and 4 years and is related to separation from familiar figures and the strange environment. There is concern about desertion or punishment. Beginning at age 4 years, there is increasing concern over the illness and treatment and about injury to one's body. Fear of death coincides with understanding of finality by age 10 years.

Immediately following hospital discharge, a child may manifest hostility, clinging, anxiety, and so on, for weeks. This is more frequent when prior parent-child relationships are problematic. There is an increased risk of emotional problems if there are multiple separations or if the hospitalization lasts longer than 1 week. **Treatment** is as follows:

1. Physician support with careful explanation of treatment plans to both parents and child is crucial.
2. Encourage familiar home routines. For the infant or toddler, overnight visits by the parents are beneficial, while in the older child, frequent visiting may be sufficient.
3. Encourage normalization of activity as much as possible. This can range from "playroom" usage to game playing to school work.
4. Consultation with a child psychiatrist can be useful for the particularly problematic or withdrawn child.
5. When hospitalization is elective, prehospitalization preparation, including visiting the hospital, can be helpful both to the child and the parents.
6. Following discharge, the parents should return to setting the same limits and discipline as they did prior to the hospitalization.

C. **Divorce.** The effect of this increasingly common event depends on the age of the child. Preschool children may be grief stricken and wonder if they themselves can be divorced. The older child will also be hurt though may be more easily reassured. The adolescent tends to separate himself or herself from the situation. At all ages, however, there is questioning about whether the child caused the divorce. Psychological difficulties will depend more on marital discord or disturbed parent-child relationships than on the separation itself. **Treatment** is as follows:

1. Encourage the parents to relate specific and honest facts about the divorce to their children. Their children often need to know that both parents still love them, that the divorce is not the children's fault, and that they will be cared for. Repeated explanations are frequently needed and requested by the child.
2. Recommend that the child be kept out of ongoing disputes between the parents. If possible, the child should not be involved in the adversary system of the court.
3. Allow ventilation of feelings about the divorce by parent or child.
4. Visitation should not be used by one parent against the other.
5. The noncustodial parent can be advised to "go where the child goes" (e.g., to a school activity) when visiting the older child who wants to be with friends.
6. A counseling referral is indicated for the child and family who are having disabling distress.

D. **Working parents.** There is a lack of evidence for a relationship between employment and maternal deprivation. Most parents work out of economic necessity. The crucial factor for the child is the quality of care. Substitute care that is caring, predictable, and meets a child's need does not appear harmful to the child. Work may be an important stress reducer for some parents, thus improving the quality of time spent with the children. It can be helpful for one parent to remain at home until an infant's behavior becomes stable.

XIV. **Sleep disorders**

A. **Non-rapid-eye movement (NREM) dyssomnia: sleep terrors and somnambulism**

1. The **etiology** is unclear. Common features include a disorder of arousal from stages III and IV (NREM) sleep; a frequently positive family history; a higher incidence in children than in adults; and increased association with early evening enuresis.

2. **Evaluation and diagnosis**
    a. **Sleep terrors**
        (1) Usually, these occur 1 to 3 hours after sleep onset.
        (2) They often begin with a scream associated with tachycardia, sweating, pupillary dilation, body movement, and irregular, deep breathing. In younger children, behavioral manifestations may be less extreme.
        (3) The child cannot be consoled or awakened until the event is complete. When awake, the child remembers little of the episode and does not remember it later.
        (4) Sleep terrors differ from nightmares, which occur during REM sleep, are frequently remembered—at least in part—and often wake the child.
    b. **Somnambulism** (sleep walking)
        (1) Approximately 15% of children have walked in their sleep at least once; it persists in 1–5%. Most who start before 10 years of age stop before 15.
        (2) The child suddenly sits up in bed glassy eyed and often will stand up and walk. Behavior may appear semipurposeful.
        (3) Episodes last 15 sec–30 min.
        (4) The child is difficult to arouse and is amnestic for the episode.
3. **Treatment**
    a. Most cases resolve over time. Therefore, it is appropriate to demystify the episodes by educating parents.
    b. Somnambulism can be dangerous. Therefore, it is advisable to make the area safe to avoid accidents.
    c. Regularizing the child's sleep schedule can be helpful.
    d. Decreasing overall stress can sometimes help.
    e. Rarely is medication necessary. In extreme cases, imipramine has been helpful in young children and diazepam in adolescents.
B. **Narcolepsy** is a syndrome consisting of excessive daytime somnolence (EDS) and abnormal manifestations of REM sleep (cataplexy, hypnogogic hallucinations, sleep paralysis). The incidence is estimated at between 0.03% and 0.05%. In families with one affected member the incidence is estimated at 5% (60 times normal).
    1. The **etiology** is unclear.
        a. Narcolepsy is associated with an abnormal transition into sleep with REM onset as the first stage.
        b. It is usually diagnosed in adulthood but may have been present (unrecognized) earlier.
    2. **Evaluation and diagnosis**
        a. One or more of the following may be present.
            (1) **Excessive daytime somnolence (EDS)** is the most common presenting symptom.
            (2) **Cataplexy**
            (3) **Hypnagogic hallucinations**
            (4) **Sleep paralysis** (while falling asleep or awakening, the patient cannot move or cry out).
            (5) **Narcoleptic tetrad.** Points **(1), (2), (3)**, and **(4)** are all present in approximately 10% of cases.
        b. It is helpful to have confirmation by an all night sleep study with multiple nap recordings.
        c. Narcolepsy may severely affect school performance as well as day-to-day lifestyle so these should be explored in the history.
    3. **Treatment**
        a. Once presumptive diagnosis is made, referral to a sleep clinic or specialist is helpful in diagnosis and monitoring therapy.
            (1) **Stimulants** (i.e., Ritalin, Dexedrine) have been used to decrease sleepiness. This may often improve school performance.

        (2) Tricyclics (e.g., imipramine, chlorimipramine) appear more effective for cataplexy, hypnogogic hallucinations, and sleep paralysis.

    b. These patients often fight sleepiness, but short naps during the day can occasionally obviate the need for medication.

    c. Driving and swimming pose a risk for these patients, and should be monitored closely until the symptoms are under control.

C. Obstructive sleep apnea syndrome is a potentially lethal condition characterized by multiple obstructive or mixed apneas during sleep, associated with repetitive episodes of inordinately loud snoring or excessive daytime somnolence.

    1. The **etiology** is unclear, but it is thought to be secondary to anatomic predisposition (e.g., large tonsils or adenoids, Pierre Robin anomaly) with possibly a CNS component.

    2. Evaluation and diagnosis

        a. The **history** should evaluate the following:

            (1) Excessive daytime somnolence

            (2) Loud intermittent snoring during sleep, with frequent episodes of apnea

            (3) Enuresis

            (4) Poor school performance

            (5) Naps that do not decrease sleepiness

            (6) Often, tape recording of sleep can be helpful.

        b. Physical examination should include an upper airway examination. An ear, nose, and throat examination and x-rays to detect upper airway obstruction are indicated when the diagnosis is suspected from the history.

        c. An ECG should be done to detect right ventricular hypertrophy, cor pulmonale, and arrhythmias.

        d. A sleep study with full monitoring of the ECG, respiratory pattern, EEG, and PO_2 should be performed.

    3. Treatment

        a. Avoid all forms of sedation, since they may exacerbate the apnea.

        b. Surgery to remove obstruction (e.g., adenoids, tonsils) has been attempted with varying success. After operation, these patients should be monitored closely in an intensive care unit until the airway is clearly stabilized.

        c. Tracheostomy cures the problem, but the cost-benefit ratio must be considered.

        d. Weight loss is often beneficial in obese patients.

        e. The use of medication is controversial and its merits unproved.

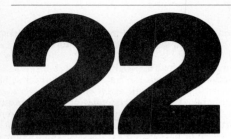

Skin Disorders

I. Specific disorders

A. Acne

1. **Etiology.** Sebaceous glands are stimulated by increased levels of androgenic steroids, particularly during adolescence. Altered follicular keratinization leads to plugging. Trapped sebum is hydrolyzed by bacterial enzymes *(Proprionibacterium acnes)* to free fatty acids which are then released into the dermis by rupture of plugged sebaceous ducts. Scarring may result. **Diet is not thought to play a role.**

2. **Evaluation**
   a. **History** includes the severity of the problem **to the patient.** Note precipitating events, particularly emotional stress or onset of menses. Note all medications taken, particularly corticosteroids, halogens, oral contraceptives, lithium, phenytoin, INH (isoniazid).
   b. Note what **topical preparations** are being used for treatment or cover-up (moisturizers, oil-based cleansing creams, hair or face grease, coal tar products, or makeup). **Occupations and hobbies** may also expose the patient to cutting greases or chlorinated hydrocarbons which may be causal.

3. **Diagnosis**
   a. **Subjective.** Flares of activity may be associated with precipitating factors in **2.b.** Patient may have pain or pruritus at sites of inflammatory lesions.
   b. **Objective.** The skin is oily. Scattered over the face, chest, and back are open and closed comedones, inflammatory papules and pustules, and, in some cases, deep cysts. Scarring may be few to many shallow "ice-pick" depressions, or larger and craterform.

4. **Therapy**
   a. **Soaps.** Drying and abrasive soaps promote superficial desquamation and may open plugged follicular orifices. **Note that these agents can be too harsh for someone also using a more effective comedolytic agent, and the two should not be combined in one therapeutic regimen.**
   b. **Comedolytic agents.** Benzoyl peroxide gel 5% or 10% or tretinoin (Retin-A) 0.05% cream or 0.01% gel is usually necessary. Begin therapy qhs with the **least** irritating agent, benzoyl peroxide 5%. As the irritation subsides, increase application to bid or tid. If the medicine is easily tolerated tid, a stronger agent should be chosen, i.e., benzoyl peroxide 10%, and used in the same way. The most irritating agent is the tretinoin cream; the tretinoin 0.01% gel can be used to minimize irritation. Patient should be instructed to apply agent to a completely dry face.
   c. **Ultraviolet light.** Either sunlight or artificial ultraviolet light (UVL) will promote faster and more complete control of acne in some but may worsen the disease in others. Thus, therapy during summertime may need adjusting. **Note that both tetracycline and tretinoin are photosensitizers,** which cause sunburn in certain individuals.
   d. **Antibiotics**
      (1) *P. acnes* organisms are extremely sensitive to **tetracycline.** However, **this drug is not to be used in infants and children.** For **inflammatory pustular and cystic acne,** start tetracycline 500 mg PO bid until

control is obtained, approximately 3–4 months. Dosage may then be gradually decreased every 4 weeks by 250 mg to the lowest effective maintenance level.

(2) Erythromycin, an alternative drug, is given in the same dosages.

(3) Topical antibiotics, erythromycin 1.5% or 2% or clindamycin 1%, are helpful when used with a comedolytic agent (although never applied simultaneously) in mild acne or with systemic antibiotics and a comedolytic agent.

  e. Estrogens. Oral contraceptives (OC) may cause an initial flare of acne and later become effective in moderating the disease. **The anovulatory effectiveness of an OC may be altered by tetracycline,** especially the low estrogen-containing pills, and concomitant therapy should be carefully considered.

  f. Oral retinoids are for severe acne but should be used only under the supervision of a dermatologist.

B. Alopecia

  1. Etiology. Interference with any phase of hair growth by an abnormality of the follicle, by systemic illness, by drugs or trauma results in a characteristic alopecia. Loss of hair may be seen in diseases intrinsic to the hair follicle (ectodermal dysplasias, alopecia areata, monilethrix). Changes in androgenic hormones will affect hair growth noticeably (puberty, pregnancy, endocrinopathies). Severe physical or psychological stress, including nutritional deficiencies, may cause a marked but reversible alopecia. Trauma to the hair, either by traction or physical agents (hot combs, hot oils, heat, hair dyes), and drugs (antimetabolites, anticoagulants) are also responsible.

  2. Evaluation

  a. History should include hair patterns of other family members, recent illnesses or trauma, medications, and systemic diseases.

  b. Physical examination should include all hair-bearing areas, nails, and skin. Look for evidence of pruritus and/or rubbing and scratching of affected areas.

  c. If **infection** is suspected, do a KOH and/or gram stain.

  d. If a scarring alopecia is evident, a 4-mm punch biopsy may be helpful.

  3. Diagnosis

  a. Subjective findings. Patients may complain of finding excessive amounts of hair in the comb. Habits or grooming techniques and hair styles where pulling or twisting are involved are important to note (tight braids, ponytails, curlers, permanents).

  b. Objective findings

  (1) Generalized alopecia. If absence of hair includes scalp, axillae, pubis, arms and legs, face, eyebrows, and eyelashes, a **systemic cause** should be sought, including intrinsic hair abnormalities, alopecia areata (which can be localized or quite extensive), drugs, or nutritional diseases.

  (2) Patchy alopecia. Distinct areas of alopecia interspersed with areas of normal hair are present. **Scales or pustules and erythema** are seen when there is infection or sometimes with skin diseases, such as **atopic dermatitis, psoriasis, lichen planopilaris, and contact dermatitis.** These patients will often have lesions characteristic of their underlying skin problem elsewhere on the body. A **smooth scalp with patchy hair loss** may be seen with **alopecia areata (AA). Exclamation point hairs** (!) at the periphery of the patch are seen with a 10× hand lens. These hairs are short, with a thick distal end, and taper to a point at the skin surface. Pitting of nail surfaces is present in some patients with AA. Traction must be considered in this category. Hair loss pattern should correspond to lines of tension obvious from the hair style worn. If the skin feels indurated and is a red or violaceous hue, an infiltrative process such as sarcoidosis, lupus erythematosus, or neoplasia should be considered in the differential diagnosis.

(3) Diffuse alopecia. Approximately 3 months after a severe physical illness, there may be a diffuse loss of hair (telogen effluvium), characterized by very easily plucked hairs all having a bulb at the proximal end. A diffuse pattern may also be seen with systemic etiologies or primary skin diseases.

(4) Scarring alopecia. If the skin in the area involved appears shiny and glassy smooth, perhaps with atrophy or fibrosis, this may indicate a permanent loss of hair.

    4. Therapy

      a. Appropriate evaluation and treatment of underlying illness. If no scarring has occurred, hair will usually regrow.

      b. If the KOH is positive for a dermatophyte, treat for tinea capitis (see **H.3.a.**). If the gram stain is positive for gram-positive cocci, treat as a pyoderma (see **J.4**).

      c. Shampoo. If there is inflammation only, use a mild shampoo qd or qod. If there is infection, shampoo qd with an antibacterial (Betadine, Hibiclens) and treat as in **b** above.

      d. Corticosteroids. For alopecia areata, a potent lotion (Betamethasone dipropionate [Diprosone] or Halcinonide) may be helpful when used qhs under occlusion for 1 month. **For inflammation without infection,** a medium-potency lotion may be used bid for 1–2 weeks only (see sec. **II.A**).

      e. For permanent hair loss, the use of wigs and hair transplantation should be considered.

C. Atopic dermatitis

    1. Etiology. Patients with atopic dermatitis tend to have elevated serum levels of IgE and decreased cell-mediated immunity. However, the role of these abnormalities in the pathogenesis of the dermatitis is still unknown.

    2. Evaluation. Allergy skin testing is unrewarding. However, **a careful history to determine the precipitants** of pruritus or dermatitis is helpful. Scratching may be done mostly during sleep and go unnoticed by parents; therefore, it is important to question how the patient looks in the morning. The disease's interference with normal activities and family dynamics is a critical diagnostic factor. A family history is positive for atopy in over 70% of cases.

    3. Diagnosis

      a. Subjective findings

        (1) The disease usually begins in infancy, although it may start in childhood or later. In 50% of all cases the disease will resolve by age 2 years; in 75% it will resolve by early childhood.

        (2) Pruritus is the major symptom.

        (3) Extremes of temperature, soap and other alkalis, chemical irritants, infection, wool, foods, and stress may worsen the disease.

      b. Objective findings. Dry roughened skin is found wherever there has been rubbing. **Acute areas** are red and scaly with papules and microvesicles. These are found most commonly in flexural areas in children, but certainly are not limited to them. In infants, the rash is usually found on cheeks and extensor surfaces. **Chronic lesions** are lichenified with prominent skin marking, scarring and hyper- or hypopigmentation. **Severe atopic dermatitis** may present with generalized erythema, excoriations, crusting and oozing. **Honey-colored crusts and pustules** represent secondary infection (usually staphylococci, sometimes herpes simplex).

    4. Therapy

      a. Avoid drying agents and irritants, e.g., soaps, wool, lanolins, and dry air.

      b. Bathe 1–2 times per day to hydrate the skin. If soaps are used, restrict to necessary areas. **All baths must be followed by application of an emollient to trap the water in the skin.**

      c. Emollients (hydrated petrolatum, Vaseline, Crisco, mineral oil, Eucerin, Aquaphor, Nivea, Alpha Keri) are used qid at a minimum. These are only effective when applied to wet skin.

      d. Oral antihistamines can be used to control pruritus. Hydroxyzine and chlorpheniramine in adequate amounts, frequently to the point of inducing drowsiness, should be started in recommended doses q4h (see sec. **II.B.**). Double doses are sometimes used at bedtime, when most pruritus occurs.

  e. Systemic antibiotics to combat gram-positive cocci are necessary when there is evidence of secondary infection, i.e., pustules, crusting, oozing (see sec. **J.4.a.(2)**).

  f. Topical corticosteroids may be necessary in severe cases. **They should not be used on infected skin.** Ointments are more emolliating than creams for dry atopic skin and should only be used bid (see sec. **II.A**).

D. Contact dermatitis

  1. Etiology. Sensitization to contact allergens. To cause contact sensitization, an antigen must penetrate the epidermis and contain reactive groups that conjugate with tissue proteins.

  2. Evaluation. The **location, distribution, and shape of the lesions** are the most useful features in determining the cause of a contact dermatitis. **Patch testing** may be done to define the etiology if not apparent by history, but should be done only *after* the acute phase of the dermatitis has resolved.

  3. Diagnosis

  a. Subjective findings. A history of contact allergy to several different substances is often obtainable. A burning sensation or pruritus may be an early symptom of the eruption.

  b. Objective findings. The first change is erythema; edema, papules, vesiculation, scale, and bullous formation follow in rapid succession. Linearly distributed vesicles, unusual shapes, and sharply demarcated borders are pathognomic of the rash in contact dermatitis. Areas of increased heat, sweating, or friction may show more florid involvement than adjacent, cooler areas.

  4. Therapy

  a. Compresses (see **II.C**) for 15 min qid relieve pruritus and loosen crusts in 2–3 days.

  b. Antipruritic lotions, applied frequently on moistened skin, help in mild cases (e.g., Calamine, any emollient with 0.25% menthol).

  c. Topical corticosteroids may be added when oozing and crusting resolve. An ointment of medium–potent strength should be selected for bid usage for a maximum of 1–2 weeks (see sec. **II.A**).

  d. Oral antihistamines should be used if pruritus is extensive and unrelieved by topical agents (see sec. **II.B**).

  e. Systemic corticosteroids may be needed for severe, widespread involvement, beginning with 0.5 mg–2.0 mg/kg/24h for 3–5 days and then tapered gradually over the next 2 weeks.

E. Diaper dermatitis

  1. Etiology. Diaper dermatitis is the result of dampness, maceration, and chemical irritation.

  2. Evaluation. Question parents regarding the use of plastic pants and detergents or disinfectants. Examine the scalp, retroauricular areas, face, and axillae for evidence of seborrhea or atopic dermatitis, psoriasis, or other dermatitides. Scrape the moist, erythematous lesion in the diaper area and examine the material for *Candida albicans* with a KOH stain.

  3. Diagnosis. Erythema, scaling, and often erosion and ulceration affect primarily convex surfaces, i.e., the buttocks, genitalia, lower abdomen, and upper thighs. The flexural folds may be spared.

  4. Therapy

  a. Stop the use of bulky diapers and occlusive plastic pants.

  b. Use cloth diapers and rinse well to remove detergent, enzymes, and chemical irritants.

  c. Leave diapers off as much as possible. Change diapers often.

  d. With each diaper change, cleanse the diaper area with tepid water or nonirritative cleanser, e.g., Cetaphil.

     e. If severe inflammation is present and the KOH stain is negative, apply hydrocortisone cream 1% bid for 1–2 weeks. If rash does not dramatically resolve, look for underlying disease.

     f. If *C. albicans* is present, add antifungal agent, e.g., nystatin cream tid and continue use for 1 week after clearing of dermatitis.

     g. If rash is oozing and crusting, use saline or aluminum sulfate (Domeboro) compresses tid for 15 min before applying any creams.

F. Erythema multiforme (EM)

  1. Etiology. Erythema multiforme is a hypersensitivity reaction to multiple agents. Among the common precipitants are infections with herpes simplex, *Mycoplasma pneumoniae,* vaccinia, adenovirus, histoplasma, and exposures to penicillin, sulfonamides, barbiturates, and butazones. However, in 50% of cases an etiologic factor cannot be determined. Severe erythema multiforme with oral and conjunctival involvement is referred to as the Stevens-Johnson syndrome.

  2. Evaluation. Review the events of the previous 3 weeks for evidence of the recognized precipitants. Determine if a similar eruption has occurred in the past. Systemic complaints may point to an infectious cause.

  3. Diagnosis

     a. Subjective findings. Successive crops of lesions may appear for 10–14 days. Mucous membrane erosions are extremely painful and debilitating.

     b. Objective findings

       (1) Painful erosions with hemorrhagic crusts may involve the mucous membranes of the mouth, lip, nose, eyes, urethra, vagina, and anus. Erythematous plaques may be seen on the back of the hands, palms, wrists, forearms, feet, and legs. The classic "target" lesion has a red rim on the outside, an inner white halo, and a dusky center. However, lesions may include papules, bullae, plaques, or all three, without target lesions.

       (2) Corneal ulcerations with subsequent opacities occur in severe cases.

  4. Therapy

     a. For mild cases, soothing baths in Oilated Aveeno, followed by application of an emollient on moistened skin (e.g., hydrated petrolatum or mineral oil), and oral antihistamines may be sufficient.

     b. Topical anesthetics applied frequently prn (Dyclone or viscous lidocaine) may be necessary for painful *mucosal* lesions.

     c. Compresses with saline or aluminum sulfate (Domeboro) for bullous and erosive lesions should be applied tid for 15 min, followed by application of emollients.

     d. Oral prednisone may be useful in recurrent erythema multiforme.

     e. Hospitalization may be necessary for supportive care if oral lesions preclude oral intake.

G. Erythema nodosum

  1. Etiology. Erythema nodosum is a hypersensitivity reaction to any one of multiple stimuli, including *Streptococcus,* drugs (oral contraceptives, sulfonamides), sarcoidosis, tuberculosis, deep fungal infections, inflammatory bowel disease, and viral infections.

  2. Evaluation includes careful history to rule out infectious and/or treatable disease.

  3. Diagnosis

     a. Subjective. Lesions are extremely painful, deep red nodules. These may be accompanied by malaise and arthralgias. Symptoms associated with underlying disease may also be present.

     b. Objective. Tender, subcutaneous red nodules, 1–5 cm in diameter, are found usually on anterior surfaces of lower extremities, although they may occur elsewhere. Borders are indistinct, but easily palpated. As they resolve, nodules turn blue, then green and yellow, and fade like an ecchymosis. Individual lesions usually last 3–6 weeks.

4. Therapy
  a. Therapy of the underlying disease usually results in spontaneous resolution.
  b. Since the disease is self-limiting, lasting for 1–2 months in two-thirds of cases regardless of underlying etiology, no treatment may be necessary.
  c. If symptoms are severe or lesions become chronic, treat with nonsteroidal anti-inflammatory agents, e.g., indomethacin (25–50 mg bid–tid for those over 14 years of age) or aspirin. Systemic steroids may be effective, but any possible underlying infectious etiologies *must* first be eliminated.

H. Fungal infections
  1. Etiology
    a. Tinea capitis, tinea corporis (ringworm), **tinea versicolor, tinea cruris, tinea pedis** (athlete's foot), and **tinea unguium** (onychomycosis) are superficial infections of the skin, hair, and nails due to keratinophilic fungi (dermatophytes).
    b. A nonpyogenic, localized hypersensitivity response to inflammatory tinea capitis results in a pustular, follicular eruption termed a **kerion**. A dry, follicular hyperkeratotic eruption on the trunk and proximal extremities may accompany kerion formation or any other severely inflamed tinea infection.

  2. Evaluation
    a. Demonstration of fungi. Scrape the active border of skin lesions and collect fine scales or hair stubs on a glass microscope slide. Apply 1 drop of KOH or Swartz-Lamkins stain, cover with a glass coverslip, and heat without boiling. Invert the slide and press onto a paper towel or gauze to express excess stain. In tinea capitis, hair stubs must be stained to demonstrate fungi. Slides may be examined immediately if the Swartz-Lamkins stain is used. For nail and hair slides, as well as when plain KOH is used, the slides should be allowed to sit for 10 min before examination.
    b. Culture of fungi may be done on Sabouraud's agar or Dermatophyte Test Media by planting scrapings of scale, hair, or nails on them. Incubation at room temperature should be a minimum of 6 weeks.
    c. In a darkened room, shine a Wood's light on the scalp. Involved hairs show brilliant green fluorescence at their bases when *Microsporum* is the agent responsible. However, most cases of tinea capitis are caused by *Trichophyton tonsorans* and will not fluoresce.

  3. Specific infections
    a. Tinea capitis
      (1) Diagnosis
        (a) Subjective findings. The incubation time is 2–3 weeks. Except in the case of painful kerion formation, the infection is slightly pruritic or asymptomatic. History is often positive in family members or schoolmates for tinea capitis.
        (b) Objective findings. Tinea capitis causes patchy, scaling alopecia with dull, lusterless hairs broken off 1–2 mm above the skin ("gray patch"). Inflammation and erythema are mild or moderate. In actively enlarging lesions, vesicles and pustules may be seen in the advancing border. Kerion formation is characterized by the appearance of one or more boggy, edematous, raised plaques with nonpyogenic, purulent material crusting on the surface of the lesion. Infected hairs pull out easily without pain.
      (2) Therapy
        Microcrystalline griseofulvin, divided doses bid for a minimum of 8–12 weeks.
        (a) For infants, 10 mg/kg/24h PO
        (b) For children weighing 30–50 lb, 125–250 mg/24h PO
        (c) For children weighing over 50 lb, 250–500 mg/24h PO
        (d) For teenagers or adults, 1000 mg/24h PO

b. Tinea corporis
  (1) Diagnosis
   (a) Subjective finding. Incubation time is 1–3 weeks.
   (b) Objective finding. Lesions begin as erythematous papules and expand centrifugally with a raised, papular, scaling, and sometimes vesicular border. They clear from the center outward and resolve spontaneously after several weeks. Occasionally a deep, inflammatory, nodular reaction occurs (Majocchi's granuloma) at the site of infection.
  (2) Therapy
   (a) Apply an antifungal agent (clotrimazole 1% or miconazole 2% cream, or solution for hairy areas) tid. Treatment should continue for 10 days after clinical resolution of lesions.
   (b) For extensive or deep involvement, **microcrystalline griseofulvin** may be necessary in dosages noted in **H.3.a.2.,** given for 2–3 weeks.

c. Tinea versicolor
  (1) Diagnosis
   (a) Subjective findings. Activity is exacerbated by warm, humid weather, or excessive sweating. The eruption may be asymptomatic or slightly pruritic.
   (b) Objective findings. Capelike area over the neck, shoulders, and proximal upper extremities are involved by round, finely scaling, hypopigmented or tan macules. The lesions may coalesce into extensive areas. Scraping with a tongue blade or surgical blade raises an abundance of fine white scales.
  (2) Therapy
   Apply **selenium sulfide suspension 2.5%** from neck down to knees. Rinse off after 15 min (may be done in shower). Repeat qd for 2 weeks. Complete retreatment may be recommended just before the hot weather begins. It may take 12–18 months after treatment for repigmentation of hypopigmented areas.

d. Tinea cruris
  (1) Diagnosis
   (a) Subjective findings. Inflammation and pruritus may be intense.
   (b) Objective findings. Sharply marginated, erythematous, scaling areas with elevated borders and little central clearing extend down the medial thighs from the crural folds. The scrotum, penis, or labia are commonly spared. In contrast, candidiasis is characterized by a bright erythematous eruption involving scrotum or labia, with satellite pustules scattered beyond the poorly marginated, central lesions.
  (2) Therapy
   Apply **antifungal cream** tid until eruption clears and continue for 10 days more. The involved areas should be kept as dry as possible by allowing air to reach the area and use of an absorbent powder (Zeasorb) after showering and frequently during the day.

e. Tinea pedis
  (1) Diagnosis
   (a) Tinea pedis is uncommon before puberty, but should be suspected in any chronic scaling eruption of the feet. Scaling, erythematous areas on the feet of children are most likely due to sweating and maceration ("sneaker dermatitis"), not infection, especially in children with an atopic diathesis.
  (2) Therapy
   (a) An **antifungal agent** is applied as in **3.b.2.** If the webs are exceedingly moist, they should be treated with a **drying agent** (aluminum chloride [Drysol] or carbol-fuchsin solution) qhs until dry before starting an antifungal cream.

      (b) Severe involvement may require use of griseofulvin (see **3.a.2.**).
- **f. Tinea unguium**
  - **(1) Diagnosis**
    - **(a) Subjective findings.** Acquisition of nail infection is probably from antecedent skin dermatophytosis. Thus, tinea pedis or tinea manus usually coexists with this entity.
    - **(b) Objective findings.** One, two, or all nails may be involved with white or yellow discoloration of the lateral nail edge. Older infections appear as a yellow or brown, thick, friable nail plate. Keratinous debris collects beneath the distal nail plate.
  - **(2) Therapy**
    Microcrystalline griseofulvin (see **3.a.2**) may be required for 6–12 months. Surgical removal of the nail plus application of a topical antifungal agent tid may help increase the probability of a cure with systemic therapy with griseofulvin. Topical therapy alone is rarely effective. Relapse is common.

I. Hemangiomas

1. **Etiology.** Hemangiomas are vascular lesions with or without endothelial cell proliferation.
   - **(a)** Forty percent of those with endothelial proliferation are present at birth. They grow rapidly, then usually slowly involute.
   - **(b)** Ninety percent of those *not* showing endothelial cell proliferation are present at birth. These lesions grow slowly as the infant grows and do not involute. Cause of these lesions is unknown.
2. **Specific lesions**
   - **a. Capillary lesions (strawberry nevus)**
     - **(1)** Diagnosis. **Hemangioma** is present at birth or shortly thereafter. The name is derived from the cobblestone or berrylike surface of the lesion. It is a bright red or purple elevated, polypoid plaque(s), often extending deep into the dermis and varying greatly in size. The lesions seldom blanch completely with pressure, and are usually found on the head and neck, but may occur anywhere. They may grow rapidly, encroaching on vital structures. However, 75% of lesions will regress by age 5–7 years. When they begin to involute, areas of hypopigmentation usually appear in the center of the lesion.
     - **(2) Therapy**
       - **(a)** Since most lesions resolve spontaneously, treatment is limited to hemangiomas that encroach on and compromise vital structures (eye, mouth), or grow rapidly, ulcerate, and become infected.
       - **(b) Systemic prednisone** (1 mg/kg/day) should cause regression in 2–3 weeks. Corticosteroids injected into the lesion have also been used.
       - **(c) Laser treatments** may slow or stop rapidly growing lesions.
       - **(d) Surgery, radiation, cryosurgery, and sclerosing agents** may be used but cosmetic results are poor.
   - **b. Cavernous lesions**
     - **(1) Diagnosis.** These malformations appear in childhood as deep blue, poorly defined nodules or plaques of varying diameter. They may exist as part of a syndrome with hemangiomas of other organ systems (disseminated hemangiomatosis), with hypertrophy of soft tissue and bone at the site of the lesion (Klippel-Trenaunay-Weber syndrome), with capillary nevi (strawberry nevus combined with cavernous component), with dyschondroplasia (Maffucci's syndrome), or with intestinal lesions (blue rubber bleb nevus). The cavernous lesions are usually compressible, but will rapidly refill. They may enlarge steadily and do not undergo spontaneous involution.
     - **(2) Therapy**
       - **(a)** Orthopedic intervention when bony structures are involved.

  (b) Surveillance for hemorrhage in other organs and rapid growth of lesions may necessitate surgical intervention.

  (c) Thrombocytopenia from platelet trapping or disseminated intravascular coagulation from consumption of clotting factors may occur in large lesions and requires standard treatment.

  (d) Prednisone therapy may be helpful as in **2.a.(2)(b).**

c. Vascular dilatations (port wine stain [face], **nevus flammeus** [back of neck], **"stork bite,"** **salmon patch)**

 (1) Diagnosis.

  Subjective findings. These lesions are pink to purple, flat, usually unilateral, commonly seen at birth on the neck, eyelids or glabella of newborns.

  Objective findings. The lesions will show some tendency to involute spontaneously, especially eyelid and glabellar lesions. They often occur in a dermatomal distribution. Older lesions may have areas of elevation. Sturge-Weber syndrome (port wine stain, mental retardation, ipsilateral cerebral calcifications, ipsilateral vascular anomalies in eye and leptomeninges, contralateral hemiparesis, and epilepsy) is associated with certain lesions when distributed in an area of trigeminal nerve innervation. Lesions on the back may signify underlying AV malformation in the spinal cord. Klippel-Trenaunay-Weber syndrome is also associated with these malformations.

 (2) Therapy

  (a) Variable success has been obtained with laser therapy.

  (b) Cover makeups are useful.

  (c) Regular eye examinations for glaucoma are indicated if lesions are in the first two divisions of the fifth cranial nerve.

J. Impetigo

1. Etiology. Impetigo is clinically and bacteriologically classified into two distinct types. The **nonbullous type** is characterized by crusted lesions caused primarily by *streptococci* and sometimes secondarily infected by staphylococci. **Bullous impetigo** is associated with a bulla or a relatively clean, eroded lesion, caused by *staphylococci* (usually bacteriophage group II). Glomerulonephritis may result from nonbullous impetigo caused by **streptococci M-type 49 or 55.** A primary cutaneous disease may underlie the impetiginous process. Rheumatic fever is not a sequela of cutaneous infection.

2. Evaluation

 a. Gram stain is helpful in bullous but not in nonbullous impetigo, since secondary infection of the latter is frequent.

 b. Laboratory evaluation. Since nephritiogenic strains are propagated by direct contact, throat and skin cultures should be done on family members and close contacts of a patient with impetigo.

3. Diagnosis

 a. Subjective findings. There is often a history of antecedent minor trauma, insect bites, or exposure to other infected children. The lesions are usually relatively asymptomatic, but occasionally pruritus may be a prominent feature.

 b. Objective findings

  (1) Nonbullous impetigo. Multiple lesions, most numerous on the face and extremities, are characterized by a thick, adherent, yellowish-brown crust. Involved areas spread centrifugally and coalesce into large, irregularly shaped lesions with no tendency for central clearing. Regional lymphadenopathy is common.

  (2) Bullous impetigo. Flaccid bullae, 1–2 cm in diameter and containing turbid fluid, occur anywhere on the body. After 2–3 days they rupture, leaving discrete, round lesions and coalescent, polycyclic areas that tend to clear centrally. On Gram's stain, fluid contains gram-positive cocci in clusters.

4. Treatment
  a. Nonbullous impetigo
    (1) Minimal disease. Local cool water soaks may be used to remove crusts. The area is washed with Betadine or Hibiclens, and a topical antibiotic (Bacitracin or Ilotycin) is applied 2–3 times daily. However, if the lesions do not resolve quickly with topical care, systemic antibiotic therapy is indicated.
    (2) Moderate or extensive disease. Penicillin G or **erythromycin** (see Tables 15-1 and 15-2) usually is effective therapy. Even if a penicillin-resistant staphylococcus is present in the lesion, treatment of the streptococci with penicillin induces cure. In rare cases, specific anti-staphylococcal therapy may be indicated.
  b. Bullous impetigo. Since the causative organism, bacteriophage group II staphylococcus, is generally penicillin-resistant, a semisynthetic, **penicillinase-resistant penicillin** must be employed (see Tables 15-1 and 15-2).
K. Infestations
  1. Scabies
    a. Etiology. Scabies is caused by infestation with the mite, *Sarcoptes scabiei.* Transmission is usually by direct personal contact; however, fomite transmission (bedclothes, towels) is possible.
    b. Evaluation. Put a drop of oil on a suspected burrow and on a glass slide. Scrape the top from a burrow tract with a No. 15 blade. Place the scraping in the oil on the slide, cover with a coverslip, and examine under low power for adult mites, ova, and feces.
    c. Diagnosis
      (1) Subjective findings include intense pruritus of patients and persons with whom they are in contact. Incubation time for first infection after contact is a minimum of 3 weeks.
      (2) Objective findings. The most frequent areas involved are the interdigital webs of the fingers, hypothenar eminences, volar surface of the wrist, elbows, periareolar skin, anterior axillary folds, intergluteal fold, penis, scrotum; and, in infants, palms, soles, head, and neck.
        (a) A fresh burrow is a 2 mm flesh-colored, linear papule with a black dot at one end.
        (b) On the genitalia, lesions are firm, 0.5 cm red nodules.
        (c) Lesions in infants are often pustular, especially on palms, soles, and scalp.
        (d) A generalized dry, red, scaly rash may accompany infestation, obscuring burrows.
    d. Therapy
      (1) For nonpregnant females, children and adults without severely excoriated skin, apply a scabicide lotion, 1% gamma benzene hexachloride (Kwell) to affected skin for 12 hr. Rinse off. Reapply once 7 days later in the same way.
      (2) Wash bedclothes, towels, and clothes in hot water, dry clean, or isolate them daily between the two treatments.
      (3) Treat close contacts.
      (4) Antihistamines are indicated for intense pruritus (see sec. **II.B**).
      (5) For severely excoriated skin, use compresses (see sec. **II.C**) to dry out the lesions, then treat as in **(1)** above.
      (6) For infants and pregnant females, use 6–10% precipitated sulfur applied at night for 3 successive nights.
  2. Pediculosis
    a. Etiology. Pediculosis is caused by *Pediculus humanus*, the body louse, and/or *Phthirus pubis*, the pubic "crab" louse. *P. humanus capitis* is transmitted via hats, combs, hairbrushes, and the backs of theater seats. *P. humanus corporis* transmission is via shared clothing and bedding. Although *P. pubis* transmission is most commonly through sexual contact, infestation is possible via clothing, bedding, and towels.

b. Evaluation. Look for the lice.
c. Diagnosis
  (1) Subjective findings include intractable pruritus and positive history in close contacts.
  (2) Objective findings
  (a) Pediculosis capitis. Oval egg capsules (nits) appear along the hair shafts as highlights that are fixed in position and do not brush away easily. Adult lice are seen on the scalp. Purulence and matting of the hair often occurs over the occiput and nape of the neck. Occipital and posterior cervical adenitis may be present.
  (b) Pediculosis corporis. Excoriated papules, parallel linear excoriations, and, in chronic cases, scaling, lichenification, and hyperpigmentation are seen across the shoulders, in the interscapular area, and around the waist. The initial lesion is a red pinpoint macule. After 7–10 days, the time required for sensitization to the louse salivary antigens, the bites become urticarial and papular. Lice and ova are found in the seams of clothing.
  (c) Pediculosis pubis. Pruritus usually dominates the clinical picture, but there may be no symptoms. The yellow, translucent, 1–3 mm adult louse is seen on close examination of the skin. Oval egg capsules (nits) are firmly attached to hair shafts 1–2 cm above the skin surface. Reddish-brown, particulate accumulations of excreted heme pigment, deposited on the skin about hair shafts, are the most apparent clinical sign. Discrete, round, bluish-gray macules (maculae caeruleae), measuring 0.5–1.5 cm in diameter, are occasionally seen on the lower abdomen and inguinal areas.
d. Therapy
  (1) Apply pediculicidal agent (pyrithrin) to affected area for 12 hours. Rinse off. Repeat once, 8 days after first application. Gamma benzene hexachloride (Kwell) may be used in the same manner, but has more reported toxicity.
  (2) If eyebrows and eyelashes are involved, petrolatum should be applied until the infestation is eliminated.
  (3) If secondary bacterial infection is prominent, prescribe an appropriate antibiotic directed against gram-positive organisms (see Table 15-1).
  (4) Wash towels, bedclothes, caps, and head scarves in hot water.
  (5) Treatment of family members and close contacts is indicated.
  (6) Although topical agents kill adult lice and nits, the nits do not fall off the hairs spontaneously. Application of a 1:1 solution of white vinegar and water, followed by a shower, will help dissolve the nits cemented to the hairs and wash off their remains.
3. Swimmers' itch (schistosoma cercaria)
  a. Etiology. Caused by the entry into the skin of nonpathogenic marine and freshwater flukes, most likely *Trichobilharzia stagnicolae,* which is found in shallow waters in endemic area in temperate and tropical regions. (Puerto Rico, Africa, Asia, and South America)
  b. Evaluation. Travel or habitation in an endemic area.
  c. Diagnosis
  (1) Subjective findings. Pruritus begins at time of exposure and continues throughout. It is worst for the first 3 days after contact.
  (2) Objective findings. A papular eruption appears on areas not protected by clothing. It lasts 1–2 weeks and clears spontaneously. Eruption is clinically indistinguishable from that caused by human blood flukes.
  d. Therapy
  (1) Antipruritic lotions (Calamine, SeaBreeze, an emollient with 0.25% menthol added) and antihistamines (see sec. **II.B**) provide symptomatic relief.

L. Melanocytic nevi
  1. **Etiology.** Collections of nevomelanocytes in the epidermis, dermis, or both appear as raised, pigmented lesions on the skin. They are present in 1% of newborns, and become more common after 2–3 years of age. The postpubertal young adult has an average of 10–20 nevi.
  2. **Evaluation.** Measure the size of the nevus. Examine for irregularity of borders, elevation, or different colors in the lesion (blue, red, or black), ulceration or any sudden or rapid change in one nevus. Ascertain the patient's feelings about the nevus. Cosmetic concerns or continued trauma as well as rapid change and atypia are indications for removal.
  3. **Diagnosis**
      a. **Subjective findings.** Inquire about family history of melanoma or multiple atypical nevi. Pruritus, bleeding, or pain are ominous signs.
      b. **Objective findings.** *Benign* lesions are small (less than 7 mm), usually round, verrucoid, polypoid, sessile, dome-shaped, minimally elevated, or papillomatous. One person may have a variety of such lesions. Each nevus is usually homogeneously tan to dark brown or evenly speckled with several shades of brown. They have sharp, symmetrical borders and a consistent surface elevation. A giant congenital nevus is one that is so large that it cannot be totally excised and primarily closed. When there is excessive hair growth within the lesion, it is termed a hairy nevus. This is common in congenital nevi. Nevi may be found anywhere on the skin surface or on mucous membranes.
  4. **Therapy**
      a. Benign nevi may be surgically removed for cosmetic reasons.
      b. If there are many nevi of varying size, shape, and color, the patient requires further evaluation for possible dysplastic nevus syndrome, which is associated with familial and sporadic melanoma.
      c. Small tan, smooth, unchanging congenital nevi may be followed and excised when the patient can have it done with local anesthesia. There is an increased risk of melanoma in congenital lesions.
      d. Giant congenital nevi have a 1 in 10 risk of developing melanoma during the first few years of life and early surgical removal should be considered.
      e. Lesions on the scalp and mucous membranes are very difficult to follow and excision should be considered.
      f. If a lesion is suspected of being malignant, an excisional biopsy should be done unless the lesion is too large for a simple closure.

M. Pityriasis rosea
  1. **Etiology.** Pityriasis rosea is a superficial, scaling, self-limiting eruption of unknown etiology.
  2. **Evaluation.** Pityriasis rosea may be virtually indistinguishable from the generalized eruption of secondary syphilis. Thus, a serologic test for syphilis is sometimes indicated.
  3. **Diagnosis**
      a. **Subjective findings.** Pruritus may be absent, mild, or severe.
      b. **Objective findings**
          (1) In 50% of cases, a single, primary lesion, the *herald patch,* precedes the generalized eruption by 7–10 days. The herald patch is oval, 2–4 cm in diameter, slightly raised, scaly, and yellowish-brown in color. It occurs on the trunk or proximal extremities.
          (2) The generalized eruption involves the neck, trunk, and proximal extremities; the face and distal extremities are spared. The lesions form a "Christmas-tree" pattern on the back, where they are oriented along skin cleavage lines.
          (3) The individual lesions are round or oval, 0.5–1.0 cm in diameter, pinkish-tan in color, and characterized by a central "cigarette-paper" crinkling of the skin, and a fine, peripheral collarette of scale. In darkly pigmented skin, the lesions may be papular and more inflammatory than in lighter skin.

(4) Inflammatory PR has numerous very red, raised plaques with the characteristic scaling pattern and papules and is quite symptomatic.

4. Therapy

　　a. Pruritus is treated with oral antihistamines (see sec. **II.B**) and soothing baths (Oilated Aveeno).

　　b. Exposure to artificial UVL or sun tanning often speeds resolution of the eruption.

　　c. Severe inflammatory PR may require a short course of systemic steroids.

N. Psoriasis is a disease of the skin characterized by thick, scaling, erythematous plaques associated with a marked increase in the rate of epidermal turnover. Two percent of patients have their onset in the first 2 years of life and 35% have their onset before age 20.

　　1. Etiology. Polygenic inheritance is the causative factor, but psoriasis is subject to environmental influences. Onset or exacerbation of the disease in children may follow pharyngeal streptococcal infection. Local lesions may be provoked by local trauma (Koebner's phenomenon).

　　2. Diagnosis

　　　a. Subjective findings. The family history is positive for psoriasis in 50% of childhood cases. Emotional stress may be associated with exacerbation of disease activity. Pruritus may be present.

　　　b. Objective findings

　　　　(1) The lesions are elevated, moderately erythematous papules and plaques that are covered with thick, silvery, loosely adherent, micaceous scale. Punctate bleeding points occur when the scale is removed (Auspitz's sign). Extensor surfaces (elbows, knees, buttocks) and the scalp are the areas most often involved. Scalp lesions stop abruptly at the hairline.

　　　　(2) An erosive, polyarticular arthritis of the distal interphalangeal joints is associated with psoriasis in 10–30% of patients.

　　3. Therapy

　　　a. Emollients for any involvement

　　　　(1) Bathe qd–bid to hydrate skin. Always follow with application of oil or cream (Vaseline, Crisco oil, Nivea, Eucerin, Aquaphor, Lubriderm, Alpha Keri) to *wet* skin bid.

　　　b. Topical corticosteroids for limited disease

　　　　(1) A medium to very potent topical agent may be used for a short period of time (1–2 weeks) (see sec. **II.A.**).

　　　　(2) For intertriginous areas, face, or genitalia, use hydrocortisone cream 1%.

　　　c. Tar for moderate to severe involvement

　　　　(1) Balnetar (1–2 cupfuls) in bath water qd

　　　　(2) Nightly application of tar to affected areas (5% crude coal tar in emollient, Psorigel, or Estargel). These medications stain clothes temporarily.

　　　d. Ultraviolet light (UVL) for extensive involvement

　　　　(1) Natural or artificial UVL in gradually incremented doses is extremely helpful in many cases. **Caution:** burning may worsen psoriasis by the Koebner phenomenon.

　　　　(2) Oral psoralens are used with UVL to enhance its effect.

　　　e. Shampoo for scalp involvement

　　　　(1) Tar shampoo qd–prn (T-gel, Zetar, Sebutone, Tiseb-T, DHS-Tar). These may be mixed or alternated with patient's regular shampoo.

　　　　(2) If scales are very thick, they should be loosened by overnight application of mineral oil under occlusion to scalp, and shampooed off in the morning.

　　　　(3) For severe involvement, a corticosteroid lotion may be added after shampooing (see sec. **II.A**).

O. Seborrheic dermatitis

　　1. Etiology. Disease activity is chronologically coincident with androgenic stimulation of sebaceous glands. Hence, seborrheic dermatitis is seen in in fancy while transplacentally acquired maternal androgens are still presen and is also seen after the onset of puberty.

2. **Diagnosis**
   a. **Infantile seborrhea.** This begins in the second or third month of life and resolves spontaneously by the fifth or sixth month. Ordinarily, the disease is limited to the scalp (cradle cap), axillae, and diaper area. Occasionally, it extends to the forehead, ears, trunk, and proximal extremities Rarely, it erupts into a generalized exfoliative erythroderma (Leiner's disease).
      (1) **Subjective findings.** There is little discomfort or pruritus. Even with widespread dermatitis, an infant will continue to eat and sleep well Diarrhea may be associated with generalized erythrodermic disease.
      (2) **Objective findings.** A thick, yellow, greasy scale (cradle cap) is present on the scalp. Confluent, scaling erythema involves the intertriginous areas (axillae, inguinal and intergluteal folds, umbilicus). Individual lesions on the extremities and trunk are erythematous papules 0.5–1.0 cm in diameter, capped by an easily removed, yellowish-tan, greasy scale.
   b. **Adult-type postpubertal seborrhea** is limited to areas of high sebaceous gland concentration (chest, retroauricular area, scalp, malar area).

3. **Therapy**
   a. **Scalp**
      (1) Shampoos containing selenium, salicylic acid, or zinc (Iosel, Zincon, Head & Shoulders, Sebulex, Danex) are used every day until scaling is controlled. Subsequently, shampooing once or twice weekly is sufficient.
      (2) If the cradle cap is thick and adherent, mineral oil should be applied to the head and occluded with cap for 3–4 hr before shampooing.
      (3) For severe inflammation, hydrocortisone lotion 1% may be applied bid for 1–2 weeks.
   b. Intertriginous areas should be left open and dry. Plastic pants should not be used, and wet diapers should be changed promptly. If *Staphylococcus* or *Candida* is present, an appropriate topical agent is added.

P. **Sunburn, photosensitivity, and sunscreens**
   1. **Etiology.** Overexposure or heightened sensitivity from cutaneous disease, drugs, and topical agents to UVL of wavelengths 290–320 nm (UVB) or 320–400 nm (UVA) will cause sunburn. UVL causes damage to cellular DNA and is carcinogenic.
   2. **Evaluation**
      a. Inquire about the ingestion of photosensitizing drugs such as the sulfonamides, sulfonylureas (Orinase, Diabinese), thiazide diuretics, phenothiazines, griseofulvin, tetracyclines, and psoralens.
      b. Other causes of photosensitivity are nutritional deficiency (kwashiorkor, pellagra); vitiligo; albinism; porphyria; phenylketonuria; systemic lupus erythematosus; dermatomyositis; xeroderma pigmentosum; and Rothmund-Thomson, Cockayne's, and Bloom's syndromes.
   3. **Diagnosis**
      a. **Subjective findings.** The initial transient erythema is relatively asymptomatic; 2–6 hr later, burning and stinging accompany the appearance of the delayed, prolonged erythema. Malaise, chills, and headache are frequent if sunburn is severe.
      b. **Objective findings.** The initial erythema limited to sun-exposed areas fades in 1–2 hr. Prolonged erythema and edema appear at 2–6 hr and reach maximum intensity (bulla formation) at 24 hr. Low-grade fever is not unusual. Hypohidrosis, hyperpyrexia, and hypotension may ensue in severe cases.

4. Therapy
   a. Prophylaxis
      (1) Para-aminobenzoic acid 5% (Total eclipse, Supershade, PreSun) provides maximum screening for the sunburn wavelengths of the spectrum 290–320 nm.
      (2) Benzophenone 10% (UVAL) provides screening over a broader spectrum 250–360 nm, but does not protect so adequately in the sunburn part of the spectrum.
      (3) Markedly sun-sensitive skin (vitiligo, albinism, porphyria) may require an *opaque screen* such as titanium dioxide or zinc oxide in a hydrophilic ointment (Reflecta, Covermark) or avoidance of sun.
   b. Sunburn
      (1) Cool baths with mineral oil or colloidal oatmeal (oilated Aveeno) are soothing.
      (2) Damp compresses with cool water relieve burning and stinging.
      (3) Aspirin in the usual doses provides symptomatic relief.
      (4) Severely affected patients, if treated early, respond rapidly to prednisone, 1–2 mg/kg/day in divided doses for no more than 2 days.

Q. Vitiligo
   1. Etiology. Vitiligo is caused by absence of melanocytes in an area of skin, producing a porcelain white appearance; a relative decrease in the normal melanin pigment leads to hypopigmentation. Melanocytes can be affected by topical chemicals or autoimmune phenomena in association with thyroiditis, Addison's disease, and pernicious anemia.
   2. Evaluation. With the use of a Wood's light in a completely darkened room, vitiligo will stand out as white in contrast to the more darkly pigmented skin surrounding it, and subtle lesions will become evident. A search for associated diseases may be indicated. Occupation, hobbies, or physical trauma may elucidate a chemical cause.
   3. Diagnosis
      a. Subjective findings. Patients will note they sunburn more easily in affected areas.
      b. Objective findings. The lesions appear as porcelain white areas of any size and shape and are accentuated under a Wood's light. They may not be symmetrical. They are often present around body orifices. Hair in the white areas need not also be white. If distribution looks artificial, consider a topically applied contactant.
   4. Therapy
      a. Repigmentation may be attempted with trimethylpsoralens and exposure to artificial or natural UVL, but improvement may take at least 1 year of treatment.
      b. Some patients may prefer to depigment surrounding skin with a hydroquinone. Repigmentation after this is virtually impossible, and should only be undertaken after careful evaluation.
      c. Sunscreens [see **P.4.(a)(3)**] should be used routinely to protect involved areas from severe burns and carcinogenesis from UVL.

R. Warts
   1. Etiology. Warts are caused by a DNA-containing virus of the papovavirus group. The localized viral infection can be spread to other sites by autoinoculation and to other people by direct contact. However, different viral strains infect different sites.
   2. Evaluation. The amount of pain and degree of disability experienced from a plantar lesion are important in deciding what treatment should be employed. Genital and perianal lesions may be spread during sexual contact. Thus, sex partners should be treated simultaneously.
   3. Diagnosis
      a. Subjective findings. Plantar warts on weight-bearing surfaces may be painful. Perianal and genital condyloma acuminatum (venereal warts) may be friable and tender.

  b. Objective findings

    (1) Common warts are firm, hyperkeratotic papules containing red and black specks of hemosiderin pigment in thrombosed capillary loops.

    (2) Periungual warts involve the lateral and proximal nail folds but usually do not cause nail plate abnormalities. Punctate, black, thrombosed capillary loops are usually apparent.

    (3) Plantar warts are hyperkeratotic, dome-shaped, or flat lesions, which may be distinguished from calluses by paring down the lesions and looking for thrombosed capillaries.

    (4) A **mosaic wart** is a superficial, nontender, confluent plaque, made up of many 2–3 mm papules, which may involve a large area of the plantar surface.

    (5) Filiform warts are small fingerlike growths seen primarily on the face and neck.

    (6) Condylomata acuminata are soft, friable, pink, elongated and filiform lesions. They may be seen in any intertriginous area, but are most often found under the prepuce, on the vaginal and labial mucosa, in the urethral meatus, and around the anal mucocutaneous junction.

4. Therapy

  a. Common warts

    (1) Apply **liquid nitrogen** with a cotton-tipped applicator. Keep the lesion frozen for 20 sec. After the lesion has completely thawed, reapply liquid nitrogen for another 20 sec freeze. In 6–10 hr a hemorrhagic bulla will form, with the wart in the blister roof. This may require repeated application for complete cure. Patient should be warned regarding subsequent pain from the blister, temporary functional loss of the involved body part, and risk of infection.

    (2) Electrocautery followed by curettage of the lesion may be used. This method may leave more noticeable hypopigmentation and scarring than other techniques.

    (3) In young children who will not tolerate the pain of the above two methods, nightly application of **16.7% salicylic acid plus 16.7% lactic acid** in flexible collodion (Duofilm) will gradually and painlessly remove the wart.

  b. Periungual warts

    (1) This area is very sensitive and Duofilm [see **4.a.(3)** above] applied qhs is effective treatment.

    (2) Liquid nitrogen should be used with caution about the nails. It is painful and freezing the nail matrix that lies beneath the proximal fold may result in permanent nail plate dystrophy. Two or three treatments at 2-week intervals may be required for adequate therapy.

  c. Plantar warts

    (1) Plantar lesions are extraordinarily difficult to eradicate. Recurrence after repeated and painful treatments is frequent. Therefore, unless the patient is suffering significant pain or disability, it is best to use only repeated daily applications of 40% salicylic acid plaster under ordinary adhesive tape, Duofilm, or applications of trichloroacetic acid 80%.

    (2) Freezing of the plantar surface with liquid nitrogen often results in a painful, tense, hemorrhagic bulla. Electrodesiccation or surgical excision may leave a tender hyperplastic scar. Both significantly interfere with ambulation.

  d. Mosaic warts. Mosaic lesions are best treated with repeated applications of 40% salicylic acid plaster [see **c.(1)**]. They are too extensive to use the more destructive methods.

  e. Filiform warts. Small filiform warts may be treated as in **4.a.**

  f. Condyloma acuminatum. The physician should apply 25% podophyllin in compound tincture of benzoin to lesions in moist, intertriginous areas. The areas should be powdered with talc to prevent smearing of podophyl-

Table 22-1. Commonly used topical corticosteroids

Potency	Chemical name	Strength	Trade name
High	Betamethasone dipropionate	0.05%	Diprosone
	Fluocinonide	0.05%	Lidex
	Fluocinonide (gel)	0.05%	Topsyn
	Halcinonide	0.01%	Halog
Medium	Betamethasone valerate	0.01%	Valisone
	Fluocinolone acetonide	0.025%	Synalar
	Flurandrenolide (tape)	0.05%	Cordran
	Triamcinolone acetonide	0.1%	Kenalog
Low	Hydrocortisone	1.0%	

lin onto surrounding normal skin. **The medication should be thoroughly washed off in 4–6 hr;** otherwise, a painful primary irritant dermatitis will follow. Never do more than a small area at one time. The recurrence rate is high, and repeated weekly applications may be required. Podophyllin will not induce resolution of verrucae on dry, nonintertriginous skin, such as the penile shaft; therefore, light application of liquid nitrogen can be used. Laser therapy is also used.

S. Molluscum contagiosum

    1. Etiology. This is caused by a DNA-containing poxvirus contracted by person-to-person contact, fomites, and autoinoculation.

    2. Evaluation. Gently nick the umbilication in the center of a papule with a No. 11 blade and squeeze out the central plug. Crush the plug onto a glass slide and put a drop of rose bengal stain onto it. Under low power, one may observe large ovoid bodies that are stained a deep pink (molluscum bodies).

    3. Diagnosis

        a. Subjective findings. Lesions are asymptomatic unless extremely large or irritated.

        b. Objective findings. Small 1–5 mm pearly papules with central white umbilication are usually scattered on the head and neck in children, but may be found anywhere. In sexually active individuals they may be limited to the genitalia.

    4. Therapy

        a. Lesions are self-limited. An individual lesion usually clears within 3 months, and a large area requires an average of 18 months to clear. Thus, any treatment which may leave marks should be undertaken with caution.

        b. Liquid nitrogen may be applied gently to each papule for 10–15 sec.

        c. Light electrodesiccation may also be used. Both **b.** and **c.** may result in pigmentary changes or scarring at the site, especially in more darkly pigmented individuals.

II. Topical corticosteroids, antihistamines, and dressings

    A. Topical corticosteroids. Commonly used corticosteroids are listed in **Table 22-1.**

        1. Application

            a. Topical corticosteroids are applied sparingly, no more than bid. Their effectiveness is enormously increased by occluding the treated area with polyethylene plastic wrap (Saran Wrap, HandiWrap). Plastic bags (Baggies) are useful on the feet, and disposable, lightweight gloves (Dispos-A-Glov) are available for use on the hands. The occlusive wrappings are applied at bedtime and removed in the morning. If using occlusion, **alert patient to stop its use if pustules occur.**

            b. Occlusion is useful in subacute, dry, nonexudative lesions, as seen in psoriasis, lichen planus, and lichen simplex. **Do not occlude acute, weeping, exudative processes** (e.g., poison ivy, contact dermatitis).

Table 22-2. Commonly used antihistamines

Chemical name	Trade name	Preparations available	Dosage
Brompheniramine maleate	Dimetane	Tablet, 4 mg Extentab, 8 mg, 12 mg Elixir, 2 mg/5 ml Parenteral, 10 mg/ml, 100 mg/ml	2–4 mg/q4–6h 0.5 mg/kg daily maximum
Chlorpheniramine maleate	Chlor-Trimeton	Tablet, 4 mg Repetab, 8 mg, 12 mg Syrup, 2 mg/5 ml Parenteral, 10 mg/ml	2–4 mg/q4–6h 0.5 mg/kg daily maximum
Cyproheptadine hydrochloride	Periactin	Tablet, 4 mg Syrup 2 mg/5 ml	2–4 mg/q4–6h 0.5 mg/kg daily maximum
Diphenhydramine		Capsule, 25 mg, 50 mg Elixir, 12.5 mg/5 ml Parenteral, 10 mg/ml	25–50 mg/q4–6h 5 mg/kg daily maximum
Tripelennamine	Pyribenzamine	Tablet, 25 mg, 50 mg Lontab, 50 mg, 100 mg Elixir, 30 mg/4 ml	25–50 mg/q4–6h 5 mg/kg daily maximum
Hydroxyzine hydrochloride pamoate	Atarax Vistaril	Tablet, 10 mg, 25 mg, 50 mg, 100 mg Syrup, 10 mg/5 ml Capsule, 25 mg, 50 mg, 100 mg Suspension, 25 mg/5 ml	25–50 mg/q4–6h 5 mg/kg daily maximum

    c. Ointments are partially occlusive because they are greasy and are used on dry, nonexudative lesions, and applied after the skin is slightly moistened. Creams are useful in intertriginous or moist areas. Lotions are good for scalp or hairy areas.

  2. Complications. The use of potent topical corticosteroids with or without occlusion or in intertriginous areas effectively occluded by skin folds can result in the development of atrophy, striae, or vascular dilatation and telangiectasia, in a rather short time. They should be used with caution on face and genitalia. **More potent agents should be reserved for the more severe cases to be used for short periods of time (1–2 weeks). Percutaneous absorption of corticosteroids through inflamed skin may be sufficient to suppress elaboration of corticotropin.**

B. Antihistamines. Antihistamines should never be used topically, because they are potent contact sensitizers. Commonly used antihistamines are listed in **Table 22-2.**

  1. Administration

    a. The oral route is the usual means of administration. IM injection is useful for rapid relief of generalized urticaria.

    b. Since sedation is an important facet of the effectiveness of these drugs in pruritic skin disease, the usual dose may have to be increased toward the recommended maximum daily dose in order to achieve the desired therapeutic result.

    c. Extentabs are useful for qhs dosage.

  2. Side effects include dizziness, tinnitus, blurred vision, nervousness, insomnia, tremors, dry mouth, nausea, tingling of the hands, and hypotension.

C. Wet dressings. Wet dressings are useful in suppressing pruritus, in drying moist and oozing lesions, and in removing crusts. Towels, washcloths, strips of bed sheets, or gauze rolls (Kerlix) are satisfactory materials for open, nonoccluded wet dressings, which allow evaporation of water and hence cool and soothe inflamed surfaces. **Do not compress extensive areas all at one time** to avoid heat loss due to evaporative cooling.

  1. Application. Strips of cotton material are soaked in the dressing solution and wrung out to a point just short of dripping wet. The dressing is wrapped about an extremity or laid on the area to be treated. Dressings are removed after 15–30 min. This process is repeated 3–4 times per day, depending on the degree of pruritus, oozing, or crusting.

  2. Precautions. Dressings should not be left in place and remoistened simply by pouring additional solution over them. The process of removal and redressing is instrumental in cooling and debriding. Wet dressings should not be wrapped with plastic or rubber sheets to prevent wetting the bedclothes. If wet dressings are occluded, they *raise* the surface temperature rather than lower it. Also, occlusion prevents evaporation and leads to maceration of tissues.

  3. Commonly used solutions

    a. Saline. One level tsp of table salt/1 pint of tap water approximates normal saline in concentration. It is a physiologic preparation for use on mild to moderate inflammation.

    b. Aluminum acetate (Burow's solution). Burow's solution 1:20 or 1:40 is prepared by adding 1 Domeboro packet or tablet to 1 pint or 1 quart, respectively, of tap water.

    c. Betadine solution. This solution has a mild antibacterial effect and can be used to wash affected areas after dressings are discontinued. The solution may stain.

23

I. Strabismus and amblyopia. The term *strabismus* refers to any abnormal deviation of the eyes from the parallel position. The eyes may be turned in (esotropia) or out (exotropia), or one eye may be higher than the other (hypertropia). *Amblyopia,* a loss of vision without evident organic defect in the visual system, will develop in over one-third of patients with strabismus. In strabismus, amblyopia occurs in the deviating eye when one eye is preferred. Amblyopia may also occur in an eye that has a worse refractive error than its fellow, as well as in visual deprivation early in infancy, as in congenital cataracts or corneal opacities.

A. Evaluation

1. Strabismus can be detected in infancy by observing the corneal light reflex when the patient fixes on a pocket flashlight. The reflexes should be approximately centered in each pupil.

2. Depending on cooperation, the **cover-uncover test** can be used in children as young as 1 year. If, when one eye is covered, the other must move to fix on a light, the patient has strabismus. This and the corneal light reflex test will reveal many cases of strabismus not obvious to gross inspection.

3. The most important single test in patients with strabismus is *visual acuity.* Amblyopia is *not* related to the amplitude of the deviation, so that a very small, inapparent strabismus may lead to profound loss of vision.

B. Therapy

1. Strabismus

a. A hyperopic (farsighted) person must accommodate to achieve clear vision, even at a distance. The patient's eyes may cross (esotropia) because of this accommodative effort, and they may be straightened with glasses that correct the hyperopia.

b. Surgery may be required to straighten the patient's eyes in nonaccommodative esotropia or in exotropia.

c. In the vast majority of patients with strabismus, straightening the eyes will be primarily of cosmetic significance, although many will achieve some partial binocularity. In a few patients, usually those whose eyes began to deviate later in childhood, normal binocular vision can be restored. In many patients with nonaccommodative congenital esotropia, surgery can restore partial binocular cooperation if the eyes are straightened before the age of 2.

d. The early school years are a difficult psychological period for the child with obvious strabismus. The eyes should be straightened by the time the child starts school.

2. Amblyopia

a. The most effective treatment of amblyopia is total occlusion of the preferred eye with an Elastoplast patch. The earlier this treatment is begun, the easier and more effective it is. A young infant may learn to use two eyes equally well with only a few days of occlusion of the preferred eye.

b. The usual period of patching in a 3-year-old is several weeks, and previously untreated amblyopia in a 4- or 5-year-old child typically requires several months of patching.

c. Beyond the age of 6, many patients will not respond to any form of treatment for amblyopia. However, some older children may still achieve near-normal vision in the amblyopic eye with prolonged occlusion of the preferred eye.

    d. Amblyopic patients should be followed into adolescence to detect and treat any recurrence of amblyopia in the successfully treated eye.

    e. Parents should never be reassured that strabismus will resolve spontaneously. Although the angle of the deviation may become less over the years, so that the patient's eyes appear straight, he or she may still be left with a profoundly amblyopic eye.

II. Inflammation. Inflammation may be infectious (bacterial, viral, or fungal) or secondary to systemic inflammatory disease.

  A. Eyelids

    1. Hordeolum (stye)

      a. Etiology. *Staphylococcus aureus*

      b. Evaluation and diagnosis. A painful swelling that points at the eyelid margin and involves the sebaceous glands of the eyelash follicle

      c. Therapy. Frequent hot soaks. Antibiotics are generally not indicated, and incision and drainage are rarely required.

    2. Chalazion

      a. Etiology. Foreign body granulomatous reaction to retained meibomian gland secretion

      b. Evaluation and diagnosis. A mass anywhere in the tarsus of the eyelid

      c. Therapy. If the lesion is small, it may involute with hot soaks; if it is large, it will usually require incision and curettage. In an older child, this can be performed under local anesthesia, but general anesthesia is required in younger children.

    3. Marginal blepharitis

      a. Etiology. Seborrhea, *S. aureus*

      b. Evaluation and diagnosis. Accumulation of yellowish scales on the eyelashes associated with erythema and thickening of the lid margins. Seborrhea is sometimes present elsewhere.

      c. Therapy. This condition can be temporarily relieved by application of hot soaks to the eyelids to soften the crusts, so that they can be removed with a soft cotton swab, and application of sodium sulfacetamide eye ointment bid–tid. Treatment of seborrhea should be carried out at the same time (see Chap. 22).

      It is important to reassure the patient that although this chronic, recurrent condition is annoying, it will not damage the eyes.

    4. Herpes simplex blepharitis

      a. Evaluation and diagnosis. Finding of either a primary or secondary infection, or a viral culture, or both

      b. Therapy. Idoxuridine (IUdR) eye ointment should be applied to the conjunctival sac prophylactically to prevent the occurrence of herpes simplex keratitis (see **E.4**). **Corticosteroids are contraindicated.**

  B. Lacrimal drainage system

    1. Congenital dacryostenosis

      a. Etiology. Congenital

      b. Diagnosis. The presence of dacryostenosis is confirmed by chronic tearing from the eye, with or without discharge, in the absence of conjunctivitis. A gush of tears, or mucus (white), or both, may be observed through the lacrimal canaliculi on digital pressure over the lacrimal sac, along the side of the nose just medial to the medial canthus of the eye.

      c. Treatment

        (1) If infection is present (see **2**), it should be treated. In any case, the mother should be taught to perform massage several times a day, with firm pressure over the lacrimal sac to empty it of accumulated tears and mucus, which form an ideal culture medium for bacteria. Massage may also help break down the membrane at the lower end of the nasolacrimal duct.

(2) Congential dacryostenosis will resolve spontaneously or with massage in the first few weeks or months of life in most infants. If it has not resolved by 8 months of age, probing of the involved nasolacrimal duct should be performed by an ophthalmologist under brief general anesthesia.

2. Dacryocystitis

a. **Etiology.** Stasis of tears and mucus in the lacrimal sac due to dacryostenosis; pneumococci; staphylococci

b. **Evaluation and diagnosis.** Purulent (yellow or green) matter regurgitates from the tear sac. If edema of the canaliculi prevents regurgitation, the sac is enlarged and may point to the skin surface inferomedial to the medial canthus of the eye. Pressure over the inflamed sac will often cause a gush of purulent material through the canaliculi and temporary relief of the swelling and discomfort. The infection is almost always localized to the area of the lacrimal sac.

c. **Therapy**

(1) Every attempt should be made to drain the sac through the normal orifices. Incision and drainage directly over the pointing area should be avoided, since this may result in a permanent lacrimal fistula to the skin. Local heat and systemic antibiotics may be indicated if the infection is severe (see Table 15-2).

(2) In nasolacrimal obstruction that has not responded to probing, resulting in recurrent dacryocystitis and chronic epiphora, dacryocystorhinostomy (surgical anastomosis of the lacrimal sac directly to the nasal mucosa) is indicated.

C. Orbital cellulitis is a serious and potentially life-threatening infection, usually occurring as a direct spread of infection from the paranasal sinuses, most commonly the ethmoids. It is characterized by proptosis and limitation of extraocular movements. Less serious is cellulitis of the lids (preseptal cellulitis or periorbital cellulitis). (See also Chap. 15, p. 383.)

D. Conjunctivitis

1. Ophthalmia neonatorum

a. **Etiology.** *Neisseria gonorrhoeae.* Any conjunctivitis beginning within the first 3 days of life should be considered gonococcal, although staphylococci, streptococci, pneumococci, and fecal organisms may occasionally cause conjunctivitis during this period.

b. **Evaluation.** Chemical conjunctivitis from the silver nitrate prophylactic drops may occasionally be confused with gonococcal conjunctivitis, but the inflammation is rarely so severe, and the characteristic copious yellow pus of gonococcal conjunctivitis is absent. A serologic test for syphilis should be obtained.

c. The **diagnosis** can be made by smear of the pus and identification of the gram-negative intracellular diplococci. In addition, culture on Thayer-Martin medium should yield positive identification.

d. **Therapy.** If untreated, corneal ulceration with permanent loss of vision or loss of the eye may occur. Treatment with systemic penicillin and frequent instillations of topical sulfacetamide drops will relieve the infection and prevent corneal ulceration and scarring (see also Chap. 6, p. 171).

2. Inclusion blennorrhea

a. **Etiology.** *Chlamydia*

b. **Evaluation**

(1) In newborns, inclusion blennorrhea starts at 5–15 days of age and is characterized by acute inflammation of the conjunctiva with swelling of the eyelids and mucopurulent discharge. It may lead to chlamydial pneumonitis (see also Chap. 6, p. 175).

(2) It may also occur in older children, in whom the follicles in the lower palpebral conjunctiva enlarge early. The infection may be contracted by swimming in a contaminated pool.

(3) The length of the course of inclusion blennorrhea is about 3 months. Permanent loss of vision does not occur, but mild corneal and conjunctival scarring may supervene.

c. The **diagnosis** is made by staining scrapings of the lower conjunctiva with Wright's or Giemsa stain and observing the typical paranuclear red- or blue-staining (or both red and blue) inclusions in epithelial cells.

d. Therapy. Treatment with oral erythromycin and topical sulfacetamide or tetracycline eye ointment qid will bring about resolution within a week.

3. Acute catarrhal conjunctivitis

a. Etiology. Common pathogens, including *S. aureus,* pneumococci, streptococci, *H. influenzae, Haemophilus aegyptius,* and, rarely, meningococci.

b. Evaluation and diagnosis reveal conjunctival injection and a mucopurulent discharge, which may accumulate on the lashes during sleep, causing them to stick together. **A gram-stained smear and culture of the conjunctival sac should be obtained before beginning therapy in any variety of bacterial conjunctivitis.** (The culture swab should be immediately placed in a tube of broth because the amount of material is very small and rapidly desiccates. If eye cultures are handled in the routine way, the organism will not grow in most cases.)

c. Treatment

(1) In general, sulfacetamide eyedrops or ointment will be effective. Since most of the causative organisms are gram positive, erythromycin is also useful.

(2) Treatment should not be delayed until the results of the culture are known.

(3) Drops or ointment containing neomycin should generally be avoided because of the toxicity of neomycin to the cornea after prolonged usage and the tendency for allergies to develop. **Antibiotic-corticosteroid combinations are especially to be avoided because of the side effects of topical corticosteroids.**

(4) Depending on the severity of the infection, the conjunctivitis will usually show some improvement within 2–3 days and will generally be completely cleared in a week. If there is no improvement, the results of the previously obtained culture will then be available, and more specific treatment can be directed at the offending organisms. The topical treatment should be continued for a full week or at least for 72 hr after the signs and symptoms of conjunctivitis have resolved. Otherwise, the infection is likely to recur.

(5) Actual failure of therapy due to bacterial resistance is unusual. The concentrations of antibiotic or chemotherapeutic agent achieved by topical therapy in the conjunctival sac are several orders of magnitude higher than that achieved by systemic treatment, so that apparently resistant staphylococci, for example, will respond to topical erythromycin or sulfonamides. However, systemic antibiotics should be added in conjunctivitis due to pneumococci, β-hemolytic streptococci, and meningococci.

4. Trachoma

a. Etiology. *Chlamydia*

b. Evaluation. Trachoma is a follicular conjunctivitis that involves the upper lid and upper portion of the globe more severely than the lower. If untreated, infiltration and vascularization of the cornea occur. There may be scarring of the eyelids, with trichiasis (inversion of the lashes rubbing against the globe), and severe visual loss may occur.

c. The **diagnosis** is made from the clinical picture and from finding typical cytoplasmic inclusion bodies in epithelial cells from conjunctival scrapings stained by Wright's or Giemsa stain.

d. Therapy. Oral sulfonamides are given for at least 10 days, and topical tetracycline eye ointment is applied qid until 72 hr after the inflammation has subsided. If photophobia is severe, the pupil may be dilated with a mydriatic-cycloplegic agent.

E. Corneal inflammation

1. Bacterial corneal ulcers

a. **Etiology.** Common gram-positive or gram-negative pathogens

b. **Evaluation.** These lesions are usually associated with infections of the lids, lacrimal sac, or conjunctiva.

c. The **diagnosis** may be attempted from a Gram stain and smear of direct scraping from the corneal ulcer itself. Cultures of the ulcer and of the conjunctival sac should also be taken.

d. **Therapy.** Topical and systemic treatment should be directed to the suspected organism.

(1) **In no case should treatment be deferred until the organism has been positively identified on culture.**

(2) When the organism cannot be reasonably identified immediately, **"shotgun" therapy with antibiotics is completely justified.**

(3) Pneumococcal corneal ulcers should be treated with systemic penicillin in addition to frequent applications of topical erythromycin or sulfonamide.

(4) *Pseudomonas* corneal ulcers should be treated with frequent instillations of polymyxin B eyedrops and systemic gentamicin until sensitivities can be obtained. Once the organism has been positively identified, systemic and topical treatment can be altered if necessary (see Table 15-2).

2. Interstitial keratitis

a. **Etiology.** Usually, congenital syphilis or tuberculosis; noninfectious varieties have been described.

b. **Evaluation and diagnosis.** It is usually a late manifestation of congenital syphilis occurring in preadolescent and adolescent children. The cornea assumes a ground-glass appearance from edema and infiltration, and corneal vascularization proceeds rapidly.

c. **Therapy.** Luetic interstitial keratitis is treated with systemic penicillin, topical corticosteroids, and mydriatic-cycloplegic drops.

3. Fungal keratitis occurs following trauma.

a. **Etiology.** The organisms most commonly involved are *Cephalosporium* and *Fusarium* species.

b. **Evaluation.** These lesions may be difficult to distinguish from bacterial ulcers, but they tend to have more raised borders with radiating lines of infiltrate in the corneal stroma, and satellite lesions often develop around the primary infection.

c. The **diagnosis** can be made by scrapings stained for fungi and fungal cultures.

d. **Therapy.** Topical treatment with **pimaricin** is most effective. Topical amphotericin B is not very effective and is irritating to the eye. Topical potassium iodide drops may have some effect in some cases. Nystatin is effective only in *Candida* infections. The patients are often left with severe scarring and may require corneal transplant. This is a serious condition. Consult an ophthalmologist for proper treatment.

4. Herpetic keratitis is the most important corneal inflammation.

a. **Etiology.** Herpes simplex virus

b. **Evaluation and diagnosis.** The disease is confirmed by the characteristic appearance of a dendritic figure, which stains with fluorescein. It is a branching, jagged linear infiltrate on the surface of the epithelium, which may resemble branching coral. The patient may be uncomfortable and photophobic, but without much evidence of inflammation.

c. **Therapy. Whenever epithelial herpes simplex keratitis is present, topical corticosteroid treatment is contraindicated.** In most cases the infection can be controlled with topical applications of idoxuridine ointment. If drops are used, they must be put in around the clock. Thus, the use of the ointment is much more convenient. Some cases of herpes have become resistant to idoxuridine. When this occurs, adenine arabinoside (AraA) or trifluorothymidine (trifluridine) or acyclovir can be used.

F. Uveitis may be **anterior,** involving primarily the iris and ciliary body; or **posterior,** involving the choroid.

   1. Anterior uveitis (iritis, iridocyclitis)

   a. Etiology. Juvenile rheumatoid arthritis (JRA). Other causes are the Reiter syndrome, Behçet's disease, and sarcoid. The disease may also be idiopathic. Herpes zoster ophthalmicus may also cause a severe iritis. Many patients will have a much more acute and symptomatic onset of iritis than those with JRA. The eye will generally be injected, more immediately around the cornea than elsewhere, and the patient often complains of severe pain and photophobia.

   b. Evaluation and diagnosis

   (1) In **JRA** the inflammation is insidious, and the first symptom is usually visual loss. Because of the insidious course and ultimately severe complications of the iritis in JRA, every child with this illness should be examined carefully with the slit lamp every 4 months in the absence of symptoms.

   (2) Sarcoid may cause a granulomatous iritis. The diagnosis depends on determining the systemic illness.

   (3) Secondary glaucoma is frequently seen in iritis.

   (4) Patients with iritis should be examined carefully for inflammation elsewhere in the body and have serologic tests for syphilis, a tuberculin test, and a chest x-ray.

   c. Therapy consists of dilation of the pupils with cycloplegic-mydriatic eyedrops (atropine, 1%, or homatropine, 5%) to prevent the formation of posterior synechiae (adhesions of the iris to the lens) and topical corticosteroid drops to control the inflammation. If band keratopathy becomes severe, the calcium can be removed with disodium edetate (EDTA) drops. Do not use Versenate, which is the calcium salt of EDTA. Cataracts may eventually require operation.

   2. Posterior uveitis (choroiditis and chorioretinitis). The most common causes are *Toxoplasma,* congenital syphilis, rubella, cytomegalic inclusion disease, visceral larva migrans, sarcoid, tuberculosis, and sympathetic ophthalmia. The cause can be determined in about 50% of cases.

   a. Toxoplasmosis

   (1) Evaluation and diagnosis

   (a) *Toxoplasma* uveitis is usually a prenatal infection, and the lesions are discrete, atrophic areas with pigmented borders and pigmented lines running through them. They may be anywhere in the retina, but are often found in the macular area in congenital toxoplasmosis.

   (b) Most commonly, the chorioretinitis is healed when the patient is first seen in the newborn period. These healed lesions contain viable parasites, and reactivation of the chorioretinitis may occur any time during life.

   (c) When active inflammation is present, the vitreous becomes cloudy, and fluffy white lesions appear, usually at the border of the old healed scar.

   (d) Presumptive diagnosis of *Toxoplasma* chorioretinitis may be made from the clinical appearance and from the Sabin-Feldman dye test or the *Toxoplasma* complement fixation test.

   (2) Therapy. Treatment of active *Toxoplasma* chorioretinitis consists of systemic and topical corticosteroids and topical mydriatic-cycloplegic drops. Treatment with combined pyrimethamine (Daraprim) and sulfonamide, although lethal to the organisms, is of questionable benefit clinically. If it is undertaken, the patient must be given folinic acid concurrently. Systemic therapy with combined clindamycin and sulfonamide seems to show more promise.

b. Congenital syphilis

(1) Evaluation consists in systemic examination and serologic tests. Syphilis typically causes a diffuse, fine pigmentary disturbance throughout the fundus.

(2) Therapy. Systemic penicillin

3. Endophthalmitis

a. Etiology. Bacterial or fungal contamination of a perforating injury of the eye, corneal ulcer, intraocular surgery, or, rarely, generalized sepsis.

b. Evaluation. Vision is lost, and the eye becomes painful and intensely inflamed, with chemosis of the conjunctiva, corneal haze, hypopyon, and vitreous opacity.

c. Therapy. If untreated, the infection may spread to the orbit. Occasionally, the globe, and even some vision, may be preserved by prompt antibiotic therapy early in the course of the disease.

III. Glaucoma

A. Etiology. Glaucoma (increased intraocular pressure) may be inherited, due to trauma, secondary to inflammation, or due to topical corticosteroid application.

B. Evaluation

1. Congential (infantile) glaucoma should be suspected in any infant with excessive tearing and photophobia, without evidence of ocular inflammation. A general pediatric examination should be performed to rule out associated primary disease.

2. A complete ophthalmic examination should also be performed, including measurement of the corneal diameters to rule out abnormal enlargement; inspection of the corneas for cloudiness; inspection of the optic nerve heads for cupping produced by an elevated intraocular pressure; and measurement of the intraocular pressures.

C. The **diagnosis** is confirmed by increased intraocular pressure.

D. Therapy

1. **Medical.** Acetazolamide (Diamox), 15 mg/kg PO daily; pilocarpine HCl, 2–4%, applied topically q6h.

2. **Surgical.** Goniotomy for infantile glaucoma, filtration surgery, and cyclocryotherapy.

IV. Retinoblastoma

A. Etiology. About 30% are dominantly inherited and about 70% are sporadic.

B. Evaluation

1. Patients present because of a white reflex in the pupil of one or both eyes, strabismus, ocular inflammation, or secondary glaucoma.

2. The patient requires examination under general anesthesia by an ophthalmologist.

C. The **diagnosis** is confirmed under general anesthesia by finding the tumor that has a typical appearance on examination.

D. Therapy

1. If useful vision can be saved in the eye, radiation therapy will achieve local control of the tumors in about 85% of cases. In bilateral tumors, this is the usual mode of therapy.

2. If the tumor is not controlled by radiation therapy, local control can usually be achieved by photocoagulation or cryotherapy directly to the tumors.

3. In cases in which useful vision cannot be preserved, the eye should be enucleated. Some surgeons would advocate enucleation for unilateral disease rather than radiation.

4. In cases in which the tumor has metastasized to bone marrow or to the CNS, palliation may be achieved by systemic chemotherapy. Chemotherapy is not helpful for the treatment of local disease in the eye.

Index

General Reference Information

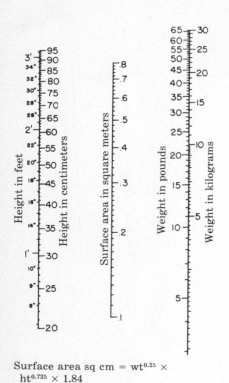

Surface area sq cm = wt$^{0.25}$ × ht$^{0.725}$ × 1.84

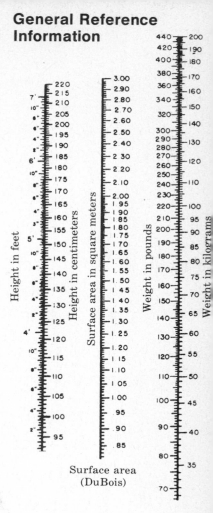

Surface area
(DuBois)

SURFACE AREA AND WEIGHT

Approximate relation, in individuals of average bodily proportions:

Weight		Area	Weight		Area
kg	lb	M^2	kg	lb	M^2
2	4.4	0.12	25	55	0.93
3	6.6	0.20	30	66	1.07
4	8.8	0.23	35	77	1.20
5	11	0.25	40	88	1.32
6	13	0.29	45	99	1.43
7	15	0.33	50	110	1.53
8	18	0.36	55	121	1.62
9	20	0.40	60	132	1.70
10	22	0.44	65	143	1.78
15	33	0.62	70	154	1.84
20	44	0.79			